WORLD HEALTH ORGANIZATION

INTERNATIONAL AGENCY FOR RESEARCH ON CANCER

IARC Handbooks of Cancer Prevention

Volume 6

Weight Control and Physical Activity

IARCPress

Lyon, 2002

Published by the International Agency for Research on Cancer,
150 cours Albert Thomas, F-69372 Lyon cedex 08, France

Distributed by Oxford University Press, Walton Street, Oxford, OX2 6DP, UK (Fax: +44 1865 267782) and in the USA by
Oxford University Press, 2001 Evans Road, Carey, NC 27513, USA (Fax: +1 919 677 1303).
All IARC publications can also be ordered directly from IARC*Press*
(Fax: +33 4 72 73 83 02; E-mail: press@iarc.fr)
and in the USA from IARC*Press*, WHO Office, Suite 480, 1775 K Street, Washington DC, 20006

IARC Library Cataloguing in Publication Data

Weight control and physical activity/
    IARC Working Group on the Evaluation of
    Cancer-Preventive Strategies (2001 : Lyon, France)

(IARC handbooks of cancer prevention ; 6)

1. Body weight – congresses 2. Exercise – congresses I. Working Group on the
    Evaluation of Cancer-Preventive Strategies II Series

ISBN 92 832 3006 X   (NLM Classification: W1)
ISSN 1027-5622

Printed in France

International Agency For Research On Cancer

The International Agency for Research on Cancer (IARC) was established in 1965 by the World Health Assembly, as an independently financed organization within the framework of the World Health Organization. The headquarters of the Agency are in Lyon, France.

The Agency conducts a programme of research concentrating particularly on the epidemiology of cancer and the study of potential carcinogens in the human environment. Its field studies are supplemented by biological and chemical research carried out in the Agency's laboratories in Lyon and, through collaborative research agreements, in national research institutions in many countries. The Agency also conducts a programme for the education and training of personnel for cancer research.

The publications of the Agency contribute to the dissemination of authoritative information on different aspects of cancer research. Information about IARC publications, and how to order them, is available via the Internet at: **http://www.iarc.fr/**

Note to the Reader

Anyone who is aware of published data that may influence any consideration in these *Handbooks* is encouraged to make the information available to the Unit of Chemoprevention, International Agency for Research on Cancer, 150 Cours Albert Thomas, 69372 Lyon Cedex 08, France

Although all efforts are made to prepare the *Handbooks* as accurately as possible, mistakes may occur. Readers are requested to communicate any errors to the Unit of Chemoprevention, so that corrections can be reported in future volumes.

Acknowledgements

The Foundation for Promotion of Cancer Research, Japan (the 2nd Term Comprehensive 10-Year Strategy for Cancer Control), is gratefully acknowledged for its generous support to the meeting of the Working Group and the production of this volume of the *IARC Handbooks of Cancer Prevention.*

Contents

List of participants

R. Ballard-Barbash
Applied Research Program
National Cancer Institute
EPN 4005
6130 Executive Blvd - MSC 7344
Bethesda, MD 20892-7344
USA

F. Berrino
Divisione di Epidemiologia
Istituto Nazionale per lo Studio e la
Cura dei Tumori
Via Venezian
20133 Milan
Italy

D. Birt
Department of Food Science and
Human Nutrition
2312 Food Sciences Building
Iowa State University
Ames, IA 50011-1061
USA

H. Boeing
German Institute of Human Nutrition
Department of Epidemiology
Arthur Scheunert Allee 114–116
14558 Potsdam Rehbrücke
Germany

P. Buffler *(Vice-Chairman)*
University of California
School of Public Health Division of
Epidemiology
140 Warren Hall
Berkeley
CA 94720
USA

T. Byers
Department of Preventive Medicine &
Biometrics
University of Colorado, School of
Medicine
Box C245
4200 East Ninth Avenue
Denver, CO 80262
USA

C. Caspersen
Division of Diabetes Translation
National Center for Chronic Disease
Prevention and Health Promotion
Centers for Disease Control and
Prevention
(mailstop K-10)
4770 Buford Highway NE
Atlanta GA 30341-3717
USA

M. Fogelholm
UKK Institute for Health Promotion
Research
Kaupinpuistonkatu 1
P.O. Box 30
FIN-33501
Tampere
Finland

C. Friedenreich
Division of Epidemiology
Prevention and Screening
Alberta Cancer Board
1331-29 St. N.W.
Calgary AB T2N 4N2
Canada

A. Hardman
Department of Physical Education
Sports Science, and Recreation
Management
Loughborough University
Ashby Road
Loughborough
Leicestershire LE11 3TU
United Kingdom

J. Kaukua
Helsinki Medical Center
Bulevardi 22 AH krs
00100 Helsinki
Finland

L. Le Marchand
Etiology Program
Cancer Research Center of Hawaii
University of Hawaii
1236 Lauhala St., Suite 407
Honolulu HI 96813
USA

A. McTiernan
Cancer Prevention Research
Program
Fred Hutchinson Cancer Research
Center
1100 Fairview Avenue N
MP 900
Seattle, WA 98109-1024
USA

J. E. Fulton, of the National Center for Chronic Disease Prevention and Health Promotion, Centers for Disease Control and Prevention, USA, also contributed to the preparation of chapters 1 and 2.

N. Owen
Associate Dean
Faculty of Health and Behavioural
Sciences
University of Wollongong
Wollongong NSW 2522
Australia

P. Pietinen*
Department of Nutrition
National Public Health Institute
Mannerheimintie 166
00300 Helsinki
Finland

J. Seidell
Department for Chronic Diseases
Epidemiology
National Institute of Public Health and
the Environment
Postbus 1
NL 372- BA Bilthoven
The Netherlands

M. Slattery
Health Research Center
Department of Family and Preventive
Medicine
University of Utah
391 Chipeta Way, Suite G
Salt Lake City
UT 84108
USA

H. Thompson
Center for Nutrition in Disease
Prevention
AMC Cancer Research Center
1600 Pierce Street
Lakewood,
CO 80214
USA

I. Thune
Norwegian Cancer Society
Faculty of Medicine
University of Tromsø
N 9037 Tromsø
Norway

A. Tjonneland
Institute of Cancer Epidemiology
Danish Cancer Society
Strandboulvarden 49
DK 2100 Copenhagen
Denmark

H. Tsuda
Experimental Pathology and
Chemotherapy Division
National Cancer Center Research
Institute
5-1-1 Tsukiji
Chuo-ku
Tokyo 104-0045
Japan

A. Turturro
Division of Biometry and Risk
Assessment
National Center for Toxicological
Research
HFT-20
3900 N.C.T.R. Rd
Jefferson
AR 72209
USA

W. Willett *(Chairman)*
Department of Nutrition
Harvard School of Public Health and
Channing Laboratory
Boston
MA 02115
USA

Secretariat

R. Baan
F. Bianchini
P. Brennan
J. Cheney
S. Franceschi
Y. Grosse
R. Kaaks
S. Lewis
A. Lukanova
E. Lund
M. Friesen
A.B. Miller
H. Ohshima
N. Slimani
E. Suonio
H. Vainio
E. Weiderpass

Technical assistance

S. Egraz
A. Meneghel
J. Mitchell
E. Perez
J. Thévenoux

* Current address: NCD Prevention and Health Promotion, World Health Organization, 20 Avenue Appia, CH-1211 Geneva 27, Switzerland

Preface

Why a Handbook on weight control and physical activity ?

Economic, social and technological developments in the second half of the 20th century have led to major changes in the lifestyle of large segments of the populations of industrialized and industrializing nations. Over the past two decades, significant gains in average weight among many human populations and within particular social groups have been observed. There are now high overall rates of overweight and obesity in the urbanized populations of industrially developed countries, in the affluent subgroups of developing nations and among socially disadvantaged groups in developed countries (Figure 1) (WHO Consultation on Obesity, 1998). For industrialized countries, it has been suggested that such increases in body weight have been caused primarily by reduced levels of physical activity, rather than by changes in food intake or by other factors (Jebb & Moore, 1999). The problem of obesity is now also becoming apparent in developing countries, due to changes in the food supply and decreasing physical activity (Zimmet, 2000).

The typical time sequence of emergence of chronic diseases following the increasing prevalence of obesity is important in public health planning for anticipation of future obesity-caused health problems (Figure 2). The first adverse effects of obesity to emerge in populations in transition are hypertension, hyperlipidaemia and glucose intolerance, while cardiovascular disease and the long-term complications of diabetes, such as renal failure, begin to

emerge several years (or decades) later. This sequence has already been observed in many developing countries (Popkin & Doak, 1998). Incidence of cancers associated in part with obesity typically increases over a longer timescale. Therefore, countries that are now seeing increasing obesity, and the sentinel events of diabetes and cardiovascular disease risk, but where rates of the obesity-related cancers are still low, should nonetheless consider prevention of future cancers as an important additional justification for controlling excess body weight in their populations.

In populations where weight gains are related to reductions in overall metabolic energy expenditure due to decreased physical activity, how does this come about? Is it due to reduced energy requirements of occupational and domestic tasks because of automation and computerization? Is it caused by reductions in leisure-time exercising and recreational energy expenditure? Are the most influential changes those in transport and commuting, with motor vehicle use replacing walking or cycling? Or is the most important influence the amount of time spent in sedentary occupations such as watching television and video, computer and Internet use? Currently, population prevalence and trend data are available primarily on leisure-time physical activity and are largely unavailable for several of these other physical activity domains, all of which can contribute to energy balance.

The expanding and strengthening evidence on the relationship between avoidance of overweight, physical activity and cancer prevention led to the initiation of this volume 6 of the *IARC Handbooks of Cancer Prevention*. Although the science of overweight, obesity and physical activity is complex and its relationship to cancer occurrence is a topic of intense research activity, much evidence already suggests that clear gains in public health can be achieved through adequate action and preventive strategies.

Current recommendations for the treatment and control of obesity and overweight are based on the recognition that this condition is a multifactorial chronic disease with strong environmental and genetic etiologies. Treatment of such a complex chronic condition requires multi-modal approaches that are maintained over years, with maintenance phases that should be continued over life. The bases of such approaches are diet, physical activity and behaviour modification. For some individuals, medication is added, most commonly for short periods of three months or less. Surgical treatment may be required for treatment of morbid obesity. The details of current recommendations for the treatment and control of obesity and overweight are summarized in the NHLBI Obesity Education Initiative Expert Panel Report (National Institutes of Health and National Heart, Lung, and Blood Institute, 1998) and are not reviewed in the present volume.

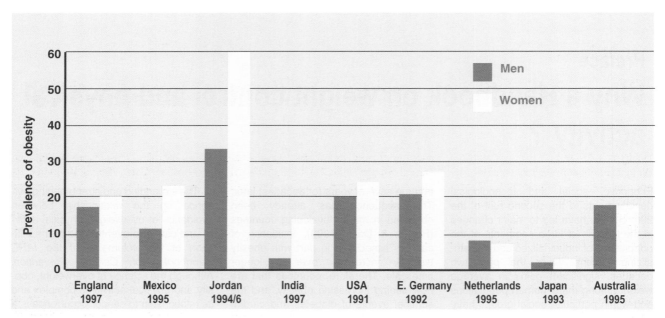

Figure 1 Prevalence of obesity in various parts of the world
Adapted from Seidell & Rissanen (2002)

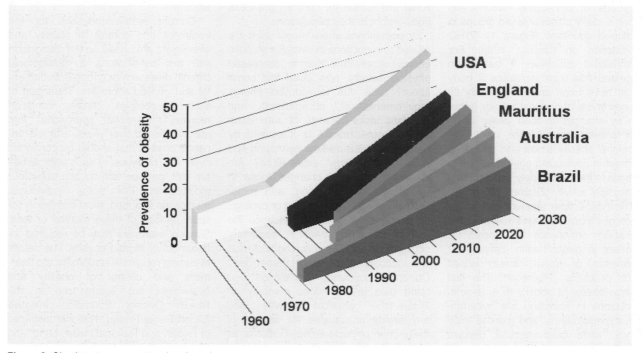

Figure 2 Obesity rates: current and projected

Chapter 1

Characteristics of weight control and physical activity

Weight control

Weight control is widely defined as approaches to maintaining weight within the 'healthy' (i.e., 'normal' or 'acceptable') range of body mass index of 18.5 to 24.9 kg/m^2 throughout adulthood (WHO Expert Committee, 1995). It should also include prevention of weight gain of more than 5 kg in all people. In those who are already overweight, a reduction of 5–10% of body weight is recommended as an initial goal.

Anthropometric measures
Body mass index

When we speak about the prevalence of obesity in populations, we mean the fraction of people who have excess storage of body fat. In adult men with weight in the acceptable range, the percentage of body fat is around 15–20%. In women, this percentage is higher (about 25–30%). Because differences in weight between individuals are only partly due to variations in body fat, many people object to the use of weight or indices based on height and weight (such as the body mass index) to discriminate between overweight and normal-weight people. Body mass index (BMI) is a measure of body mass relative to height, calculated as weight (kg) divided by height squared (m^2). Examples can of course be found to illustrate inappropriate use of BMI to compare certain individuals, such as an identical body mass index in a young male body builder and a middle-aged obese woman. In general, however, there is a very good correlation between BMI and the per-

centage of body fat in large populations. Deurenberg *et al.* (1991) showed that, in Dutch adults, the following equation can be used to estimate the body fat percentage:

Percentage body fat = 1.2 x BMI + 0.23 x (age) – 10.8 x (gender) – 5.4

In this equation the value for gender is one for men and zero for women.

About 80% of the variation in body fat between individuals can be explained by this formula, with a standard error of about 4%. It follows from the equation that for a given height and weight, the body fat percentage is about 10% higher in women than in men. Also, people get fatter when they get older even when their body weight is stable. The good correlation between BMI and fat percentage implies that, at the population level, BMI can be used to classify people in terms of excess body fat. In practice, people or populations are usually not classified on the basis of their body fat percentage but of their BMI. Usually, the same cut-points are applied for men and women and for different age-groups, because the relationships between BMI and mortality are similar (i.e., the relative mortality associated with obesity is similar in men and women). However, in most age-groups, the absolute mortality is much lower in women, implying that the effect of excess body fat is less in women than BMI in men. This may be because in women the excess body fat is usually distributed as subcutaneous fat and mainly peripherally (thighs, buttocks,

breasts), while in men there is a relative excess of body fat stored in the abdominal cavity and as abdominal subcutaneous fat. It has been suggested that the optimal body mass index (i.e., the BMI associated with lowest relative risk) increases with age (Andres, 1985).

Fat distribution patterns

Fat can be stored in adipose tissue as subcutaneous fat and as intra-abdominal fat. The pattern of subcutaneous fat can differ greatly with age, sex and ethnicity. Women tend to store subcutaneous fat in the gluteal and femoral regions and breasts, whereas men tend to store subcutaneous fat more in the truncal region. Intra-abdominal (or visceral) fat is formed by fat deposition in the omentum and mesentery and as retro-peritoneal fat. The omental and mesenteric adipose tissues are drained by the portal vein and are sometimes labelled as 'portal fat' (Björntorp, 1990). Apart from their unique location and venous drainage, the portal tissues have several other characteristics that make them liable to involvement in the metabolic disturbances associated with obesity. The fat cells here are more responsive to lipolytic stimuli (such as epinephrine and norepinephrine) and less responsive to the anti-lipolytic effect of insulin. The result can be overproduction of free fatty acids which are released into the portal vein and thus expose the liver to relatively high concentrations of free fatty acids, implicated in the development of heart disease and diabetes (Björntorp, 1990).

Since the pioneering work of Jean Vague in the 1940s, it has slowly become accepted that different body morphology or types of fat distribution are independently related to the health risks associated with obesity (Vague, 1956). Starting with Vague's brachio-femoral adipo-muscular ratio as an index of fat distribution (which was based on ratios of skinfolds and circumferences of the arms and thighs), more recent indices were designed specifically to be good predictors of intra-abdominal fat. The most popular is the waist to hip circumference ratio (WHR). The simplest measure is the waist circumference, which may be predictive of intra-abdominal fat at least as accurately as the WHR (Pouliot et al., 1994) and levels of cardiovascular risk factors and disease as well as BMI and WHR (Han et al., 1995). It has been suggested that waist circumference could be used to replace classifications based on BMI and the WHR (Lean et al., 1995; Booth et al., 2000) and this has been agreed by the WHO. More complex measures, such as the sagittal abdominal diameter, the ratio of waist/thigh circumference, the ratio of waist/height or the conicity index, have also been proposed to perform even better than waist circumference for one or more of these purposes. However, the differences between these measures are small and the use of ratios may complicate the interpretation of associations with disease and their consequences for public health. For instance, the waist/height ratio may be a better predictor of morbidity because the waist circumference is positively associated with disease, and because height, for reasons unrelated to body composition or fat distribution, is inversely associated with cardiovascular disease risk.

Replacing BMI and WHR by simple cut-points which are optimal for each sex, age-group, population and relationship with specific diseases may, however, be too simple. Still, as suggested by Lean et al. (1995), some cut-points may provide guidance in interpreting values of waist circumference for adults (Table 1). Other cut-points, based on classification of subjects on a 'critical level' of intra-abdominal fat, have been proposed (Lemieux et al., 1996).

Definition of obesity, overweight and underweight

Cut-points of BMI, that apply to both men and women and to all adult age-groups, have been proposed by a WHO Expert Committee for the classification of overweight (WHO Expert Committee, 1995) (Table 2). The BMI cut-points for degrees of under- and over-weight are largely arbitrary. The cut-points for overweight (25, 30, 40 kg/m^2) were initially based on the monotonic increase in the risk of mortality throughout the range of 20 to 40 kg/m^2. The cut-point for under-weight (18.5 kg/m^2) was largely based on health-related problems associated with malnutrition in developing countries.

There are limitations in the interpretation of BMI in very old subjects as well as in certain ethnic groups with unusual body proportions (e.g., populations where stunted growth is common or those with relatively short leg length compared to sitting height).

Causes of obesity

Obesity is always caused by an excess of energy intake over energy expenditure, referred to as a positive energy balance. Factors influencing this are biological (e.g., age, sex, genes), environmental and behavioural (including diet and physical activity). It has been argued that the prevalence of obesity in populations is determined mainly by the physical, economical and socio-cultural environment (Egger & Swinburn, 1997), which may act at a macro-level (i.e., on nations or large populations) or at a micro-level (a local or household level). These factors determine what percentage of the population is or will become

Table 1. Sex-specific cut-points for waist circumference

	Level 1[a]	Level 2[b]
Men	≥ 94 cm (~ 37 inches)	≥ 102 cm (~ 40 inches)
Women	≥ 80 cm (~32 inches)	≥ 88 cm (~ 35 inches)

[a] Level 1 was initially based on replacing the classification of overweight (BMI ≥ 25 kg/m^2) in combination with high WHR (≥ 0.95 in men and ≥ 0.80 in women)
[b] Level 2 was based on classification of obesity (BMI ≥ 30 kg/m^2) in combination with high WHR (Han et al., 1995; Lean et al., 1995).

Table 2. Cut-points of body mass index for the classification of weight

BMI	WHO classification	Popular description
< 18.5 kg/m^2	Underweight	Thin
18.5–24.9 kg/m^2	–	'Healthy', 'normal' or 'acceptable' weight
25.0–29.9 kg/m^2	Grade 1 overweight	Overweight
30.0–39.9 kg/m^2	Grade 2 overweight	Obesity
≥ 40.0 kg/m^2	Grade 3 overweight	Morbid obesity

Source : WHO Expert Committee, 1995

obese, but do not explain which individuals are likely to become obese; at the individual level, the biological and behavioural factors are the primary determinants of obesity.

Diminished physical activity, changing dietary patterns, energy-dense diets and inadequate adjustment of energy intake relative to diminished energy requirements are all likely to be major determinants of the observed changes in the prevalence of obesity over time. Prentice and Jebb (1995) proposed that, at the population level, limited physical activity was more important than energy or fat consumption in explaining the time trends of obesity in the United Kingdom. Their analysis was based on aspects of physical activity (such as number of hours spent watching television) and household consumption survey data. Although such ecological correlations seem compelling, they may also be misleading. One could, for example, find very impressive correlations over time when plotting the density of mobile

phones versus the prevalence of obesity, without any likely mechanism.

The influence of dietary intake on the prevalence of obesity in populations and individuals is a very difficult subject to study, as it is usually necessary to rely on self-reporting of diet. In particular, energy and fat consumption are known to be underreported with increasing degrees of overweight (Seidell, 1998).

Changes in smoking behaviour may also contribute to changes in body weight at a population level. Data from the United States show that, although smoking cessation can explain some of the increase in the prevalence of overweight, it cannot on its own account for the major portion of the increase (Flegal et al., 1995). Other studies have suggested that the increase in prevalence of obesity may be independent of smoking status (Boyle et al., 1994; Wolk & Rössner, 1995).

Epidemiological methods based on self-reporting, used to assess energy intake and energy expenditure, are not

only subject to bias but also have a high ratio of within- to between-subject variation. Even subtle disruptions in energy balance can explain weight gain over time in individuals or populations (Figure 3). In populations, an increase of one unit in BMI corresponds to an increase of about 5% in the prevalence of obesity. Assuming height remains constant, an average weight increase of slightly less than 3 kg corresponds to an increase in one unit of BMI. If this occurs over a ten-year period, the excess number of calories ingested need only be of the order of 87 000 kJ (21 000 kcal) over ten years (i.e. about 21 kJ (5 kcal) per day). In this theoretical calculation, we ignore the effect of the increased energy expenditure that results from a weight increase (about 190–250 kJ (45–60 kcal) per day for a 3-kg weight increase). Nevertheless, an energy imbalance of about 210 kJ (50 kcal) per day is easily achieved. It is clear that such small persistent changes in energy balance over several years are not detectable

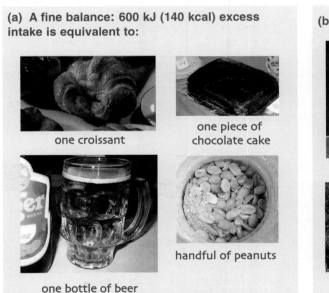

(a) A fine balance: 600 kJ (140 kcal) excess intake is equivalent to:

one croissant

one piece of chocolate cake

one bottle of beer

handful of peanuts

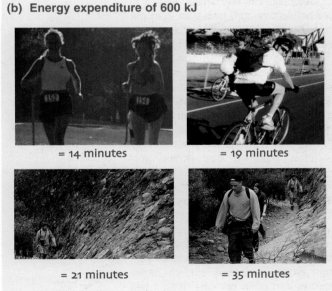

(b) Energy expenditure of 600 kJ

= 14 minutes

= 19 minutes

= 21 minutes

= 35 minutes

Figure 3 A fine balance: examples of (a) intake and (b) expenditure of 600 kJ (140 kcal)

by existing methods for measuring energy expenditure and energy intake in populations (WHO Expert Committee, 1995).

At the population level, some other characteristics are associated with the prevalence of obesity, which in individuals is the result of a long-term positive energy balance. These include:

♦ Age: obesity increases at least up to age 50 to 60 years in men and women
♦ Gender: women generally have a higher prevalence of obesity compared with men, especially above 50 years of age
♦ Ethnicity: there are large, usually unexplained, variations between ethnic groups
♦ Educational level and income: in industrialized countries, prevalence of obesity is higher in those with lower education and/or income
♦ Marital status: obesity tends to increase after marriage
♦ Parity: BMI may increase with increasing number of children. Although this contribution seems to be, on average, less than 2 kg per pregnancy (Williamson et al., 1994), pregnancy-related weight gain may be a significant contribution to weight gain for some women, especially those not lactating.
♦ Smoking: smoking lowers body weight and cessation of smoking leads to an increase. The associations between smoking and obesity may, however, vary considerably between populations (Molarius et al., 1997).
♦ Alcohol consumption: the effect is unclear in most populations

Obesity also has a strong familial component. By combining evidence from twin studies, adoption studies, family studies and other relevant data, it has been calculated that the heritability of overweight is in the range 25–40%

(Bouchard, 1994) (Figure 4). Studies in animal models of genetic obesity have revealed important pathways of energy homeostasis, e.g., the role of leptin (Friedman & Halaas, 1998), and gene mutations have been identified that are rare causes of human obesity. For common human obesity, however, the evidence for genetic factors is still fragmentary and incomplete (Chagnon et al., 2000). It is very likely that obesity is a multifactorial polygenic trait. Gene–environment and gene–gene interactions are likely to play an important role.

Timing of obesity
Although it is clear that obesity can develop at any age, there are several critical periods when humans seem to be more liable to accumulate body fat (Dietz, 1994).

♦ Prenatal growth: there is evidence that low birth weight is associated with abdominal fatness in middle-age (Dietz, 1994)
♦ Adiposity rebound period: when BMI is plotted against age, there is first a sharp reduction of BMI from birth until about six years of age. There is then a levelling off followed by an increase of BMI with age. Dietz (1994) has proposed that an early adiposity rebound is predictive of obesity in adults.
♦ Adolescence: physical activity in affluent societies declines rapidly with age in adolescents, the decline being especially pronounced between 15 and 18 years (Caspersen et al., 2000).
♦ Young adulthood: a period of rapid weight gain is often observed in young adults aged 25–40 years. This is usually a period of great behavioural change. People become settled, have children, buy a car and work long hours to build a career.

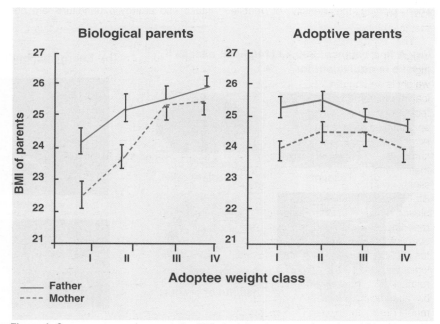

Figure 4 Genes versus environment: the BMI of adults who were adopted as children is clearly correlated with that of their biological parents but not that of the adoptive parents (I, thin; II, median, III, overweight; IV, obese)
Adapted from Stunkard et al. (1986)

Such changes all may reduce physical activity levels.

♦ Menopause: BMI tends to level off in men by the age of 50–60 years but continues to increase in women. Women tend to continue to gain weight after menopause and to accumulate more fat as abdominal fat compared to their premenopausal period.

Measures of weight (critical assessment of the various measures used)

BMI, WHR and waist circumference (Figure 5) are the most common measures used to estimate overweight, obesity and relative body composition in epidemiological studies. The only widely accepted criteria for obesity are based on BMI. New methods based on electrical resistance and impedance, magnetic resonance imaging and computer-assisted tomography are also used, but are expensive and seldom applicable in epidemiological studies. This chapter therefore concentrates on simple anthropometric methods.

The reproducibility and validity of weight and height measurements are high (Willett, 1998). In general, body weight is among the most precise biological measurements, even under imperfect conditions. However, in many epidemiological studies, weight and height are based on self-reports and it is known that people tend to underreport their weight and overreport their height slightly (Figure 6). As a consequence, BMI based on self-reported data will be biased downward. The degree of underreporting is proportional to the degree of overweight, age, and socioeconomic status (Niedhammer *et al.*, 2000). Epidemiological measures of association, such as relative risks, however, are not appreciably affected by this degree of measurement error. In contrast, comparisons of obesity prevalence between populations will be invalid if some data are based on actually measured weight and height while others are based on self-reported values. For instance, a study in Australia showed that 62% of men and 47% of women were classified as overweight or obese based on measured height and weight compared with 39% and 32%, respectively, based on self-reported height and weight (Flood *et al.*, 2000). Even recalled weight from many years earlier is highly valid, although the error is greater than for self-reported current weight. Correlations between measured weight at 18–30 years of age and recalled weight 20–30 years later usually are about 0.80 (Rhoads & Kagan, 1983; Stevens *et al.*, 1990; Must *et al.*, 1993; Troy *et al.*, 1995).

The validity of BMI as a measure of obesity is generally high. In studies where the reference method has been underwater weighing, the correlation between BMI and densitometry-estimated body fat has generally been 0.60–0.70 in adults (see Willett, 1998). Although BMI is primarily thought of as an estimate of percentage body fat, it is more correctly a measure of absolute fat mass adjusted for height. Thus, considerably higher correlations (0.82–0.91) between BMI and absolute fat mass adjusted for height have been found (Spiegelman *et al.*, 1992).

Even though BMI is an excellent measure of adiposity in young and middle-aged adults, it is less useful in older adults. Many elderly people lose lean body mass, so that for the same BMI, the percentage of fat mass increases (Gallagher *et al.*, 1996). Thus other measures of adiposity may be more appropriate for the elderly (Willett, 1998). For example, changes in abdominal circumference reflect adipose rather than muscle tissue and may thus be a better indicator of overall adiposity than weight alone or BMI.

There are also differences between populations in body build. For example, the relationship between percentage body fat and BMI is different between Singaporeans and Caucasians and also

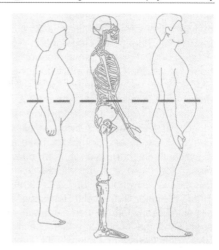

Figure 5 Waist circumference measurement. To measure waist circumference, locate the upper hip bone and the top of the right iliac crest. Place a measuring tape in a horizontal plane around the abdomen at the level of the iliac crest. Before reading the tape measure, ensure that the tape is snug, but does not compress the skin, and is parellel to the floor. The measurement is made at the end of a normal expiration.

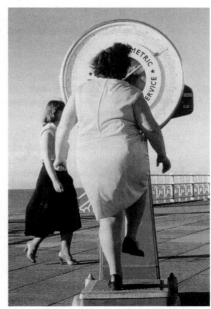

Figure 6 Studies have demonstrated that obese people have a tendency to underreport their weight

between the Chinese, Malaysians and Indians in Singapore (Deurenberg-Yap *et al.,* 2000). For the same amount of body fat as for Caucasians who have BMI 30 kg/m² or over, the cut-points for obesity would have to be about 27 for Chinese and Malays and 26 for Indians. In contrast, Polynesians living in New Zealand (Maoris and Samoans) have a significantly higher ratio of lean body mass to fat mass compared with Europeans (Swinburn *et al.,* 1999). Thus, at higher BMI levels, Polynesians are significantly leaner than Europeans, suggesting the need for ethnic-specific BMI definitions of overweight and obesity.

With the increasing evidence on the health risks associated with a predominance of abdominal (visceral) fat, numerous anthropometric indicators of abdominal obesity have been proposed (Molarius & Seidell, 1998). Of these indicators, waist circumference and WHR are widely used in epidemiological studies as well as in screening persons at risk of chronic diseases.

The WHR is difficult to measure in a strictly standardized way and also difficult to interpret biologically. The waist circumference predominantly measures visceral organs and abdominal (both subcutaneous and intra-abdominal) fat. The hip circumference may reflect various aspects of body composition, such as muscle mass, fat mass and skeletal frame. When these two circumferences are combined in a ratio, it is difficult to interpret differences between or within individuals (Molarius & Seidell, 1998). In addition, a reduction in weight usually results in a reduction in both waist and hip circumference, so will not necessarily result in a change in WHR.

Waist circumference is strongly correlated with visceral fat areas and can easily be measured and interpreted. This makes it a suitable candidate for an indicator of abdominal obesity. It is also well correlated with overall fatness.

Waist circumference is strongly correlated with BMI and adding waist measurements to age and BMI does not much improve the explanation of the variance in visceral fat, especially in women (Seidell *et al.,* 1988). Waist circumference is also strongly correlated with abdominal subcutaneous fat, total abdominal fat and total body fat (Lean *et al.,* 1996).

Cut-points have been suggested for both waist circumference and WHR (Molarius & Seidell, 1998), based on results obtained in Caucasian populations. A detailed analysis of 19 populations in the WHO MONICA study showed that the optimal screening cut-points for waist circumference may be population-specific (Molarius *et al.,* 1999). At waist action level 2 (waist circumference 102 cm or more in men and 88 cm or more in women, respectively; BMI 30 kg/m² or more), sensitivity varied from 22% to 64% in men and from 26% to 67% in women, whereas specificity was >95% in all populations. Sensitivity was in general lowest in populations in which overweight was relatively uncommon and highest in populations with a relatively high prevalence of overweight.

Even though criteria for waist circumference and WHR to be used in the public health setting are difficult to determine, these measurements should be applied in epidemiological studies, as the use of different measures of adiposity may give further insight into the etiology of disease.

Physical activity
Definition of physical activity
Physical activity is defined as bodily movement that is produced by the contraction of skeletal muscle and that substantially increases energy expenditure (US Department of Health and Human Services, 1996) (Figure 7). It has three main components:
- Occupational work
- Household, garden and other domestic activities
- Leisure-time physical activity (including exercise and sport)

By the terms physical inactivity or sedentary behaviour, we mean "a state in which body movement is minimal and energy expenditure approximates the resting metabolic rate".

Measurement of physical activity
To determine the relationship between physical activity and cancer, it is necessary to obtain valid and reproducible measurements of exposure and outcome variables. This can be difficult, since physical activity is a very complex behaviour that can be measured in many ways. Further, methods for measuring human energy expenditure are either precise but very restrictive – and thus limited to use over a short period of time – or are less restrictive and usable over longer periods but of lower precision.

Available methods to estimate physical activity and total energy expenditure include:
- Calorimetry (direct and indirect)
- Physiological markers (e.g., using doubly labelled water)
- Mechanical and electronic monitors (e.g., of heart rate, pedometers)
- Behavioural observation

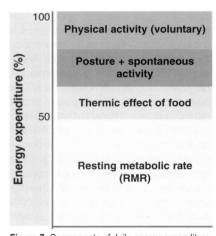

Figure 7 Components of daily energy expenditure
Adapted from: US DHHS, 1996

- Job classification
- Surveys (indirect calorimetric diaries, recall questionnaires, quantitative histories, and lifetime individual histories)

The operational definition of physical activity will vary not only according to the measurement method used, but also according to the type of research being done.

The biological and physiological approaches to assessment of physical activity, i.e., calorimetry, physiological and mechanical monitors, are not applicable in large population studies, but provide objective data for validating population surveys. The method using doubly labelled water has potential to bridge the gap. This involves measuring integral production of carbon dioxide for up to three weeks by the difference in elimination rates of the stable isotopes deuterium and oxygen-18 from doubly labelled water after ingestion of a quantity of water enriched with both isotopes. At present, however, such labelled water is expensive and not widely available.

The most convenient and commonly used measures of physical activity in cancer epidemiology have been job classification and surveys. Questionnaires and interviews used in such surveys are usually unrestricted but imprecise. Because of the low costs involved, they remain the most frequently used methods for assessment of physical activity, especially in epidemiological studies. The validity and test–retest reproducibility of questionnaires and/or interviews concerning physical activity have not been extensively studied. In general, strenuous physical activity appears to be recalled with greater accuracy than light or moderate-intensity activity, whether the recall is for recent periods or earlier periods of time (Slattery & Jacobs, 1995). It is useful to include both weekdays and weekend days and to include seasonal variation in the assessment.

A number of factors need to be taken into account in choosing methods for assessing physical activity:
- Accuracy (reliability and validity)
- Time frame
- Nature and details of the physical activity. Physical activity is commonly considered to have three dimensions: duration, frequency and intensity (or "strenuousness").
- The performance of an activity or group of activities such as in a job activity questionnaire.
- Mode of data collection (personal interview, telephone interview, self-administered questionnaire or mail survey)
- Summary estimate of physical activity for an individual (or a group), i.e., a summary estimate or score that can be used for ranking individuals according to level of physical activity)

Intensity of physical activity

Many terms have been used to characterize the intensity of physical activity such as light, moderate, hard or very hard. These terms can be related to the absolute amount of energy expenditure or oxygen consumption associated with specific types of physical activity. An example is the amount of oxygen consumed in walking at 5 km/h, which may be expressed in multiples of resting oxygen consumption. One metabolic equivalent (MET) is set at 3.5 mL of oxygen consumed per kilogram body mass per minute – an amount associated with sitting in a rested state. Walking at 5 km/h requires about 3 METs or 630 mL of oxygen consumed per minute by a 60-kg person. It should be noted that the amount of oxygen consumed by a young or old 60-kg person while walking at 5 km/h will have the same absolute level, but this constitutes a greater relative demand for the older person because maximal oxygen consumption declines with age.

Another way of characterizing intensity of activity is to describe the effect of participating in a specific type of activity relative to an individual's maximal oxygen consumption. This approach has been valuable in prescribing safe levels of exercise for cardiac patients and for otherwise healthy adults in whom exercise may produce untoward consequences (American College of sports Medicine, 1990). Because oxygen consumption and heart rate during physical exercise are highly correlated, the percentage of maximal heart rate has often been used to reflect the relative effect on maximal oxygen consumption (American College of Sports Medicine, 1990).

Finally, on a subjective level, a person may rate the intensity of an activity him/herself. For example, a person may be asked to report the frequency and duration of participation in vigorous activity that results in increased breathing or heart rate. As noted above, this would closely parallel the relative demands on a person.

Summary scores in physical activity measures

Physical activity can be described in a variety of ways, as evidenced by the many different summary scores used in various countries for large representative surveys or as part of epidemiological studies, notably in relation to monitoring cardiovascular disease risk. One way of characterizing physical activity is estimation of energy expenditure, expressed either as total energy expenditure (kilojoules, kJ) per day or week, or relative to an individual's body mass (kJ/kg/day). In addition, specific patterns of frequency and duration of physical activity can be established to clarify the particular categories and specific amounts of behaviours being reported. Some combinations of parameters have been used to reflect energy expenditure (e.g., regular moderate physical activity such as walking five times per week for 30 minutes). Another pattern reflects the

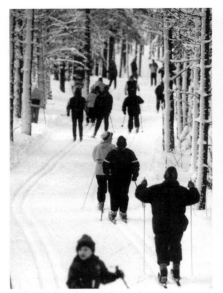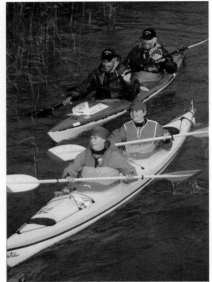

Figure 8 Examples of leisure-time physical activity (cross-country skiers and canoeists)

activity needed to improve or maintain aerobic capacity (e.g., vigorous activity performed three times per week and lasting for 20 minutes) – the traditional exercise prescription for cardiovascular disease prevention (Caspersen *et al.*, 1994). Other summary scores have been created by combining data on the frequency, duration and intensity of all or even specific types of physical activity. Such scores have often been inferred to reflect energy expenditure.

Critical assessment of the various measures used

Measures of cardiorespiratory fitness have been considered as a surrogate of physical activity and have been employed in some prospective studies of cancer mortality (Oliveria *et al.*, 1996). However, because genetic aspects dictate both cardiorespiratory fitness level and its response to physical activity, and because fitness measures are influenced by age, gender and other health habits, cardiorespiratory fitness level is inadequate as a measure of physical activity (Ainsworth *et al.*, 1994).

These measures have rarely been used in epidemiological studies of cancer, and are not considered further.

Job classification

Because employed adults spend many hours at work and have the opportunity for considerable expenditure of energy, occupational titles and related approaches have been used to define levels of physical activity in cancer studies. In a study of breast cancer, Calle *et al.* (1998a) asked about the current and longest-held job over a woman's lifetime and identified and compared separate risks for 13 occupational groups, using housewife as a reference group. Another study used occupational titles to compare cancer risks for four occupational groupings as part of three industries, using farmworkers/agriculture as the referent group (Hsing *et al.*, 1998a). Some studies have gone beyond using titles alone to further delineate tasks, by using resources such as the US Department of Labor's *Dictionary of Occupational Titles* (1993), which uses the intensity and duration of lifting,

pushing and pulling, the body's position during exertion, as well as the estimated rate of energy expenditure for work tasks, to create sedentary, light, medium and heavy groupings (Coogan *et al.*, 1997; Coogan & Aschengrau, 1999). Others have used similar approaches to create three (Fredriksson *et al.*, 1989) or five occupational activity groupings (Moradi *et al.*, 1998; Bergström *et al.*, 1999), while Dosemeci *et al.* (1993) created two separate indices, one for job-related energy expenditure (< 8, 8–12, >12 kJ/min) and one for sitting time (< 2, 2–6, > 6 h/day), to compare cancer risks in their population. While occupational titles and related classifications can be valuable, they are unreliable if misclassification is known to exist, or in populations where work-related energy expenditure is less prevalent. In such instances, other types of physical activity must be assessed and in some cases combined with occupational measures to yield measures of exposure.

Questionnaires

Recall questionnaires for occupation, leisure, household or other activity generally require less respondent effort and are less likely to affect the respondent's physical activity. Because recall questionnaires have time frames of one week (Sallis *et al.*, 1985) to one year (Taylor *et al.*, 1978) or even a lifetime (Friedenreich *et al.*, 1998), the respondent may have to expend considerable effort in remembering details of past participation in physical activity. Recall questionnaires can be either self- or interviewer-administered, the latter entailing more interviewer training, quality control and study costs. Recall questionnaires may ask for precise details on physical activity or may solicit general reports of usual participation in physical activity over a given time frame; they can generally be characterized as global, single-item and comprehensive questionnaires.

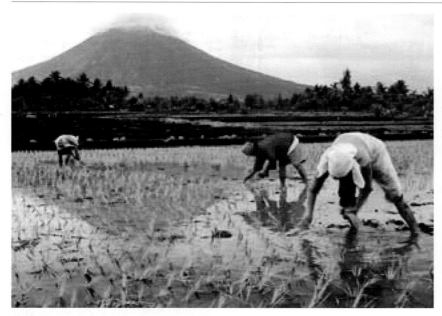

Figure 9 Rice planting in the Philippines

Global questionnaires require comparison of one's physical activity with that of other people in general. The global self-report is very easy to use and has at least some evidence of validity (Sternfeld *et al.*, 2000). Several cancer studies have used global questionnaires (Andersson *et al.*, 1995; Kotake *et al.*, 1995; Neugut *et al.*, 1996; Marcus *et al.*, 1999; Verloop *et al.*, 2000). However, it has been questioned what precise physical activity profiles form the basis of comparison when groups differing in age, gender, or racial/ethnic status report the same self-assessment rating (Sternfeld *et al.*, 2000).

Single-item questionnaires allow rapid assessment of general patterns of physical activity. For example, among Iowa women aged 55–69 years, physical activity was measured as the weekly frequency of moderate-intensity and vigorous activity and responses to the two questions were used to group women into low-, moderate- and high-activity categories (Mink *et al.*, 1996;

Moore *et al.*, 2000a), though the repeatability and validity of these two items have yet to be reported. In prospective studies of physicians in the United States, investigators assessed the frequency of vigorous physical activity likely to promote sweating (Lee *et al.*, 1997a; Liu *et al.*, 2000). Correlations between answers to the sweat question and oxygen uptake were reported to be 0.54 for males, 0.26 for females and 0.46 for the total group (Siconolfi *et al.*, 1985).

The Godin questionnaire assesses the frequency per week of exercise lasting at least 15 minutes or more for three categories of effort: strenuous (heart beating rapidly), moderate (not exhausting) and mild (minimal effort) (Godin & Shephard, 1985). For each category, examples of activities that produce the level of effort are proposed, while an additional question asks "how often do you engage in any regular activity long enough to work up a sweat?". Coefficients for 2–4-week repeatability have ranged from 0.24–0.48 for light effort to 0.84–0.94 for strenuous effort

and 0.69–0.80 for the sweat question (Godin & Shephard, 1985; Jacobs *et al.*, 1993). Correlations of 0.54–0.61 with other physical activity surveys (Miller *et al.*, 1994), with indices of maximal cardiorespiratory fitness (0.52–0.57) and with body fat (–0.43) (Jacobs *et al.*, 1993) constitute indices of validity for this approach. Friedenreich and Rohan (1995) modified the Godin questionnaire to assess total time per week at each level of effort and multiplied each by 5-, 7.5-, and 10 kcal/min to create a summary score in kcal/week. Thune *et al.* (1997) and Gram *et al.* (1999) used one question for work and one for leisure, each graded from 1 to 4, as part of the Second and Third Tromsö Studies (Thune *et al.*, 1998). These two questions demonstrated some aspects of validity (Wilhelmsen *et al.*, 1976; Holme *et al.*, 1981; Løchen & Rasmussen, 1992). Many other single-item questionnaires have been used in cancer studies (Garfinkel & Stellman, 1988; Gerhardsson de Verdier *et al.*, 1990a; Hirose *et al.*, 1995; Fraser & Shavlik, 1997; Hartman *et al.*, 1998; John *et al.*, 1999; Terry *et al.*, 1999; Stessman *et al.*, 2000), but neither their repeatability nor validity have been reported.

Comprehensive questionnaires. In studies of college alumni, Lee *et al.* (1999a) used a recall questionnaire to assess the distance and pace of walking, flights of stairs climbed, and frequency and duration of sports or recreational activities typically performed during the past year, in order to create a kilocalorie summary score. For this questionnaire, the short-term repeatability (four weeks) for the total score was 0.76 (Washburn *et al.*, 1991), while Rauh *et al.* (1992) found two-week repeatability to be greater for flights climbed (0.68) and sports participation (0.67) than for blocks walked (0.23), again revealing better recall of participation in more intense activity. Long-term repeatability

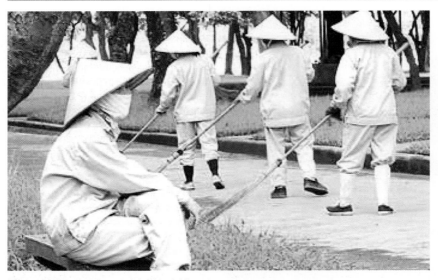

Figure 10 Workers in a park in Hanoi, Vietnam

(9–12 months) was between 0.50 and 0.73, with coefficients ranging between 0.39 and 0.42 for flights climbed, between 0.30 and 0.54 for blocks walked and 0.63 for sports (LaPorte *et al.*, 1983; Jacobs *et al.*, 1993). As indices of validity, the College Alumni questionnaire has shown favourable correlations (> 0.50) with other instruments (Albanes *et al.*, 1990) and reasonable correlations with a four-week activity history (0.31), indices of cardiorespiratory capacity (0.52) and body fat (–0.30) and motion sensor counts (0.30) (Jacobs *et al.*, 1993).

As part of the Framingham Study, Dorgan *et al.* (1994) used an interviewer-administered recall questionnaire to assess hours spent per day in sleep, work and extracurricular activities in a typical day, and then multiplied the time estimates by weighting factors of 1.1, 1.5, 3.4 and 5.0, corresponding to increasing levels of oxygen uptake. Modest repeatability coefficients of 0.30–0.59 between reports two to three years apart have been found for this instrument (Garcia-Palmieri *et al.*, 1982), while validity has been assessed by correlations with other physical activity questionnaires (0.48–0.72) and with total

energy intake (0.43) (Albanes *et al.*, 1990).

Le Marchand *et al.* (1997) used the Stanford seven-day physical activity recall questionnaire (Sallis *et al.*, 1985) to assess usual work and leisure averaged over a three-year period. The Stanford recall questionnaire asks subjects to report time spent in sleep, moderate, hard and very hard activities for each of the past five weekdays and two weekend days, differentiating between work and leisure. Repeatability coefficients for the total report have ranged from 0.34 (Jacobs *et al.*, 1993) to 0.86 (Gross *et al.*, 1990), while subtotals for very hard activity and sleep have correlations as high as 0.86 and 0.76, respectively (Rauh *et al.*, 1992). However, moderate-intensity activity had correlations of 0.08–0.12 (Sallis *et al.*, 1985; Jacobs *et al.*, 1993) to 0.52 (Rauh *et al.*, 1992). Validity coefficients for weekend and weekday physical activity logs were as high as 0.70 and 0.75 for moderate-intensity activity and 0.66 and 0.39 for hard and very hard activity, respectively (Taylor *et al.*, 1984). Validity correlations were low (having an absolute value of 0.36 or less) between the survey score

and a four-week activity history, indices of cardiorespiratory capacity and body fat, and motion sensor counts (Jacobs *et al.*, 1993).

Sandler *et al.* (1995) used a telephone-administered version of the Baecke questionnaire (Baecke *et al.*, 1982). This particular physical activity recall questionnaire consists of sections for work activity, sports activity and non-sports leisure activity. Each section has questions scored on a five-point Likert scale ranging from "never" to "always" or "very often", except that for reports of the two most frequently played sports, the number of months per year and hours per week of participation are solicited. The repeatability, in terms of correlation coefficients, has been between 0.70 and 0.90 for the three sections, regardless of the study population of men and women, and whether for short (1–5 months) (Baecke *et al.*, 1982; Jacobs *et al.*, 1993) or longer time periods (11 months) (Pols *et al.*, 1995). Validity for the Baecke questionnaire has been demonstrated by favourable correlations with data from other physical activity questionnaires (0.56–0.78) (Albanes *et al.*, 1990; Miller *et al.*, 1994) and physical activity diaries (0.33–0.66) (Pols *et al.*, 1995; Richardson *et al.*, 1995). Richardson *et al.* (1995) reported correlations of 0.46 and 0.57 comparing the survey results with cardiorespiratory fitness, and of –0.51 and –0.30 with indices of body fat for women and men, respectively.

The CARDIA (Coronary Artery Risk Development in Young Adult Study) questionnaire (Jacobs *et al.*, 1989) consists of a set of 13 activity categories (eight for strenuous and five for non-strenuous activities). For each set, the respondent provided the total number of months of participation, with further probing for the number of months in which activities were performed for at least one hour, and additionally for activities performed for at least two hours, during any of the preceding

12 months. Slattery and Jacobs (1995) found, for a subsample of 81 CARDIA participants, that recalled activity two to three years earlier was highly associated with activity reported during the examination of the corresponding time. Spearman correlations were 0.84 for vigorous, 0.64 for moderate, and 0.81 for total activity. Distantly recalled activity was less well associated with contemporary activity reports, with correlations being 0.57, 0.45 and 0.59, respectively, suggesting that activity was not completely stable over time. As an index of validity, Slattery and Jacobs (1995) found that distantly recalled activity was significantly correlated with resting pulse rate as measured during the examination at the corresponding time (−0.21). The CARDIA questionnaire has been used in several cancer studies (Slattery et al., 1997a, 1999).

Comprehensive questionnaires have been used in large prospective studies of health professionals. Men participating in the Health Professionals Follow-up Study recalled the average time per week spent over the past year in six vigorous (jogging, running, bicycling, swimming, tennis/squash/racket-ball, calisthenics/rowing) and two non-vigorous activities (walking/hiking, flights of stairs climbed) (Giovannucci et al., 1995, 1998). Time spent in each activity was multiplied by a specific intensity code (Ainsworth et al., 1993) to derive an estimate of energy expenditure in physical activity (MET-hours/week). Two-year repeatability coefficients were 0.52 for vigorous, 0.42 for non-vigorous and 0.39 for lack of activity, while, as an index of validity, correlations with data from four one-week seasonal diaries were 0.58, 0.28 and 0.41, respectively (Chasan-Taber et al., 1996). The close correspondence between the averages and distributions for the four diaries and the recall suggested that respondents had effectively incorporated seasonal information over the preceding year to create the average weekly estimate as

part of their recall. In the Nurses' Health Study (in even years, beginning in 1986) and the Nurses' Health Study II (in 1989), women completed a physical activity questionnaire similar to that used by men in the Health Professionals Follow-up Study (Giovannucci et al., 1996; Martinez et al., 1997; Rockhill et al., 1998, 1999). The two-year repeatability of the Nurses' Health Study II questionnaire was 0.59 for activity and 0.52 for inactivity, while validity coefficients, as assessed with the four one-week seasonal diaries, were 0.56 and 0.41, respectively (Wolf et al., 1994).

The European Prospective Investigation into Cancer and Nutrition (EPIC) included physical activity recall among other lifestyle assessments in its core questionnaire (Riboli & Kaaks, 1997). Subjects were asked to describe their participation in various types of activity: work (sedentary, standing, manual, heavy manual); walking, cycling, gardening, do-it-yourself activity, exercise, and housework (hours/week); stairs climbed (flights/day). Five-month and 11-month repeatability coefficients for energy expenditure were 0.86 and 0.75 for men and 0.63 and 0.68 for women, respectively (Pols et al., 1997). The correlation between energy expenditure estimated from the questionnaire with that from four three-day seasonal diaries was 0.43 for men and 0.51 for women.

Histories

Quantitative history. The retrospective quantitative history is the most thorough physical activity enquiry because it requires detailed recall of physical activity for time frames of up to one year or longer. The immense detail associated with the quantitative history implies a very large memory burden for the respondent and has high costs for administration, interviewer training, quality control and data-processing (Caspersen, 1989). Quantitative history questionnaires that cover at least one

year can assess seasonal physical activity. For example, McTiernan et al. (1996) asked respondents to report months, average frequency, and duration of participation for individual activities, identified from listed activity groupings, over the preceding two years, modelling their questionnaire on the Minnesota Leisure-Time Physical Activity Questionnaire (MLTPAQ) (Taylor et al., 1978). The time reported for each activity in the MLTPAQ was multiplied by an activity metabolic index (AMI, work metabolic rate divided by basal metabolic rate) to create a summary score approximating energy expenditure per week. The summary score has been further reported according to total, light (AMI < 4), moderate (AMI 4–6), and heavy (AMI > 6) activity following a convention that applies almost solely to men aged 35–57 years participating in that study. The short-term repeatability (about four weeks) for total, light, moderate and heavy activity was 0.92, 0.73, 0.80 and 0.95, respectively, while values for long-term (one year) repeatability were 0.69, 0.60, 0.32, and 071, respectively (Richardson et al., 1994). As a reflection of validity, the MLTPAQ has compared favourably with other physical activity questionnaires, showing correlations of greater than 0.47 (Albanes et al., 1990). In addition, the MLTPAQ has shown reasonable correlations with a physical activity record (0.47), an index of aerobic capacity (0.47) and body fat measurements (−0.24) (Richardson et al., 1994).

Lifetime history. To overcome part of the problem of memory burden, one lifetime physical activity questionnaire (Friedenreich et al., 1998) used cognitive interviewing techniques for women aged 34–65 years, noting a high test–retest repeatability (Pearson correlation ≥ 0.72) for a 6–8-week repeat questionnaire for occupational, household, exercise/sports and total activities for women. Repeatability was generally highest for

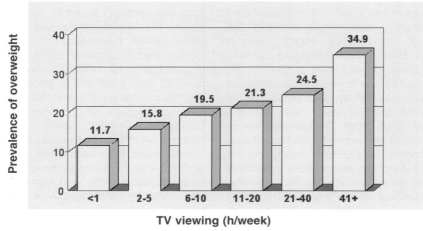

Figure 11 Relationship between overweight and TV viewing
Data from Ching *et al.* (1996)

occupational activity, for high-intensity activities, and for each type of activity reported for time periods earlier than for the year preceding the interview. On the other hand, repeatability of lifetime physical activity recall may vary by gender. A comparison of recalled physical activity with data from essentially the same questionnaire administered 30–35 years earlier found intraclass correlations of 0.43 for light and 0.45 for moderate weekday (occupational) activity for both men and women, and 0.38 for hard free-day (leisure) activity for women only (men had a correlation of 0.26) (Falkner *et al.*, 1999). In addition, while under-estimation occurred for both men and women who reported time spent in past weekday activities; only men over-estimated hard free-day activity. Otherwise, estimated time did not vary by gender when examined by intensity level of activity. Cognitive interviewing techniques hold promise for lifetime quantitative questionnaires in terms of both the quantity and precision of responses, compared with traditional standardized interviews, but they entail

additional costs for interviewer training, time spent in conducting interviews and difficulties in coding the responses. While they may be an excellent way to assess activity in a specific population, their specificity may limit the possibility of comparing different populations or use in other settings (Fisher *et al.*, 2000).

Concluding comments
Physical activity takes many forms, which explains, in part, why it is difficult to measure and why it has been measured in so many ways as part of experimental, intervention and epidemiology research. While some measures such as calorimetry and use of doubly labelled water are precise, they tend to restrict the physical activity behaviour being measured. On the other hand, job classification and recall measures (global, general, comprehensive and quantitative histories) are less precise but do not restrict physical activity measurement and are most often used for epidemiology and survey research.

One area of particular interest is *sedentary behaviour* as a distinct entity.

Sedentary behaviour needs to be seen as different from simple non-participation in physical activity. There is evidence that time spent in sedentary behaviour (particularly television viewing) is significantly associated with being overweight, even among people who are quite physically active in their leisure time (Figure 11) (Salmon *et al.*, 2000), but data on the health impact of such behaviour, its prevalence in populations and trends over time are sparse (Jebb & Moore, 1999; Pratt *et al.*, 1999; Owen *et al.*, 2000).

Many questionnaires that have been used in cancer epidemiology have been tested for reliability and validity. In general, strenuous physical activity appears to be recalled with greater accuracy than either light or moderate-intensity activity, while recent activities are recalled more accurately than those performed at earlier times. However, so many different samples of persons varying in age, gender and other important sociodemographic characteristics have been studied, so many different validation measures have been applied, and so many different correlational statistics have been used to assess their quality that it is not possible to determine what type of questionnaire is best or even qualitatively better than another.

A programme of new research to establish a broader set of reliable and valid measures is gaining momentum (Macera & Pratt, 2000). The use of objective tools such as accelerometers (motion sensors), heart rate monitors and direct observation of physical activities is also being explored (Sallis & Saelens, 2000). These assessment procedures may help to validate the self-report measures that are used because of the practical and financial constraints inherent in carrying out large-scale population surveys.

Chapter 2

Occurrence, trends and analysis

Weight profiles

Prevalence of obesity in developing and developed countries

This overview on the prevalence of obesity is based on adult population surveys in which both weight and height have been measured. The WHO classification of obesity as BMI 30 kg/m^2 or over (see Chapter 1) is systematically used to allow comparison of different studies. Although extensive data exist on self-reported weight and height, since this information is often requested in questionnaires, they are known to be unreliable, especially in the obese, and thus would give an underestimate of the prevalence of obesity. Most of the data presented are from the last 10–15 years, since the prevalence of obesity has been changing rapidly all over the world and old data without time-trend information are not very useful. The surveys are arranged according to the six WHO Regions, with the exception of the MONICA Project.

The MONICA Project (Monitoring trends and determinants in cardiovascular disease) covered 54 study populations in 26 countries, mainly in Europe. Risk factor surveys were carried out through two or three independent cross-sectional surveys, each five years apart, ranging from the early 1980s to the 1990s. These surveys included random samples of at least 200 persons of each gender and for 10-year age groups for the age range 35–64 years, and optionally 25–34 years. Common standardized methods were applied for data collection and analyses, making these data an invaluable source for comparison between populations.

In this section, the data for each country had to have been drawn from some sort of representative national sample. Table 3 summarizes the prevalence of obesity (BMI 30 kg/m^2 or more) in all MONICA centres where 10-year trend data were available (http://www. ktl.fi/publications/monica). In men, the prevalence of obesity was lowest in China (3–4%) and highest (at least 20%) in Finland, Glasgow (United Kingdom), rural Germany, Strasbourg (France), Kaunas (Lithuania), Warsaw (Poland), the Czech Republic and Stanford (United States). There was an overall increase in the prevalence of obesity in men in most populations. The biggest increases in ten years (by at least 10 percentage points) took place in Glasgow and in Stanford. The only centres where the prevalence of obesity decreased were Ticino (Switzerland) and Moscow (Russian Federation). The overall prevalence of obesity in men in most European populations was 15–25%. In women, the prevalence of obesity was lowest (10% or lower) in Gothenburg (Sweden), Toulouse (France), Fribourg (Switzerland) and Beijing (China). A high prevalence of obesity (at least 20%) was found in 14 centres out of 29, the highest prevalences being in eastern Europe. There was an overall tendency of increasing prevalence of obesity over ten years also in women, the biggest increases being in Glasgow and in Stanford, while the prevalence of obesity in women decreased in the Russian Federation and Lithuania. The prevalence of obesity varies in women more than in men, from 10 to 35% within European populations.

Other survey data from European populations are summarized in Table 4. The Health Surveys for England show an extraordinary increase in the prevalence of obesity (Seidell, 2001) (Figure 12). In the late 1980s, 7% of men and 12% of women were obese, while the respective numbers in 1997 were 17% and 19%. The age ranges in the other studies vary and, thus, the prevalence data are not necessarily comparable. The low prevalence in the Netherlands (Seidell et al., 1995) and Belgium (Moens et al., 1999) are influenced by the inclusion of young people, the prevalence being about 10%. There is an increasing trend in the Netherlands. The EURALIM Project, covering six European countries (Beer-Borst et al., 2000), shows big differences within countries such as Italy, where the prevalence of obesity is 37% in women in the Latina area and only 19% in Naples. However, the age ranges differ, which explains at least part of the difference.

In the United States, the prevalence of obesity is increasing rapidly (Table 5). The secular trends are based on national representative surveys: NHES I (1960–62), NHANES I (1971–74), NHANES II (1976–78) and NHANES III (1988–94). There are also racial differences in the prevalence of obesity (Flegal et al., 1998). In the early 1990s, 20% of non-Hispanic white men, 21% of non-Hispanic black men and 23% of Mexican-American men were obese. The respective numbers for women were 22%, 37% and 34%. Of particular public health concern is the high prevalence (over 40%) of class II obesity (BMI 40 kg/m^2 or more) among non-Hispanic

Table 3. Prevalence (%) of obesity (BMI 30 kg/m² or more) in the WHO MONICA populations in the early 1980s (baseline) and the early 1990s

Area	Country	Centre	Men		Women	
			1980s	1990s	1980s	1990s
Northern Europe	Denmark	Glostrup	11	13	10	12
	Finland	Kuopio Province	18	24	19	26
	Finland	North Karelia	17	23	24	24
	Finland	Turku-Loimaa	19	22	17	19
	Iceland	Iceland	11	16	11	18
	Sweden	Gothenburg	7	13	9	10
	Sweden	Northern Sweden	11	14	14	14
Western Europe	United Kingdom	Glasgow	11	23	16	23
	United Kingdom	Belfast	11	14	14	16
	Germany	Bremen	14	16	18	19
	Germany	Augsburg	18	17	15	21
	Germany	Augsburg, rural	20	24	22	23
	Belgium	Ghent	11	13	15	16
	France	Lille	14	17	19	22
	France	Toulouse	9	13	11	10
	France	Strasbourg	22	22	23	19
	Switzerland	Ticino	20	13	15	16
	Switzerland	Vaud-Fribourg	13	17	13	10
Eastern Europe	Russian Federation	Novosibirsk	14	17	44	35
	Russian Federation	Moscow	13	8	33	22
	Lithuania	Kaunas	22	20	45	32
	Poland	Warsaw	18	22	26	29
	Poland	Tarnobrzeg V.	13	15	32	36
	Czech Republic	Czech Republic	21	23	32	30
Southern Europe	Spain	Catalonia	9	16	24	25
	Italy	Area Brianza	11	14	15	18
	Italy	Friuli	16	17	19	19
North America	United States	Stanford	10	20	14	23
Asia	China	Beijing	3	4	10	8

Source: www.ktl.fi/publications/monica

black women in the middle-aged groups.

In Canada, the prevalence of obesity is lower than in the United States, being about 15% in 1991 (Reeder *et al.*, 1992). An increasing trend, however, may have occurred from the late 1970s to the early 1990s, especially in men (Table 5).

Data from Brazil are also based on nationally representative nutrition surveys showing that increases in adult obesity have been occurring in both men and women. The most recent data show that about 7% of men and 13% of women are obese (Monteiro *et al.*, 2000). The prevalence is high in the Caribbean, especially in women in Barbados, Cuba, Jamaica and St Lucia (Forrester *et al.*,

1996). However, since these data were not reported using the cut-off value of BMI 30 kg/m², the numbers are not comparable with those from other countries. In the Dutch Caribbean Island of Curaçao, 36% of women older than 18 years are obese (Grol *et al.*, 1997).

Obesity is still uncommon (1–3%) in Japan and China, but slightly more

Table 4. Prevalence (%) of obesity (BMI 30 kg/m² or more) in European populations

Population	Period	Age (yrs)	Men	Women	Reference
United Kindom, national surveys	1987/89	16+	7	12	Seidell, 2001
	1993		13	16	
	1994		14	17	
	1995		15	17	
	1996		16	18	
	1997		17	19	
Belgium (Flanders and Brussels)	1994	18–64	11	9	Moens *et al.,* 1999
The Netherlands, national surveys	1987–91	20–59	7	9	Seidell *et al.,* 1995
	1993		8	10	
	1994		10	11	
Sweden	1963	> 50	6	–	Rosengren *et al.,* 2000
	1994	> 50	11	–	
Euralim study					Beer-Borst *et al.,* 2000
The Netherlands	1990–92	20–59	12	14	
France	1995–96	35–65	8	7	
Italy (Naples)	1993–96	30–69	–	19	
Italy (Latina)	1993–96	20–84	20	37	
Switzerland (Geneva)	1993–96	29–83	11	9	
UK (Belfast)	1991–92	25–65	15	16	
Spain (Catalonia)	1992	25–75	11	22	

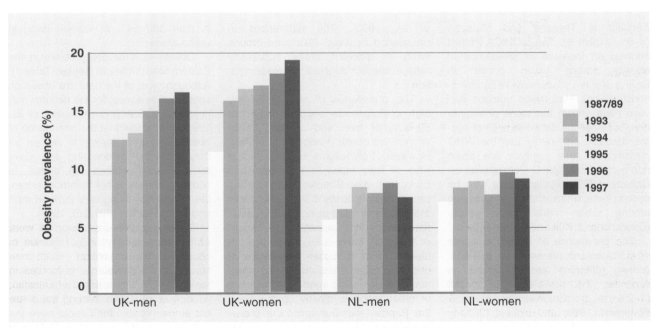

Figure 12 Time trends in the prevalence (%) of obesity in the United Kingdom (UK) and the Netherlands (NL)

Table 5. Prevalence (%) of obesity (BMI 30 kg/m² or more) in the American region

Population	Period	Age (yrs)	Men	Women	Reference
United States					
NHES I	1960–62	20–74	10	15	Flegal *et al.*, 1998
NHANES I	1971–74		12	16	
NHANES II	1976–78		12	17	
NHANES III	1988–94		20	25	
– non-hispanic white	1976–78	20–74	12	15	
	1988–94		20	22	
– non-hispanic black	1976–78	20–74	15	30	
	1988–94		21	37	
– Mexican-American	1976–78	20–74	15	25	
	1988–94		23	34	
Canada	1978	20–70	6.8	9.6	WHO Consultation on Obesity, 1998
	1981	20–70	8.5	9.3	
	1988	20–70	9.0	9.2	
National survey	1986–92	18–74	13	14	Reeder *et al.*, 1992
	1991	18–74	15	15	
Brazil, national surveys	1975	25–64	2.4	7.0	Monteiro *et al.*, 2000
	1989		4.7	12.0	
	1997		6.9	12.5	
Curaçao	1993–94	>18	19	36	Grol *et al.*, 1997

frequent in Thailand and Malaysia (4–8%) (Table 6). The MONICA Project showed an increase in prevalence of obesity among urban people in Beijing over ten years (www.ktl.fi/publications/monica). Nationwide nutrition surveys have shown the same phenomenon, but since the data-sets are not age-standardized and rarely use the WHO classification, the numbers are again non-comparable (WHO Consultation on Obesity, 1998). Similar trends can be seen in India, where obesity is increasing among urban middle-class people (Dhurandhar & Kulkarni, 1992).

The prevalence of obesity is about 10–15% in Australia and New Zealand. Among different ethnic groups in Australia, the prevalence is lowest (1–2%) in the Chinese (Hsu-Hage & Wahlqvist, 1993) and highest (25% in men and 38% in women) in the Aboriginals in the south-east (Guest

et al., 1993). The differences in prevalence between Aboriginal groups living in different areas apparently reflect different degrees of westernization.

The prevalence of obesity is very high in Polynesian populations. About 50–60% of men and up to 77% of women are obese (Hodge *et al.*, 1995). However, Polynesians have a higher ratio of lean mass to fat mass than Europeans (see Chapter 1) and so the prevalence of obesity is somewhat lower than that estimated using the BMI criteria developed for Caucasians (Swinburn *et al.*, 1999). There is an urban–rural difference, with a higher prevalence of obesity in urban areas, as well as a pronounced increasing trend. The influence of urbanization is clearly seen among the Papua New Guineans: the prevalence of obesity is only about 5% among those still living in the highlands but 36%

in men and 54% in women living in urban areas.

Obesity is a severe problem in the Eastern Mediterranean Region (Table 7). Although most of the data are based on small studies except for the national surveys in Saudi Arabia (Al-Nuaim *et al.*, 1996), they show that the prevalence of obesity increases rapidly in women as they enter the childbearing age. Over 40% of adult women are obese. In contrast, obesity is not common in Iran, the prevalence being only 2.5% in men and 8% in women (Pishdad, 1996).

Obesity is still uncommon in most African countries (Table 8). However, in countries in transition such as Mauritius, the prevalence is increasing rapidly with increasing urbanization (Hodge *et al.*, 1996). Among the different ethnic groups, the Creole have the highest prevalence (8% in men and 21% in women) and the Chinese the

Table 6. Prevalence (%) of obesity (BMI 30 kg/m² or more) in the Western Pacific Region and India

Population	Period	Age (yrs)	Men	Women	Reference
Japan, national surveys	1976	20+	0.7	2.8	WHO Consultation on Obesity, 1998
	1982		0.9	2.6	
	1987		1.3	2.8	
	1993		1.8	2.6	
Japan, national surveys	1990–94	35–64	1.9	2.9	Asia-Pacific Perspective, 2000
China, Beijing		35–64	3	4	www.ktl.fi/publications/monica
			10	8	
China, national survey	1992	20–45			Asia-Pacific Perspective, 2000
Urban			1.0	1.7	
Rural			0.5	0.7	
Thailand, national survey	1991	20+	4.0	5.6	Asia-Pacific Perspective, 2000
Malaysia		18–60	4.7	7.9	Ismail et al., 1995
Urban			5.6	8.8	
Rural			1.8	2.6	
Indian				17.1	
Chinese				4.3	
New Zealand, national survey	1989	18–64	10	12	Ball et al., 1993
Australia					
National surveys	1980	25–64	9.3	8.0	Bennett & Magnus, 1994
	1983		9.1	10.5	
	1989		11.5	13.2	
Australians	1990	20–64	9	11	Hsu-Hage & Wahlqvist, 1993
Melbourne Chinese	1989	25–69	0.8	2.3	
Newcastle	1986	35–65	15	16	Molarius et al., 1997
Perth	1986	35–65	9	11	
South-east		25–64			Guest et al., 1993
Aboriginals			25	38	
Europids			17	18	
Non-aboriginal	1980		6	9	Jones & White, 1994
Central aboriginal	1985		22	51	
West Kimberley aborig.	1986		–	17	
Yologu	1991		2	4	
Philippines		20+	1.7	3.4	Asia-Pacific Perspective, 2000
Nauru	1987	25–69	65	70	Hodge et al., 1995

Table 6 (contd)

Population	Period	Age (yrs)	Men	Women	Reference
Samoa, urban	1978	25–69	39	59	Hodge et al., 1995
	1991		58	77	
Samoa, rural	1978	25–69	18	37	
	1991		42	59	
Papua New Guinea	1991	25–69			Hodge et al., 1995
Urban coastal			36	54	
Rural coastal			24	19	
Highlands			5	5	
Rodrigues, creoles	1992	25–69	10	31	Hodge & Zimmet, 1994
India, Bombay, middle class	1991	15–30	0.3	2.5	Dhurandhar & Kulkarni, 1992
		31–50	6.5	9.6	
		50+	8.1	9.8	

lowest (only 2% in men and 6% in women) (Hodge & Zimmet, 1994).

Age, sex, social class and education
A recent analysis of data from the MONICA Project shows that socioeconomic inequalities in health consequences associated with obesity may be widening in many countries (Molarius et al., 2000). Among women, there was a statistically significant inverse association between educational level and BMI in almost all 26 populations. The difference between the highest and the lowest educational tertiles ranged from –3.1 to 0.4 kg/m² in the initial survey and from –3.3 to 0.6 kg/m² in the final survey. In men, the difference in BMI between the educational tertiles ranged from –1.2 to 2.2 kg/m² and from –1.5 to 1.2 kg/m² in the two surveys, respectively. In about two thirds of the populations, the differences in BMI between the educational groups increased over the 10-year period. There was no geographical pattern in women. In men, the association between educational level and BMI was positive in some eastern and central European populations and in Beijing, China. BMI was positively associated with education in populations with a low prevalence of

obesity and negatively in affluent populations with high prevalence of obesity.

A strong educational gradient has been found in almost all western populations besides the MONICA centres. The prevalence of obesity is higher among those with low education compared with the highly educated groups, especially among women. In many countries (e.g., Denmark, Sweden), the prevalence is not increasing only in women with high education, whereas among men it is increasing in all educational groups (Peltonen et al., 1998; Stam-Moraga et al., 1998; Moens et al., 1999; Heitmann, 2000; Lahti-Koski et al., 2000). The same phenomenon is seen in Brazil, where a very recent trend is a decrease in the prevalence of obesity in urban women (Monteiro et al., 2000). Highly educated women are more resistant to gradual weight gain with ageing than are other population groups.

Although surveys with self-reported height and weight are not generally included in this review, a recent survey among 15 239 individuals aged 15 years and over in the European Union is worth quoting since it has information on determinants of obesity (Martinez et al., 1999a). The results concerning over-

weight (BMI 25–29.9 kg/m²) are also quoted because self-reporting of weight and height leads to underestimation of BMI. Subject selection was quota-controlled to make the sample nationally representative following a multi-stage stratified cluster sampling. Self-reporting and inclusion of persons from age 15 years explain the lower prevalence rates, which were highest in the United Kingdom (12%) and lowest in France, Italy, Sweden and Switzerland (about 7%). Individuals of higher social class and younger age in all groups had a lower risk for obesity. People with a higher level of education also had lower risk, and the interaction between educational levels and obesity was weaker for men than women.

Among males, the highest prevalence of overweight was found in those aged 45–54 years who had primary school education and those aged 65+ years who had tertiary education. For all educational levels, obesity was more prevalent among the older age groups, particularly among those with a low level of education. A strong inverse association between levels of obesity and education was apparent, with 55–64-year-old primary-educated women having four times

Table 7. Prevalence (%) of obesity (BMI 30 kg/m² or more) in the Eastern Mediterranean Region

Population	Period	Age (yrs)	Men	Women	Reference
Israel (Jerusalem)	1970	50–84	12	29	Gofin et al., 1996
	1986	50–84	16	33	
	1986	50–64	18	36	
Cyprus	1989–90	35–64	19	24	Berrios et al., 1997
Saudi Arabia	1990	18–25[a]	–	4.5	Rasheed et al., 1994
		18–35[b]	–	20	
		15–35[b]	–	11	
National survey	1990–93	17+			Al-Nuaim et al., 1996
Total			16	24	
Urban			18	28	
Rural			12	18	
	1992	Adults[b]	–	47	Ghannem et al., 1993
Kuwait		Adults[b]	–	42	Rasheed et al., 1994
	1994	18+[b]	32	44	Al-Isa, 1995
Bahrain	1991–92	20-65	10	30	Al-Mannai et al., 1996
Iran	1989	20–59[c]	5	5	Ayatollahi & Carpenter, 1993
	1993–94	20–74	2.5	8	Pishdad, 1996
Morocco	1984/85		5.2		WHO Expert Committee, 1995
Tunisia, suburban	1991	20+	12	26	Ghannem et al., 1993
Tunisia	1990		8.6		WHO Expert Committee, 1995

[a] Female medical students
[b] Adults attending primary health care or private clinics
[c] Parents of schoolchildren

Table 8. Prevalence (%) of obesity (BMI 30 kg/m² or more) in the African region

Population	Period	Age (yrs)	Men	Women	Reference
Congo	1986/87		3.4		WHO Expert Committee, 1995
Ghana	1987/88		0.9		
Mali	1991		0.8		
Tanzania	1986–89	35–64	0.6	3.6	Berrios et al., 1997
Mauritius	1987	25–74	3.4	5.3	Hodge et al., 1996
	1992		5	15	
Asian Indian	1992	25–69	5	16	Hodge & Zimmet, 1994
Creole			8	21	
Chinese			2	6	
Rodrigues, creoles	1992	25–69	10	31	Hodge & Zimmet, 1994

the level of obesity of those in the same age group with tertiary education.

Risk of obesity rose steeply with increasing age, especially for the lowest social class, up to 45–64 years and declined among those over 65 years for all social classes. The highest risk of obesity was observed in 45–64-year-olds of low social class.

Survey data from Jerusalem show that in women the prevalence of obesity was lowest in the more educated and lower in those born in Europe or America than among those born in Israel (Gofin et al., 1996).

Martorell et al. (2000a) have summarized the prevalence of overweight and obesity in women from population surveys carried out in 32 developing countries in the 1990s (Table 9, Figures 13 and 14). All the surveys were cross-sectional surveys of nationally representative samples (sample sizes from 773 to 10 747 women). Most were demographic health surveys in which women of child-bearing age (15–49 years) were interviewed and measured using standard survey instruments. These data are available through the Internet (http://www.macroint. com.dhs/). South Asian women were the leanest, with about 97.7% having a BMI less than 25 kg/m^2 and only 0.1% a BMI of 30 or over. The percentages of obese women were 2.5% in sub-Saharan Africa, 9.6% in Latin America and the Caribbean, 15.4% in the Central Eastern Europe/-Commonwealth of Independent States (CEE/CIS) region and 17.2% in the Middle East and North Africa. In very poor countries, mostly in sub-Saharan Africa, obesity is concentrated among urban and highly educated women. In more developed countries, such as those in Latin America and the CEE/CIS region, levels of obesity are more equally distributed across subgroups in each country.

For comparison, the authors also analysed the prevalence of obesity in different educational groups from the United States NHANES III survey (Martorell et al., 2000a). Women were divided into four groups depending on the number of years of education completed: middle school or less (0–9 y), high school (10–12 y), university (13–16 y) and graduate work (>16 y). The prevalence of obesity in these groups was 20.1%, 24.1%, 18.9% and 9.2%, respectively.

Overweight and underweight people may co-exist in countries in transition, with underweight children living in families with overweight adults (Doak et al., 2000). Data from three large national surveys from Brazil, China and the Russian Federation show that the prevalence of such households was 8% in China and Russia and 11% in Brazil. Even more important from the public health perspective is the finding that these 'underweight/overweight' households accounted for a high proportion of all households that had at least one underweight member (China, 23%; Brazil, 45%; Russian Federation, 58%). The prevalence of such underweight/overweight households was highest in urban areas in all three countries. The underweight child co-existing with an overweight non-elderly adult was the predominant pair combination in all three countries.

It is to be expected that increasing migration between countries and from rural to urban environments all around the world, and the consequent increasing urbanization, will create wider differences in the prevalence of obesity within populations as the mixture of cultural and educational factors come into play. The findings on the high prevalence of obesity in certain social groups raise questions about the possible structural causes – the roles of social, economic, cultural or environmental factors. How such factors may be acting to curtail physical activity and/or influence food habits remains unclear.

Obesity during childhood and adolescence

It is not possible to give an overview of the global prevalence of obesity in children or adolescents because there is no common agreement on the classification of obesity in different periods of growth. BMI cut-points for different ages have recently been proposed (Cole et al., 2000). Obesity is mostly acquired during adulthood and its role in the etiology of cancer usually concerns middle-aged and older adults. However, childhood obesity seems to be increasing in all countries that have data on time trends and it usually persists into adulthood (Rudolf et al., 2001).

Cross-sectional studies in Europe indicate that overweight and obesity are a growing problem (Livingstone, 2000). The prevalence varies in a complex manner with time, age, sex and geographical region. The prevalence of obesity in young children is lower than among adolescents. Gender differences in prevalence are inconsistent. The highest rates of obesity are observed in eastern and southern European countries, particularly in Greece, Hungary, Italy and Spain. In contrast, northern European countries tend to have lower rates that are broadly similar across countries.

In the United States between 1963 and 1994, prevalence of obesity in 6–17-year olds (defined as a BMI at or above the NHANES II 95th percentile) has increased from approximately 4% to 11%. A further 14% are currently at risk of becoming overweight (BMI between the 85th and 95th percentiles) and these rates are continuing to increase (Livingstone, 2000) (Figure 15). The prevalence of overweight and obesity has increased among young inner-city schoolchildren, for example this was reported in Montreal from the early to late 1990s (O'Loughlin et al., 2000). Primary school children in Australia have also become more obese between 1985 and 1997 (Lazarus et al., 2000). Similar

Table 9. Prevalence (%) of overweight (BMI 25–29.9 kg/m^2) and obesity (BMI 30 kg/m^2 or more) in women 15–49 y in developing countries

Country (period)	% Overweight	% Obese				
		Total	Urban	Rural	High education	Low education
Sub-Saharan Africa						
Benin (1996)	6.9	2.1	3.5	1.4	8.7	1.7
Burkina Faso (1992/93)	5.9	1.0	3.5	0.6	7.1	0.8
Central African Republic (1994/95)	5.5	1.1	2.0	0.5	3.1	0.8
Comoros (1996)	15.9	4.4	9.6	2.7	7.0	4.0
Cote d'Ivoire (1994)	11.0	3.0	6.2	1.3	5.4	2.7
Ghana (1993)	9.3	3.4	8.1	1.5	12.2	2.9
Kenya (1993)	11.4	2.4	5.4	2.0	3.6	2.1
Malawi (1992)	8.1	1.1	–	–	8.3	0.8
Mali (1996)	7.2	1.2	3.5	0.4	6.5	1.0
Namibia (1992)	13.8	7.1	13.4	3.4	9.6	5.7
Niger (1992)	6.2	1.2	6.4	0.3	9.6	1.1
Senegal (1992/93)	12.0	3.7	7.2	1.9	9.7	3.4
Tanzania (1992/92)	9.3	1.9	4.1	1.2	9.6	1.6
Tanzania (1996)	10.8	2.6	6.0	1.7	8.4	2.3
Uganda (1995)	7.3	1.2	4.2	0.7	2.6	1.0
Zambia (1992)	11.8	2.4	4.5	0.4	3.9	1.9
Zambia (1996/97)	10.5	2.3	4.3	0.8	3.4	1.9
Zimbabwe (1994)	17.4	5.7	12.5	3.4	7.3	4.8
Middle East and North Africa						
Egypt (1992)	33.9	23.5	35.8	14.8	29.6	21.7
Egypt (1995/96)	31.7	20.1	30.0	26.1	13.0	17.0
Morocco (1992)	22.3	10.5	18.3	5.5	16.4	9.8
South Asia						
Bangladesh (1995/96)	2.2	0.6	2.7	0.4	1.9	0.3
Nepal (1996)	1.5	0.1	1.0	0.1	0.0	0.1
Latin America and Caribbean						
Bolivia (1994)	26.2	7.6	9.8	5.1	8.0	7.4
Brazil (1989)	25.0	9.2	9.4	8.0	13.4	8.7
Brazil (1996)	25.0	9.7	9.9	8.9	8.8	11.0
Colombia (1995)	31.4	9.2	9.2	9.1	8.7	9.9
Dominican Republic (1991)	18.6	7.3	8.8	4.7	7.8	6.9
Dominican Republic (1996)	26.0	12.1	13.4	9.6	10.0	13.8
Guatemala (1995)	26.2	8.0	12.9	5.2	13.1	7.1
Haiti (1994/95)	8.9	2.6	4.8	1.4	9.5	1.5
Honduras (1996)	23.8	7.8	13.0	4.8	6.6	8.1
Mexico (1987)	23.1	10.4	10.0	10.4	5.4	15.8
Peru (1992)	31.1	8.8	11.2	4.6	9.5	8.1
Peru (1996)	35.5	9.4	12.1	4.6	10.4	8.2
Central Eastern Europe/Commonwealth of Independent States (CEE/CIS)						
Kazakstan (1995)	21.8	16.7	17.5	15.6	–	–
Turkey (1993)	31.7	18.6	19.5	17.1	10.5	20.5
Uzbekistan (1996)	16.3	5.4	7.4	4.2	–	–

Source: adapted from Martorell *et al.*, 2000a

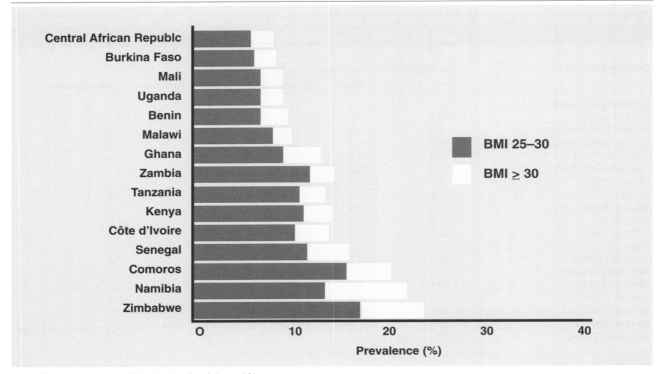

Figure 13 Obesity in women (15–49 yrs) in Sub-Saharan Africa
Adapted from Martorell *et al*., 2000a

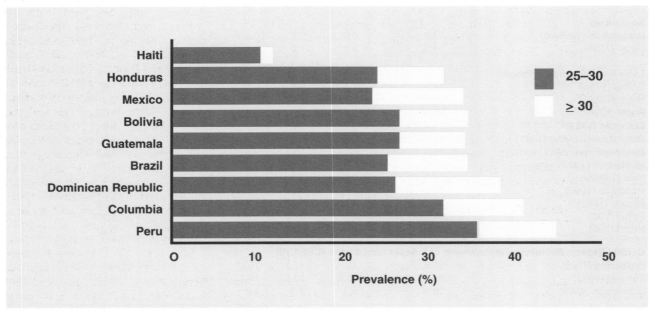

Figure 14 Obesity in women (15–49 yrs) in Latin America/Caribbean
Adapted from Martorell *et al*., 2000a

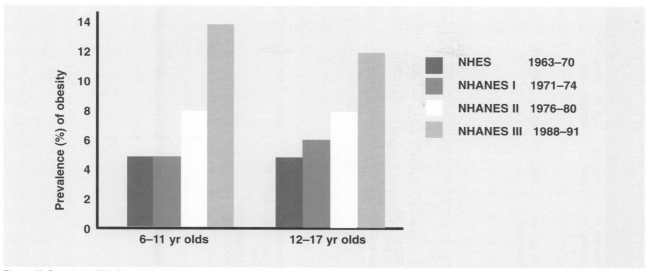

Figure 15 Prevalence (%) of obesity in 6–11-year-old and 12–17-year-old children in surveys in the United States from the 1960s to the late 1980s

trends have been reported from Denmark (Sørensen *et al.,* 1997; Thomsen *et al.,* 1999), the Netherlands (Fredriks *et al.,* 2000) and Portugal (de Castro *et al.,* 1998).

In a large analysis on overweight and obesity in preschool children in developing countries, 71 national nutrition surveys since 1986 from 50 countries were used (Martorell *et al.,* 2000b). For this analysis, overweight and obesity were defined as values >1 or >2 standard deviations above the WHO/NCHS mean weight-for-height. The prevalence of overweight and obesity was lowest in Asia and sub-Saharan Africa. Overweight was more common in urban areas, in children with mothers with high education, and in girls. In a number of countries in Latin America and the Caribbean, the Middle East and North Africa, and the CEE/CIS region, levels were as high as in the United States. A recent study of Bahraini school children found that the mean BMI for girls aged 13 years and above exceeded that of their American counterparts (Musaiger & Gregory, 2000).

Since fatness can change at a constant BMI, it is possible that children may be getting fatter at the expense of lean tissue, which may be decreasing as a result of diminishing physical activity.

Physical activity

Because physical activity is important in the prevention of a variety of diseases and conditions (US Department of Health and Human Services, 1996), it has been included as part of health behaviour monitoring in many countries.

Many countries monitor only leisure-time physical activity because national policies assume that individuals find this type of activity most amenable to intervention, and because occupational physical activity is now uncommon in westernized countries, which are the source of most comparative national data (Caspersen, 1994). However, individuals who perform large amounts of occupational activity would be misclassified as inactive if they performed little or no leisure-time activity. Even though countries may not employ a common survey assessment methodology, there is value in comparing existing data while carefully examining factors that may be responsible for differences in the estimates. Little

information from developing countries is available.

National surveys

Seven countries have included questions on physical activity as part of national surveys during the 1990s. (1) Australia conducted a National Physical Activity Survey in 1997 and 1999 (Armstrong *et al.,* 2000); (2) Canada conducted a National Population Health Survey in 1994–95 and 1996–97 (Health Canada, 1999); (3) England conducted a National Health Survey in 1994–95 and 1998–99 (Prior, 1999); (4) Finland conducted a National Health Monitoring Survey annually from 1978 through 1999 (Helakorpi *et al.,* 1999); (5) Ireland conducted the Happy Heart National Survey in 1992 (Irish Heart Foundation, 1994); (6) New Zealand conducted the Life in New Zealand Survey in 1989–90 (Hopkins *et al.,* 1991; Russell & Wilson, 1991); and (7) the United States conducted the National Health Interview Survey (NHIS) in 1985, 1990 and 1991 (US Department of Health and Human Services, 1996). In addition, one multinational comparison of physical activity was conducted in 1997 among the 15

Table 10. Characteristics of national survey systems which include physical activity, their modes of administration, their samples and response rates

Country, survey name (reference) year(s) of survey	Sponsor	Type of survey sample	Mode of administration	Months of survey	Sample size	Age of sample	Response rate
Australia							
National Physical Activity Survey (Armstrong *et al.*, 2000), 1997, 1999	Australia Institute of Health and Welfare, Department of Health and Aged Care	Households randomly selected using electronic White Pages directory. Individuals of the household with the most recent birthdate were asked to participate.	Telephone interview	November–December	3841	18–75	49–58%
Canada							
National Population Health Survey (Health Canada, 1999), 1994–95, 1996–97	Health Canada	Target population was provincial residents aged 12 years and older, except those living on Indian reserves, Canadian Forces bases, and in remote areas of Ontario and Quebec	Household interview	June 1994–August 1995 and June 1996–August 1997	69 524	> 12	NR[a]
England							
National Health Survey for England (Prior, 1999), 1994–95, 1998–99	National Centre for Social Research, Department of Health	Multi-stage stratified random sample with households drawn from Postcode Address File. Sampled addresses selected from 720 postal sectors.	Computer-assisted household interview	January 1994–April 1995 and January 1998–April 1999	1908	≥ 16	63%
European Union[b]							
Pan-European Union Survey (European Commission, 1999; Kearney *et al.*, 1999), 1997	European Commission, Directorate-General for Employment, Industrial Relations and Social Affairs	Multi-stage stratified cluster sample with quota samples in 15 countries based on age, sex and social class	Household interview	March–April	1239	≥ 15	NR

Table 10 (Contd)

Country, survey name, (reference) year(s) of survey	Sponsor	Type of survey sample	Mode of administration	Months of survey	Sample size	Age of sample	Response rate
Finland							
National Health Behaviour Monitoring System (Helakorpi et al., 1999), 1978–99	National Public Health Institute	Random sample selected from the National Population Register	Postal survey	April	3371	15–64	68%
Ireland							
Happy Heart National Survey (Irish Heart Foundation, 1994), 1992	Irish Heart Foundation	Household address chosen at random from Electoral Register. Interviewers chose remainder of households within the cluster. Additional sample quotas by age and sex.	Household interview	November	1798	30–69	N/R
New Zealand							
Life in New Zealand Survey (Hopkins et al., 1991; Russell & Wilson, 1991), 1989–90	Hillary Commission for Recreation and Sport	Random sample drawn from 97 electoral rolls of 1988. Mailing sent to about 10 persons per month	Phase I: Postal survey Phase II: Interviewer-administered survey at health examination	April 1989–March 1990	11 295	≥ 15	45%
United States							
National Health Interview Survey (USDHHS, 1996), 1985, 1990, 1991	National Center for Health Statistics	Stratified multi-stage probability design with oversampling of African-Americans and Hispanics	Household interview	January–December	36 399–43 732	≥ 18	83–88%

a NR, not reported.
b The 15 countries included in the European Union survey were Austria, Belgium, Denmark, Finland, France, Germany, Greece, Ireland, Italy, Luxembourg, the Netherlands, Portugal, Spain, Sweden and the United Kingdom.

Table 11. Characteristics of physical activity surveys, data collection and resulting data

Country, survey name (reference), year(s) of survey	Recall period	Total survey items	Method of activity probing	Type of physical activity and nature and detail of survey data	Activity summary score
Australia					
National Physical Activity Survey (Armstrong et al., 2000), 1999	Past week Average week in past 6 months	8 3	Open-ended Open-ended	Recall of number of times and total time spent doing: 1. walking for recreation/ exercise or transport ($\geq$ 10 minutes) 2. moderate-intensity activities (gentle swimming, social tennis, golf) 3. vigorous activities (jogging, cycling, aerobics, competitive tennis) to make one breathe hard, puff or pant 4. vigorous gardening and heavy yard work	Sufficient time ($\geq$ 150 minutes/week) and sessions ($\geq$ 5 sessions/ week) Sum of minutes/week spent doing walking and moderate activity plus vigorous activity (weighted by 2)
Canada					
National Population Health Survey (Health Canada, 1999), 1996–97	Past 3 months	NR[a]	List-specific	Recall of average frequency and average duration from list of activities using a modifed version of the Minnesota Leisure Time Physical Activity Questionnaire (Taylor et al., 1978) Leisure (non-working activity) Non-leisure time (at work, commuting to/from work or school, doing daily chores)	Physical activity index: Inactive: < 1.5 kcal/kg/day Moderate: 1.5–2.9 kcal/kg/day Active: $\geq$ 3.0 kcal/kg/day
England					
National Health Survey for England (Prior, 1999), 1998	Past 4 weeks	24	Close-ended	Non-work Recall of frequency (days/4 weeks) and usual duration in heavy housework, gardening, heavy manual work, walking, and sports/exercise. Used cards showing examples of types of activity	Group I (low activity) $\leq$ 3 occasions/4 weeks of moderate or vigorous activity for $\geq$ 30 minutes Group 2 (medium activity) 4–19 occasions/4 weeks of moderate or vigorous activity for $\geq$ 30 minutes Group 3 (high activity) $\geq$ 20 occasions/4 weeks of moderate or vigorous activity for $\geq$ 30 minutes

Table 11 (contd)

Country, survey name, (reference), year(s) of survey	Recall period	Total survey items	Method of activity probing	Type of physical activity and nature and detail of survey data	Activity summary score
	Past 4 weeks	5	Close-ended	Work. Combination of Standard Occupational Classification code and perception of degree of physical activity on the job (mainly sitting down/standing up/walking about, doing any climbing (excluding climbing stairs), lifting/carrying heavy loads. Work coded as vigorous if on a selected list of vigorous occupations.	Three non-independent groups: 1. Mainly sitting or standing 2. Climbing 3. Lifting/carrying heavy loads
European Union[b] Pan-European Union Survey (European Commission, 1999; Kearney et al., 1999), 1997	Average week	18 activities (17 listed, 1 'other')	List-specific	Leisure. Recall of hours/week in 18 activities spent in 7 categories of duration: ≤ 0.5, 1, 1.5, 2, 3, 4 ≥ 5 h/week	Sum of time/week spent in 18 activities. Summarized into 4 groups: none, < 1.5, 1.5–3.5, > 3.5 h/week
	Typical day at work, college, in office or at home	3 activities	List-specific	Work. Recall of hours/day spent in 3 intensity levels of work activity (sitting, standing/walking, physical work) for 10 categories of duration ranging from 0–≥ 8 h/day	Time/day spent in each of 3 work intensity levels. Summarized into 4 groups: none, < 2, 3–6, > 6 h/day
Finland National Health Behaviour Monitoring System (Helakorpi et al., 1999), 1999	Past year	1	Close-ended	Leisure. Physical activities performed for at least one half hour and that at least causes light sweating or breathlessness	Categories of a few times a year or less, 2–3 times a month, once a week, 2–3 time/week, 4–6/per week, and daily (noted those who cannot exercise)
	Usual work day	1	Close-ended	Work. 'How physically demanding is respondent's job?'	Categories included: 'Job mainly involves sitting', 'Work involves quite a lot of walking,' 'Work involves much walking and lifting,' and 'Work is very physically demanding'
	Usual work day	1	Close-ended	Transportation[c]. Time spent travelling to and from work by walking or cycling	Categories of 15, 15–30, 30–60, ≥ 60 minutes/day

Table 11 (contd)

Country, survey name, (reference), year(s) of survey	Recall period	Total survey items	Method of activity probing	Type of physical activity and nature and detail of survey data	Activity summary score
Ireland					
Happy Heart National Survey (Irish Heart Foundation, 1994), 1992	NR	NR	NR	Leisure NR	Times/week
	Usual work day	NR	NR	Work NR	Times/week
	NR	NR	NR	Outside of work NR	Times/week
	N/R	NR	NR	Watching television, playing video games NR	Hours/day spent viewing television and playing video games
New Zealand					
Life in New Zealand Survey (Hopkins et al., 1991; Russell & Wilson, 1991), 1990	Past 4 weeks	2	Close-ended	Mild/moderate and vigorous/strenuous activity Usual time spent (hours/day) in these intensity groupings	High ≥ 2 occasions/week in high-intensity activity for total of ≥ 1 h/week Moderate Not in high group but had ≥ 21 h/week of medium/low-intensity activity Low Not in moderate or high group
		2	Close-ended	Selected activities and sports Times/week spent in selected activities (lawn mowing, gardening, chopping wood, house repair, washing car, walking, running/jogging, cycling, fitness classes, fitness exercises at home) and as many as seven 'other' activities	
		1	Close-ended	Work Days/week and time/day spent in physical work or labour	
		1	Close-ended	Transportation Days/week and time/day spent walking to or from work	
		1	Close-ended	Housework Houses/day spent in 'on the move' housework	

Table 11 (contd)

Country, survey name, (reference), year(s) of survey	Recall period	Total survey items	Method of activity probing	Type of physical activity and nature and detail of survey data	Activity summary score
United States National Health Interview Survey (USDHHS, 1996), 1991	Past 2 weeks	24 activities (22 listed, 2 'other')	List-specific	Leisure Recall of average frequency, average duration, and perceived degree of increase in breathing or heart rate (i.e., none, small, moderate or large)	No leisure-time physical activity No reported activity during the previous 2 weeks Regular, sustained activity $\geq$ 5 times per week and $\geq$ 30 min per occasion of physical activity of any type and at any intensity Regular, vigorous activity $\geq$ 3 times per week and $\geq$ 20 min per occasion of physical activity involving rhythmic contractions of large muscle groups (e.g., jogging or running, racket sports, competitive group sports) performed at $\geq$ 50% of estimated age- and sex-specific maximum cardiorespiratory capacity[d]

[a] NR = not reported

[b] The 15 countries included in the European Union survey were Austria, Belgium, Denmark, Finland, France, Germany, Greece, Ireland, Italy, Luxembourg, the Netherlands, Portugal, Spain, Sweden and the United Kingdom.

[c] Response included those who did not work or worked at home.

[d] The two regression equations used to estimate the respondent's maximum cardiorespiratory capacity (expressed in metabolic equivalents, METs) are: [60−0.55 x age (years)] 3.5 for men, and [48−0.37 x age(years)] 3.5 for women (Jones & Campbell, 1982).

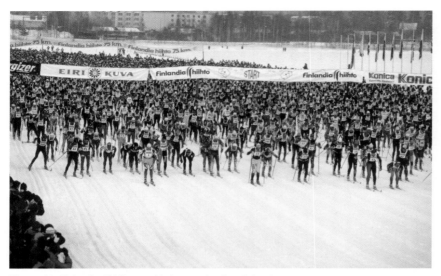

Figure 16 Finlandia Ski Race, with thousands of participants

member states of the European Union (EU) (European Commission, 1999; Kearney *et al.*, 1999; Margetts *et al.*, 1999; Vaz de Almeida *et al.*, 1999). To be considered in this section, the data for each country had to have been drawn from some sort of representative national sample and had to offer sufficient details of the physical activity survey and mode of administration to allow to understanding of the summary scores that were presented.

The methods used for these surveys are summarized in Table 10 and show the following common features: the surveys in most countries except Ireland had governmental sponsors; each country used some form of random sampling strategy to derive a population sampling frame; and the most common mode of survey administration was a household interview, except for a telephone interview (Australia) and postal surveys (Finland and New Zealand). Many countries conducted surveys in several different seasons of the year, although Canada, England, New Zealand and the United States collected data for 12-month periods. Although

countries had different sample sizes that paralleled the sizes of their populations, they tended to have different lower age bounds for their samples but generally no upper age bound, except for Australia (age 75), Finland (age 64) and Ireland (age 69). Overall survey response rates varied from 49–58% for Australia to 88% for the United States.

The summary of the characteristics of physical activity surveys in Table 11 shows that the recall period varied from a usual work day to the prior year (both for Finland); the total survey items ranged from four single-item queries with closed-ended responses (Finland) to batteries of listed activities with questions on average frequency, duration and intensity of activity participation (United States). Each country assessed leisure-time physical activity, while four countries (England, Finland, Ireland and New Zealand) and the EU assessed work activity, and two countries (Finland and New Zealand) assessed transport to and from work. The wording of the activity questions varied in many ways from survey to survey. Although countries had collected physical activity data via

self-reported questionnaires having less than ideal reliability and validity (see also Chapter 1), more accurate, meaningful and cost-effective physical activity measures are not available for representative, population-based samples.

Physical activity summary scores ranged from selecting one or combining several closed-ended response options (Finland), to scoring specific patterns of frequency and duration of leisure-time physical activity (England and the United States) or estimating daily expenditure of energy (per kg body weight) (Canada). At the highest levels of activity (see Table 12), summary scores usually reflected energy expenditure (regular activity at least five times per week and lasting ≥30 minutes duration) or the likelihood of enhancing and maintaining aerobic capacity (vigorous activity performed at least three times per week and lasting ≥20 minutes duration) – the traditional exercise prescription (Caspersen *et al.*, 1994). Most countries could be compared according to the lowest levels of physical activity, which ranged from physical inactivity in leisure time to ≤6.3 kJ (1.5 kcal)/kg/day of total estimated energy expenditure (Canada). Summary scores for work activity focused on prolonged times spent sitting on the job (EU and Finland) to participation in jobs requiring a lot of walking, lifting or physically demanding tasks (Finland). Generally, higher prevalence of the lowest levels of activity, regardless of whether this reflected leisure, work or transportation activities, were most likely to be considered as risk factors for disease or as detrimental to health.

Total prevalence of physical activity
In the surveys, the country-specific prevalence of the lowest activity levels in leisure time varied greatly (Table 12). The lowest prevalence was associated with restrictive activity definitions that were hard to meet, such as performing leisure-time activity for only a few times a year or

being unable to exercise (10.7% for Finland), or performing absolutely no physical activity during the previous week (14.6% for Australia) or during leisure-time (24.3% for the United States). The prevalence was highest for Canada (56.7%), where the definition (<6.3 kJ (1.5 kcal)/kg/day) could be easily satisfied by either doing no activity or even small amounts of physical activities. All other country-specific prevalence estimates were intermediate between those from these countries with extremes in definitions.

The country-specific prevalence for the highest activity levels in leisure time also varied widely (Table 12), being lowest for large amounts of vigorous activity such as running for ≥3 hours per week (12.7% for Ireland). The prevalence of regular participation in vigorous physical activity during the prior two weeks was 16.4% in the United States. In contrast, the highest prevalence was 59.0% (EU countries) for those reporting >3.5 hours/week in 18 leisure

activities and 62.8% (Finland) for those participating in as little as two episodes per week of physical activity producing light sweating or breathlessness lasting ≥30 minutes (Figure 17). The prevalence for other countries varied between 20.6% (Canada) and 45.2% (Australia). Estimates of persons who reported that they did not participate in any recreational activities were compiled for the 15 individual member countries of the EU (Figure 18). The lowest prevalence (8.1%, average for men and women) was in Finland and the highest (59.8%) in Portugal, a nearly three-fold difference. The average for all EU countries was 30.9%, with countries of more northerly latitude having lower prevalence and Mediterranean countries and those of more southerly latitude having higher prevalence than the average.

Four countries assessed work-related physical activity (Table 12); the lowest prevalence (19.0%) for the lowest work levels was noted for EU countries report-

ing at least six hours of sitting at work. The highest prevalence was for Finland (50.9%) for work that involves mainly sitting. The prevalence of the highest levels of work-related physical activity that had definitions most indicative of more physically demanding jobs was 31.6% for active or very active work in Ireland, and 45.0% for lifting and/or carrying heavy loads in England.

Only Finland assessed activity associated with travel to or from work (Table 12), with 46.0% of employed adults reporting the use of car or bus for transport and 39.0% walking or cycling for at least 15 minutes per day.

Prevalence of physical activity according to sociodemographic characteristics

Within a data-set, differences in cross-sectional prevalence between sexes (Table 12), age groups (Figure 19) or levels of socioeconomic status (Table 13) are described by the absolute size of the difference in percentage points (in

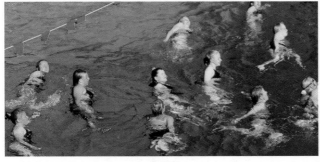
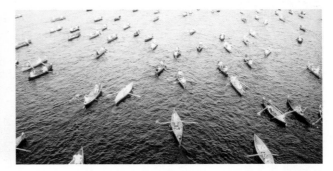
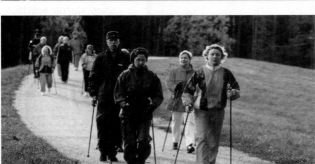
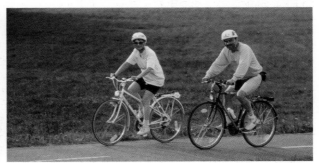

Figure 17 Examples of recreational activities (practised in Finland)

Table 12. Prevalence of physical activity for leisure, work and transport among the total population, males and females in national physical activity surveys

Type of activity, country, survey name (reference), year of survey	Lowest activity — Definition of activity level	Prevalence (%)[a] T	M	F	Moderate activity — Definition of activity level	Prevalence (%) T	M	F	Highest activity — Definition of activity level	Prevalence (%) T	M	F
Leisure activity												
Australia												
National Physical Activity Survey (Armstrong et al., 2000), 1999	Sedentary No physical activity during previous week	14.6	14.6	14.7	Insufficiently active > sedentary and < sufficiently active	40.2	38.3	41.9	Sufficiently active ≥ 150 min/week and ≥ 5 sessions/week in walking, moderate, or vigorous activity	45.2	47.1	43.4
Canada												
National Population Health Survey (Health Canada, 1999), 1996–97	Inactive < 1.5 kcal/kg/day	56.7	53.8	59.5	Moderately active 1.5–2.9 kcal/kg/day	22.7	22.3	23.0	Active ≥ 3.0 kcal/kg/day	20.6	23.9	17.5
England												
National Health Survey for England (Prior, 1999), 1998	Group 1 ≤ 3 occasions/4 weeks of moderate or vigorous activity for ≥ 30 min	38.0	35.0	41.0	Group 2 4–19 occasions/4 weeks of moderate or vigorous activity for ≥ 30 min	31.0	28.0	34.0	Group 3 ≥ 20 occasions/4 weeks of moderate or vigorous activity for ≥ 30 min	31.0	37.0	25.0
European Union[b]												
Pan-European Union Survey (Vaz de Almeida et al., 1999), 1997	Leisure time No time spent in 18 leisure time activities	31.0	NR[c]	NR	Leisure time > 0–3.5 h/week spent in 18 leisure time activities	10.0	NR	NR	Leisure time > 3.5 h/week spent in 18 leisure time activities	59.0	NR	NR
Finland												
National Health Behaviour Monitoring System (Helakorpi et al., 1999), 1999	Leisure time ≤ a few times a year of physical activity to produce light sweating or cannot exercise	10.7	12.1	9.4	Leisure time 1 time/week or 2–3 times/month of physical activity to produce light sweating	26.6	25.0	28.0	Leisure time ≥ 2 times/week and ≥ 30 min/occasion of physical activity to produce light sweating	62.8	62.9	62.6
Ireland												
Happy Heart National Survey (Irish Heart Foundation, 1994), 1992	Sedentary Sedentary at leisure	39.0	36.1	42.0	Moderate (walking, etc., ≥ 4 h/week)	48.3	47.2	49.4	Active/very active Active (running, etc > 3 h/week) and very active (regular training, competitive sports)	12.7	16.7	8.6
New Zealand												
Life in New Zealand Survey (Hopkins et al., 1991; Russell & Wilson, 1991), 1990	Low Not in moderate or high group	31.0	37.0	25.0	Moderate Not in high group but had ≥ 21 h/ week of medium/ low-intensity activity	41.0	31.0	51.0	High ≥ 2 occasions/week in high-intensity activity for total of ≥ 1 h/week	28.0	32.0	24.0

Table 12 (contd)

Type of activity, country, survey name (reference), year of survey	Lowest activity				Moderate activity				Highest activity			
	Definition of activity level	Prevalence (%)[a]			Definition of activity level	Prevalence (%)			Definition of activity level	Prevalence (%)		
		T	M	F		T	M	F		T	M	F
United States												
National Health Interview Survey (USDHHS, 1996), 1991	No leisure-time activity	24.3	21.4	26.9	100% – (prevalence of lowest plus highest activity levels)	52.2	52.2	52.4	Regular, sustained ≥ 5 times/week and ≥ 30 min/occasion	23.5	26.6	20.7
Work activity												
England												
National Health Survey for England (Prior, 1999), 1998	Mainly sitting or standing Not in any of the 3 groups (e.g., mainly walking about, climbing, or lifting and/or carrying heavy loads)	36.0	32.0	40.0	Climbing 100% – (prevalence of lowest plus highest activity)	19.0	19.0	19.0	Carrying heavy loads Lifting and/or carrying heavy loads	45.0	49.0	41.0
European Union												
Pan-European Union Survey (European Commission, 1999), 1997	Sitting ≥ 6 h/day	19.0	20.0	18.0	Sitting < 2–6 h/day	75.0	74.0	76.0	Sitting 0 h/day	6.5	6.0	7.0
Finland												
National Health Behaviour Monitoring System (Helakorpi et al., 1999), 1999	Work activities Job mainly sitting	50.9	48.9	52.6	Work activities NR	NR	NR	NR	Work activities Work involves quite a lot of walking, much walking and lifting, or is very physically demanding	49.1	51.1	47.5
Ireland												
Happy Heart National Survey (Irish Heart Foundation, 1994), 1992	Sedentary Sedentary during usual working day	27.0	25.2	32.1	Moderate Moderately active, walking quite a lot	41.4	35.4	58.8	Active/very active Active/very active during a usual working day	31.6	39.4	9.1
Transport												
Finland												
National Health Behaviour Monitoring System (Helakorpi et al., 1999), 1999	Transport Travel to work by car or by bus	46.0	55.8	37.5	Transport < 15 min/day of walking or cycling to work	15.0	14.0	15.9	Transport ≥ 15 min/day of walking or cycling to work	39.0	30.0	46.5

[a] T, = total, M = male, F = female. Total prevalence represents a simple, unweighted average of male and female prevalences for England (for all types of activity) and the European Union (for work activity only).

[b] The 15 countries included in the European Union survey were Austria, Belgium, Denmark, Finland, France, Germany, Greece, Ireland, Italy, Luxembourg, the Netherlands, Portugal, Spain, Sweden and the United Kingdom

[c] NR, not reported

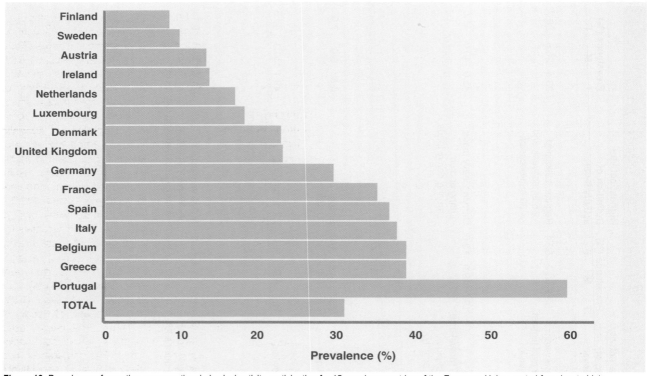

Figure 18 Prevalence of reporting no recreational physical activity participation for 15 member countries of the European Union, sorted from low to high European Commission, 1999

parentheses) as: small (<5.0%), moderate (5.0–9.9%), large (10.0–14.9%), and very large (≥15.0%) (Caspersen *et al.*, 2000). The differences between sexes for the lowest levels of leisure-time physical activity were small for Australia (0.1%) and Finland (2.7%), but large for New Zealand (12.0%), with all other countries having moderate differences of 5.5–6.0%. For the highest activity levels, the same countries showed similar small and moderate differences between the sexes to those noted for the lowest activity levels, except that the largest sex difference (12.0%) was noted for England, where the definition of highest activity included participation in moderate and vigorous physical activity. Because 'vigorous' was defined in absolute terms in England, e.g., ≥31 kJ (7.5 kcal)/min, it may have been harder for women to reach this intensity than for

men, who have a higher average maximal cardiorespiratory capacity at any given age (Caspersen, 1994). Although not tabulated, the sex difference for regular, vigorous physical activity participation was small (3.2%) in the United States, where the definition of "vigorous" was standardized according to age and sex. Otherwise, sex differences were mainly of moderate magnitude (e.g., 5.9–8.0%).

Sex differences for individual EU countries were quite variable. Women usually had lower prevalence of physical activity than men, the differences being small for Austria (–2.5), Denmark (–2.5) and Ireland (–1.0), moderate for Germany (–5.6), Italy (–6.9), Spain (–7.2) and Sweden (–7.2), large for France (–12.6) and Greece (–12.8), and very large for Portugal (–20.5). Men had lower prevalence than women for

Belgium (9.4), Finland (1.5), and the United Kingdom (5.0). There was essentially no sex difference for Luxembourg (–0.1) and the Netherlands (0.9).

For Finland, sex differences were small (3.7%) for prolonged time spent sitting on the job, while differences were moderate (8.0%) for lifting and/or carrying heavy loads in England, but very large (30.3%) for active and/or very active work in Ireland (Table 12). For Finland, sex differences were very large (≥15%) for transport to or from work, with men being more likely to use a car or bus, and women more likely to walk or cycle for ≥15 minutes per day.

Most countries showed increases in the lowest levels of physical activity as cross-sectional age increased (Figure 19(*a*)). Canada had a curvilinear increase essentially reaching an asymptotic plateau for the oldest ages,

(a)

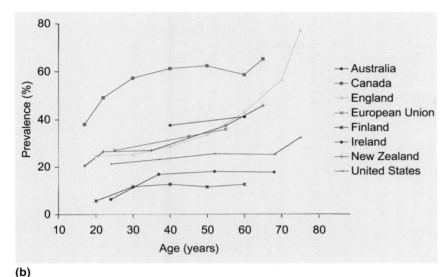

(b)

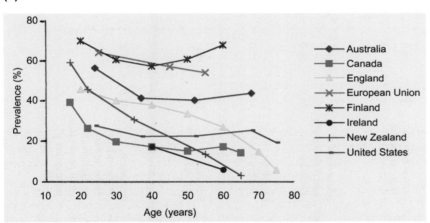

Figure 19 Changes in the (a) lowest and (b) highest levels of physical activity by cross-sectional age, by country
Data from Vaz de Almeida *et al.* (1999)

while Australia, Finland and the United States had plateaus across broad age spans following an initial increase at the youngest ages, or which was followed by an increase in prevalence in the oldest age group. The increases in prevalence were nearly identical for England and New Zealand between the ages of 20 and 60 years. The decreases in prevalence with increasing age for the highest levels of physical activity (Figure 19(*b*)) often corresponded to the increases in the lowest activity levels (Figure 19(*a*)). Australia and the United States had plateaus that corresponded to increases noted for the lowest activity levels, although Finland's plateau for the lowest activity level became a notable U-shaped curve. The other countries showed varying forms of decreasing prevalence with increasing age.

Each country provided data on prevalence of physical activity levels according to levels of socioeconomic status (Table 13) that suggest not only existing health disparities but also areas needing intervention. In terms of level of education, the differences in prevalence for the lowest leisure-time physical activity levels were moderate for Australia (8.6% comparing <12 and ≥12 years of education) and for New Zealand (9.0% comparing primary school with university or technical school education), and very large for the United States (22.9% comparing <12 years with college education or higher). The differences for the highest levels of physical activity were large for Australia (13.7%) and for the United States (10.4%), and very large for New Zealand (23.0%), but almost non-existent for Finland (1.0% comparing <10 years and ≥13 years of education). Three countries used different constructs to assess socioeconomic status. For the lowest and highest activity levels, respectively, Canada reported a large (10.7%) and a moderate (5.9%) difference comparing the lowest and highest quartiles of income adequacy; England reported a small (4.0%) and a moderate (9.5%) difference when comparing social class I with class V; and Ireland reported moderate differences (5.4% and 6.8% when comparing persons engaged in unskilled, semiskilled, and skilled manual professions with those engaged in professional and non-manual professions). Hence, there was a tendency, though not uniform, towards larger differences for the highest leisure-time activity levels compared with the lowest levels, regardless of the construct used to assess socioeconomic status. The converse was seen for socioeconomic contrasts for work activity, where differences were larger for the lowest activity levels compared with the highest activity levels for countries of the EU (15.0% and 6.0%, respectively when comparing primary and tertiary

Table 13. Prevalence of physical activity for leisure, work and transport for the lowest and highest socioeconomic groups in national physical activity surveys

Type of activity, country, survey name (reference), year of survey	Definition of socioeconomic status		Physical activity level[a]					
			Lowest (%)		Moderate (%)		Highest (%)	
			Socioeconomic status		Socioeconomic status		Socioeconomic status	
	Lowest	Highest	Lowest	Highest	Lowest	Highest	Lowest	Highest
Leisure activity								
Australia								
National Physical Activity Survey (Armstrong *et al.*, 2000), 1999	Education < 12 years	Education > High school	19.5	10.9	41.9	36.8	38.6	52.3
Canada								
National Population Health Survey (Health Canada, 1999), 1996–97	Income adequacy[b] Lowest quartile	Income adequacy Highest quartile	59.5	48.8	20.8	25.6	19.7	25.6
England								
National Health Survey for England (Prior, 1999), 1998	Social class of head of household[c] Class V	Social class of head of household Class I	34.0	38.0	40.5	26.5	25.5	35.0
European Union								
Pan-European Union Survey (Vaz de Almeida *et al.*, 1999), 1997	Education Primary level	Education Tertiary level	41.0	23.0	11.0	10.0	48.0	68.0
Finland								
National Health Behaviour Monitoring System (Helakorpi *et al.*, 1999), 1999	Education < 10 years	Education ≥ 13 years	NR[d]	NR	NR	NR	64.0	63.0
Ireland								
Happy Heart National Survey (Irish Heart Foundation, 1994), 1992	Profession Unskilled, semi-skilled, and skilled manual professions	Profession Higher professional, lower professional, other non-manual professions	41.6	36.2	49.1	47.7	9.4	16.2

Table 13. (contd)

Type of activity, country, survey name (reference), year of survey	Definition of socioeconomic status		Physical activity level[a]					
			Lowest (%)		Moderate (%)		Highest (%)	
			Socioeconomic status		Socioeconomic status		Socioeconomic status	
	Lowest	Highest	Lowest	Highest	Lowest	Highest	Lowest	Highest
New Zealand Life in New Zealand Survey (Hopkins *et al.*, 1991; Russell & Wilson, 1991), 1990	Education Primary school	Education University, technical school	46.0	37.0	49.0	35.0	5.0	28.0
United States National Health Interview Survey (USDHHS, 1996) 1991	Education < 12 years	Education College (≥ 16 years)	37.1	14.2	44.8	57.3	18.1	28.5
Work activity								
European Union Pan-European Union Survey (European Commission, 1999) 1997	Education Primary level	Education Tertiary level	13.0	28.0	78.0	69.0	9.0	3.0
Ireland Happy Heart National Survey (Irish Heart Foundation, 1994), 1992	Profession Unskilled, semi-skilled, and skilled manual professions	Profession Higher professional, lower professional, other non-manual professions	15.9	35.3	48.6	47.5	35.6	22.4
Transport								
Finland National Health Behaviour Monitoring System (Helakorpi *et al.*, 1999), 1999	Education < 10 years	Education ≥ 13 years	NR	NR	NR	NR	45.0	37.0

[a] Prevalence represents a simple, unweighted average of male and female prevalences for England (for all types of activities) and New Zealand (for all types of activity).
[b] Income adequacy is based on household income and number of persons living in the household.
[c] Social class of head of household is defined as Class I and II = professional and intermediate occupations, Class III = manual skilled occupations, Class IV and V = partly-skilled and unskilled occupations.
[d] NR, = not reported

37

(a)

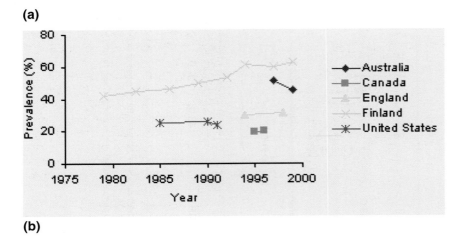

(b)

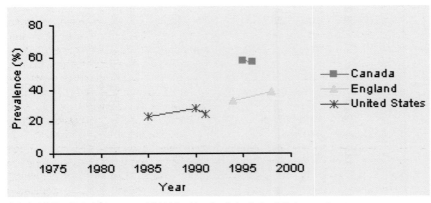

Figure 20 Trends in (a) lowest and (b) highest levels of physical activity by country

educational levels) and for Ireland (19.4% and 13.2%, respectively). For transport to and from work, there was a moderate difference (8.0%) in Finland. From these data, it is clear that socio-economic status usually has a moderate to very large association with prevalence of physical activity.

Trends in physical activity prevalence

Physical activity trends are described by the absolute size of the average annual rate of change in prevalence (in parentheses) as: small (<0.5%/yr), moderate (0.5–2.9%/yr), large (3.0–4.9%/yr) and very large (≥5.0%/yr) (Caspersen *et al.*, 2000). Trends in the lowest levels of

physical activity are inconsistent (Figure 20(*a*)), with a moderate decrease for Canada (–0.5%/yr from 1995 to 1996), a moderate increase for England (+1.4%/yr) from 1994 to 1998), and a small decrease for the United States (–0.2%/yr) from 1985 to 1990). A decrease for the United States from 1990 to 1991 reflected a survey change (Pereira *et al.*, 1997; US Department of Health and Human Services, 1996), so that further trend determination is not possible.

Trends in the highest levels of physical activity (Figure 20(*b*)) were also inconsistent, showing small decreases for Canada (–0.2%/yr) from 1995 to 1996), for England (+0.4%/yr from 1994

to 1998) and for the United States (+0.2%/yr) from 1985 to 1990). Although not shown in Figure 20, there was a small decrease in regular, vigorous physical activity in the United States (–0.1%/yr) over the same time period. Conversely, there was a quite large decrease for Australia (–2.9%/yr) from 1997 to 1999) which would be truly alarming for this country if continued over an extended period.

Children and adolescents

Childhood is generally the most physically active time during life, although in westernized countries, both cross-sectional and longitudinal studies have shown levels of physical activity to decline dramatically during adolescence and early adulthood (Anderssen *et al.*, 1996; van Mechelen *et al.*, 2000; Telama & Young, 2000). However, there have been few surveys of nationally representative samples of children and adolescents which can be compared (Caspersen *et al.*, 2000). This may arise in part from the difficulty in reliably and validly measuring physical activity in children and adolescents ranging in age from 4 to 17 years (Kohl *et al.*, 2000), while physical activity assessment for children aged 3–5 years is even more problematic.

Concluding comments

Data from these national surveys reveal that many countries have high prevalence of the lowest physical activity levels in their adult populations, suggesting that many adults are at risk for chronic diseases. This is reinforced by the often low prevalence of the highest physical activity levels – levels that would be likely to confer health benefits. However, existing surveys have not normally been designed to determine physical activity levels to address population-based cancer risks.

The differences in physical activity prevalence by sex and age, and for contrasting levels of socioeconomic

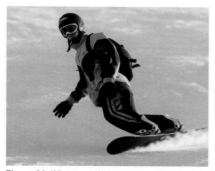 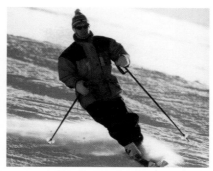

Figure 21 Winter sporting recreational physical activity

indices, reveal that disparities prevail for physical activity participation between population groups in these countries. Such differences suggest foci for intervention efforts. The few available trend data are, however, inconsistent from country to country and mostly relate to short time frames (with the exception of Finland), highlighting the need for longer-term, immutable surveillance systems that use questionnaires having high reliability and validity (Caspersen *et al.*, 1994).

In conclusion, national population prevalence data, primarily on participation in leisure-time physical activity, exist for only a small number of industrialized nations. Earlier comparisons of population surveys from various countries concluded that the extent of participation by adults in leisure-time physical activities

of the moderate and vigorous type is not at a satisfactory level (Stephens & Caspersen, 1994).

♦ Over half the adult populations of industrialized countries are insufficiently active in their leisure time to yield health benefits.

♦ One quarter to one third of adults may be classified as totally inactive in their leisure time.

♦ Less than 15% of adults participate in regular, vigorous activity.

♦ There is a clear social-class gradient for leisure time physical activity in most industrialized populations; those who are socially and economically disadvantaged are less active.

More recent data on trends in leisure-time physical activity participation show these patterns to have been relatively stable over the past two decades. There are several examples of significant regional (Bauman *et al.,* 1999; US Department of Health and Human Services, 1996), seasonal (Uitenbroek, 1993) and latitudinal (Centers for Disease Control, 1997) variations in participation in leisure-time physical activity. However, leisure-time activity is just one component of overall energy expenditure – other aspects of physical activity need to be better understood.

For the vast majority of countries worldwide, population data on physical activity participation are unavailable. This is the case for most of the world's developing nations. In these countries, economic transition involves large numbers of people moving from traditionally active rural lifestyles to cities and other urban environments. In such settings, they are likely to be much less physically active. It is plausible that such changes in physical activity are occurring and affecting an increasing proportion of the world's population, but to what extent they are taking place cannot be quantified, in the absence of population surveillance systems. Even in many developed countries, relevant data are unavailable, and where available, often address only leisure-time physical activity.

Chapter 3
Preventing weight gain and promoting physical activity

Preventing weight gain and changing the physical activity habits of individuals and populations present a formidable set of challenges. Patterns of food intake and physical activity in individuals and populations are subject to a plethora of influences at several levels (see Chapter 1). What people eat and how active or inactive they are can be influenced by genetic and biological factors; by psychological states, traits and learned habit patterns; by family, community and other proximal social influences; by organizational structures at work and other formal and informal social systems; by barriers and opportunities in people's physical environments; by economic factors that influence access to private and public resources; and by the broad political, economic and social processes that ultimately shape the patterns of behavioural choice in whole populations. It is therefore not surprising that even the best planned and most carefully implemented efforts to prevent weight gain and promote physical activity have shown only modest results.

As the body of scientific evidence in this Handbook makes clear, preventing weight gain and promoting physical activity should be central to the cancer-preventive agendas of all countries. Thus, we have a strong imperative for preventive action, but still only limited knowledge of the likely effectiveness of different types of intervention. Most interventions for weight gain prevention or for promotion of physical activity have shown only modest changes that usually were not well maintained over time after the intensive intervention phase. The way forward for cancer-prevention initiatives based on weight gain prevention and physical activity promotion must be guided by both realism and by the best use of the available scientific information.

Diet and prevention of weight gain

This Handbook has a primary focus on prevention of weight gain and promotion of physical activity. However, energy balance can also be maintained by limiting energy intake. Optimal ways to prevent weight gain by dietary modification are largely unknown. Epidemiological studies tend to suffer from increasing under-reporting of food intake with increasing body weight (Seidell, 1998). Intervention studies usually have too limited duration and too few participants to allow proper evaluation of the long-term effects on body weight in populations. There are also many dimensions of food intake other than just energy intake that may play a role (Table 14). These include macronutrient composition, energy density, food palatability and pleasure of eating, portion sizes and meal patterns (e.g., nibbling versus gorging) (Table 15).

Physical, economic and sociocultural factors also influence dietary intakes at the levels of populations, households and individuals (Egger & Swinburn, 1997).

Influences of diet on weight gain always interact with that of physical activity. For example, regular physical activity influences fat and substrate balance. This effect is considerable when an activity is maintained over a long period; physically trained individuals metabolize more fat at equivalent levels of energy expenditure than untrained individuals (Hurley et al., 1986). Stubbs et al. (1995) showed that volunteers who were moderately active were able to

Table 14. Energy content of macronutrients

Macronutrient	Energy content	
	kJ/g	kcal/g
Carbohydrate	16	4
Fat	37	9
Protein	17	4
Alcohol	29	7

Table 15. Characteristics of consumption of the major macronutrients: fat is easy to eat, but difficult to shift

	Protein	Carbohydrate	Fat
Ability to end eating	High	Moderate	Low
Ability to suppress hunger	High	High	Low
Storage capacity	Low	Low	High
Pathway to transfer excess to alternative compartment	Yes	Yes	No
Ability to stimulate own oxidation	Excellent	Excellent	Poor

consume *ad libitum* diets with 40% energy from fat, whereas the same individuals when sedentary gained weight on the same diet. It is therefore thought that people who sustain moderate or high levels of physical activity are less likely to gain weight when they eat diets with a high fat content (35–40% of energy). Because fat is a major contributor to overall energy intake, lower fat intake (e.g., 20–25% of energy) may be needed to minimize energy imbalance and weight gain in sedentary individuals. Physical activity not only influences food metabolism. It also interacts with food choice and may also affect energy balance through its effects on food intake and preferences. Information on this is rather limited.

Prevention of weight gain through physical activity

Because both weight gain and weight loss are functions of energy balance, prevention of weight gain could theoretically be achieved by changes in either dietary energy intake or physical activity (energy expenditure). Weight reduction resulting from increased physical activity without restricted energy intake is only modest (Garrow & Summerbell, 1995; National Institutes of Health and National Heart, Lung, and Blood Institute, 1998 (Figure 22). In contrast, many recent reviews have underscored the importance of physical activity in prevention of weight gain (Saris, 1998; Ravussin & Gautier, 1999; Wing, 1999; Jeffery et al., 2000). However, because of the narrative and non-systematic nature of most available reviews, a systematic review was undertaken to evaluate all research reports with data on physical activity and weight gain, published between 1980 and early 2000 (Fogelholm & Kukkonen-Harjula, 2000). The following section is based on that review. It is important to note that the review was restricted to Caucasian (white) adults, because comprehensive data were available only for this group.

The following criteria were applied in selecting prospective, observational studies for inclusion in the review:

♦ data on physical activity and change of weight (or BMI) were provided;
♦ duration of follow-up was at least two years;
♦ no intervention was performed;
♦ studies on weight change during special circumstances, e.g., after smoking cessation or during pregnancy, were excluded.

Seventeen prospective observational studies (Rissanen et al., 1991; Klesges et al., 1992; Owens et al., 1992; Williamson et al., 1993; Taylor et al., 1994; Bild et al., 1996; Haapanen et al., 1997a; Heitmann et al., 1997; Kahn et al., 1997; Parker et al., 1997; Barefoot et al., 1998; Coakley et al., 1998; Thune et al., 1998; French et al., 1999a; Guo et al., 1999; Crawford et al., 1999; Fogelholm et al., 2000a) fulfilled these criteria (Table 16). The mean duration of follow-up was approximately seven years, with a range from 2 to 21 years. All studies used a retrospective questionnaire to assess the habitual (usually over the past year) level of physical activity. Three studies (Rissanen et al., 1991; Parker et al., 1997; Thune et al., 1998) used a rough, subjective classification into 2–4 activity classes. Most studies assessed physical activity of both moderate intensity and more intense activities. Two studies focused on vigorous exercise activities (Barefoot et al., 1998; Coakley et al., 1998). Three studies also assessed occupational (or non-recreational) activity (Klesges et al., 1992; Williamson et al., 1993; Guo et al., 1999). Finally, Coakley et al. (1998) and Crawford et al. (1999) asked specifically about television and video use.

The outcomes of the studies may be grouped according to when physical activity data were collected, that is, whether baseline, follow-up or change (from baseline to follow-up) in physical activity was compared against change in weight. The studies using baseline physical activity data yielded inconsistent results. In three (Klesges et al., 1992; Owens et al., 1992; Haapanen et al., 1997a), an inverse relationship between baseline physical activity and weight change was seen, i.e., a large amount of physical activity was associated with smaller weight change. However, Haapanen et al. (1997a) reported this inverse relationship for men, but not for women. High baseline activity at work was associated with less weight gain in the study by Klesges et al. (1992). In contrast, two studies reported that a large amount of vigorous physical activity at baseline was associated with greater weight gain (Klesges et al., 1992; Bild et al., 1996). Finally, three studies did not find a significant association between baseline total physical activity (Williamson et al., 1993; Parker et al., 1997) or television and video watching (Crawford et al., 1999) and the magnitude of weight change.

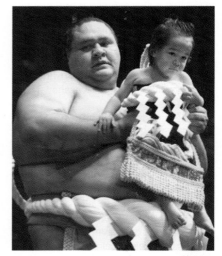

Figure 22 Difference in weight: The body weight of a person doing physical activity also affects the amount of energy used. A person weighing 220 kg will expend more energy walking for 30 minutes than a 90-kg person (Sumo wrestler Akebono and his son Hiroshi)

Table 16. Physical activity and weight gain: a summary of prospective, observational studies

Reference	Subjects, sex (age at entry)	Follow-up	Assessment of physical activity	Statistical adjustments	Main effects of PA	Results
Rissanen et al., 1991	6165 M, 6504 W (25–64 y)	5.7 y (median)	Leisure PA at follow-up (questionnaire, 3 categories: frequent, occasional, rare)	Age, BMI, education, marital status, parity, smoking, alcohol, coffee, health status	+	PA at follow-up was inversely associated with wt gain in men and women
Klesges et al., 1992	142 M, 152 W (mean 34 y)	2 y	Leisure sports activity and occupational PA score (Baecke PA scale) (data collected annually)	Baseline wt, diet, pregnancy, smoking, alcohol, family risk of obesity	+/ns/–	Baseline work ($\beta = -3.5$) and leisure ($\beta = -6.2$) activity predicted wt loss in W, but not in M. Baseline sports activity predicted wt gain in W ($\beta = 3.0$) and M ($\beta = 1.9$).
Owens et al., 1992	500 W (42–50 y)	3 y	Leisure habitual PA (Paffenbarger questionnaire; kcal/wk)	Sex-hormone use, smoking, change in menopausal status	+	Both baseline PA and increased PA were associated with less wt gain
Williamson et al., 1993	3515 M, 5810 W (mean 47 y)	10 y	Non-recreational and recreational PA (three-point scale)	Age, BMI, race, education, smoking status, alcohol, physician-diagnosed health conditions, parity	+	Wt change was inversely associated with PA at follow-up. Decreased PA was associated with wt gain. Baseline PA was not associated with wt change.
Taylor et al., 1994	568 M, 668 W (20–60 y)	7 y	Moderate and heavy PA. TV watching (h/day)	Age, smoking, sex	+	Increased PA (compared to stable or decreased PA) was associated with less wt gain
Bild et al., 1996	1100 M, 1096 W (18–36 y)	2 y	PA score (intensity and duration of PA at leisure and work)	Age, BMI, perception of fatness, physical fitness, education, smoking, diet, alcohol	ns/–	Low baseline PA predicted wt loss (OR = 0.05) in M. Change in PA was not associated with wt change.
Haapanen et al., 1997a	2564 M, 2695 W (19–63 y)	10 y	Leisure PA (scores, grouped into tertiles) and single-item self-assessment of total PA (4 classes)	Age, perceived health status, smoking status and socioeconomic status	+/ns	No regular PA at baseline was associated with ≥ 5 kg wt gain in W (OR = 1.6), but not in M (vigorous activity twice a wk was used as reference). Inactivity at follow-up was inversely associated with wt gain in both genders (OR = 2.6–2.7). Becoming physically inactive was also associated with wt gain (OR = 2.0–2.5).
Heitmann et al., 1997	2110 M, 2490 W (twin pairs) (18–39 y)	6 y	PA during leisure (classified into 3 classes by tertiles of total MET values) at follow-up	Age, smoking, zygosity, BMI at entry, change in BMI of the twin pair	ns	PA at follow-up was not associated with wt change (multiple regression)

43

Table 16 (contd)

Reference	Subjects, sex, (age at entry)	Follow-up	Assessment of physical activity	Statistical adjustments	Main effects of PA	Results
Kahn et al., 1997	35156 M, W 44080 (mean 40 y)	10 y	Jogging, aerobics, tennis, gardening and walking (h/wk). Both baseline and follow-up data were queried at follow-up.	Age, education, region of the country, BMI at age 18 y, marital status, diet, alcohol, smoking, meno-pausal status, estrogen use, parity	+	Compared with no activity, jogging > 1 h/wk (M,W), aerobics > 1 h/wk (M) or > 4 h/wk (W), tennis 1–3 h/wk (W) gardening > 1 /wk (W) or >4 h/wk (M) and walking > 4 h/wk were associated with significant BMI loss (mean −0.08 to −0.49 kg/m²).
Parker et al., 1997	176 M, 289 W (mean 47 y)	4 y	Participation in aerobic activity (dichotomous) at baseline.		ns	No association between baseline aerobic exercise and subsequent weight change (tertiles)
Barefoot et al., 1998	3885 M, 841 W (mean 19 y)	21 y	h/wk (questionnaire) at follow-up	BMI at entry, smoking, gender, depression	+	Exercise was negatively correlated with wt gain (β = −0.88).
Coakley et al., 1998	10 272 M (44–54 y)	4 y	Vigorous PA (min/wk), TV/VCR watching (h/wk) (questionnaire)	Age, diet, smoking, baseline values (including PA and TV/VCR use)	+	Vigorous PA (β = −0.16) and TV/VCR use (β = 0.02) at follow-up (adjusted to base-line values) were associated with wt change.
Thune et al., 1998	5220 M, 5869 W (20–49 y)	7 y	Leisure PA at baseline and follow-up (questionnaire, PA graded in four groups)	Age, smoking, coffee, dietary fat, menopausal status	+	Sustained high or increased PA was associated with less weight gain during the follow-up period.
French et al., 1999a	228 M, 892 W (mean 35 y)	4 y	Leisure PA score (annual questionnaire)	Age, diet, baseline values	ns	The cumulative duration of increased PA was not significantly associated (β = −0.035) with wt loss.
Guo et al., 1999	102 M, 108 W (mean 44 y)	9.1 y (mean)	Leisure and occupational PA score; individuals divided into three PA groups (biannual questionnaires)	Age, menopausal status, duration of estrogen use	+/ns	Compared with high PA (throughout the entire study period), low and medium PA were associated with wt increase (2.8 and 1.8 kg, respectively) in M, but not in W.
Crawford et al., 1999	176 M, 705 W (20–45 y)	3 y	TV watching (h/day)	Baseline BMI, obesity prevention treatment, age, education, baseline smoking, diet (multiple regression)	ns	TV viewing at baseline, average TV viewing and change in TV viewing were not associated with wt change.
Fogelholm et al., 2000a	442 M (36–49 y)	10 y	Leisure PA score (intensity x duration x frequency)	Age, weight at age 20, weight at entry, chronic diseases, smoking, occupa-tional class, diet, alcohol, marital status, former sports training	+/ns	Increased PA was negatively associated (β = −2.23) with wt change. No association for decreased PA, continuous high PA or continuous low PA vs. wt change.

Abbreviations: β, beta coefficient in multiple regression; BMI, body mass index; h, hour(s); M, men; MET, metabolic equivalents; ns, = no association between physical activity and weight maintenance; OR, odds ratio; PA, physical activity; W, women; wk, week(s); wt, weight; y, year(s); +, physical activity associated with better weight maintenance; −, physical activity associated with poorer weight maintenance.

The results using data on physical activity at follow-up were more consistent. Four studies found that a large amount of physical activity or exercise (Rissanen *et al.*, 1991; Williamson *et al.*, 1993; Haapanen *et al.*, 1997a; Barefoot *et al.*, 1998) at follow-up was associated with less weight gain. Only Heitmann *et al.* (1997) did not find such an association.

Many studies used data on physical activity from both baseline and follow-up. An increase in physical activity was associated with less weight gain in seven studies (Owens *et al.*, 1992; Williamson *et al.*, 1993; Taylor *et al.*, 1994; Haapanen *et al.*, 1997a; Coakley *et al.*, 1998; Thune *et al.*, 1998; Guo *et al.*, 1999; Fogelholm *et al.*, 2000a). Two studies did not find any association between changes in physical activity (Bild *et al.*, 1996) or in television and video watching (Crawford *et al.*, 1999) and weight change. In one study (Fogelholm *et al.*, 2000a), increased but not decreased physical activity was associated with weight change. French *et al.* (1999a) did not find an association between the cumulative duration of increased physical activity (annual recording) and weight change.

Both studies with data on only vigorous exercise (Barefoot *et al.*, 1998; Coakley *et al.*, 1998) found an inverse association between exercise and weight change. However, the different types and intensities of physical activity cannot be compared from these data. The two studies using data on television watching yielded contradictory results (Coakley *et al.*, 1998; Crawford *et al.*, 1999).

The findings that a larger amount of physical activity, assessed at the end of follow-up, was associated with less weight gain may be interpreted in three different ways: first, physical activity may really prevent weight gain; second, less weight gain may lead to better exercise adherence; third, participation in physical activity may be a proxy for a generally healthier lifestyle or psychological profile (e.g., better self-regulation).

The studies cited above did not generally include data that would allow calculation of the level of energy expenditure associated with prevention of weight gain. Data from studies examining prevention of weight relapse after prior weight reduction suggest that an increase in weekly energy expenditure of approximately 6300 to 8400 kJ/week (1500–2000 kcal/week, corresponding to about 1 h of brisk walking daily) is associated with improved weight maintenance (Fogelholm & Kukkonen-Harjula, 2000). This would correspond to an increase in daily energy expenditure of approximately 10%. However, the increase in energy expenditure needed for primary prevention of weight gain may be slightly lower.

Community interventions for prevention of weight gain

Only a few controlled community interventions have had physical activity as a central behavioural component and BMI as an outcome (Fortmann *et al.*, 1990; Murray *et al.*, 1990; Brownson *et al.*, 1996; Tudor-Smith *et al.*, 1998). These interventions were designed to decrease mortality and morbidity of cardiovascular heart diseases, but all had increased physical activity and decreased prevalence of obesity as means to achieve this main objective. Three projects (Heartbeat Wales (Tudor-Smith *et al.*, 1998), the Minnesota Heart Health Program (Murray *et al.*, 1990; Kelder *et al.*, 1993; Luepker *et al.*, 1994; Jeffery *et al.*, 1995) and the Stanford Five City Project (Fortmann *et al.*, 1990; Taylor *et al.*, 1991; Young *et al.*, 1996)) included both intervention and control communities, whereas the Bootheel Heart Health Project (Brownson *et al.*, 1996) had the state as a comparison area. The duration in the interventions was 4–7 years. The subjects were obtained by random cross-sectional sampling at the beginning and the end of the follow-up (Brownson *et al.*, 1996; Tudor-Smith *et al.*, 1998) or through a combination of

cohort and independent cross-sectional surveys (Fortmann *et al.*, 1990; Murray *et al.*, 1990).

These projects based their intervention on widespread educational approaches, that is, face-to-face counselling by health professionals and peers, and use of mass media (television, radio, newspapers, print materials). Moreover, the use of social support (organized groups, such as walking clubs), physical activity contests, opinion leaders and models, and risk-factor screening were common to these interventions. Changes in the physical environment (e.g., building of walking and fitness paths) were reported in one project only (Brownson *et al.*, 1996), whereas policy changes, with special labelling of foods in grocery stores and restaurants, were described in two interventions (Kelder *et al.*, 1993; Tudor-Smith *et al.*, 1998).

Out of the four projects, two (Brownson *et al.*, 1996; Tudor-Smith *et al.*, 1998) did not detect any significant effect of intervention on physical activity, although there was a tendency for increased physical activity in the intervention areas of the Bootheel Heart Health Project (Brownson *et al.*, 1996). The residents of the intervention communities of the Minnesota Heart Health Study were somewhat more physically active (self-reported) at the end of the follow-up (Kelder *et al.*, 1993), an increase apparently due to an increase in activities of low intensity. In the Stanford Five-City Project, the intervention had a positive effect on physical activity in the independent, cross-sectional samples, but not in the cohort survey (Fortmann *et al.*, 1990; Young *et al.*, 1996). The observed increase was seemingly due to increased amounts of daily usual activities, rather than to vigorous exercise (Young *et al.*, 1996).

Although the results on physical activity were somewhat positive in most projects, the effects on body weight change were disappointing. Three projects did not find any effect of intervention on BMI (Jeffery *et al.*, 1995; Brownson *et al.*, 1996; Tudor-Smith *et al.*, 1998). In the Stanford Five-City Project, BMI increased less in the treatment than the control communities, but this effect was observed only by using cross-sectional, independent surveys (Taylor *et al.*, 1991).

Despite the fact that a majority of cross-sectional and observational studies have shown that high physical activity is associated with smaller weight gain, the success of community studies in preventing weight gain was not very good. The failure to show clear intervention effects could be due to methodological problems. Multifaceted interventions are difficult to evaluate in general and methods of assessing physical activity in large groups are quite crude and imprecise (Wareham & Rennie, 1998). Moreover, favourable secular trends in dietary choices as well as in smoking cessation may not only dilute intervention effects but also confound the effect of physical activity in prevention of weight gain.

Another obvious reason for the above discrepancy is that physical activity and energy expenditure in the intervention communities did not increase enough to counterbalance secular changes in food intake and daily activity (Fogelholm *et al.*, 1996a). In the most successful intervention (The Stanford Five-City project; Taylor *et al.*, 1991) the difference in estimated daily energy expenditure between the intervention and control communities was 250 kJ/day (60 kcal/day), a weekly difference of 1750 kJ (420 kcal). This is much less than has been associated with prevention of weight regain (Fogelholm & Kukkonen-Harjula, 2000). Moreover, it is probable that the three other community interventions were even less successful in increasing total energy expenditure. There are several potential explanations for the difficulty in increasing physical activity in intervention communities:

- The focus has been too much on traditional physical activity, rather than usual daily activities (lifestyle activity). The same problem is also seen in controlled obesity treatment trials. It is likely that large population segments may more readily accept increased lifestyle activity than more structured exercise training.

- There was too little priority for physical activity in the interventions. All interventions cited above had a decrease in cardiovascular disease mortality and morbidity as primary objective. This meant that the approaches were very broad and physical activity was just one focus of the intervention plan.

- The interventions were too general and hence important subgroups were lost. For instance, Jeffery *et al.* (1995) noted that the intervention effects were more clearly seen in residents with elevated serum cholesterol concentration or a history of obesity-related disease. Other potential subgroup targets for physical activity interventions could be people of lower social status, minority groups and older adults.

- A high-profile health promotion programme extended even to the control area (Luepker *et al.*, 1994; Tudor-Smith *et al.*, 1998). The intervention and control communities were not isolated, both areas being targets of health promotion through mass media and from physicians and other health professionals. If the educational environment is already saturated with health promotion material, any additional efforts may have only marginal effects (Jeffery *et al.*, 1995).

- All interventions had a strong emphasis on education, their basic assumption being that increasing the level of knowledge about obesity-related risks, dietary choices and exercise behaviour would enable people to improve weight

maintenance (Jeffery *et al.*, 1995). Only the Bootheel Heart Health Project reported deliberate efforts to change the physical environment by construction of walking and fitness paths (Tudor-Smith *et al.*, 1998).

Prevention of weight regain after prior weight reduction

The challenge in weight reduction is not really to lose enough weight, but rather to maintain the reduced weight. Most studies show very poor weight maintenance, regardless of the technique used to reduce body weight (Glenny *et al.*, 1997). The role of physical activity in prevention of weight regain was studied in the review by Fogelholm and Kukkonen-Harjula (2000) of both observational studies and randomized clinical interventions. The main results are summarized below.

A total of 19 non-randomized weight-reduction interventions with an observational follow-up were reviewed. The duration of the follow-up was typically between one and three years. Most of the studies used a retrospective questionnaire or an interview to assess physical activity. Only Schoeller *et al.* (1997) measured total activity level by the doubly labelled water technique, focusing on vigorous exercise, rather than total physical activity.

The results from the above studies were quite consistent: a total of 12 studies found that a large amount of physical activity at the follow-up measurement was associated with less weight regain after weight reduction. Four studies used the change in physical activity from baseline (immediately after weight reduction) to the end of the follow-up: they all reported that increased physical activity was associated with a smaller weight regain. Using only baseline (after weight reduction) data on physical activity, however, gave less consistent results: Schoeller *et al.* (1997) found that more physical activity was associated with better weight maintenance,

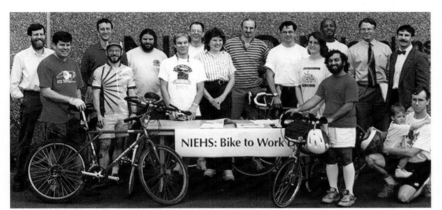

Figure 23 Bike to Work Day: promotion of physical activity at the National Institute of Environmental Health Sciences (NIEHS) in the United States

although McGuire et al. (1999) did not find such an association. Jeffery et al. (1984) reported that physical activity immediately after weight reduction, but not one year later, was associated with less weight regain at two years' follow-up.

Eight randomized interventions with exercise and control groups and a prospective follow-up of at least one year's duration (Perri et al., 1986; Sikand et al., 1988; King et al., 1989; Pavlou et al., 1989; van Dale et al., 1990; Skender et al., 1996; Wadden et al., 1998; Wing et al., 1998) were reviewed (Table 17). The duration of weight reduction varied between eight weeks and 12 months. Three studies used a very low-energy diet (Sikand et al., 1988; Pavlou et al., 1989; van Dale et al., 1990) during the weight-reduction phase, while the other studies used a more conventional diet with restricted energy intake. Only Perri et al. (1986) reported use of behaviour therapy. All studies used aerobic exercise (walking or ergometer cycling) with a target duration of approximately 1.5 to 3 h/week. In addition, Wadden et al. (1998) had one group with strength training.

Only one study (Pavlou et al., 1989) found clearly that exercise training during weight reduction led to less weight gain during the follow-up than in non-exercising groups. Sikand et al. (1988) reported a similar but non-significant difference. King et al. (1989) found that weight regain was smallest in exercising subjects randomized to supportive telephone contacts during the follow-up. However, those exercising subjects who were randomized to no extended support showed a tendency to regain even more weight than the diet-only subjects. van Dale et al. (1990) reported better weight maintenance in one physical exercise group ($N = 5$), but the finding was apparently caused by one outlier. In contrast to the above results, four studies did not find exercise training to improve maintenance of reduced body weight (Perri et al., 1986; Sikand et al., 1988; Wadden et al., 1998; Wing et al., 1998).

Very few studies (Perri et al., 1988; Leermakers et al., 1999; Fogelholm et al., 2000b) have used a design with randomization to exercise and control groups after weight reduction (Table 18). Perri et al. (1988) used several weight-maintenance techniques, including aerobic exercise in two groups (men and women). All groups participating in the six-month weight-maintenance intervention had less weight gain compared with the controls, who were not contacted after the weight reduction. Nevertheless, the exercise groups did not succeed any

better or worse than the other weight-maintenance groups. Leermakers et al. (1999) randomized 67 subjects (men and women) into exercise-focused and weight-focused groups after a six-month weight-reduction period. The exercising subjects met bi-weekly in supervised exercise session and were also trained in relapse prevention strategies to avoid or cope with lapses in exercise. The weight-focused group learned problem-solving for weight-related difficulties, without emphasis on physical activity. During the unsupervised follow-up (six months), the exercise-group gained more weight than the weight-focused group. Finally, in the study of Fogelholm et al. (2000b), weight-reduced, but still overweight or obese, premenopausal women were randomized into control, moderate walking (target activity energy expenditure 4.2 MJ/week (1000 kcal/week)) and heavy walking (8.4 MJ/week (2000 kcal/week)). All groups received diet counselling. Compared with the end of weight reduction, weight regain at the two-year follow-up was 3.5 (95% confidence interval 0.2–6.8) kg less in the moderate walking group than in control subjects. The heavy walking group did not differ from the controls.

Inadequate amounts of physical activity may help to explain why it has been so difficult to find an effect of physical activity on weight maintenance in clinical trials. The weekly amount of prescribed exercise in the randomized trials varied from 80 min to 300 min, which corresponds to an increase in weekly energy expenditure by 2300 to 8800 kJ (560 to 2100 kcal). However, adherence to the exercise prescription is much less than 100%, and in particular long-term adherence may be poor.

According to four studies (Hartman et al., 1993; Ewbank et al., 1995; Schoeller et al., 1997; Jakicic et al., 1999), the estimated difference in energy expenditure from physical activity between the highest and the lowest exercise group was more than 5500 kJ/week (1300

Table 17. Physical activity and weight regain: a summary of randomized controlled trials with or without exercise during weight reduction. All subjects were overweight or obese initially

Reference	Subjects	Weight reduction trial design (method, amount)	Exercise prescription	Follow-up	Results
Perri et al., 1986	14 M, 76 W	20 wk. BT only, BT + EX. Mean wt loss 9.4 kg.	4 x 20 min aerobic EX weekly	18 mo, including 6 mo maintenance support by mail and phone. 67 measured (74%)	Wt regain was similar in BT (3.1 kg) and BT + EX (3.3 kg) groups
Sikand et al., 1988	30 W	4 mo. VLED only, VLED + EX. Mean wt loss 19.8 kg.	Aerobic EX, 2 supervised weekly sessions (about 60–90 min/wk)	24 mo. 21 measured (70%).	Wt regain tended to be less in EX subjects (58% vs. 96%)
King et al., 1989	103 M	12 mo. Diet only, EX only. Mean wt loss 6.0 kg.	3 x 40–50 min brisk walking weekly + encouragement to increase lifestyle activity (120–150 min/wk)	12 mo. Randomized into support contacts by mail and phone vs no contact. 72 measured (70%); 48 in maintenance support.	2-y wt regain was smallest (17%) in EX subjects with maintenance support. EX without support gained 71% and the diet groups 41–42% of wt loss.
Pavlou et al., 1989	160 M	8 wk. 4 different VLEDs (420–1000 kcal/d). Diet only, diet + EX (4 x 2 groups). Mean wt loss 13.3 kg.	3 x 90 min EX weekly, including 35–60 min aerobic EX per session (270 min/wk)	18 mo. 110 measured (69%).	EX groups regained about 10% of the wt loss, whereas the diet groups regained 92%
van Dale et al., 1990	15 M, 39 W	Duration 12–14 wk. VLED only, VLED + EX. Mean wt loss 12.2 kg.	Aerobic (2–3 h/wk) and fitness (2 h/wk) training (240–300 min/wk)	18–42 mo. 36 measured (67%).	In one study, EX improved wt maintenance at 42 mo, but the difference was apparently caused by one outlier. No other effects of EX were reported for the other two studies.
Skender et al., 1996	66 M, 61 W	12 mo. Diet only, EX only, diet + EX. Mean wt losses 6.8, 2.9, 8.9 kg.	Walking; target goal 5 x 45 min/wk (225 min/wk)	12 mo. 61 measured (48%)	Wt regain was similar in diet + EX vs. diet only groups. EX only lost and regained less.
Wadden et al., 1998	99 W	48 wk. Aerobic EX + diet, strength training + diet, aerobic EX + strength training + diet, diet only. Mean wt loss 15.6 kg.	2–3 weekly sessions. Aerobic = step aerobics; strength = Universal Gym or Cybex equipment; combination = 40% aerobic, 60% strength (120–180 min/wk).	12 mo. 77 measured (78%).	EX did not affect maintenance of wt loss.
Wing et al., 1998	32 M, 122 W	6 mo. CON, diet only, EX only, diet + EX. Mean wt losses 1.5, 9.1, 2.1, 10.3 kg.	Brisk walking etc., 5 days/wk, target energy expenditure 6.3 MJ (1500 kcal) per wk.	18 mo. 129 measured (84%).	EX did not affect maintenance of wt loss.

Abbreviations: BT, behavioural therapy; CON, control subjects (no treatment); EX, exercise; M, men; mo, month(s); PA, physical activity; VLED, very-low-energy diet; W, women; wk, week(s) wt, weight

Table 18. Physical activity and weight regain: randomized controlled trials with or without exercise training after weight reduction

Reference	Subjects	Weight reduction	Maintenance intervention	Follow-up (method, amount)	Results
Perri et al., 1988	26 M, 97 W	BT. 12.4 kg in 20 wks	6 mo. Extended therapist contact (C) vs C and social influence (S) vs C and 4 x 20 min aerobic EX weekly vs C, S and EX vs no maintenance support	12 mo. 91 measured (74%)	All 4 conditions with maintenance support yielded better long-term wt loss than BT alone. EX did not significantly affect the results
Leermakers et al., 1999	13 M, 54 W	Diet + BT, 8.8 kg in 6 mo.	6 mo. EX vs wt-focused. EX = 150 min/wk, biweekly sessions, contingencies, relapse prevention training. 57 (85%) completed	6 mo. 48 completed (72%)	EX subjects gained more (4.4 kg) than the wt-focused subjects (0.8 kg) during mo 6 to 12.
Fogelholm et al., 2000	85 W	VLED, 13.1 kg in 3 mo.	9 mo. Randomized into walking (2 groups, EX-1 = target energy expenditure 4.2 MJ/wk, EX-2 = 84 MJ/wk) and CON. All received diet instruction.	24 mo. 74 measured (87%)	The mean wt regain after WR was 8.3 kg. Compared with the end of WR, wt regain at the end of follow-up was 3.5 (95% CI 0.2–6.8) kg less in EX-1 vs CON.

Abbreviations: BT, behavioural therapy; CI, confidence intervals; CON, control subjects (no treatment); EE, energy expenditure; EX, exercise; M, men; mo, month(s); VLED, very-low-energy diet; W, women; WR, weight reduction intervention; wt, weight

kcal/week), but less than 8400 kJ/week (2000 kcal/week). The difference in yearly weight regain (high versus low exercise groups) in the above studies was 5 to 8 kg. Hence, it seemed that an increase in energy expenditure of physical activity of approximately 6300 to 8400 kJ/week (1500–2000 kcal/week, corresponding to 1 h of brisk walking daily) was associated with improved weight maintenance. This is more than most randomized trials aimed at, and certainly more than the exercisers actually achieved. Keeping up increased regular exercise is believed to be particularly problematic among obese subjects, who may have both physiological and psychological barriers to physical activity (Fogelholm & Kukkonen-Harjula, 2000).

All randomized trials used traditional structured training prescription with walking, jogging or ergometer cycling as the modes of exercise. Only King et al. (1989) encouraged subjects also to increase daily lifestyle activity. Since the introduction of health-related exercise (Pate et al., 1995), interest in lifestyle activity (with several short bouts of exercise daily) has increased, but few groups have studied the effects of lifestyle activity (Andersen et al., 1999; Dunn et al., 1999) or of multiple short-bout exercise (Jakicic et al., 1999) on weight change in overweight persons. None of these studies found any statistically significant difference between the effects of different kinds of activity on weight.

Some groups have studied different strategies to improve adherence to exercise programmes. Three papers have reported that adherence to a home-based exercise programme is at least as good as a supervised group programme among overweight persons (King et al., 1991; Perri et al., 1997; Jakicic et al., 1999). Exercise prescribed in multiple short bouts rather than as one continuous daily bout may or may not improve exercise adherence (Jakicic et al., 1995, 1999). Although one might suppose that adherence would be easier for a lifestyle activity than for a more fixed exercise regimen, two studies (Andersen et al., 1999; Robinson, 1999) found adherence to be equal for both approaches.

How to increase physical activity

The first US Surgeon General's Report on Physical Activity and Health (United States Department of Health and Human Services, 1996) has established the importance of the overall physical activity and health agenda. It is not known to what extent it will be feasible to integrate systematic and cost-effective exercise

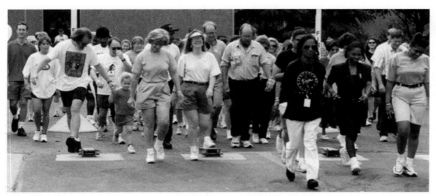

Figure 24 Organized walking day for NIEHS staff members and family

counselling into routine primary care and other health services. It is also not yet clear what effects might be achieved by mass-reach, ubiquitous public health strategies that offer 'passive' protection to populations by creating (or recreating) environments in which physical activity is a natural and enjoyable part of people's lives.

Trials of interventions to increase physical activity typically lead to modest initial changes in behaviour and any changes tend not to be maintained after the intensive initial intervention phase.

Controlled intervention trials in health-care settings that yielded the strongest and best-maintained effects on behaviour have revealed several important elements, including multiple and continuing contacts with participants and multiple behavioural intervention components (Simons-Morton *et al.,* 1998). For such individual or small-group interventions, the most effective programme elements appear to be the use of structured behaviour-change techniques; educational, health-risk appraisal and verbal persuasion methods have been found to be far less effective (Dishman & Buckworth, 1996).

Workplace, community and mass-media intervention studies have typically found modest or no actual effects on behaviour and, where it has been assessed, poor maintenance of behav-

ioural changes (Dishman *et al.,* 1998; Marcus *et al.,* 1998).

The conduct of physical activity intervention trials on which to base large-scale, comprehensive strategies has inherent scientific difficulties. Meta-analyses and qualitative reviews of published studies have identified several areas of methodological limitation. These include lack of standardized outcome measures, lack of rigorous experimental controls and compromises in the implementation of interventions (Dishman *et al.,* 1998). Studies that meet rigorous methodological criteria and that demonstrate strong and sustained effects on physical activity behaviour are few. However, behavioural scientists, epidemiologists, exercise and sport scientists and others are developing improved, standardized and objectively validated measures of physical activity behaviours and are applying these in population studies (Sallis & Saelens, 2000). New studies of physical activity determinants, including environmental influences, are being developed (Baker *et al.,* 2000; Owen *et al.,* 2000). Particular issues for higher-risk or traditionally neglected groups are being identified and addressed systematically (Taylor *et al.,* 1998; Ainsworth, 2000; Ainsworth *et al.,* 2000). Trials of innovative approaches to increasing energy expenditure through incidental and

lifestyle activities are under development (Dunn *et al.,* 1998).

The major need is to develop evidence-based mass-reach interventions, along with environmental and policy changes that can be demonstrated to have a positive impact on rates of participation in physical activity (Jebb & Moore, 1999; Sallis *et al.,* 1998). For example, there are now opportunities to conduct trials of mass-reach behavioural-change services that use combinations of traditional broadcast media with the new capacities provided by the Internet and other information technology innovations. Such strategies can potentially provide automated, individually tailored physical activity assessments and structured, interactive advice to large numbers of people at very low cost (Marcus *et al.,* 1998).

It may be helpful for interventions to focus on sedentary behaviour as an entity in its own right (Jebb & Moore, 1999; Owen *et al.,* 2000). Prolonged periods of sedentary behaviour at work may in future be regarded as an occupational health risk.

Trials of interventions to influence physical activity have focused on individuals. The challenge is to influence whole populations effectively. The extensive social changes and strategies needed to promote physical activity will require strong interactions between science, advocacy and public health policy. Environmental and policy initiatives require research on new ways to assess putative macro-level influences on physical activity. Such environmental and policy interventions include, for example, the provision of walking and cycling paths, restrictions on automobile access to city centres and provision of showers and changing facilities at workplaces. Systematic trials are needed to demonstrate the extent to which such changes can influence people's choice to be more active (Sallis *et al.,* 1998).

Lessons to be learned from other successful public health campaigns

Campaigns that have been successful in dealing with public health problems include those to discourage smoking and drink-driving or to promote immunization and the wearing of seatbelts. Analyses of these campaigns have helped to identify features that can be applied in public health interventions to control obesity (Egger & Swinburn, 1997). For example, it appears that programmes which involve government, the community, the food industry and the media, and which are of long duration, lead to positive and sustainable change (WHO Consultation on Obesity, 1998).

Public health programmes to prevent weight gain are unlikely to achieve the same spectacular rates of success as those associated with the control of infectious disease. Unlike the case of pathogens, it is not feasible to remove totally the causes of obesity. Nor is it a simple process to isolate and manage exposure to major disease-promoting factors in the way that the control of smoking and hypertension has contributed to the reduction in rates of chronic heart disease. Overweight, the consequence of energy imbalance, is more tightly controlled physiologically than other risk factors are and is subject to many environmental influences that shape food choices and physical activity behaviours (Figure 25). Nevertheless, with concentrated efforts, particularly along the lines recommended in Chapter 10, successes in weight gain prevention and in physical activity promotion can be achieved.

There are good reasons to believe that well conducted preventive initiatives with adequate resources will succeed. For example, large numbers of people in many populations do maintain habits of regular physical activity and maintain a healthy body weight. While this is more likely in higher socioeconomic groups, it should nevertheless be seen as realistic and achievable. Regular physical activity and maintaining a healthy body weight will be more possible if people have supportive environments. Where governments and community bodies provide facilities and settings for physical activity, or where there are well organized programmes with adequate resources, people are better able to maintain regular activity. For societies to provide such support and services, significant commitments of funding and well developed policies and organizational systems are required. Given the extent of cancer-related risk and other health risks associated with overweight and inactivity including heart disease and diabetes, such serious commitments should be made.

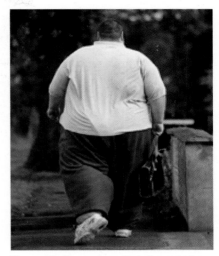

Figure 25 Keep on moving! A person loses 25% of his or her lean body mass and 75% of his or her fat when losing weight through reduction of energy intake alone. Weight loss that is achieved with a combination of dietary restriction and physical activity is more effective !

For maintenance of desirable body weight a maintenance level of energy intake alone with physical activity is recommended to preserve lean body mass and muscle tone.

Chapter 4

Metabolic consequences of overweight, underweight and physical activity/inactivity

Humans

Both body weight and physical activity can have marked effects on several physiological systems that may subsequently affect cancer risk. These include in particular effects on hormonal milieu and immune function. In this section, results from cross-sectional and human intervention studies on the relationships of weight, weight loss and physical activity with hormonal and immunological variables are reviewed. Both acute effects of physical activity sessions and long-term effects of training are covered.

Results on the association of selected hormones and binding globulins with obesity and weight reduction, and with physical activity are summarized in Tables 19 and 20, respectively.

Insulin resistance

An essential action of insulin in the body is control of the uptake, synthesis and use of glucose. The action of insulin is reflected in the glycaemic curve, which is a plot of plasma glucose level against time after an oral glucose dose (the oral glucose tolerance test, OGTT, as used routinely for diabetes diagnosis). The area under the glycaemic curve provides a measure of the rate of disposal of glucose; insulin levels can be similarly plotted during the test and the area under the insulinaemic curve is also an indication of insulin sensitivity. Obesity and lack of physical activity are major determinants of insulin resistance.

Insulin resistance is a state of reduced responsiveness of muscle, liver and adipose tissue to insulin. One major effect of insulin resistance is a rise in

blood glucose levels, due to lower glucose uptake from blood by skeletal muscle and liver, as well as to reduced insulin-related inhibition of hepatic gluconeogenesis (DeFronzo, 1988; Mandarino, 1999; Radziuk & Pye, 1999). This chronic increase in blood glucose concentration is also reflected in higher levels of glycosylated haemoglobin (Larsen, 1989). At the extreme, insulin resistance may cause glucose intolerance and lead to the development of (type II) diabetes mellitus (Unger & Foster, 1998). In insulin-resistant states, fasting and non-fasting plasma insulin levels increase so as to maintain blood glucose levels within acceptable limits.

Elevated fasting and postprandial insulin concentrations, increased glycosylated haemoglobin and decreased glucose tolerance are indisputably associated with obesity (Haffner et al., 1994a; Strain et al., 1994; Ivandic et al., 1998; Boeing et al., 2000). The relationship between BMI and fasting insulin level is continuous and linear: for example, in the study of Strain et al. (1994), fasting insulin concentration increased by 1 U/mL per unit increase in BMI. There is also good evidence that an increase in intra-abdominal (visceral) fat is especially related to the development of insulin resistance (Krotkiewski et al., 1983; Seidell et al., 1990a; Leenen et al., 1994; Rasmussen et al., 1994; Cigolini et al., 1995; Björntorp, 1997; Anderssen et al., 1998; Ivandic et al., 1998; Haffner, 2000).

One central mechanism linking particularly visceral fat accumulation to insulin

sensitivity is an increase in plasma concentrations of free fatty acids (Figure 26). (Seidell et al., 1990a; Haffner, 2000). Intra-abdominal fat is mobilized more easily than most fat deposits elsewhere in the body, because it is more sensitive to lipolytic stimuli (e.g., through β3-adrenergic receptors), leading to a constantly increased release of free (non-esterified) fatty acids into the circulation. Elevation of free fatty acid levels causes liver and skeletal muscle to shift towards greater oxidation of fatty acids for energy production, and a relative inhibition of enzymes in the glycolytic cascade (Krebs cycle) (Randle, 1998). As a consequence, the capacity of these tissues to absorb and metabolize glucose and to store glucose in the form of glycogen decreases (Ebeling & Koivisto, 1994) and cells accumulate more triglycerides instead of glycogen as a local energy reserve. In addition to the altered activities of glucose and fatty acid-metabolizing enzymes, insulin-resistant cells generally have lower membrane levels of insulin receptors (Flier, 1983).

Insulin resistance and fasting plasma insulin concentrations reach peak levels during the pubertal growth spurt (Amiel et al., 1986; Bloch et al., 1987; Smith et al., 1988; Caprio et al., 1989). This may be due to the rise in pituitary secretion of growth hormone, which has strong lipolytic effects and increases plasma concentrations of free fatty acids (Bratusch-Marrain et al., 1982; Rizza et al., 1982; Hindmarsh et al., 1988; Martha & Reiter, 1991). During puberty and adolescence, as at adult age, insulin resistance is

Table 19. Associations of obesity and weight reduction with selected hormones and binding globulins

Hormone or binding globulin	Obesity (cross-sectional)	Weight reduction
Insulin	↑	↓
Insulin-like growth factor-I (IGF-I)	↓ or NE; ↑ (free IGF-I)	↑ or NE
IGF binding protein-1	↓	↑ ?
IGF binding protein-3	↑ or NE	↑ ?
Human growth hormone	↓	↑
Sex-hormone binding globulin	↓	↑
Total testosterone	↑ (PCOS); ? (F); ↓ (M)	↓ or NE (F); ? (M)
Free testosterone	↑ (F) ; ↓ (M)	↓ or ↑ or NE
Estradiol	↑ (M, postmenopausal F)	↓
	NE ? (premenopausal F)	↓ or NE
Dehydroepiandrosterone (sulfate)	↓ or NE	↑ or NE
Prolactin	NE	NE

↑, increased levels; ↓, decreased levels; NE, no observed effect; ?, very uncertain; M, males; F, females.

Table 20. Associations of physical activity with selected hormones and binding globulins

Hormone or binding globulin	Acute effects	Chronic effects
Insulin	↓	↓
Insulin-like growth factor-I (IGF-I)	↑ or NE	↑ or NE
IGF binding protein-1	↑	?
IGF binding protein-3	↑ or NE	↑ or NE
Human growth hormone	↑	↑ ?
Sex-hormone binding globulin	↑	?
Testosterone	↑ (also for free testosterone)	↓ or NE
Estradiol	↑ or ↓	↓ ? (F); NE (M)
Dehydroepiandrosterone (sulfate)	?	NE
Prolactin	↑	NE

Acute effects: assessment made during or immediately after physical activity; chronic effects: assessment made cross-sectionally (physically active vs inactive subjects) or longitudinally (effects of increased activity levels).
↑, increased levels; ↓, decreased levels; NE, no observed effect; ?, very uncertain; M, males; F, females.

generally aggravated by obesity (Travers et al., 1995; Attia et al., 1998).

Weight reduction, and particularly loss of visceral fat mass, leads to improved insulin sensitivity and to decreased serum insulin concentration, especially in subjects with impaired glucose tolerance (Leenen et al., 1994; Strain et al., 1994; Colman et al., 1995; Rasmussen et al., 1995; Dengel et al., 1996; Torjesen et al., 1997; Turcato et al., 1997; Fogelholm et al., 2000b; Ross et al., 2000a). Weight regain, often observed after weight reduction, is followed by an impairment in insulin action (Fogelholm et al., 2000b). A few studies have shown a decrease in insulin levels along with weight loss during or shortly after the intervention period, but a rebound of insulin concentrations afterwards, even though weight was maintained at a reduced level (Fogelholm et al., 2000b).

Independently of the effect of excess body fat, lack of physical activity level may also contribute to the development of insulin resistance. Relationships between physical activity and indices of insulin sensitivity have been extensively investigated and reviewed (e.g. Schwartz, 1990; Bonen, 1995; Ivy, 1997;

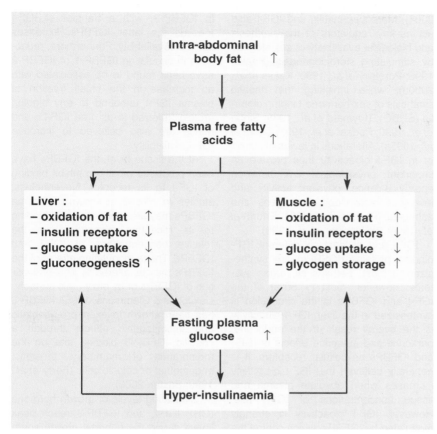

Figure 26 Effects of obesity on insulin sensitivity
Modified from Kaaks (1996)

Godsland *et al.,* 1998; Thune *et al.,* 1998; Grimm, 1999; Kelley & Goodpaster, 1999; van Baak & Borghouts, 2000; Raastad *et al.,* 2000). Cross-sectional studies have shown that regular physical activity and aerobic fitness are associated with better insulin sensitivity. In non-insulin-dependent diabetes mellitus (NIDDM) patients, physical fitness is inversely related to modest but favourable changes in glycosylated haemoglobin and glucose tolerance (Albright *et al.,* 2000).

To some extent, the effects of regular physical activity on insulin sensitivity may be mediated by reductions in body fat deposits. Regular aerobic exercise has been shown in a few studies to cause a preferential reduction in intra-abdominal fat in both men and women (Després *et al.,* 1991; Schwartz *et al.,* 1991; Buemann & Tremblay, 1996), but these data are not conclusive. However, apart from any such effect, physical activity has been shown to decrease insulin resistance and plasma insulin levels by more rapid mechanisms that may be relatively independent of changes in body weight and composition (Borghouts & Keizer, 2000; van Baak & Borghouts, 2000). Cross-sectional studies have shown inverse associations between physical activity levels and indices of insulin sensitivity independent of body size (Lindgarde & Saltin, 1981; Wang *et al.,* 1989; Regensteiner *et al.,*

1991; Feskens *et al.,* 1994; Borghouts & Keizer, 2000). Possible mechanisms unrelated to changes in overall adiposity include reduction of intramuscular stores of triglycerides (Pan *et al.,* 1997a), increased muscular phosphatidylinositol-3 kinase activity (Houmard *et al.,* 1999) and an increased capacity of skeletal muscle to metabolize or store glucose (Perseghin *et al.,* 1996; Hargreaves, 1998; Goodyear & Kahn, 1998). In addition, there are increases in insulin receptor density (Ivy, 1997) and in the number of glucose transporters (e.g., GLUT-4) in muscle cell membranes, and improved intrinsic activity of the glucose transporters (Bonen, 1995; Perseghin *et al.,* 1996; Grimm, 1999; van Baak & Borghouts, 2000).

Human intervention studies show both acute and long-term effects of physical activity on insulin sensitivity and plasma insulin concentrations. Because impaired glucose tolerance is more prevalent in the aged, it is not surprising that many interventions on the effects of exercise training and insulin action have been conducted with elderly subjects (Grimm, 1999; Kelley & Goodpaster, 1999). Even a single session of sustained submaximal physical activity improves insulin sensitivity and reduces plasma insulin levels for up to 48 hours (Perseghin *et al.,* 1996; Kraemer *et al.,* 1999; van Baak & Borghouts, 2000). However, although insulin action is improved acutely following an exercise session, long-term improvements in glucose tolerance due to moderate physical activity accrue only slowly (Bonen, 1995).

Randomized controlled trials have shown that a programme of aerobic exercise (three times weekly), with a duration of 6–10 months and without a concomitant decrease in body weight, improves insulin action, as shown by decreased area under the glycaemic curve during an oral glucose tolerance test. Many, but not all (Poehlman *et al.,* 1994), studies also show decreased fasting serum insulin concentrations. Most non-randomized trials with obese, insulin-resistant subjects used aerobic exercise as the training mode (Kelley & Goodpaster, 1999), with results similar to those from randomized trials. Eriksson *et al.* (1997) showed that resistance training also may improve glucose tolerance.

Because of the wide diversity of types of exercise, training volume and subject characteristics, it is not possible to draw firm conclusions on, for instance, a possible dose-dependence of the response. The effect of exercise intensity is also uncertain, but the present view is that even exercise of moderate intensity is beneficial in terms of insulin sensitivity (van Baak & Borghouts, 2000).

It should be noted that the effects of exercise *per se* on insulin action, without a concomitant weight change, are more modest than the changes seen after weight reduction (Torjesen *et al.*, 1997; Ross *et al.*, 2000a). However, the effects of exercise and diet together on insulin action may be more effective than the effects of diet alone (Dengel *et al.*, 1996), even though the added exercise programme usually does not increase the loss of body weight. In a study by Ross *et al.* (2000a), the improvement in glucose disposal after a 7.5-kg weight reduction was slightly, but not significantly, better when weight reduction was achieved solely by exercise, compared with a traditional low-energy diet. These results indicate that weight loss and exercise affect insulin metabolism through different mechanisms (van Baak & Borghouts, 2000).

IGF-I and IGF-binding proteins

Insulin and insulin-like growth factor (IGF)-I are central to the regulation of anabolic (growth) processes as a function of available energy and essential nutrients (e.g., amino acids) from body reserves and diet (Straus, 1994; Thissen *et al.,* 1994; Estivariz & Ziegler, 1997; Yu & Berkel, 1999; Kaaks & Lukanova,

2001). Moreover, insulin and IGF-I also act as key regulators of the synthesis and biological availability of sex steroids by stimulating steroidogenesis (Kaaks, 1996; Poretsky *et al.*, 1999; Kaaks *et al.,* 2000a), while inhibiting the hepatic synthesis of sex-hormone-binding globulin (SHBG) (Plymate *et al.,* 1988; Singh *et al.,* 1990; Pugeat *et al.,* 1991; Crave *et al.,* 1995a). Alterations in levels of insulin or in IGF-I bioactivity thus provide an important physiological link between energy balance, physical activity and levels of bioavailable androgens and estrogens (Pugeat *et al.*, 1991; Erfurth *et al.,* 1996; Pfeilschifter *et al.,* 1996).

IGF-I and at least six different IGF-binding proteins (IGFBPs) are synthesized in most, perhaps all, organ systems; however, most (> 80%) of the IGF-I and IGFBPs in the circulation is synthesized in the liver. IGF-I bioactivity is the overall result of the endocrine, paracrine and autocrine effects of IGF-I and IGFBPs on cellular receptors. It is generally believed that IGF-I bioactivity increases when absolute plasma and tissue concentrations of IGF-I rise. However, IGF-I bioactivity is strongly modulated by IGFBPs, which control the efflux of IGF-I from the circulation towards target tissues and, within tissues, regulate binding of IGF-I to its tissue receptors (Jones & Clemmons, 1995; Wetterau *et al.*, 1999).

In the circulation, more than 90% of IGF-I is bound to IGFBP-3, plus another glycoprotein called acid-labile subunit (ALS). Another small fraction is bound to IGFBP-5, which also forms a ternary complex with ALS, or to the IGFBPs -1, -2, -4 and -6. Because of the very high affinities of IGFBP-3 and IGFBP-5 for IGF-I, and their large complexes with ALS, IGF-I bound to IGFBP-3 or IGFBP-5 cannot diffuse through the endothelial barrier. The IGFBPs -1, -2, -4 and -6 are smaller (hence can diffuse from the circulation into the extravascular space), and have lower affinity for IGF-I. Therefore, it is believed that a reduction

in IGFBP-3, with a transfer of IGF-I towards the latter IGFBPs, increases IGF-I bioavailability. Furthermore, reductions in circulating IGFBP-1 or IGFBP-2 have been found to be associated with an increase in the small fraction of plasma IGF-I unbound to any binding protein (referred to as 'free IGF-I'), and hence are also believed to increase IGF-I availability.

At the tissue level, the IGFBPs have been proposed mostly to inhibit binding of IGF-I to its receptor. Nevertheless, studies *in vitro* have shown that some IGFBPs may also enhance IGF-I binding to its receptors, depending on the relative concentrations of IGF-I and IGFBPs. These modulating effects of the IGFBPs may be altered by phosphorylation of IGFBPs or by enzymatic proteolysis (Jones & Clemmons, 1995). IGFBP-3 has been shown to exert pro-apoptotic and antimitogenic effects through a specific IGFBP-3 binding site on the membranes of mammary, prostatic, endometrial or colonic cells (Ferry *et al.*, 1999; Baxter, 2000).

Circulating levels of growth hormone (GH), IGF-I, and IGFBP-3 reach peak levels during the pubertal growth spurt, but then gradually decrease with age. Conversely, levels of IGFBP-1 and IGFBP-2 are lower during puberty than at later ages.

Levels of IGF-I and of IGFBPs -1, -2 and -3 vary strongly with changes in energy intake and body energy (fat) stores. Nutritional regulation of levels of IGF-I and IGFBPs -1, -2 and -3 is effectuated largely along two relatively independent physiological axes – one for GH and one for insulin (Straus, 1994; Thissen *et al.*, 1994; Kaaks & Lukanova, 2001). GH provides the principal stimulus for synthesis of IGF-I and of IGFBP-3 (Figure 27). This stimulatory effect by GH, however, is modulated by insulin, which stimulates the synthesis of GH receptors (Baxter & Turtle, 1978; Leung *et al.*, 1997, 2000) and favours cellular amino acid uptake for protein synthesis.

Furthermore, insulin directly inhibits the synthesis of IGFBP-1 (Suikkari *et al.*, 1988; Conover & Lee, 1990; Jones & Clemmons, 1995) and is also inversely related to circulating IGFBP-2 levels (Wabitsch *et al.*, 1996; Argente *et al.*, 1997a; Nam *et al.*, 1997).

Through these mechanisms, conditions of low pancreatic insulin production, such as chronic fasting (Clemmons *et al.*, 1981; Caufriez *et al.*, 1984), energy-protein malnutrition (Clemmons & Underwood, 1991; Thissen *et al.*, 1994), anorexia nervosa (Tanaka *et al.*, 1985; Counts *et al.*, 1992; Hochberg *et al.*, 1992; Golden *et al.*, 1994), but also insulin-dependent diabetes mellitus (IDDM) (Bereket *et al.*, 1995, 1999) cause resistance of liver and other tissues to the GH stimulus, and hence a dramatic drop in absolute levels of IGF-I and IGFBP-3. In addition, levels of IGFBP-1 and IGFBP-2 rise. As an overall result, the bioavailability of IGF-I to tissue receptors decreases, and this is also reflected by a reduction of plasma free IGF-I (Thissen *et al.*, 1994; Kaaks & Lukanova, 2001).

In contrast, under conditions of elevated endogenous insulin production, such as obesity, NIDDM and other insulin-resistant states, tissues are optimally responsive to the GH stimulus, so that smaller amounts of GH are needed to stimulate IGF-I synthesis. Furthermore, conditions related to chronic hyperinsulinaemia reduce levels of IGFBP-1 (Clemmons & Underwood, 1991; Thissen *et al.*, 1994; Frystyk *et al.*, 1995; Wabitsch *et al.*, 1996; Argente *et al.*, 1997b; Nam *et al.*, 1997) and IGFBP-2 (Wabitsch *et al.*, 1996; Argente *et al.*, 1997b; Nam *et al.*, 1997). As a consequence, plasma free IGF-I levels increase (Frystyk *et al.*, 1995; Nam *et al.*, 1997; Nyomba *et al.*, 1997; Attia *et al.*, 1998).

Paradoxically, however, obesity does not increase absolute plasma IGF-I levels, but generally does not change or leads to a mild reduction in IGF-I concentrations compared with those in the normally nourished but non-insulin-resistant state (Copeland *et al.*, 1990; Conover *et al.*, 1992; Rasmussen *et al.*, 1995; Morales *et al.*, 1996; Goodman-Gruen & Barrett-Connor, 1997; Attia *et al.*, 1998; Saitoh *et al.*, 1998). Three studies have shown that low IGF-I levels are more strongly related to visceral than to subcutaneous or total fat mass (Mårin *et al.*, 1993; Rasmussen *et al.*, 1994; De Pergola *et al.*, 1998). However, more data are needed to confirm the relationships between fat distribution and IGF-I.

The mild decrease in absolute IGF-I concentrations in obese and hyperinsulinaemic subjects can be explained by an increased negative feedback of plasma free IGF-I on pituitary GH secretion (Tannenbaum *et al.*, 1983; Chapman *et al.*, 1998). Basal GH levels, as well as

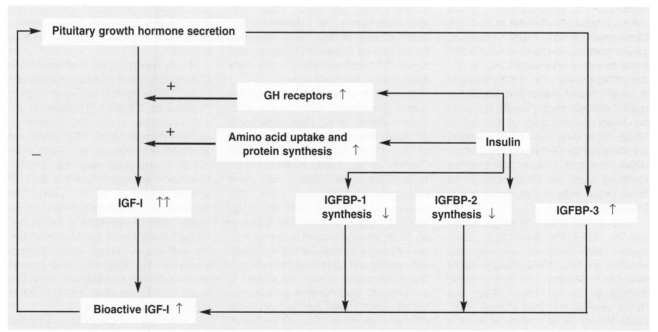

Figure 27 Regulation of the bioactivity of insulin-like growth factor (IGF)-I by growth hormone (GH) and insulin.
+, stimulating effect; −, inhibitory effect; ↑, increased; ↓, decreased
Kaaks *et al.* (2000b)

GH secretion stimulated by various physiological stimuli, have been shown to be lower in obese subjects (Iranmanesh et al., 1991; Veldhuis et al., 1995; Rasmussen et al., 1995; Morales et al., 1996; Bona et al., 1999; Micic et al., 1999). This decrease appears to be due to reductions both in growth hormone burst frequency (Veldhuis et al., 1991; Morales et al., 1996) and in burst mass (Veldhuis et al., 1995). In addition, GH levels may also be decreased by an increased rate of clearance (Iranmanesh et al., 1991; Veldhuis et al., 1991; Langendonk et al., 1999).

Data on the relationship between IGFBP-3 and obesity are conflicting, so that no firm conclusions can be drawn. Overall, there appears to be no strong association of obesity with IGFBP-3 levels (Rasmussen et al., 1994; Morales et al., 1996; Falorni et al., 1997; Attia et al., 1998; Saitoh et al., 1998).

Weight reduction leads to increased serum GH levels and to restored responses to physiological stimuli (Gama et al., 1990; Tanaka et al., 1990; Rasmussen et al., 1995). Moreover, growth hormone-binding protein (GHBP) levels decrease after weight loss. In one study (Rasmussen et al., 1996), changes in waist circumference and abdominal sagittal diameter during weight loss were the major determinants of the fall in GHBP. Short-term hypo-energy feeding did not affect GHBP (Rasmussen et al., 1996), suggesting that the changes observed were due to changes in fat mass rather than, for example, insulin availability.

Data on the effects of weight reduction on IGF-I are conflicting. Some studies have showed an expected increase in total IGF-I during weight reduction (Poulos et al., 1994; Rasmussen et al., 1994, 1995), but others saw no response (Gama et al., 1990; Falorni et al., 1997) or even a decrease (Smith et al., 1995; De Pergola et al., 1998). The conflicting findings may be caused partly by varying IGF-I

responses to large variations in energy and protein intake (Smith et al., 1995; De Pergola et al., 1998; Ross, 2000). In addition, results may vary according to whether one measures an acute effect during the weight reduction phase or afterwards, and may depend on the subject's degree of obesity at start. Weight reduction has been shown to increase plasma concentrations of IGFBP-1 (Kiddy et al., 1989; Musey et al., 1993; Hellénius et al., 1995) and IGFBP-2 (Clemmons et al., 1991; Thissen et al., 1994; Wabitsch et al., 1996).

Cross-sectional studies comparing baseline (resting) levels of IGF-I between trained and untrained individuals are few, and do not allow any firm conclusions. They have covered both aged and young adult subjects, but the results do not indicate any age-by-physical-activity interactions. After proper adjustment for age and body composition, these studies did not show any difference between IGF-I levels of trained and untrained participants (Goodman-Gruen & Barrett-Connor, 1997; Walker et al., 1999). However, Poehlman and Copeland (1990) reported higher IGF-I concentrations in physically active than in inactive subjects.

Numerous small human intervention studies (Bang et al., 1990; Cappon et al., 1994; Koistinen et al., 1996; Schwarz et al., 1996; Hornum et al., 1997; Nguyen et al., 1998; Bermon et al., 1999; Chadan et al., 1999; Wallace et al., 1999; Elias et al., 2000), with some exceptions (Kraemer et al., 1992, 1995; Hopkins et al., 1994; Schmidt et al., 1995; Di Luigi et al., 1997; Bonnefoy et al., 1999), have shown an acute but transient increase in levels of IGF-I immediately during and after a bout of exercise. The IGF-I response may be related to the intensity and duration of exercise: Nguyen et al. (1998) reported increased IGF-I after short-term (20 min) ergometer exercise, a decrease after prolonged (3 h) endurance exercise and no change after interval training. The increase in

IGF-I may be explained by an acute rise in pituitary GH secretion (Cappon et al., 1994; Kraemer et al., 1995; Schmidt et al., 1995; Di Luigi et al., 1997; Hornum et al., 1997; Wideman et al., 1999). Nevertheless, one study in peripubertal children and adolescents, who have the highest plasma IGF-I levels compared to other age groups, showed a significant reduction in IGF-I after a short bout of exercise (Scheett et al., 1999) or after an increase in physical activity levels for three days. The serum concentration of the main binding protein of IGF-I, namely IGFBP-3, seems to increase during exercise, if a simultaneous rise in IGF-I is observed (Schwarz et al., 1996; Nguyen et al., 1998).

More prolonged episodes of intense exercise for several hours, such as running a marathon, have also been found to decrease circulating IGF-I as well as IGFBP-3 levels (Koistinen et al., 1996). This suggests that decreases in absolute IGF-I levels may be achieved only by more prolonged exercise, and possibly this is so only when exercise leads to a (transient) negative energy balance.

A very consistent acute effect of more prolonged bouts of physical exercise is a large (up to tenfold or even higher) increase in IGFBP-1 (Hopkins et al., 1994; Koistinen et al., 1996; Schwarz et al., 1996; Nguyen et al., 1998; Wallace et al., 1999; Scheett et al., 1999). The IGFBP-1 response may be smaller, however, if exercise intensity is not high enough (Schwarz et al., 1996). The increase in IGFBP-1 appears to be independent of variations in insulin but, instead, is most likely due to an exercise-induced rise in cortisol levels. Cortisol increases the synthesis and plasma levels of IGFBP-1 (Unterman, 1993; Lee et al., 1997b; Katz et al., 1998), an effect opposite to that of insulin.

Longer-term increases in physical exercise (regular training) over periods of weeks to several months have also led to increases in IGF-I levels in elderly subjects (Poehlman *et al.*, 1994; Bonnefoy *et al.*, 1999), as well as in younger men and women (Roelen *et al.*, 1997; Koziris *et al.*, 1999), although several other studies in elderly men showed no clear effect on IGF-I (Nicklas *et al.*, 1995; Vitiello *et al.*, 1997). In a weight-reduction study, inclusion of exercise prevented a diet-induced decrease in IGF-I concentration (Hellénius *et al.*, 1995). The effects of resistance training on IGF-I seem to be negligible (Kraemer *et al.*, 1999).

Data on the effects of regular training on IGFBP-3 levels are limited: both increased (Koziris *et al.*, 1999) and maintained (Poehlman *et al.*, 1994) IGFBP-3 concentrations have been reported.

Taken together, although physical activity leads to an acute increase in absolute IGF-I levels, its effect on long-term average IGF-I concentrations is less clear. Furthermore, the effects of physical activity on IGFBP-3 concentrations and on IGF-I levels relative to IGFBP-3 are unclear.

Total and bioavailable sex steroids

Sex steroid hormones are essential for the growth, differentiation and function of many tissues in both men and women. This section covers the main human androgens (Δ4-androstenedione, testosterone, dehydroepiandrosterone (DHEA) and its sulfate (DHEAS)), estrogens (estrone, estradiol) and SHBG. In women, androgens are produced by the ovary (testosterone, androstenedione) as well as by adrenal glands (DHEA, DHEAS, androstenedione) (Stanczyk, 1997); in men the androgens are also produced both by the testes and adrenal glands. Estrogens (estrone, estradiol) are produced by the ovary in premenopausal women. After menopause, ovarian production of estrogens and of progesterone falls to very low levels, whereas that of androgens decreases more gradually with age. In postmenopausal women, the principal estrogen is estrone, produced by peripheral

aromatization of androstenedione, mainly within adipose tissue. Adipose tissue is also an important source of estrogens in men.

Both overall and central adiposity have been associated with differences in total and bioavailable plasma sex steroid levels, in pre- and postmenopausal women as well as men. These relationships are mediated by a number of mechanisms (Figure 28). First, obesity leads to a state of relative insulin resistance, chronic hyperinsulinaemia and an increase in IGF-I bioactivity, due to insulin-mediated decreases in IGFBP-1 and IGFBP-2. Insulin and increased bioactive IGF-I, in turn, inhibit the hepatic synthesis of SHBG (Plymate *et al.,* 1988; Pasquali *et al.*, 1990; Singh *et al.*, 1990; Pugeat *et al.,* 1991; Crave *et al.*, 1995a; Nestler, 2000), a globulin that specifically binds sex hormones in the circulation. It is generally agreed that the unbound fraction determines the actual biological activity of androgens and estrogens (Enriori *et al.*, 1986). Second, insulin and

IGF-I enhance the synthesis of sex steroids (androgens and estrogens) by the gonads and adrenal glands (Kaaks, 1996; Poretsky *et al.*, 1999; Kaaks *et al.*, 2000a). Third, in the adipose tissue compartment, androgens (Δ4-androstenedione, testosterone) are converted into estrogens (estrone, estradiol) by the enzyme aromatase (Siiteri, 1987; Azziz, 1989). Fourth, an increase in bioavailable androgens, unbound to SHBG, may lead to increased estrogen synthesis in adipose tissue. Fifth, for a given level of SHBG, an increase in plasma testosterone concentration tends to raise the level of bioavailable estradiol, because SHBG has a greater affinity for testosterone than for estradiol. One general consequence of these mechanisms, in both women and men, and irrespective of menopausal status, is a decrease in plasma SHBG level, which generally correlates inversely with plasma fasting insulin and IGF-I. However, the final consequences of these actions for levels of total and bioavailable sex steroids are

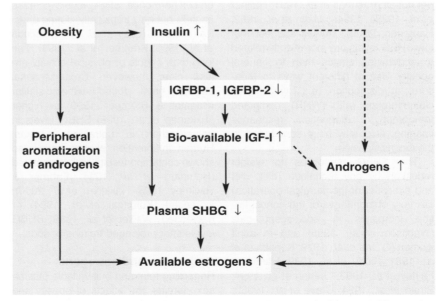

Figure 28 Mechanisms underlying relationships between overall and central adiposity and differences in total and bioavailable plasma sex steriod levels

↑ Increased levels, ↓ decreased levels, ------------, observed only in PCOS not identical in men and women, and in women may also depend on the presence of genetic background factors that predispose to development of ovarian hyperandrogenism.

Sex hormone-binding globulin

The amount and distribution of body fat has very clear associations with blood SHBG concentration. In children and adolescents, obesity may be associated with low SHBG levels (Wabitsch et al., 1995), although not all studies have found a significant relationship (de Ridder et al., 1990). For girls, the inverse correlation is stronger with abdominal than gluteal obesity (Wabitsch et al., 1995). Similar inverse correlations between BMI and SHBG are observed in both adult women (Kirschner et al., 1990; Leenen et al., 1994; Bernasconi et al., 1996; Pasquali et al., 1997a; Turcato et al., 1997) and men (Field et al., 1994; Haffner et al., 1994a, 1997; Hautanen, 2000). Many (Kirschner et al., 1990; Pasquali et al., 1990; Kaye et al., 1991; Leenen et al., 1994; Ivandic et al., 1998), but not all (Pasquali et al., 1991; Haffner et al., 1993a, 1994a; Mårin et al., 1993; Hautanen, 2000), studies suggest that low SHBG levels are more tightly related to abdominal fatness than to general obesity. Use of different ways to measure fat distribution (e.g., waist-to-hip circumference ratio (WHR), computed tomography, magnetic resonance imaging, etc.) may have contributed to the inconsistencies.

The SHBG responses to weight reduction by any technique (diet, diet and exercise, drugs, surgical operation) are very straightforward: the concentration increases in adolescent girls (Wabitsch et al., 1995) and in adult women (O'Dea et al., 1979; Kopelman et al., 1981; Kiddy et al., 1989; Hamilton-Fairley et al., 1993; Leenen et al., 1994; Strain et al., 1994; Crave et al., 1995b; Turcato et al., 1997) and men (Harlass et al., 1984; Strain et al., 1988, 1994; Guzik et al., 1994; Leenen et al., 1994;

Vermeulen, 1996; Jakubowicz & Nestler, 1997; Tymchuk et al., 1998). The reverse is also true: SHBG decreases in anorexia nervosa patients during refeeding and weight gain (Barbe et al., 1993). Strain et al. (1994) estimated that SHBG levels increased by 0.43 nmol/L per unit decrease in BMI. They also noted that the slope of the change in SHBG versus change in BMI was steeper than the slope of the cross-sectional inverse relationship between BMI and SHBG. These findings may indicate that part of the increased SHBG is an acute response to the weight reduction technique (e.g., diet). An alternative explanation could be that during the dynamic phase of weight loss, SHBG is temporarily increased further than one would expect on the basis of the cross-sectional relationship, perhaps because of a stronger reduction in insulin levels during the intervention period than in the subsequent weight-maintenance phase.

The relationships between physical activity and SHBG are important in order to interpret the effects of physical activity on sex hormones. SHBG levels increase acutely, but only transiently, during physical exercise (Gray et al., 1993; Zmuda et al., 1996; Kraemer et al., 1998). The long-term effects of physical activity are less clear, however. Cross-sectional studies have found either similar (Bagatell & Bremner, 1990) or higher (Tikkanen et al., 1998) SHBG levels in trained than in untrained subjects. Human intervention studies have also shown conflicting results, with unchanged (Houmard et al., 1994; Fahrner & Hackney, 1998; Häkkinen et al., 2000), increased (Kumagai et al., 1994) or decreased (Walker et al., 1999) SHBG levels after prolonged training periods.

Androgens and estrogens

Regarding total and bioavailable plasma sex steroids, the effects of obesity and physical activity vary between men and women. In women, these effects depend also on menopausal status and on the

presence or absence of functional ovarian hyperandrogenism or polycystic ovary syndrome (PCOS), a relatively frequent syndrome characterized by elevated plasma androgen levels, oligomenorrhoea and frequent anovulatory cycles, that affects 4–8% of premenopausal women (Figure 29).

Most studies of normo-androgenic premenopausal women have not shown any clear association between plasma insulin and absolute androgen concentrations (Evans et al., 1983; Pasquali et al., 1987; Amemiya et al., 1990; Seidell et al., 1990b; Weaver et al., 1990; Austin et al., 1991). Nevertheless, because of the decrease in plasma SHBG, obesity does increase levels of bioavailable androgens, unbound to SHBG, also in these women (de Ridder et al., 1990; Kirschner et al., 1990; Leenen et al., 1994; Bernasconi et al., 1996; Ivandic et al., 1998; Penttilä et al., 1999). In contrast, in normo-androgenic premenopausal women, obesity and chronic hyperinsulinaemia appear to have no or only little effect on levels of estradiol, measured either as absolute concentrations or as bioavailable levels unbound to SHBG. This might be explained by the relatively low estrogen production by adipose tissue, compared to the ovarian production. Another possible explanation is that in premenopausal women, total estrogen levels are maintained at relatively constant levels through feedback of estradiol on pituitary secretion of follicle-stimulating hormone (FSH). Kirschner et al. (1990) and Leenen et al. (1994) found that free estradiol levels in premenopausal women with abdominal (android) obesity were higher than in subjects with lower-body (gluteal) obesity. Moreover, abdominal obesity may be associated with higher estrone concentration (Pasquali et al., 1990) in premenopausal women. Underweight, anorectic and eating-disordered premenopausal women have reduced concentrations of estradiol (Soygür et al., 1996).

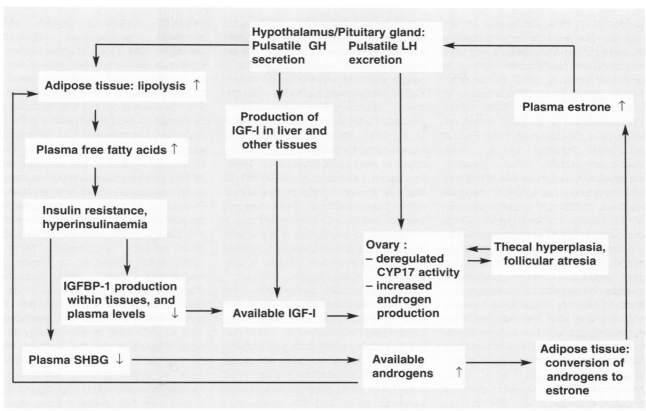

Figure 29 Role of hyperinsulinaemia in the development of functional ovarian hyperandrogenism (polycystic ovary syndrome, PCOS). Modifed from Kaaks (1996)

In premenopausal women with PCOS, obesity and chronic hyperinsulinaemia lead to markedly increased ovarian production and plasma levels of Δ4-androstenedione and testosterone (Burghen *et al.*, 1980; Chang *et al.*,1983; Pasquali *et al.*, 1983; Shoupe *et al.*, 1983; Evans *et al.*, 1988; Wajchenberg *et al.*, 1988; Lanzone *et al.*, 1990; Holte *et al.*, 1994; Pasquali *et al.*, 1994; Ehrmann *et al.*, 1995). A very high proportion of women with PCOS are obese, and insulin resistance appears to play a central role in the development of the syndrome (Ehrmann *et al.*, 1995). In women with PCOS, the degree of obesity (BMI) correlates with the frequency of anovulatory cycles, as indicated by frequency of oligomenorrhoea/amenorrhoea, and in

these women is thus also a clear negative determinant of ovarian progesterone production (Kiddy *et al.*, 1992; Robinson *et al.*, 1993). Women with PCOS generally have normal to mildly elevated plasma estrogen levels, which may derive in part from increased aromatization of androgens (mostly to estrone) in adipose tissue. Since SHBG levels are reduced, women with PCOS also have increased levels of bioavailable androgens and estrogens, unbound to SHBG (Lobo *et al.*, 1981; Waldstreicher *et al.*, 1988; Ehrmann *et al.*, 1995; Rosenfield, 1999).

After menopause, ovarian production of estrogens stops and conversion of the androgen precursor androstenedione to estrone in adipose tissue becomes the primary source of estrogens in women

(Siiteri, 1987; Azziz, 1989). In postmenopausal women, BMI has been frequently associated with increased levels of total and bioavailable estrogens (Austin *et al.*, 1991; Kaye *et al.*, 1991; Katsouyanni *et al.*, 1991), but not with total or free testosterone (Cauley *et al.*, 1989; Kaye *et al.*, 1991; Newcomb *et al.*, 1995; Turcato *et al.*, 1997). The increase in serum estrone and estradiol is linearly related to the degree of obesity (Kaye *et al.*, 1991).

In men, in contrast to postmenopausal women and premenopausal women with PCOS, obesity and chronic hyperinsulinaemia generally correlate inversely with plasma total testosterone levels (Seidell *et al.*, 1990a; Pasquali *et al.*, 1991, 1995; Haffner *et al.*, 1993b, 1994b; Vermeulen *et al.*, 1993, 1996;

Giagulli *et al.,* 1994; Tibblin *et al.,* 1996), and do not lead to any noticeable increase but generally rather a decrease in bioavailable testosterone unbound to SHBG (Strain *et al.,* 1982; Seidell *et al.,* 1990a; Zumoff *et al.,* 1990; Pasquali *et al.,* 1991; Haffner *et al.,* 1993b, 1994b, 1997; Vermeulen *et al.,* 1993; Andersson *et al.,* 1994; Giagulli *et al.,* 1994; Field *et al.,* 1994; Tchernof *et al.,* 1995; Vermeulen, 1996). The generally accepted explanation for this is that free testosterone causes long-loop negative feedback inhibition of pituitary secretion of luteinizing hormone (LH). Thus, decreases in SHBG are accompanied by a decrease in pituitary LH secretion and hence by a decrease in testicular androgen production, while bioavailable testosterone remains approximately constant. In severely obese men, however, not only are total testosterone levels decreased, but also bioavailable testosterone levels are lower, due to additional mechanisms that are less well understood (Veldhuis *et al.,* 1992). Δ4-Androstenedione levels show a negative correlation with BMI in men (Field *et al.,* 1994; Tchernof *et al.,* 1995). Many studies have found a positive relationship between obesity and serum estrogens in males (Brind *et al.,* 1990; Tchernof *et al.,* 1995; Soygür *et al.,* 1996; Hsieh *et al.,* 1998), although some studies show no obesity-related association (Haffner *et al.,* 1993b, 1994b), whereas such an association has not been reported for women (Kirschner *et al.,* 1990; Austin *et al.,* 1991; De Pergola *et al.,* 1994; Bernasconi *et al.,* 1996).

A few intervention studies have been conducted to examine the effects of weight loss on serum testosterone levels. In hyperandrogenic women, weight reduction leads to decreased total and free testosterone concentrations (Pasquali *et al.,* 1989; Guzick *et al.,* 1994; Leenen *et al.,* 1994; Strain *et al.,* 1994; Crave *et al.,* 1995b). A similar response has been found in adolescent girls (Wabitsch *et al.,* 1995), among whom the reduction of free testosterone was more significant in those with initially more abdominal-type obesity. There are very few recent studies on effects of weight reduction on testosterone in men. Earlier data showed that serum total and free testosterone concentrations increased after weight reduction (Stanik *et al.,* 1981; Strain *et al.,* 1988). The increase may be proportional to the magnitude of weight loss (Strain *et al.,* 1988). In contrast, Leenen *et al.* (1994) did not find any change in total or free testosterone concentration in obese men and women, despite a 13.5-kg weight loss. A more detailed description of the effects of weight loss on endogenous hormones in human intervention studies is presented later in this chapter.

Serum estradiol concentration has been reported to decrease in obese men (Leenen *et al.,* 1994) and in obese adolescent girls (Wabitsch *et al.,* 1995) during successful weight reduction, while no change in levels in postmenopausal women was reported by Turcato *et al.* (1997). The effect of weight reduction on hormonal status and the regularity of menstrual cycles are dependent on the baseline hormonal profile and on the magnitude of weight loss. Although large weight losses (>20% of body weight) and reduced estradiol concentration may induce amenorrhoea, weight reduction in massively obese women, with menstrual disturbances caused by hyperandrogenicity, will normalize the menstrual cycle (Pasquali *et al.,* 1989). In this study, the change in fasting estradiol concentration in plasma was inversely related to change in WHR.

Plasma androgen levels of women with PCOS can be reduced to approximately normal levels by weight loss (Kopelman *et al.,* 1981; Bates & Whitworth,1982; Kiddy *et al.,* 1989; Pasquali *et al.,* 1997b) or by insulin-lowering drugs (Ehrmann, 1999; Pugeat & Ducluzeau, 1999).

Girls participating in vigorous sports such as ballet dancing and running frequently experience primary and secondary amenorrhoea, delayed menarche and more irregular cycles, compared with non-athlete girls (Frisch *et al.,* 1980, 1981; Fogelholm *et al.,* 1996b; Fogelholm & Hiilloskorpi, 1999). The late menarcheal age may be caused by intense physical activity and/or dietary restriction, but selection bias (girls with early menarche drop out) cannot be ruled out. Moreover, the low BMI of athletic girls may also contribute to menstrual irregularities (Maclure *et al.,* 1991; Petridou *et al.,* 1996). Late menarche is associated with a prolonged period of anovulatory cycles after menarche and lower estradiol concentrations (Apter, 1996), which is reflected by menstrual irregularities even after puberty (Fogelholm *et al.,* 1996b). A cross-sectional study of 174 girls aged 14–17 years found that those who expended 2500 kJ (600 kcal) or more energy per week (described by the authors as comparable to two or more hours per week in activities such as aerobic exercise classes, swimming, jogging or tennis) were two to three times more likely than less active girls to have anovulatory menstrual cycles (Bernstein *et al.,* 1987).

High physical activity measured by self-reporting and by movement monitors has been found to be associated with decreased serum concentrations of estradiol, estrone and androgens in postmenopausal women (Cauley *et al.,* 1989). This significant association persisted after adjustment for BMI.

Cross-sectional evaluations of baseline testosterone levels have given somewhat conflicting results. Several studies have reported that high physical activity is associated with lower total and free fasting serum testosterone concentrations in men (Arce *et al.,* 1993; De Souza *et al.,* 1994; Tikkanen *et al.,* 1998), but others found no difference in total or free testosterone concentration between male athletes and controls (Bagatell & Bremner, 1990; Tegelman *et* al., 1990) or between non-athletes with different levels of recreational exercise (Handa et al., 1997). Moreover, serum testosterone levels at rest may be higher in aged male runners compared with controls of similar age (Hurel et al., 1999).

Exercise-induced increases in estradiol and metabolites have been found in adult women (de Crée et al., 1997a) and men (Gray et al., 1993). In contrast, Montagnani et al. (1992) found decreased estradiol levels, together with increased metabolic clearance rate, after a 2-h treadmill run in premenopausal women. It should be noted, however, that any hormonal response following an exercise session is difficult to interpret, because of wide between-study variation in, for instance, subjects' age, body composition and training status, mode, intensity and duration of exercise, dietary status and phase of menstrual cycle.

The increase in testosterone levels during an acute exercise session in men is well documented (Jürimäe et al., 1990; Zmuda et al., 1996; Fahrner & Hackney, 1998; Häkkinen et al., 2000). The response in women is less clear (Häkkinen et al., 2000). However, the increase is very short-lasting and baseline levels are reached within 1–2 hours (Zmuda et al., 1996). If the exercise session has been strenuous, serum testosterone concentration in men may even drop below preexercise levels (Kraemer et al., 1998).

A high-intensity exercise intervention in 28 untrained college women with normal ovulation and luteal adequacy resulted in reversible abnormal luteal function in two thirds and loss of LH surge in over half of the subjects (Bullen et al., 1985). The most marked disturbances were observed during the periods of most intense training and among those women who had been randomized to a weight loss (vs weight maintenance) group.

Indirect evidence also supports the view that among athletes estrogen metabolism is affected more by training intensity than by volume: the prevalence of menstrual disorders is higher in endurance than in aesthetic (gymnastics, ballet, etc.) athletes, despite clearly more weekly training hours in the latter group (Fogelholm & Hiilloskorpi, 1999). Interventions in previously untrained subjects have mostly shown unchanged testosterone levels after increased physical activity in men (Oleshansky et al., 1990; Houmard et al., 1994) and postmenopausal women (Häkkinen et al., 2000).

Dehydroepiandrosterone and its sulfate

Data on other sex hormones are scarce. DHEA and DHEAS concentrations in obese women are lower than those of normal-weight controls (De Pergola et al., 1994) or similar (Azziz et al., 1994; Bernasconi et al., 1996; Denti et al., 1997; Ivandic et al., 1998). Subnormal concentrations of DHEA (Field et al., 1994) and DHEAS (Field et al., 1994; Tchernof et al., 1995; Hsieh et al., 1998) have also been observed in men, but not consistently (Denti et al., 1997). In women, a high DHEAS/free testosterone ratio is a positive predictor of lower fasting and postprandial insulin concentrations (Ivandic et al., 1998).

DHEAS levels have been reported to be inversely related to WHR in some studies (Haffner et al., 1993b, 1994b; De Pergola et al., 1994) but not in others (Ivandic et al., 1998; Kirschner et al., 1990; Denti et al., 1997). Moreover, the free testosterone/DHEAS ratio is more closely (positively) related to visceral adipose tissue than to BMI (De Pergola et al., 1994).

Leenen et al. (1994) found increased DHEAS levels after weight reduction, but Pasquali et al. (1989) reported that they were unchanged.

De Souza et al. (1994) did not find any difference between athletes' and controls' DHEAS concentrations, and baseline DHEAS levels do not seem to be affected by long-term exercise training (Houmard et al., 1994; Häkkinen et al., 2000).

Other hormones
Obesity seems to have very little effect on prolactin metabolism. Cross-sectional comparisons have not revealed any difference in serum prolactin concentration between obese and normal-weight subjects (Coiro et al., 1990; Scaglione et al., 1991). In agreement with these cross-sectional findings, serum prolactin concentration was also found to remain unchanged after weight reduction (Hainer et al., 1992).

Physical exercise acutely increases serum prolactin concentration in both males and females (Jürimäe et al., 1990; Oleshansky et al., 1990; Gray et al., 1993). The increase may be more than 200% above resting levels. However, Arce et al. (1993) and De Souza et al. (1994) reported no difference in baseline prolactin level between well trained male athletes and untrained controls.

Immune function
The immune system has been hypothesized to modulate the likelihood of tumour formation by inhibiting cell growth and countering the action of tumour growth promoters (Shephard & Shek, 1998). The most often studied immunological outcomes are numeration of immune cells and tests of their functional capacity (Stallone, 1994). Neutrophil, monocyte and total lymphocyte counts, as well as phenotypic analyses of lymphocyte and immunoglobulin populations, are common measures. Phenotypic analysis of lymphocytes may give more information than the total count. However, the interpretation of the results is complicated by the increased number of variables. Lymphocyte activation by mitogens in vitro provides specific information about cellular functions. Some studies have used less specific functional tests, such as measurement of delayed-type hypersensitivity.

Several studies have shown impaired immune function in obese children (Chandra & Kutty, 1980) and adults

(Weber *et al.,* 1986; Tanaka *et al.,* 1993), but results have been inconsistent. Moriguchi *et al.* (1995) reported impaired immune function (natural killer (NK) cell cytotoxic activity, mitogenic stimulation of lymphocytes) in obese elderly subjects (60–69 years), whereas immune function in younger obese subjects tended to be better than in normal-weight controls. Nieman *et al.* (1996) also found indications of improved immunity in obese subjects.

The acute effects of weight reduction on immune function are more straightforward: most indices show impaired immune status. Several papers report decreased leukocyte, neutrophil, monocyte, NK cell counts and/or immunoglobulin concentration after weight reduction (mean 7–32 kg) by very low-energy diet or other protein-modified fasts (Merritt *et al.,* 1980; Field *et al.,* 1991; Nieman *et al.,* 1996) or after a low-energy diet (Kelley *et al.,* 1994). Decreased delayed-type hypersensitivity (Stallone *et al.,* 1994), mitogen-induced lymphocyte proliferation (Field *et al.,* 1991; Tanaka *et al.,* 1993; Nieman *et al.,* 1996) and bacterial killing and chemotaxis of granulocytes (McMurray *et al.,* 1990) are other findings of impaired immune function during weight reduction. It is not possible to tell whether the observed changes are caused by inadequate intake of nutrients or by negative energy balance and weight reduction *per se.*

Two studies examined the effects of additional exercise training during weight reduction by dietary techniques. Nieman *et al.* (1998) reported that moderate aerobic exercise training did not affect immune function during weight reduction, but the number of days with symptoms of upper respiratory tract infections was lower in exercising than in diet-only subjects. In another study (Scanga *et al.,* 1998), exercise training prevented a weight-reduction-induced decrease in NK cell cytotoxicity. However, leukocyte and lymphocyte counts decreased during weight reduction, with or without added exercise training.

Decreased immune cell counts have also been observed in anorexia nervosa (Marcos *et al.,* 1997a) and bulimia nervosa (Marcos *et al.,* 1997b) patients. Among bulimic patients, those with low weight had the most deteriorated status. A decrease in NK cell count was the most consistent finding in both studies. Partial weight regain in anorexia nervosa patients was followed by a partial recovery in the immunological indices, except for NK cell count, which remained low (Marcos *et al.,* 1997a).

Several potential mechanisms could explain, at least partly, the observed associations between obesity and immune function (Kumari & Chandra, 1993; Stallone, 1994). An excess dietary intake of certain lipids may impair immune status. Both inadequate and very high intakes of several micronutrients (e.g., vitamins A and E, carotenoids, iron, zinc and selenium) may have negative effects on immune status. Ketosis, an almost inevitable consequence of a very low-energy diet, may also inhibit immune cell function by inhibiting glucose uptake and utilization.

A session of physical activity has marked acute effects on the immune system. Several types of immune cell have been observed to increase acutely in response to exercise, including neutrophils, monocytes, eosinophils and total lymphocytes (Eliakim *et al.,* 1997; Gabriel & Kindermann, 1997; Robson *et al.,* 1999; Moldoveanu *et al.,* 2000), but the levels may remain unchanged after eccentric exercise (Miles *et al.,* 1999). After a strenuous exercise session, the increased levels of indicators of immune function may still be observable after 24 h (Eliakim *et al.,* 1997; Gabriel & Kindermann, 1997).

The number of NK cells increases sharply during high-intensity activity, but decreases during very prolonged moderate-intensity activity (Tvede *et al.,* 1993;

Eliakim *et al.,* 1997; Gabriel & Kindermann, 1997). After exercise, NK cell number decreases more rapidly subpopulation (Eliakim *et al.,* 1997; Gabriel & Kindermann, 1997). A suggested reason for post-exercise suppression of NK cell activity is inhibition by prostaglandins released by monocytes (Tvede *et al.,* 1993). NK cell count does not seem to be affected by eccentric exercise (Miles *et al.,* 1999).

Pedersen *et al.* (2000) recently reviewed the effects of an acute bout of exercise on cytokine production. The plasma levels of various cytokines (TNF-α, IL-1β, IL-6) increase during intense exercise. The increase of IL-6 is proportionally much greater than that of other cytokines. In a systematic review on mucosal immunity in élite athletes, Gleeson (2000) identified 25 studies on the effects of an acute exercise bout on salivary concentration of immunoglobulin (Ig)A. Sixteen studies showed decreased levels and only two reported increased IgA after exercise. IgA concentration in saliva returns to basal levels within 1 h after physical activity.

Very few functional tests have been used to study immune response to physical activity. However, Bruunsgaard *et al.* (1997) studied cell-mediated immunity evaluated by skin tests in 22 males after intense, long-duration exercise (triathlon). The results indicated impaired immunity in the first few days after the exercise.

Studies on immune function during long-term training have yielded somewhat inconsistent results. Many have found depressed immune function following intense physical training, using NK cell count, neutrophil oxidative capacity, T-cell responses *in vitro* or saliva IgA concentration as a marker (Pyne *et al.,* 1995; Kramer *et al.,* 1997; Gleeson, 2000). Nine out of 12 studies identified in the review by Gleeson (2000) reported decreased salivary IgA concentration in athletes after long-term training, indicating cumulative mucosal immune suppression over training periods. In contrast, moderate exercise training does not seem to have any negative effect on IgA level (Mackinnon, 2000).

In contrast to the above studies, others have suggested that physical activity may be related to improved immune function. Kumae et al. (1999) found increased lymphocyte and eosinophil counts, but decreased neutrophil generation of reactive oxidative species in runners. Moderate exercise training has been shown to lead to increased immunoglobulin levels (Nehlsen-Cannarella et al., 1991), elevated NK activity or cell count (Watson et al., 1986; Nieman et al., 1990; Rhind et al., 1994, 1996; Hoffman-Goetz et al., 1998), changes in lymphocyte subsets (LaPerriere et al., 1994; Host et al., 1995), IL-2 production and IL-2 receptor expression (Rhind et al., 1994, 1996) and immunoglobulin levels (Nehlsen-Cannarella et al., 1991).

Nieman et al. (1993) conducted a randomized controlled trial (walking vs calisthenics) among 32 sedentary, elderly Caucasian women (67–85 years). Although the exercise training programme (5 × 30–40 min/wk for 12 weeks) resulted in no significant improvement in either NK cell or T-lymphocyte function, the incidence of upper respiratory tract infections was significantly lower in the walking group (21%) than in the calisthenics group (50%), and was lowest in a comparison group of highly trained elderly people (8%). These results are consistent with those from a trial in younger obese women (mean age 35 years) in which exercise subjects (45 min of walking, 5 d/wk) experienced half the number of days with symptoms of upper respiratory tract infection during a 15-week period compared with a sedentary control group (5.1 vs 10.8, $p < 0.05$) (Nieman et al., 1990). Nieman et al. (1995) also reported higher NK cell cytotoxic activity in marathon runners compared with sedentary controls. In contrast,

extremely heavy exertion (such as a 90 km run) has been shown to increase the incidence of upper respiratory tract infections (Peters, 1997).

In a recent review, Mackinnon (2000) presented a summary of resting values of immune function variables in athletes, compared with those of non-athletes or with clinical norms. Many indices (leukocyte, granulocyte and lymphocyte number, serum specific antibody) were similar in athletes and controls. NK cell number and cytotoxic activity, and lymphocyte activation and proliferation, were normal or higher in athletes. In contrast, neutrophil function and immunoglobulin concentration in serum and mucosa were clearly suboptimal in athletes. Hence, compared with studies on moderate training (Nieman et al., 1990; Nehlsen-Cannarella et al., 1991), athletic training seems to have more deleterious effects on immune function.

In summary, immune responses to an acute exercise bout include increased immune cell counts and cytokine production, but decreased saliva IgA concentration, immediately after intense activity. After strenuous exertion, the immune cell counts decrease rapidly and may reach levels that are clearly below pre-exercise values 1–3 h after cessation. This has been referred to as an "open window of decreased host protection" (Nieman, 1997). Most immune variables reach normal or slightly elevated levels 24 h after exercise. Responses are less clear after moderate-intensity and short-duration activity. Cross-sectional comparisons between trained and untrained subjects have yielded inconclusive results (Nieman, 1997; Jonsdottir, 2000). However, many authors hold the view that moderate physical activity has a positive effect on the immune system (Peters, 1997; Shephard & Shek, 1998; Jonsdottir, 2000). The inconsistencies in study results described above may be due to the use of different immune measures, differences in exercise regimen, small sample sizes with insufficient

statistical power to detect changes, characteristics of the participants, or effects of unmeasured confounding factors, such as nutritional factors, smoking or alcohol intake and stress levels. It is unclear to what extent the results in young adults or athletes pertain to exercise in the elderly.

Intervention trials
Weight reduction

Table 21 summarizes many weight reduction studies that have been carried out with different intervention strategies in obese patients, pre- and post-menopausal women, men, children and adolescents.

The overall picture is that, with weight loss, insulin resistance decreases, and basal and postprandial glucose and insulin levels are similarly reduced. Reduced fasting glucose and insulin levels have been consistently observed, whether weight was lost with a low-energy diet (usually 4200–6300 kJ (1000 to 1500 kcal)/day) or a very low-energy diet (1700–3400 kJ (400 to 800 kcal)/day), with or without associated physical activity or pharmacological treatment. Glucose and insulin areas after glucose tolerance test and blood lipid patterns improved as well. Plasma levels of SHBG were also consistently shown to increase with weight reduction, while the effects on sex steroid hormones were less clear-cut and were different in men and women. It is not clear, however, if the improvement in insulin sensitivity which has been demonstrated in short-term studies is sustained over longer periods. On average, it appears that a 15-week diet or diet-and-exercise programme can achieve an approximately 11-kg weight loss, with a 6–8-kg maintained loss after one year. Few studies appear to have been continued for longer than a year and those few show generally disappointing results (reviewed by Mann, 2000). It does not seem necessary, however, to achieve the ideal body weight to improve the metabolic profile – in most instances a 5–10% weight reduction is sufficient to induce a clinically beneficial effect (Weinstock *et al.*, 1998).

Some of the randomized controlled trials and the largest uncontrolled intervention studies are presented below in some detail, but several other trials are summarized in Table 21.

Premenopausal women. Fujioka *et al.* (1991) investigated 40 premenopausal Japanese obese women, aged 38 years, with mean BMI 35 kg/m² at recruitment, in whom substantial weight reduction was obtained by means of a low-energy diet. In 14 women with predominantly visceral fat tissue (as determined by computed tomography scan), BMI decreased from 34.3 to 29.4 kg/m² and in 26 women with predominantly subcutaneous adipose tissue, BMI decreased from 36.0 to 30.9 kg/m². Fasting plasma glucose and insulin levels, plasma glucose and insulin areas after an oral glucose tolerance test and total cholesterol and triglycerides levels decreased significantly. The changes in plasma glucose area and in triglyceride levels were significantly correlated with changes in the ratio of visceral to subcutaneous fat volume ($r = 0.307$ and 0.486, respectively).

Guzick *et al.* (1994) randomized 12 obese, hyperandrogenic, anovulatory women to a 12-week weight loss programme or a 12-week 'waiting list': in the intervention group, body weight decreased from 108.0 ± 5.3 to 91.8 ± 6.0 kg, and SHBG increased from 0.60 ± 0.09 to 0.73 ± 0.09 mg/dL. Crave *et al.* (1995b) randomized 24 obese (BMI > 25 kg/m²) hirsute patients with high fasting insulin and low SHBG levels into a metformin and a placebo group, and both were treated with a low-energy diet (6300 kJ (1500 kcal)/day with 30% fat) for four months. SHBG increased significantly in both groups (from 19.1 ± 1.9 to 26.0 ± 3.3 nmol/L in the placebo group and from 17.6 ± 1.6 to 21.6 ± 2.1 in the

metformin group). Both studies showed decreases in free testosterone corresponding to the increase in SHBG and a decline (though in the study by Guzick not statistically significant) in fasting insulin after the dietary intervention. Androstenedione decreased and DHEAS increased (Crave *et al.*, 1995b), but there was no reduction in serum total testosterone. Nevertheless, several studies showed that energy restriction reduced total testosterone level, especially in obese, infertile hyperandrogenic women with polycystic ovaries. The results on total serum estradiol were inconsistent, with some studies showing a significant reduction and some others no effect.

Weinstock *et al.* (1998) randomized 45 obese non-diabetic women (aged 43.3 ± 1.1 years; mean baseline weight 96.9 ± 2.2 kg and BMI 35.9 ± 0.9 kg/m²) to one of three treatment groups: diet alone, diet and aerobic training, diet and strength training. All subjects received the same 48-week group behaviour modification programme and diet (3900 kJ (925 kcal)/d for the first 16 weeks, 6300 (1500 kcal)/d thereafter). During weeks 48 to 96, subjects were unsupervised. Subjects on all three treatments achieved a mean weight loss of 13.8 kg by week 16, which was associated with decreased fasting insulin levels (from 15.4 ± 1.0 to 10.6 ± 0.6 mU/L) and insulin area after an oral glucose tolerance test (61.8% of baseline), without significant differences among groups and without further improvement with further unsupervised diet. Fasting glucose and the area under the glycaemic curve after an oral glucose tolerance test decreased slightly after weight loss, but this change was not significant. Only 22 out of the initial 45 subjects were studied at week 96. They maintained a loss of approximately 10% of the initial weight (–9.9 kg), but insulin levels had returned to pretreatment levels.

Postmenopausal women. Svendsen *et al.* (1995) carried out a clinical interven-

tion study on 98 healthy, overweight, postmenopausal women aged 49–58 years, with BMI 25–42 kg/m², who were given a 4200 kJ (1000 kcal) diet daily for three months. Increased SHBG was significantly correlated with reduction in weight and loss of fat determined by total body dual-energy X-ray absorptiometry (DXA) scanner ($r = -0.4$ to -0.5, $p < 0.01$) and with reduction in waist circumference, visceral adipose tissue and WHR ($r = -0.3$ to -0.4, $p < 0.01$). There was no reduction in serum levels of total testosterone or estradiol.

Kasim-Karakas *et al.* (2000) modified the diet of 64 healthy postmenopausal women with a mean age of 61 ± 11 years and a mean baseline weight of 75 ± 2.4 kg. For the first four months, participants followed a controlled-energy diet with stepwise reduction of fat intake from 35% to 25% to 15% of energy. They were then requested to follow a self-selected 15% fat diet *ad libitum* for eight months. Mean carbohydrate consumption increased from 200 g/day at baseline to 377 g/day at four months and 256 g/day at 12 months. The actual food composition of the diet was not published. During the *ad libitum* diet, the mean weight loss was 4.6 ± 0.5 kg, fasting plasma glucose decreased significantly (down to 4.77 ± 0.11 mmol/L from 5.44 ± 0.11 at baseline and 5.16 ± 0.11 at four months), insulin decreased non-significantly, triglycerides increased during the euenergetic treatment and returned to baseline values after the *ad libitum* period, total, high- and low-density lipoprotein (HDL and LDL) cholesterol decreased in the first four months but LDL returned to baseline values after the *ad libitum* period. Similar weight loss with an *ad libitum* low-fat diet without increasing triacylglycerolaemia was observed in other studies (Berrino *et al.*, 2001; Schaefer *et al.*, 1995).

Studies in NIDDM patients. Wing *et al.* (1991) randomly assigned 36 type-II diabetic subjects (10 men and 26 women, age 35–70 years), 30% or more above ideal body weight, either to a low-energy diet for 20 weeks or to the same programme that included, however, an eight-week period of very low-energy diet (1700 kJ (400 kcal) of lean meat, fish and fowl). Both diets were associated with behaviour therapy and an exercise programme. 33 subjects completed the 20-week programme and complied with the one-year follow-up. The very low-energy group had greater weight loss at week 20, but weight losses from pretreatment to one year were similar (from 102.1 to 93.5 kg and from 104.5 to 97.7 kg on average). The very low-energy diet produced a greater decrease in fasting glucose at the end of the 20-week programme (-6.5 mmol/L vs -3.5, $p = 0.035$) and at one year (-3.8 vs $+0.7$ mmol/L, $p = 0.001$) and greater long-term reduction of glycosylated haemoglobin. The very low-energy group, however, had a greater rise in insulin during the oral glucose tolerance test carried out at 20 weeks, suggesting to the authors that the improved glycaemic control could be due to an increase in insulin secretion. The change in average fasting insulin from baseline to 20 weeks to one year was from 141 to 120 to 133 pmol/L in the low-energy group, and from 163 to 104 to 205 pmol/L in the very low-energy group. A similar biphasic effect on plasma insulin was previously observed by Stanik and Marcus (1980), who placed seven severely hyperglycaemic obese patients (men and postmenopausal women) on severe energy restriction for 4–12 weeks. On entry, mean fasting plasma glucose level was 326 ± 23 mg/dL. The insulin response to oral glucose was completely flat. After initiating caloric restriction, fasting plasma glucose rapidly fell, reaching 150 ± 21 mg/dL by two weeks, and remained low throughout the diet period. At restudy, improved oral glucose tolerance was accompanied by significant increases in the insulin secretory responses to both glucose and tolbu-

tamide. These results support the concept that control of plasma glucose concentration allows recovery of insulin secretion. The degree of weight loss necessary to achieve this effect was modest.

Treatment of NIDDM patients (10 males aged 40–70 years, WHR > 0.9 and mean BMI 26 kg/m²) with dexfenfluramine (and low-energy diet) for three months resulted in a significant decrease in visceral (from 484 ± 230 to 333 ± 72 cm²) rather than subcutaneous adipose tissue. This specific decrease in visceral adipose tissue was accompanied by a remarkable increase in insulin sensitivity, as assessed by the minimal model technique (from 0.29 ± 0.13 to 0.54 ± 0.21 min⁻¹ mU/L, $p = 0.01$), significantly decreased levels of C-peptide (from 0.77 ± 0.24 to 0.58 ± 0.15 mmol/L, $p = 0.002$), total cholesterol and triglycerides ($p < 0.001$ and $p = 0.021$) and non-significantly decreased fasting glucose and glycosylated haemoglobin (Marks et al., 1996).

Further studies showing improved glucose control in diabetic patients are cited in Chapter 6.

Studies in men and both sexes together. Stanik et al. (1981) investigated the effects of weight reduction on reproductive hormones in 24 moderately obese men, 18–108% above ideal body weight. Serum estrone, estradiol, testosterone, percentage free testosterone, SHBG binding capacity, and, in nine subjects, androstenedione were measured serially before and during an outpatient supplemented fasting programme (1300 kJ (320 kcal)/day) for 8–20 weeks. At the baseline, mean estrone was elevated to 100 ± 7 pg/mL (normal, 30–60 pg/mL). Estradiol was slightly elevated to 36 ± 3 pg/mL (normal, 8–35 pg/mL). The mean testosterone level of 400 ± 20 ng/dL was at the lower end of the normal range (400–1000 ng/dL) but the mean % free testosterone was elevated to 4.1 ± 0.2% (normal 1.6–3%). The calculated free

testosterone level was normal. The mean SHBG binding capacity was 0.99 ± 0.05 µg dihydrotestosterone bound/dL (normal, 1.0–1.8 µg/dL). The mean androstenedione level of 52 ± 5.8 ng/dL was normal. These data were consistent with previous findings in much heavier men. Weight loss (mean, 19.5 kg) after eight weeks was associated with normalization of all the measured parameters: mean estrone decreased to 48 ± 23 pg/mL ($p < 0.01$), estradiol to 28 ± 2.1 pg/mL ($p < 0.05$), testosterone increased to 536 ± 35 pg/dL and % free testosterone fell to 3.2 ± 0.2% (both $p < 0.01$). Data on 16 men remaining on the programme for 16 or 20 weeks showed a continued fall of estrogens and stabilization of testosterone and % free testosterone. However, unlike the findings of increased SHBG binding capacity with weight loss in obese women, SHBG did not change significantly over the entire time period.

Tymchuk et al. (1998) measured the levels of insulin, SHBG, prostate-specific antigen (PSA) and serum lipids in 27 obese men (mean age 57 ± 2.6 years) undergoing a three-week low-fat (< 10% of calories) high-fibre and high complex carbohydrate diet and exercise programme. BMI decreased from 35 ± 1.9 to 33.4 ± 1.8 kg/m². Insulin decreased from 222 ± 30 to 126 ± 21 pmol/L and SHBG increased from 18 ± 2 to 25 ± 3 nmol/L. PSA decreased but not significantly (all the three men with slightly elevated levels showed a decrease). Triglycerides and total and LDL and HDL cholesterol decreased significantly (average 41, 49, 37, and 5.3 mg/dL, respectively), as did the total/HDL cholesterol ratio (all $p \leq 0.01$). Sex steroids were not measured, but in a previous study on 21 men, the same intervention for 26 days decreased serum estradiol levels from 47.2 ± 4.6 to 23.8 ± 2.5 pg/mL whereas serum testosterone levels were unchanged (5.1 ± 0.3 versus 5.1 ± 0.2 ng/mL). Total serum cholesterol levels decreased from 229 ± 9 to 181 ± 7

Table 21. Hormonal and metabolic effects in weight reduction trials on obese subjects

(a) Studies on premenopausal women

Reference	Mean age or range	No.	Type (daily energy) and duration of intervention	Initial BMI or % IBW*, weight	Weight change
Low-energy diet					
Bates & Whitworth, 1982	NR	7[b]	Unspecified caloric restriction	141*	−15%
Grenman et al., 1986	35	25	1200 kcal, 12 mo	43, 121	−11%
Pasquali et al., 1989	22	20	1000–1500 kcal, 6–12 mo	32, 86	−11%
Leenen et al., 1994	39	33	4.2 MJ deficit, 3 mo	31, 87	−14%
Slabber et al., 1994[d]	35	30	Low glycaemic index vs balanced diet, both 1000–1200 kcal, 12 wk	35, 94 / 35, 97	−10% / −7%
Crave et al., 1995b	NR	24[e]	1500 kcal, 4 mo	34, 87.5	−4%
Turcato et al., 1997	34	26	1286 kJ, 4 wk	38, 101	−8%
Weinstock et al., 1998	43	45	925–1500 kcal ± EX, 58 wk	36, 97	−14%
Very low-energy diet					
Harlass et al., 1984	NR	6[e]	500 kcal 4–6 mo	>30, 103	−11%
Kiddy et al., 1989	NR	5[f]	330 kcal, 4 wk	36	−5.2 kg
Fujioka et al., 1991	38	40[f]	800 kcal, 8 wk	35, 86	−14%
Wing et al., 1992[g]	38	101	1000–1500 kcal + EX, 20 wk	31, 83	−8%
Hamilton-Fairley et al., 1993	NR	6[b,e]	350 kcal, 4 wk	34	−7%
Zamboni et al., 1993	39	16	1286 kJ x 2 wk + 4200 kJ x 14 wk	38, 104	−15%
Guzick et al., 1994[g]	32	12	400–1200 kcal + EX, 12 wk	178*, 108	−15%
Holte et al., 1995[h]	NR	13[f]	1200 kcal, up to stable weight	32, 89	−14%
Jacubowicz & Nestler, 1997	30	11	1000–1200 kcal, 8 wk	32	−7% (BMI)
Jacubowicz & Nestler, 1997	29	12[f]	1000–1200 kcal, 8 wk	32	−7% (BMI)
De Pergola et al., 1998	32	21	318 kcal, 3 wk	39	

(b) Studies on postmenopausal women

Reference	Mean age or range	No.	Type (daily energy) and duration of intervention	Initial BMI or % IBW*, weight	Weight change
Low-energy diet					
Svendsen et al., 1995	49–58	98	4.2 MJ ± EX, 3 mo	> 25, 78	−13%
Kasmin-Karakas et al., 2000	61	64	15% fat, 1 y	28, 75	−8%
Very low-energy diet					
O'Dea et al., 1979	50–63	12	Supplemented fast, 12–17 wk	124–193*, 105	−23%
Turcato et al., 1997	58	15	1286 kJ, 4 wk	35, 88	−6%

fG	fl	IGF	BP[a]	Ga	la	CP	IS	SH	E1	E2	T	fT	A	D	tri	chl	Other relevant effects
											↓	↓					
								(↑)[c]	↑	=	=	↑					C↓, PRL↓
					↓				(↓)	(↓)	↓	=	(↓)	(↓)			LH↓, P↓
								↑	=	↓	↓	↓	↓	↑			fE2↓
=	↓					=											
=	(↓)					↑											
=	↓							↑			=	↓	↓	↑	(↓)	(↓)	
↓	↓							↑	(↑)		(↑)	↓	(↓)				LH↓ C↓
(↓)	↓[c]		(↓)	↓													
								↑			↓						LH↓
	↓	↓	1↑					↑			=	↓					
↓	↓			↓	↓										↓	↓	
↑				(↓)											=	↓	
			1=	=	↓			↑									
↓	↓			↓	↓										↓	↓	
(↓)	(↓)							↑			(↓)	↓					
=	↓	=		(↓)	↓	(↓)	↓	↑				↓	=	=			LH =
=	↓							↑			=	=	=	↑			LH =
=	↓							↑			↓	↓	=	=			17αOHP↓, LH =
	↓	↓	3↑														

fG	Hb	fl	SH	E2	T	fT	A	D	tri	chl	Other relevant effects
			↑	=	=		=				
↓	=	(↓)							=	↓	FFA ↓
			↑	↓	=	↓					LH ↑
↓		=	(↑)		=	(↑)	(↓)				LH ↑, C↓

Table 21 (contd)

(c) Studies in children and adolescents

Reference	Sex	Mean age or range	No.	Type (daily energy) and duration of intervention	Initial BMI or % IBW*, weight	Weight change
Pintor *et al.*, 1980	Girls	7–11	12	1000 kcal until IBW	175–220*	NR
Knip & Nuutinen, 1993	Both	6–16	32	Hypocaloric, 1 y	29, 69	−16%
Wabitsch *et al.*, 1995	Girls	15	92	4321 kJ + EX, 6 wk	31, 87	−10%

(d) Studies on men and both sexes together

Reference	Sex	Mean age or range	No.	Type (daily energy) and duration of intervention	Initial BMI or % IBW*, weight	Weight change
Low-energy diet						
Rosenthal *et al.*, 1985	M	57	21	LF-HF + EX, 26 d	NR, 99	−5%
Strain *et al.*, 1988	M	20–50	11	Individual low-cal diet, 17 mo	167*	26–130 kg
Wing *et al.*, 1992[g]	M	37	101	1000–1500 kcal + EX, 20 wk	31, 96	−10%
Leenen *et al.*, 1994	M	40	37	4.2 MJ deficit, 3 mo	31, 97	−14%
Rasmussen *et al.*, 1994	B	36	60	1200 kcal, 16 wk	34, 96	−8%
Colman *et al.*, 1995[h]	M	60	35	LED, 9 mo	30, 91	−10%
Rasmussen *et al.*, 1995	NR	NR	9	1.6 MJ[i]	39, 111	−27%
Dengel *et al.*, 1996[g]	M	59	47	300–500 kcal deficit ± EX, 10 mo	120–160*, 92	−10%
Torjesen *et al.*, 1997[g]	B	40	219[j]	Low-fat, high fish ± EX, 1 y	29	−9%
Goodpaster *et al.* 1999	B		32	800–1200 kcal, 13 wk[k]	35, 100	−13%
Ross *et al.*, 2000a[g]	M	45	52	700 kcal deficit ± EX, 12 wk	31, 96	−8%
Very low-energy diet						
Stanik & Marcus, 1980	B	48–67	7	600 kcal, 4–12 wk	169*, 107	−10%
Stanik *et al.*, 1981	M	30–63	24	320 kcal, 8 wk	154*, 112	−17%
Gama *et al.*, 1990	B	41	7	445 kcal, 3 wk	35, 97	−5%
Tanaka *et al.*, 1990	B	16–29	15[f]	VLED, over 1 wk	34, 87	−13%
Wing *et al.*, 1991[g]	B	51	33[l]	VLED programme, 20 wk	38, 103	−7%
Megia *et al.*, 1993	B	43	20	Fasting or VLED, 29 d	46	−12% (BMI)
Strain *et al.*, 1994	M	NR	17	LF-HF low cal, 6 wk–39 mo	51	−19%
Vermeulen *et al.*, 1996	M	25–62	50	PSMF, 6 wk	41, 124	−12%
Tymchuk *et al.*, 1998	M	57	27	LF-HF + EX, 3 wk	35	−5%
Fogelholm *et al.*, 2000a	M	40	74	VLED programme, 12 mo	34, 92	−14%

fl	CP	SH	E2	T	fT	A	D	tri	Other relevant effects
			=	↓	↓				C =, PRL =, P ↓
↓								↓	
↓	↑	↑	↓	↓	↓	=	↓		fC ↑

fG	Hb	fl	IGF	Ga	la	CP	IS	SH	E1	E2	T	fT	A	D	tri	chl	Other relevant effects
=									↓	=					↓	↓	
=			(↓)					↑	(↑)	=	↑	↑			↓	↓	
		↓						↑	↑	↓	=	=	↓	↑			fE2↓
↓		↓	↑c														GH = , BP-3 =
=		↓	↓	↓													
		↑															GH↑, BP-3 =
=		↓		↓	↓												
↓		↓	↓			↓	↑								↓		
=		↓					↑								↓	↓	Leptin ↓
=		(↓)	=	(↓)			↑										
↓							↑										
								=	↓	↓	↑	%↓	=				
=		↓	=	↓													GH ↑
=		↓															GH ↑
↓	↓	↓c													(↓)	(↓)	
↓		↓	↓														GH ↑
		↓						↑									
		↓	↑					↑	↓	↑	=	(↓)	=		↓		GH(↑)
		↓						↑							↓	↓	
		↓															

Table 21 (contd)

(e) Intervention trials with drugs or surgery

Reference	Sex	Mean age or range	No.	Type (daily energy) and duration of intervention	Initial BMI or % IBW*, weight	Weight change
Kopelman et al., 1981	Wp	30	12	Bypass surgery, 1 y	225*, 126	−31%
Poulos et al., 1994	NR	42	50	Bypass surgery, 1 y	45, NR	−29%
Marks et al., 1996	M	40–70	10[l]	Dexfenfluramine, 12 wk	26, 78	−4%
Van Gaal et al., 1998[g]	NR	43	55	600 kcal deficit, EX, ± sibutramine, 6 mo	36	−11 kg
Sjöström et al., 1998[g]	B	45	688	600 kcal deficit ± orlistat, 1 y	36, 99	−10% vs −6%
Davidson et al., 1999[g]	B	44	892	2100–3360 kJ deficit ± orlistat, 2 y	36, 100	−9% vs −6%
James et al., 2000[g]	B	40	467	600 kcal ± sibutramine, 2 y	37, 102	−10% vs −5%

Arrows indicate a statistically significant increase or decrease; arrows in brackets indicate a non-statistically significant increase or decrease greater than 10%; =, no change, IBW, ideal body weight; LED, low-energy diet; VLED, very low-energy diet; LF-HF, low-fat, high complex carbohydrates and fibre; PSMF, protein-sparing modified fast; EX, exercise; y, years; mo, months; wk, weeks; d, days; NR, not reported
Wp, women, premenopausal; M, men; B, both men and women
fG, fasting glucose; Hb, glycosylated haemoglobin; fI, fasting insulin; IGF, insulin-like growth factor-I; BP, IGF-binding protein; Ga, glucose area (or glucose at 2 h) under glucose tolerance test; Ia, insulin area; CP, C peptide; IS, insulin sensitivity; SH, sex-hormone binding globulin; E1, estrone; E2, estradiol; T, testosterone; fT, free testosterone; A, androstenedione; D, dehydroepiandrosterone sulfate; tri, triglycerides; chl, cholesterol; FFA, free fatty acids; GH, growth hormone; C, cortisol; PRL, prolactin; P, progesterone; LH, luteinizing hormone; fC, free cortisol; fE2, free estradiol; 17αOHP, 17α-hydroxyprogesterone

Energy values are given in calories or joules as in the publication cited: 1 kcal = 4.19 kJ

fG	Hb	fl	IGF	CP	IS	SH	E1	E2	T	A	tri	chl
						↑	(↑)	↑	↓	↓		
↓	↓	↓	↑									
(↓)	(↓)			↓	↑						↓	↓
↓		↓									↓	
↓		↓									=	↓
=		↓									=	↓
=		↓		↓							↓	=

[a] IGFBP-1 or IGFBP-3 as indicated
[b] PCOS patients (the study by Kiddy included also six normal-weight women, with the same results; in particular IGF-I decreased significantly in two weeks)
[c] Early decrease followed by an increase to baseline values (or vice versa)
[d] Cross-over trial
[e] Hirsute patients
[f] Japanese subjects
[g] Randomized trial
[h] Controlled trial
[i] The intervention continued up to when body weight was 30% above IBW
[j] All subjects aged 40 years
[k] Ascertainment at 17 weeks
[l] NIDDM patients

mg/dL, whereas triglyceride levels fell from 301 ± 66 to 151 ± 13 mg/dL. HDL cholesterol levels fell from 41 ± 3 to 35 ± 1 mg/dL, whereas the total/HDL cholesterol ratio was unchanged (5.5 ± 0.4 versus 5.1 ± 0.3) (Rosenthal et al., 1985).

Goodpaster et al. (1999) examined the relationship between weight loss-induced change in regional adiposity and improvement in insulin sensitivity. 32 obese sedentary women and men completed a four-month weight loss programme and had repeat determinations of body composition (DXA and computed tomography) and insulin sensitivity (euglycaemic insulin infusion). 15 lean men and women served as control subjects. The intervention achieved significant decreases in weight (100.2 ± 2.6 to 85.5 ± 2.1 kg), BMI (34.3 ± 0.6 to 29.3 ± 0.6), total fat mass (36.9 ± 1.5 to 26.1 ± 1.3 kg), percentage body fat (37.7 ± 1.3 to $31.0 \pm 1.5\%$) and fat-free mass (FFM) (59.2 ± 2.3 to 55.8 ± 2.0 kg). Abdominal subcutaneous and visceral adipose tissue were reduced (494 ± 19 to 357 ± 18 cm^2 and 157 ± 12 to 96 ± 7 cm^2, respectively). Insulin sensitivity improved from 5.9 ± 0.4 to 7.3 ± 0.5 mg $\times$ FFM^{-1} $\times$ min^{-1}. Rates of insulin-stimulated non-oxidative glucose disposal accounted for the majority of this improvement. Serum levels of leptin, triglycerides, cholesterol and insulin all decreased ($p < 0.01$). After weight loss, insulin sensitivity continued to correlate with generalized and regional adiposity but, with the exception of the percentage decrease in visceral adipose tissue, the magnitude of improvement in insulin sensitivity was not correlated with the various changes in body composition.

Several randomized controlled trials have addressed the issue of adding an aerobic exercise programme to a low-energy diet for weight reduction and improvement of metabolic parameters in obese subjects. Studies with a factorial design have usually shown that a low-energy diet is more effective than aerobic exercise, but the combination of both may improve insulin-linked parameters (Dengel et al., 1996; Torjesen et al., 1997; Ross et al., 2000a).

Studies with drugs. James et al. (2000) reported on the efficacy of treatment with sibutramine (an inhibitor of serotonin and adrenalin uptake that increases satiety) for weight maintenance after weight loss in otherwise healthy obese patients of both sexes, aged 17–65 years, with initial BMI between 30 and 45 kg/m^2. 467 patients who succeeded in losing more than 5% of their weight over six months of low-energy diet and sibutramine treatment (weight loss phase) were randomly assigned to sibutramine or placebo for 18 months (weight maintenance phase). At 24 months, the mean weight loss from baseline was -10.2 ± 9.3 and -4.7 ± 7.2 kg, respectively. Weight loss was accompanied by substantial decreases in the concentrations of serum triglycerides (-25% and -6%, respectively, in the sibutramine and placebo group), insulin (-22% and -3%) and C-peptide (-26% and -12%). Similar results were reported by Van Gaal et al. (1998) from an ongoing randomized study.

Two large randomized placebo-controlled trials of treatment with orlistat (an intestinal lipase inhibitor) in subjects on a slightly hypocaloric diet showed some improvement in body weight reduction (about 10% vs 6% in the placebo group), glucose and lipid levels and blood lipids (Sjöström et al., 1998; Davidson et al., 1999).

Dietary modification in female volunteers aiming at reducing estrogen levels. Several studies showed statistically significant reductions of total serum estradiol levels in (mostly) non-obese pre- (Williams et al., 1989) or postmenopausal women (Rose et al., 1987, 1993; Boyar et al., 1988; Prentice et al., 1990) who lost weight (3–4 kg) by following a low-fat diet. Similar results were reported with a low-fat high-fibre diet among pre- (Bagga et al., 1995) and postmenopausal women (Heber et al., 1991). A further study reported a significant reduction in body weight, increased SHBG and decreased total testosterone after a comprehensive dietary modification aiming to increase insulin sensitivity and consumption of phytoestrogens (Berrino et al., 2001). [The Working Group noted that these studies could not distinguish between a possible effect of weight reduction and an independent effect of dietary modification]. Only the three largest studies are summarized here.

Rose et al. (1993) randomized 93 postmenopausal breast cancer patients (63 under adjuvant treatment: 50 with tamoxifen alone, 6 chemotherapy alone and 7 with both treatments) to either a dietary intervention group, for which the goal was to reduce total fat intake to 15–20% of total energy, or a control group. The intervention group actually reduced fat intake to about 21% of energy intake and maintained the reduction for 18 months. Control patients showed a sustained increase in body weight (over 1 kg in 18 months), while patients assigned to the low-fat diet showed a reduction in body weight of about 2 kg, which was maintained over the 18-month dietary intervention. Among the 30 patients who did not receive any adjuvant therapy, the 12 in the dietary intervention group exhibited average weight losses of 4.1 and 4.3 kg after 12 and 18 months, respectively, while the 18 patients in the control group did not change their body weight. In the latter group, body weight was significantly correlated with serum estrone sulfate levels ($r = 0.49$). Correlations with other hormone levels were not given. Overall, there was no change in serum estradiol levels over the study period. In 21% of the patients, however, estradiol levels were below the detection limit of the assay (5 pg/mL). Restricting the analysis to patients with initial estradiol levels above 10 pg/mL, those allocated to the low-fat diet showed average reductions of 20% at six months and 15% at 18 months ($p < 0.005$), while control women did not show any significant change. [The Working Group noted that part of this apparent hormonal effect could be due to regression towards the mean.] There was no significant difference between the serum estrone and estrone sulfate concentrations of the low-fat and control groups. Serum SHBG levels were, as expected, increased by tamoxifen, but were reduced significantly after 12 months (−17%, $p < 0.01$) and 18 months (−23%, $p < 0.05$) on the low-fat diet in patients not receiving tamoxifen (despite a significant weight reduction).

Within the framework of the Women's Health Trial, Prentice et al. (1990) studied 73 postmenopausal healthy women (median age 60 years) not using exogenous estrogens, who agreed to reduce dietary fat from customary levels of about 40% energy to a target level of 20%. The duration of dietary intervention was at least 10 weeks (median 14 wk, max. 22 wk). Estimated fat intake decreased from 68.5 g/day to 29.5 g/day (from 37.3% to 20% of their average daily energy intake). Total cholesterol decreased from 234 to 222 mg/dL and the average weight reduction was 3.4 kg, from a mean weight of 69.6 before the intervention to 66.2 kg ($p < 0.001$). Serum concentrations of estrone and estrone sulfate did not change significantly following intervention. On the other hand, total estradiol concentrations were significantly reduced (from 0.71 to 0.63 pg/mL on average, $p < 0.001$), as were the concentrations of bioavailable (unbound and albumin-bound) estradiol (from 0.46 to 0.39 pg/mL, $p = 0.01$) and, to a lesser extent, of SHBG-bound estradiol (from 0.28 to 0.18 pg/mL, $p = 0.03$). Women with high pre-intervention estradiol levels experienced relatively greater reduction, but the authors noted that measurement error in the pre-intervention determinations and consequent regression to the mean in the post-intervention determinations may partially

explain this observation. Notwithstanding a significant weight reduction, the serum concentration of SHBG was also reduced after dietary intervention, but not significantly (from 0.07 to 0.02 mg/dL, $p = 0.14$).

It has been hypothesized that the lack of increase in SHBG levels associated with low-fat diets may be attributable to simultaneous increased intake of high glycaemic index carbohydrates, which would prevent the improvement in insulin sensitivity that would be expected following weight reduction (Berrino et al., 2001).

Bagga et al. (1995) studied 12 healthy premenopausal women over two months on a very low-fat (10% of energy) and high-fibre (25–35 g/day, provided by whole grain cereals and legumes) ad libitum diet. There was a small but statistically significant overall weight loss (−2.0 ± 1.4 kg), a significant reduction in serum levels of estrone (−19 and −18% in the follicular and luteal phase, respectively) and estradiol (−25 and −22%), and no significant change in serum estrone sulfate, SHBG and progesterone. [The Working Group noted that most trials of dietary fibre supplementation show a reduction in estrogen levels, probably due to reduced enterohepatic circulation, suggesting that the effect observed in this study may be independent of weight loss.]

Berrino et al. (2001) randomized 104 healthy and mostly non-obese postmenopausal women whose serum testosterone was above the upper tertile of the distribution (> 0.38 ng/mL) to either a dietary intervention or a control group (DIANA study). The diet was available ad libitum and designed to reduce plasma insulin levels by lowering animal fat and refined carbohydrates and increasing low-glycaemic index foods and monounsaturated and n–3 polyunsaturated fatty acids; phytoestrogen-rich foods, such as soy foods and various seeds, were also increased. The intervention included intensive dietary counselling and specially prepared

group meals twice a week over 4.5 months. Control women were not informed of the dietary goals of the study but received a standard recommendation to increase fruit and vegetable consumption. Body weight decreased significantly (4.06 kg vs 0.54 in the control group, $p < 0.0001$). Mean BMI in the intervention group decreased from 26.9 to 25.3 kg/m². Waist circumference and hip circumference also decreased significantly (−3.9 and −2.5 cm, respectively, $p < 0.0001$) together with WHR (from 0.82 to 0.80, $p = 0.0045$). SHBG increased from 36.0 to 45.1 nmol/L (25% vs 4% in the control group, $p < 0.0001$) and serum testosterone decreased from 0.41 to 0.33 ng/mL (−20% vs −7% in the control group, $p = 0.0038$). Serum estradiol decreased (−18% vs −6%) but not significantly. Fasting glucose (−5.7% vs −1.2%, $p = 0.026$) and insulin area after an oral glucose tolerance test (−7.7% vs +9.4%, $p = 0.04$) also changed significantly. After adjustment for change in body weight, the differences in changes in hormonal levels between the intervention and control groups were no longer statistically significant (only the difference in fasting glycaemia remained of borderline significance), suggesting that the hormonal effects of dietary intervention were largely mediated through changes in body weight. The increase in consumption of fibre and phytoestrogens, however, may have contributed to the overall effect. Other studies that achieved a similar weight reduction in normal-weight women, in fact, did not observe any effect on SHBG (Rose et al., 1993; Prentice et al., 1990).

Physical activity

Sex hormones in premenopausal women. A few intervention studies have tested effects of chronic exercise on menstrual factors or sex hormones in premenopausal women (Table 22). Sample sizes ranged from 6 to 28 in six of the studies and one study randomized

132 subjects but only 57 completed the study. Thus, the information available from carefully controlled studies is scarce. Most reports on sex hormones in pre-menopausal women or of an association between physical activity and menstrual disorders have been case reports or observational studies. Most of the latter have been cross-sectional studies of convenience samples, although there have been a few population-based cohort studies.

In a randomized clinical trial of control of energy intake for weight-loss vs weight maintenance (Bullen et al., 1985; Beitins et al., 1991), 28 untrained college-aged women all received the same exercise prescription of 10 miles/-day running plus 3.5 hours/day of sports. All activities took place during eight weeks at a college training camp. Food intake was carefully prescribed and controlled by camp dieticians. Overnight urine was collected daily. During the intervention, eighteen women developed loss of LH surge, 13 experienced delayed menses and 18 developed luteal phase defects. Among women in the weight-loss arm, 75% had delayed menses vs 8% of women in the weight-maintenance arm ($p < 0.005$). Similarly, 81% of women in the weight-loss arm experienced loss of LH surge vs 42% of women in the weight-mainte-nance group ($p < 0.05$). There was no difference in the incidence of luteal phase defects between the two groups. Six months after termination of the inter-vention, all subjects were experiencing normal menstrual cycles. The authors interpreted their study as suggesting that vigorous exercise, especially in conjunction with weight loss, can result in reversibly disturbed reproductive function.

In the largest published clinical trial, Bonen (1992) randomized 132 women aged 18–40 years to one of six jogging exercise programmes for either two or four months: < 10 miles/week; 10–20 miles/week; or 20–30 miles/week. There was no control group. Women were fol-lowed for nine menstrual cycles. Results

were presented only for the 57 who com-pleted the entire study. There was no change in LH concentration, menstrual cycle length or luteal phase length, nor any trend towards increased change in FSH or progesterone with increasing physical activity. There was no change in body weight or percentage body fat, despite a significant increase in maximal aerobic capacity (VO$_2$max) in all study arms ($p < 0.05$). The authors concluded that recreational running of up to 30 miles/week for four menstrual cycles had no deleterious effect on menstrual cycle. [This study had the benefit of a random-ized controlled design with long follow-up, but the considerable drop-out rate (75 out of 132) limits the interpretation of the results.]

In a later study by Williams et al. (1999), 15 women were randomly assigned to one of four groups: seden-tary control, active control (jogging or cycling 45 minutes/day, 2–3 days/week), training during the follicular phase of the menstrual cycle, or training during the luteal phase of the cycle. The training consisted of twice-daily running or cycling for five days/week. The exercise bouts consisted of running 3.2 km per exercise bout, increasing by 1.2 km per bout each week. The training lasted through two menstrual cycles. Diet was controlled to maintain weight within ± 2 kg of baseline weight. At the end of the intervention, almost half of the trained women showed evidence of abnormal luteal function, including short luteal defects and low urinary progesterone. None experienced loss of LH surge and none had delayed menses or abnormal bleeding. The changes in luteal function were observed in both training groups, suggesting that exercise at any time in the cycle can affect menstrual function.

In the HERITAGE Family Study (An et al., 2000), parents and their adult sons and daughters completed a 20-week endurance training programme (three days/week gradually increased to 75% VO$_2$max for 50 minutes) on cycle ergo-

meters. On average, SHBG increased by 3.4 nmol/L in the daughters (mean age 25.5 years), but decreased by an aver-age of 7.9 nmol/L in their premenopausal mothers (mean age 48.6 years). Change in SHBG with training was minimal in both fathers and sons.

Insulin-like growth factor (IGF) and insulin-like growth factor binding protein (IGFBP). Information on exercise effects on the IGF system is limited to that gained from a few small intervention studies. An eight-week aerobic exercise programme (three times per week cycling, 1260 kJ (300 kcal) expended) in previously sedentary older subjects (mean age 66 years) increased IGF-I by 19% ($p < 0.01$) in ten men and by 8% in eight women ($p = 0.10$) (Poehlman et al., 1994). No controls were included in this study. The participants did not lose body fat or weight, because the study was designed to maintain energy balance. In a randomized controlled clin-ical trial in older individuals (31 men, 21 women, mean age 67 years), six months of endurance training three times per week (30–45 minutes/session, gradually increasing intensity to 80–85% heart rate reserve) resulted in a non-significant increase in mean IGF-I from 122.4 ± 8.0 to 131.1 ± 7.6 µg/L (Vitiello et al., 1997). In comparison, IGF-I decreased non-significantly in stretching control subjects from 129.2 ± 11.3 to 125.2 ± 9.3. This result was in spite of a significant decrease in body weight and fat mass in exercisers (compared with no change in controls). A 16-week progressive resistive training programme produced a non-significant decline in IGF-I, from 200.4 ± 60.4 to 190.8 ± 57.6 mg/L in 13 older men (mean age 60 years) (Nicklas et al., 1995). Among nine con-trols, there was a non-significant increase in IGF-I levels. The assignment to intervention or control group was made by the investigators, based on a judgement of likely success in the inter-vention.

Table 22. Intervention studies of the association between exercise and menstrual factors in premenopausal women

Reference	Study design	No. of subjects	Mean age or range	Length of follow-up	End-points	Results	Energy balance
Bullen et al., 1984	Cycle ergometry 2 d/wk + running 4 d/wk up to 45 min per session	7	25	2 months	LH, FSH, E2, E3, P, PRL	Decreased urine E3 (4); decreased urine luteal P (2)	
Bullen et al., 1985	Randomized trial weight-loss vs weight-maintenance training – all ran 10 miles/day + 3.5 h/day sports	28	22	2 menstrual cycles, 6 months follow-up	Menstrual cycles, urine LH, FSH, E3, P	Loss of LH surge (18); delayed menses (13); luteal phase defects (18)	75% of weight-loss vs 8% of weight-maintained groups had delayed menses.
Bonen, 1992	Randomized trial of six exercise programmes, no control group	57	20–36	9 menstrual cycles	LH, FSH, P, menstrual cycle characteristics	No effect	No change in body weight or % body fat
DeCrée et al., 1997a	Progressive training programme, no controls	6	19	3 menstrual cycles	4-OHE, 4-MeOHE, E2, P, LH, PRL	4-MeOHE/4-OHE ratio increased with progressive training ($p < 0.01$)	
DeCrée et al., 1997b	Five-day exercise inter-vention, no controls	15	18.7	2 menstrual cycles	RBC-COMT activity; 2-MeOHE and 4-MeOHE	Increased COMT activity after intense training	
Loucks et al., 1998	Randomized cross-over trial, energy balance vs restriction, all exercised at intense level	9	21	2 menstrual cycles	LH pulsatility and amplitude	No effect of exercise alone	Low-energy group had 10% ($p < 0.01$) decrease in LH pulse frequency and 36% ($p = 0.03$) increase in LH pulse amplitude
Williams et al., 1999	Randomized controlled trial (active control, passive control, follicular exercise luteal exercise)	15	20	3 menstrual cycles	Luteal abnormalities; urine, LH, P, FSH, E3	Luteal phase defects (4 of 9 exercisers vs 0 of 6 controls); decrease in urinary LH and P	Changes in energy intake may have explained luteal defects

E1, estrone; E2, estradiol; E3, estriol; COMT, catechol-O-methyltransferase; 4-OHE, 4-hydroxyestrogen; 2-MeOHE, 2-methoxyestrogen; 4-MeOHE, 4-methoxyestrogen; P, progesterone; PRL, prolactin; FSH, follicle-stimulating hormone; LH, luteinizing hormone

Two weeks of intense endurance training in 10 healthy, young, non-obese men caused a significant increase in IGF-I and GHBP plasma levels with respect to 10 control subjects matched for sex, age and prestudy activity (mainly recreational) (Roelen et al., 1997). In a study of 28 athletes belonging to three swimming teams, four months of increasing training volume (distance swum increased from 5500 to 10 300 m or from 4500 to 6900 m) caused a two-fold increase in IGF-I and IGFBP-3 levels. Free IGF was also increased, but the ratio of IGF-I to IGFBP-3 did not change. IGFBP-1 did not change (Koziris et al., 1999).

Diet in cancer patients. There have been few exercise or weight-loss intervention studies in cancer patients. Studies targeting weight loss in breast cancer patients have had limited evaluation and mixed results.

De Waard et al. (1993) randomized 102 postmenopausal women (BMI > 27 kg/m^2) with a recent breast cancer diagnosis to a weight-loss programme in volving stepwise reduction in energy intake versus a control group. After one year, median weight loss was 6.0 kg with the intervention ($p < 0.001$).

Using a non-intensive approach, the Mayo Clinic conducted a randomized trial of monthly dietician counselling versus control beginning in the period immediately following breast cancer diagnosis in 107 patients. Median weight increase six months after the start of chemotherapy was 2 kg in the dietary-counselling group versus 3.5 kg in the control group, a non-significant difference (Loprinzi et al., 1996).

Goodwin et al. (1998) evaluated a multidisciplinary weight management approach incorporating group dietary sessions, psychological support groups and nutrition and exercise programmes in a non-controlled 61 patient intervention. In breast cancer patients with BMI ≥ 25 kg/m^2, weight loss was 1.63 ± 4.11 kg,

and increased aerobic exercise was strongly correlated with successful weight loss.

In a small pilot study, an eight-week exercise–low-fat diet intervention resulted in significant reductions in weight, waist circumference, hip circumference and percentage body fat in nine breast cancer patients aged 40–74 years (McTiernan et al., 1998). Slight, non-significant decreases were observed in serum concentrations of total and free estradiol, estrone sulfate, total testosterone, androstenedione, dehydroepiandrosterone and SHBG.

No multicentre studies aiming at weight reduction with or without exercise as an integral component have been successfully conducted among women with resected breast cancer (Pinto & Maruyama, 1999).

Experimental models

The physiological and hormonal changes that occur with lowering energy intake and/or increasing physical activity affect virtually all organ systems. Qualitatively, the changes seem to readily extrapolate across genotypes and species, presumably because the systems effected are so basic to survival. However, the quantitative extent of the responses may differ with species.

Methodological issues
Controls

One problem in comparing different rodent experiments is the variability observed among animals used as controls in different experiments (Turturro et al., 1995, 1996, 1998). For instance, in the United States National Toxicology Program, chronic bioassay experiments with tight environmental controls are routinely performed so that studies can be compared, but spontaneous liver tumour incidences in the male B6C3F1 mouse have been observed to vary from 20 to 90% (see for example National Toxicology Program, 1997). The control animals are almost always fed *ad libitum*,

and similar changes in intake or activity can have very different consequences depending upon the control body weight, complicating interpretation (Turturro et al., 1993). For example, an experimental procedure that results in a 10% lower body weight, either due to exercise or a decrease in food intake, can have adverse effects in control mice with low initial body weight, but when applied to a mouse with a heavy initial body weight can have minimal consequences. This may result from the non-linear relationship between body weight and parameters relevant to the whole animal, such as survival or spontaneous tumour incidence (Turturro et al., 1996; 1998), or specific organs and cells, such as liver cell proliferation and apoptosis (Turturro et al., 2000).

Diets

Research on the physiological and metabolic consequences of underfeeding animals has primarily used dietary restriction protocols where lower levels of all dietary constituents are fed. While this approach does not provide information on the dietary components responsible for a change, dietary restriction studies using laboratory diets do not result in overt malnutrition since standard diets are generous in vitamins and minerals. Malnutrition, such as zinc malnutrition, can be devastating for normal animal physiological function (Good et al., 1982).

Evidence for suboptimal intake of nutrients in some dietary restriction studies has come from studies by Birt et al. (1991). In this experiment, dietary restriction was directly compared to energy restriction (the selective reduction of energy-providing components of the diet) in the inhibition of skin papilloma induction (7,12-dimethylbenz[a]anthracene-initiated/O-tetradecanoylphorbol 13-acetate-promoted) in SENCAR mice. While dietary restriction and energy restriction similarly reduced the incidence and multiplicity of skin tumours, energy restriction resulted in extremely small lesions, while with dietary restriction the lesions became as large as those observed in control mice. Similarly, in a comprehensive analysis of the studies conducted in another laboratory, it was found using purified diets and selectively reducing single components that only restriction of total energy and not any specific macronutrient (i.e., protein, fat or carbohydrate) or protein source was effective in suppressing spontaneous neoplasms (Shimokawa et al., 1996). These experiments were conducted using semi-purified diets, since similar studies are not possible with cereal-based diets.

Finally, although decreases in dietary intake in dietary restriction studies can be greater than the decreases usually used to control body weight, dietary restriction studies have used such a wide range of models and approaches that they can give only general insights. When short-term (20 days) and chronic (15 months) dietary restriction (of 40%) were compared, many of the consequences for metabolism (e.g., plasma glucose level, plasma insulin, etc.) were qualitatively similar (Dean et al., 1998) if the animal at the beginning of the experiment was not obese. The effects that occur with dietary restriction appear to represent a gradient of responses related to the extent of dietary intake (Turturro et al., 2000).

Decreasing dietary intake for weight control

Many studies on physiological, hormonal and metabolic effects of underfeeding have used dietary restriction. When all components are reduced, it cannot be determined which one is responsible for any particular observation in a model. It is known that significant changes in dietary composition can alter physiological and hormonal parameters (e.g., Iwasaki et al., 1988), but in the present review, the focus is on using diets that do not result in malnutrition.

Size

In rodents, the most prominent effect of lowering dietary or energy intake is decreased body weight gain during growth, resulting in lower body weight and reduced adiposity (i.e., percentage body fat) or fat mass. Using a dietary restriction of 40% (with vitamin supplementation) with cereal-based diets, fat is lost at a higher rate than lean body mass (Duffy et al., 1989, 1990a,b), with emergence of a stable lower body weight after a few weeks, unless the animal was very obese at the start of the study. Rodents grow throughout much of their lifespan, so diet-restricted animals tend to be smaller as well as less fat than those fed ad libitum.

Lifespan

One of the most consistent effects of dietary restriction is increased lifespan. For example, using a dietary restriction (with supplementation) of 40%, lifespan, measured as either mean or maximal (average lifespan of the 90th percentile survivors), was extended by 15–30% in four different genotypes of mice and three of rat (Turturro et al., 1999).

Water consumption, body temperature and activity

In animals of average body weight with a dietary restriction (with supplementation) of 40%, daily water consumption is at least twice that of animals fed ad libitum (Duffy et al., 1989, 1990a,b; Mittal et al., 2000). Urinary output increases 2–4-fold (depending on age) in male mice using a similar protocol (Taylor et al., 1995). Average body temperature is decreased by approximately 1.5°C in mice and 0.8 °C in rats and the daily range is wider than in animals fed ad libitum. Thermotolerance to hot temperatures (measured by ability to survive heat stress) is improved with dietary restriction (Hall et al., 2000a), while ability to withstand cold is decreased. Activity is increased around feeding time, but decreased for the rest of the day in diet-restricted animals.

Cardiac parameters

Blood pressure decreases with dietary restriction (e.g., Haddad et al., 1993, using a 50% dietary restriction), especially in old rats subjected to lifelong dietary restriction of 40% (with supplementation) (Thomas et al., 1993). Short-term 50% dietary restriction or long-term dietary restriction (40%, with supplementation) (Thomas et al., 1993) leads to bradycardia. Short-term intense (50%) dietary restriction decreases the rate of cardiac contraction and relaxation (Hilderman et al., 1996). These decreases are consistent with a smaller heart resulting from dietary restriction, which has been reported with long-term 30% dietary restriction (Oscai & Holloszy, 1970).

Puberty

Puberty can be delayed if intense dietary restriction is started early. For example, in rats maintained at 80–90 g body weight by dietary restriction, puberty was delayed for at least 13 days (Messer & l'Anson, 2000). Refeeding of different dietary intakes allowed puberty to proceed in a dose-dependent manner (time to puberty being inversely related to amount of food consumed). It has been suggested that delay of puberty involves insulin receptor substrate 2 (IRS-2) (a part of the insulin signalling cascade system) in female animals (Burks et al., 2000).

Overall metabolic effects

Overall metabolic parameters, such as oxygen consumption, follow the pattern of physical activity, rising when activity is elevated and falling when it is decreased. Overall metabolism, per gram lean body mass, is approximately the same with dietary restriction and ad libitum feeding in mice and rats (Duffy et al., 1989, 1990a,b). Diurnal rhythms of metabolic and most physiological parameters appear to be coordinated to feeding time rather than time of day, while activity is related to light rhythm (Duffy et al., 1995).

Intermediary metabolism

With 40% dietary restriction (with supplementation), the activity of key regulatory enzymes associated with glycolysis decreases, whereas the activities of those associated with gluconeogenesis and with the disposal of ammonia by-products increase. For instance, key glycolytic enzymes, such as pyruvate kinase and alcohol dehydrogenase, decrease in terms of both mRNA expression (Dhahbi et al., 1999) and activity (Feuers et al., 1989; Dhahbi et al., 1999). Increases are also seen in both mRNA expression (Dhahbi et al., 1999) and enzyme activity (Feuers et al., 1989; Dhahbi et al., 1999) of gluconeogenic enzymes, such as phosphoenolpyruvate carboxykinase and liver glucose-6-phosphatase and in insulin-mediated muscle glycogen synthesis activity (Banerjee et al., 1997). mRNA expression of genes important for ammonia detoxification, such as hepatic glutaminase, carbamyl phosphate synthase I and tyrosine transferase, also increases (Dhahbi et al., 1999).

Certain enzymes associated with lipid metabolism, such as malic enzyme and glycerokinase, decrease with 40% dietary restriction (with supplementation), as does the formation of fatty acid epoxides (Allaben et al., 1990). However, there is enhancement of the lipoprotein lipase response in adipocytes to a meal with dietary restriction as well as increased utilization of circulating fatty acids (Sugden et al., 1999).

Although the effects of 40% dietary restriction (with supplementation) on blood glucose and cholesterol levels appear to be modest at best, the effects of dietary restriction on insulin levels are more consistent. Levels of circulating insulin are lowered with dietary restriction (e.g., Feuers et al., 1995), while insulin clearance is increased (Wetter et al., 1999) and the phosphorylation of insulin receptor substrate-1 (IRS-1) in muscle is increased (Dean & Cartee, 2000). Insulin sensitivity increases with dietary restriction in rodents (e.g., Koohestani et al., 1998).

These changes, especially those in the effectiveness of IRS-1, suggest that energy metabolism operates more efficiently in diet-restricted animals compared with those fed ad libitum, effectively producing substrates to be utilized in the near term.

Endocrine effects

Studies of the effects of dietary restriction and energy restriction on endocrine status are complicated by the diurnal rhythms seen in hormones, the pulsatile nature of some endocrine phenomena and the sensitivity of hormonal levels to environmental stimuli. This is particularly a problem with studies involving restriction of diet, since the animal may associate the investigator with meals. The animal may then respond with the burst of activity seen at feeding time (Duffy et al., 1989).

A 40% dietary restriction can have such severe effects on the pituitary gland that this treatment has been studied as a model of hypophysectomy (Everitt et al., 1980). One of the most affected pituitary functions involves the lactotrope (Engelman et al., 1993). This also results in inhibition of mammary gland growth and tumorigenesis (Engelman et al., 1994). Growth hormone was 95% inhibited by an energy restriction of 40% after one month, resulting in lowered weight gain; IGF-I was lowered by 12% (Oster et al., 1995). However, with long-term dietary restriction, the ability to produce growth hormone is retained in old animals (Shimokawa et al., 1997).

Leptin, produced by adipocytes, is also reduced by dietary restriction (40%). The lowered level may activate the pituitary–adrenal axis and suppress the gonadal somatotropic and thyroid axes (Aubert et al., 1998; Shimokawa & Higami, 1999). Use of a 40% dietary restriction (with supplementation) of a cereal-based diet also decreased sex-specific steroids and many of the sex differences these steroids support. For example, female- and male-specific cytochrome P450s are inhibited in rats (Leakey et al., 1995). Energy restriction of up to 60% for a month did not appear to affect parathyroid hormone (Ndiaye et al., 1995), except to inhibit its age-related increase. A 40% dietary restriction did not affect calcitonin (Salih et al., 1993). However, a long-term 40% dietary restriction (with supplementation) results in decreased cortical bone mass and mineralization (Banu et al., 1999).

Glucocorticoid levels appear, on the whole, to increase with dietary restriction (Leakey et al., 1998); the major reason for this increase may be the glucogenic role of this hormone rather than a stress response. Plasma glucose and insulin levels fall with a 40% dietary restriction, and free fatty acid metabolism supplies much of the energy for muscle, as noted above. Glucocorticoids, by stimulating apoptosis, provide lipid for this metabolism. This is consistent with the 2–3-h delay in raising plasma glucose levels seen when increasing glucocorticoids (e.g., Shamoon et al., 1981).

Physical activity

Like the effects of restriction of dietary intake, those of physical activity depend upon the system used, as well as the body weight of the animal at the start of the study. For example, in the same rat strain and laboratory, when the control animals weighed approximately 400 g (Holloszy et al., 1985), voluntary wheel-running diminished the beneficial long-term effects on survival expected from the decreased body weight due to this activity. However, when the initial control animal weighed 325 g, the effect on survival of the lower body weight appeared to be overwhelming (Holloszy, 1997). Studies have shown some positive effect of voluntary exercise on survival if the activity began early in life (1–4 months of age). Voluntary exercise started later seems to have little effect on survival or can even have adverse consequences

(Goodrick, 1974). This indicates that timing and level of exercise may be important, as also seen with dietary restriction.

In terms of studying physical activity, because rodents are kept in cages, almost all research has been conducted on relatively inactive animals, particularly for rats. Thus, the following discussion focuses on increases in physical activity rather than inactivity.

Size

One common, though not universal, consequence of exercise is loss of body weight and adiposity (e.g., Garthwaite et al., 1986, using voluntary wheel-running). Fat is lost and there can be an increase in lean body mass that is assumed to be mostly muscle. There seem to be lower levels of basal lipolysis in adipocytes from trained animals, which increase to a greater extent when catecholamines are present (Toode et al., 1993).

Lifespan

The effects of physical activity on rodent lifespan are unclear; there appears to be an increase in mean lifespan but little or no effect in extending maximal lifespan (Poehlman et al., 2001).

Water consumption and body temperature

Since exercise often causes animals to have lower body weight, it will have some of the same effects as dietary restriction or energy restriction. Other than this body weight effect and the immediate need to increase water intake to prevent dehydration, it is not known how exercise affects water consumption, excretion or clearance. Similarly, except for body weight-related effects and the immediate consequences of exercise, little is known of the impact of exercise on body temperature or thermo-tolerance.

Cardiac parameters

Exercise training (by treadmill for 22 weeks) reduced the tendency for blood pressure to rise in obese rats and reduced blood pressure in normotensive rats (Arvola et al., 1999). This effect appeared to be mediated through vasodilation. There appears to be an increase in heart weight with long-term voluntary exercise (Oscai & Holloszy, 1970), which might be a reaction to increased blood flow during the exercise. Training (treadmill exercise) is reported to maintain cardiac size as animals lose weight (Dowell et al., 1976).

Puberty

Puberty can be suppressed by forced exercise. Comparing voluntary exercise, which does not suppress puberty, and forced wheel-running, only the forced exercise suppressed LH production and interfered with the release of gonado-tropin-releasing hormone (Manning & Bronson, 1991).

Overall metabolic effects

There are few reports of resting metabolic rate, which was unaffected by exercise training per se in female rats in a study which evaluated the effect over a 23-h period (Ballor, 1991). This approach eliminates the effects of diurnal variation on measurements, which can confound results.

Intermediary metabolism

Chronic exercise appears to have a major effect on glycogenolysis, with increasing fat oxidation as the intensity is increased. In animals trained by either treadmill or a swimming tank, glycogenolysis is inhibited and glycogen levels increase in cardiac and skeletal muscle (Bhagavathi & Devi, 1993). Endurance training increases translocation into muscle of glucose by the glucose transporter protein GLUT-4 and increases gluconeogenesis (Cartee, 1994). These effects may be stimulated by exercise-induced (one hour of swimming) brady-kinin, which may enhance the effect of insulin (Taguchi et al., 2000). Blood glucose levels fall, with blood glucose replenished from fat stores and from proteins (if the exercise is prolonged). Muscle has a large capacity to produce ammonia (from protein and amino acid metabolism), alanine and glutamine (Felig et al., 1970). Levels of intramuscular glutamate drop during exercise and stay low even through prolonged exercise, despite increased glutamate uptake (Graham & MacLean, 1998). Additionally, chronic training seems to result in higher glutamate levels, both when resting and with exercise.

The main function of metabolism appears to be getting substrate to the muscle, for tension development (Stanley & Connett, 1991), without dropping blood glucose so low that there is a problem with brain function.

Endocrine effects

The major endocrine effects of exercise appear to be on growth hormone, catecholamines and the sex steroids.

Plasma levels of growth hormone can increase 100-fold acutely with exercise (especially heavy resistance) in humans (Kraemer et al., 1993) and to a lesser extent in other species such as horse (Golland et al., 1999), sheep (Bell et al., 1983) and trout (Kakizawa et al., 1995). In rodents, this hormone and its metabolites can be inhibited with both acute and chronic involuntary exercise (e.g., Butkus et al., 1995). It is not known what factors are most important in these differences. One speculation is that rodents, whose physical activity is entrained by light, have been fasting since the previous night, and thus are more likely to be affected by the lower levels of nutrients in plasma than other species that have usually eaten a few hours before exercising. An example of the importance of the relationship between feeding and physiological response is that time-of-day of feeding has a significant effect on bone growth in rats (Okano et al., 1999).

Forced swimming exercise elevates levels of catecholamines and glucocorticoids acutely (e.g., Axelson, 1987), but may also lower the level of response to further activity (so that the activity is not as stressful in trained animals).

Testosterone level is reduced by acute exhausting exercise, but chronic training had no effect on serum and testicular concentrations and seems to only affect the capacity of a testicular interstitial cell suspension to produce testosterone (Harkonen *et al.*, 1990). Moderate forced exercise reduced ovarian steroids and disrupted vaginal cycles in rats (Axelson, 1987). An interesting metabolic effect of estrogen is that it increases fatty acid utilization in male and female rats (Hatta *et al.*, 1988) and improves resistance to fatigue.

Combined exercise and decreased energy intake

Many studies of exercise are actually evaluating exercise combined with uncontrolled weight loss. Because this factor is often overlooked, the attribution of effects to exercise *per se* is often not definitive. Similarly, there can be changes associated with physical activity in some dietary and energy restriction experiments. Surprisingly, few long-term experiments have combined measure-ment or control of physical activity with controlled dietary intake in rodents, although there are many such combinations that could be tested.

The combination of even voluntary wheel-running and approximately 30% dietary restriction resulted in increased mortality throughout much of the lifespan of rats (Holloszy & Schechtman, 1991). The cause of death of these animals was not evaluated, but further studies using the same model suggested an increase in cardiomyopathy in exercised animals (Holloszy, 1997).

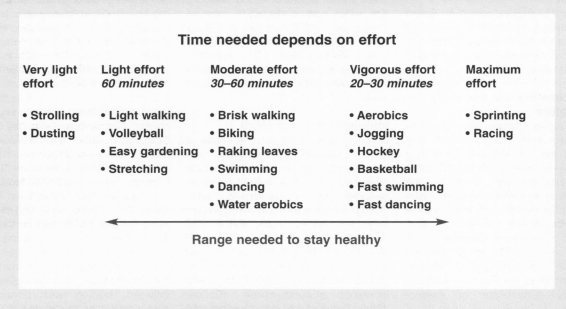

How do I know if I'm doing enough physical activity to stay healthy ?

If you are not sure you're probably doing activities in the light to moderate range on the chart below. You need to work towards adding up 60 minutes of activities a day in periods of at least 10 minutes each.

Time needed depends on effort

Very light effort	Light effort *60 minutes*	Moderate effort *30–60 minutes*	Vigorous effort *20–30 minutes*	Maximum effort
• Strolling	• Light walking	• Brisk walking	• Aerobics	• Sprinting
• Dusting	• Volleyball	• Biking	• Jogging	• Racing
	• Easy gardening	• Raking leaves	• Hockey	
	• Stretching	• Swimming	• Basketball	
		• Dancing	• Fast swimming	
		• Water aerobics	• Fast dancing	

Range needed to stay healthy

Extracted from Handbook for Physical Activity Guide to Health active Living. Canadian Society for Exercise Physiology

Chapter 5
Cancer-preventive effects

Human studies

In view of the large number of epidemiological studies of effects of body weight and adiposity on cancer, the following review focuses on what the Working Group deemed to be the most informative ones. In general, they are those in which the analysis was based on larger numbers of cases (usually over 100), though the cut-off used varies from 200 cases for the most studied cancer sites to only 50 for some others.

A single cohort study has often generated a number of publications over many years, with longer follow-up and thus more cases. Likewise, data from case–control studies are often further analysed to examine new measures or address new issues. Only the latest follow-up from cohort studies is generally discussed or presented in the tables and further analyses of case–control data are considered only if they provide important new information.

Methodological considerations

Epidemiological studies are critical to the evaluation of weight control and physical activity in relation to cancer incidence because they address the effects of these variables, over a realistic range of exposures, on the endpoints of direct interest to humans. Randomized trials, which in theory might provide superior data, have not been conducted and may never be, due to the difficulty of maintaining informative contrasts in exposure among large populations for many years. This section highlights some of the methodological issues surrounding study design, sources of bias, measurement of adiposity and physical activity, and the interpretation of findings.

Positive energy balance cannot be measured directly in large epidemiological studies but in theory can be estimated by examining its components: energy intake and expenditure. However, neither of these components can be well estimated by existing self-reporting methods, and one of the most valid measures of recurrent positive energy balance in humans remains adult weight gain.

Recall bias

Many factors can influence the recall or reporting of weight and physical activity. This is potentially most serious in case–control studies, because even small differences in over- or under-reporting by cases compared with controls can seriously influence the observed associations.

Selection bias

Biased associations can also occur if persons who participate as controls are more likely to be health-conscious, and thus more likely to be physically active and lean, than those who do not participate. This would tend to produce erroneous positive associations with obesity and inverse associations with physical activity. If potential control subjects are truly a representative sample of the population from which the cases arose and participation rates are high, selection bias is minimal. However, participation rates have declined progressively over time in many countries, so that the potential for selection bias has become increasingly serious. Both recall and selection biases are avoided in prospective studies.

Detection bias

For some cancers that can be detected by a screening test, such as early prostate cancer diagnosed by screening for prostate-specific antigen (PSA), bias may exist in either case–control or cohort studies if the likelihood of screening is associated with other health-conscious behaviour. Studies of only fatal end-points, rather than incident cancers, can be misleading if body weight or activity affects prognosis or is correlated with behaviours that lead to earlier diagnosis or better compliance with treatment. These concerns are not important for cancers that are almost always fatal, such as cancers of the pancreas or lung or for which early diagnosis and treatment have little effect.

Publication bias

Failure of investigators to report or of journals to publish negative findings on physical activity or weight could result in a biased conclusion based on the available literature. Pooled analyses in which the studies were selected for reasons other than having data on weight or activity should not be susceptible to this form of bias.

Confounding

People who conscientiously exercise and successfully control their weight often have healthier lifestyles than those who do not. Furthermore, high physical activity is associated with low socioeconomic status, which, in turn, is correlated with increased or decreased cancer risk, depending upon site. Cigarette smoking is a particularly important confounding variable, as it is a strong cause of many cancers and is less common among exercising individuals but more frequent among lean persons, in part due to its mild anorectic effect. Thus, if smoking is not taken into account, physically active and overweight persons appear to have lower rates of many cancers, even if weight and physical activity have no direct effect. In evaluating the results of epidemiological studies, the degree to which the results have been adjusted for potentially confounding variables is an important consideration.

In this report, the independent effects of body weight and physical activity are of particular interest. Because regular physical activity is an important method of controlling weight, these variables tend to be inversely correlated. While it is often of interest to mutually control the effects of weight and physical activity for each other to determine the degree to which they are independently associated with cancer risk, the results should be interpreted cautiously. For example, an observation that physical activity was associated with cancer risk before, but not after, controlling for body weight would not mean that physical activity has no effect. The most likely interpretation would be that the effect of physical activity is mediated by its influence on weight.

Reverse causation

In evaluating associations between weight or physical activity and cancer incidence, the direction of causality should be carefully considered. Preclinical cancer is a well-known cause of weight loss and may also lead to a reduction in physical activity. In addition, factors such as cigarette smoking or occupational factors that cause both chronic lung disease and some cancers can lead to changes in weight and activity years before the diagnosis of cancer. Merely controlling statistically for smoking may not be adequate to

account for reverse causation, because nuances of smoking habits or susceptibility to cigarette smoke are not taken into account. Analytical strategies such as restriction to never-smokers or allowing a long lag time between the assessment of weight or activity and diagnosis of cancer can be helpful.

Studies of weight loss and risk of cancer are particularly problematic because relatively few healthy persons in a population successfully lose weight and maintain their loss, so that statistical power is low. More seriously, in epidemiological studies, these healthy persons are usually impossible to distinguish from those who have lost weight due to cancer or chronic disease that may be the result of smoking or other factors.

Generalizability

Most reported studies of weight and physical activity in relation to cancer incidence have been based on Caucasian populations of Europe and North America. Part of the incompleteness of information from other areas of the world is due to a lack of tested methods for assessing physical activity in different cultures. Also, the lack of knowledge about personal weight and height in societies where scales are not widely available can make case–control studies of these relationships impossible, because they typically depend on self-reported measures several years before diagnosis. This is unfortunate because, as is discussed in the section on breast cancer, some relationships with body weight appear to differ between high- and low-risk populations. These differences are unlikely to be the result of genetic factors, because rates of most cancers converge when various ethnic groups live in similar environments. A more likely explanation is that the relationship of body weight and physical activity to cancer risk depends on the range of these variables present in a population and interactions with other aspects of lifestyle and diet.

Measurement of weight and physical activity

Studies of weight and physical activity depend directly on valid measures of these variables. Issues of validity are discussed in detail in Chapter 1, but some issues particularly relevant to epidemiological studies are mentioned below.

Measurement of weight : Weight is commonly used in epidemiological studies among adult populations as an indirect measure of adiposity. Adjustment for height, most often by calculating BMI, removes variation in weight due to height and thus improves the correlation with body fat mass. Although use of BMI does not allow distinction between lean and fat mass, in most general populations, the majority of the variation is due to adiposity. Thus, correlations of BMI with body fat mass adjusted for height measured by underwater weighing have been approximately 0.9 (Spiegelman *et al.,* 1992; Willett, 1998). In populations where scales are widely available, self-reported weights are commonly used in epidemiological studies. There is some tendency for overweight persons to under-report weight and for underweight persons to over-report weight. However, self-reported weights have been shown to be highly valid, being strongly correlated with measured weights (correlations typically over 0.95), and to be consistently predictive of diseases known to be related to excessive adiposity (Willett, 1998). Even when referring to periods many years in the past, self-reported weight and height have been shown to retain a high degree of validity. Because use of self-reported data on weight and height is necessary in most case–control studies to avoid the influence of cancer on weight, and these are the only feasible measures in some prospective studies, the majority of information on adiposity and cancer risk is obtained in this way. In populations engaged in heavy physical labour, as in some developing countries, it is possible that BMI may reflect adiposity less well.

Other measures of adiposity used in epidemiological studies include changes in weight, skinfold and abdominal and hip circumferences, each of which provides somewhat different information. Changes in weight from, for example, age 20 years to midlife, can be particularly useful because they take into account possible differences in frame size, and increases are largely due to changes in body fat unless a person has consciously engaged in body-building. Changes in weight also are simple and readily interpretable by the public.

Measurement of physical activity: Physical activity involves many components, including the *type* of activity (i.e., occupational, recreational, household), the *dose* of the activity (i.e., frequency, intensity and duration) and the *time period* in life when it is measured. These components of physical activity have been measured using widely different methods in epidemiological studies. Some of the inconsistencies in results obtained by these studies may be attributable to these differences in the methods used. Furthermore, since the underlying biological mechanisms involved in the disease process were largely unknown when these studies were conducted, the relevant types of activity and time periods in life when these activities were performed may not have been adequately captured.

Errors in measuring physical activity tend to lead to underestimation of the strength of associations with cancer risk. Many early studies used crude methods for assessing activity and were sometimes only based on occupation. Most recent studies have used physical activity questionnaires that are more detailed and comprehensive in the types of activity evaluated. Differences in the degree of validity of various questionnaires lead to differences in estimates of associations with cancer risk. However,

even a highly valid questionnaire that is directed to a time period not relevant to the development of cancer may fail to detect an important effect of physical activity. Thus, questionnaires that assess activity at various periods in life, and repeated assessments of physical activity in prospective cohort studies, can be particularly informative.

Studies that have evaluated the validity of recalled activity have shown that more intense activities are recalled with greater accuracy than moderate activities. Consequently, the ability to detect stronger associations for intense activity, as shown in some studies particularly of colon cancer, may reflect more accurate measurement of these activities. However, it is also possible that associations with vigorous activity reflect important biological mechanisms.

Measures of physical activity assessed by standardized questionnaires as used in recent epidemiological studies have been shown to be correlated with biological measurements such as resting pulse and treadmill assessments of fitness (see Chapter 1). Moreover, these measurements have been associated with future risks of cardiovascular disease and diabetes in prospective studies. When physical activity as assessed by questionnaires has been compared with that recorded in detailed activity diaries, correlations have been approximately 0.5 to 0.6 (Wolf *et al.*, 1994; Chasan-Taber *et al.*, 1996). Thus, it is clear that the methods of assessing activity in epidemiological studies are providing informative data, but the magnitude of the associations tends to be underestimated. The correlations with detailed diaries suggest that the strength of an observed relative risk will be about half of the true relative risk (Willett, 1998).

Modification of associations by other factors

In this evaluation, we consider evidence that associations between physical

activity or weight and cancer incidence may be modified by other variables including gender, age or family history. Ideally, genetic factors based on DNA markers might be examined as modifiers, but little such work has been done up to now. In general, an ability to examine these interactions requires large sample sizes, which have often not been available. However, the evaluation of associations within population subgroups can also provide insight on possible mechanisms. For example, the finding that the association between BMI and post-menopausal breast cancer is largely absent among women currently using estrogen replacement treatment (which results in high blood estrogen levels in all women regardless of their BMI) adds to evidence that the effect of obesity on post-menopausal breast cancer is largely mediated by endogenous estrogens.

Considerations in assessing causality

Whether associations observed in epidemiological studies should be considered to be causal has been much discussed (Tomatis, 1990). Here we do not consider international correlations (ecological studies) relating population average values of weight or physical activity to cancer rates, because these associations are likely to be seriously confounded by a multitude of factors associated with economic development. In reviewing the case–control and cohort studies, particular attention is paid to the consistency of findings across a range of populations, the statistical robustness of associations as reflected by confidence intervals, and the degree to which potentially confounding factors have been accounted for.

Weight and weight control
Colorectal cancer

This review summarizes what is known about the relationships between body weight and the risk for both colorectal cancer and colorectal adenomas, the pre-malignant lesion for colorectal cancer. The evidence for an overall association is examined, as well as the patterns by gender, by colorectal subsite and by stage of carcinogenesis. The possible biological mechanisms underlying such an association and how the interrelated risk factors of physical activity and dietary energy intake (Potter, 1996; Hill, 1998) might contribute independently or along the same causal pathway with obesity are discussed later in this chapter.

Colorectal cancers arise predominantly from adenomas, a process that in most people takes at least 10 years (Vogelstein et al., 1988; Kronborg & Fenger, 1999). Small adenomas first develop from mutated normal colonic epithelium, then some of the small adenomas grow in size and become more histologically abnormal with successive mutations, until finally invasive cancer develops. Body weight may have effects on colorectal cancer risk at any of these stages, including initiation, promotion and progression, over a 10–15-year period or longer. Inferences about point(s) in the development of colorectal cancer at which obesity might be relevant can be made by examining not only the existence of an association between body fatness and colorectal cancer, but also the pattern of association with lifetime weight history, and whether that association differs by adenoma size.

Several very large case–control and cohort studies have reported not only on the overall association between measures of body fatness and colorectal cancer but also, with substantial power, findings stratified by subsite within the colorectum and by gender. Some have also added measures of body fat distribution, often as the WHR, in order to investigate whether body fat distribution acts as a cancer risk factor independent of overall adiposity, as is often estimated by the BMI. There is extensive literature on body fatness indicators near the time

of diagnosis, but much less evidence concerning lifetime weight patterns.

This review does not attempt to describe all published studies. Only the larger studies are included and only those that have presented evidence regarding a dose–response relationship between BMI and colorectal neoplasia. Studies that presented only average BMI levels for case and comparison groups are not included. For studies that have generated several reports, the report presenting the greatest detail on body weight or the most recent update (e.g., from ongoing cohort studies) has been reviewed. Studies relating body weight to adenomas are less numerous, so the review is less selective. Thus for colorectal cancer, only studies with more than 200 cases were included, while for adenomas, studies with as few as 100 cases are included.

Body mass index
The associations between BMI, body weight changes and body fat distribution are summarized separately for colon and rectal cancer, but there are only a small number of studies of rectal cancer (Table 23). Several studies have presented findings by subsite of the colon in which the cancer arose. Findings from studies of BMI and adenomas are also presented in Table 23, since they can provide evidence regarding the time(s) in colorectal carcinogenesis when factors associated with body weight might be most important.

Cohort studies
Despite some variation, cohort studies generally show positive associations between body fatness, as indicated by the BMI, and risk of colorectal cancer. Across the cohort studies, there is about a 50–100% higher risk in the highest quartile of BMI compared with the lowest quartile. Different BMI cut-points have been used, but the strength of the association corresponds in most studies to nearly a doubling of risk in those with

BMI of 30 kg/m^2 or over compared with those having a BMI under 23 kg/m^2. Most studies have found a trend of increasing colon cancer risk with increasing BMI across a wide range, with no clear evidence for a threshold effect. The cohort study by Chyou et al. (1994), which found the smallest relative risk (RR = 1.2; 95% CI 0.87–1.7), was conducted among Asian men living in Hawaii, and the difference in BMI between the groups compared was narrow (>26 vs <22 kg/m^2). Whether the weaker association was due to this lower distribution of BMI values in that population or to other factors is unknown.

The observed association between BMI and colorectal cancer risk is generally more consistent and of higher strength for men than for women. The strength of the association is nearly twice as high for males as for females in studies that have presented results for both. For example, in a large cohort study of cancer mortality conducted by the American Cancer Society (Murphy et al., 2000a), the relative risks associated with a BMI in the obese range (above 30 kg/m^2) compared with a BMI below 25 kg/m^2 were 1.8 for men and 1.2 for women. There is also a pattern of a positive association of about the same strength between BMI and colon adenomas. A cohort study of male health professionals (Giovannucci et al., 1995) reported no association between adenomas and BMI, but the findings were not presented in detail. Among the adenoma studies, the differences between the genders seem less than for cancer, although there are too few such studies to allow a firm conclusion to be drawn. For studies that assessed the association with BMI separately for larger and smaller adenomas, the pattern suggests that the association is stronger for larger adenomas. For example, in a cohort study of US nurses (Giovannucci et al., 1996), the relative risk for overweight was 2.2 (95% CI 1.2–4.2) for large adenomas, but only

Table 23. Studies of body mass index and risk of colorectal neoplasia

Author, date, study location	Study dates	No. of cases	BMI range contrasts (no. of categories)	Relative risk (95% CI)	Trend*	Adjustment for confounding	Comments
Colon cancer, cohort studies							
Lee & Paffenbarger (1992a), USA	1962–88	M 290	≥26 vs < 22.5 (5)	1.5 (1.1–2.1)	Yes	Age, physical activity, family history	Harvard alumni
Bostick et al. (1994), USA	1986–90	F 212	>30.6 vs < 22.9 (5)	1.4 (0.90–2.2)	Yes	Age, energy intake, height, parity, two nutrients	Age 55–69 years
Chyou et al. (1994), USA	1965–92	M 289	≥26 vs < 22 (4)	1.2 (0.87–1.7)	Yes	Age	Japanese living in Hawaii
Giovannucci et al. (1995), USA	1986–92	M 203	≥29 vs < 22 (5)	1.5 (0.89–2.5)	Yes	Age, height, physical activity, screening, family history, smoking, NSAIDs, five foods/nutrients, alcohol	Health professionals
Martinez et al. (1997), USA	1980–92	F 393	≥29 vs <21 (5)	1.4 (1.0–2.1)	Yes	Age, smoking, family history, physical activity, hormone replacement therapy, NSAIDs, alcohol, red meat	Nurses
Ford (1999), USA	1971–92	M 104 F 118	≥30 vs <22 (6)	3.0 (0.99–8.7) 2.7 (1.0–7.2)	Yes Yes	Age, race, smoking, education, cholesterol, physical activity, alcohol	Age 25–74 years
Murphy et al. (2000a), USA	1982–94	M 1792 F 1616	≥30 vs <25 (3)	1.8 (1.5–2.0) 1.2 (1.1–1.5)	Yes No	Age, race, education, smoking, physical activity, alcohol, NSAIDs, family history, hormone replacement therapy, three foods/nutrients	Mortality study
Rectal cancer, cohort studies							
Le Marchand et al. (1992), USA	1972–86	M 203	Highest vs lowest tertile	0.8 (0.5–1.2)	No	Age, socioeconomic status	Hawaii residents
Colorectal adenoma, cohort studies							
Giovannucci et al. (1996), USA	1976–92	F 178 F 125	≥29 vs < 21 (5)	1.4 (0.86–2.4) 2.2 (1.2–4.2)	No Yes	Age, family history, screening, smoking, NSAIDs, four foods/ nutrients, alcohol	Small adenomas Large adenomas By colonoscopy

87

Table 23 (contd)

Author, date, study location	Study dates	No. of cases	BMI range contrasts (no. of categories)	Relative risk (95% CI)	Trend	Adjustment for confounding	Comments
Colon cancer, case–control studies							
Graham et al. (1988), USA	1975–84	M 205 F 223	Highest vs lowest quartile	2.2 (1.2–4.0) 1.8 (1.0–3.4)	Yes Yes	Age, race	Population-based
Gerhardsson de Verdier et al. (1990b), Sweden	1986–88	M 233 F 271	>26.5 vs < 21.4 (5)	2.8 (1.3–6.0) 1.5 (0.9–2.7)	Yes Yes	Age	Population-based
Kune et al. (1990), Australia	1980–81	M 388 F 327	> 31 vs 20–25 (3) > 31 vs 19–24 (3)	1.2 (0.50–2.9) 0.73 (0.30–1.6)	Yes No	Age, dietary risk index	Population-based
Dietz et al. (1995), USA	1990–91	F 758	Weight > 72.6 kg vs <58.1 kg (4)	1.3 (1.0–1.7)	Yes	Height, age, family history, screening	Population-based
Le Marchand et al. (1997), USA	1987–91	M 698 F 494	>26 vs <22 (4) >26 vs <21 (4)	2.2 (1.5–3.2) 1.2 (0.8–1.9)	Yes No	Age, family history, alcohol, smoking, energy intake, three foods/nutrients, physical activity	Colorectal cancer Population-based
Caan et al. (1998), USA	1991–94	M 1095 F 888	Highest vs lowest quintile	2.0 (1.5–2.6) 1.4 (1.1–1.9)	Yes Yes	Age, NSAIDs, energy intake, fibre, calcium, family history, physical activity	Population-based
Russo et al. (1998), Italy	1992–96	M 687	≥25 vs < 25 (2)	1.2 (1.0–1.5)	NE	Age, education, physical activity, energy intake	Colorectal cancer Hospital-based
Rectal cancer, case–control studies							
Gerhardsson de Verdier et al. (1990b), Sweden	1986–88	M 106 F 109	>26.5 vs <21.4 (5)	1.7 (0.7–4.0) 1.0 (0.5–1.9)	No No	Age	Population-based
Dietz et al. (1995), USA	1990–91	F 239	Weight > 72.6 kg vs < 58.1 kg (4)	1.1 (0.7–1.7)	No	Height, age, family history, screening	Population-based
Le Marchand et al. (1997), USA	1987–91	M 221 F 129	Highest vs lowest tertile	2.9 0.8	Yes No	Age, family history, alcohol, smoking, energy intake, three foods/nutrients, physical activity	Population-based

Table 23 (contd)

Author, date, study location	Study dates	No. of cases	BMI range contrasts (no. of categories)	Relative risk (95% CI)	Trend	Adjustment for confounding	Comments
Russo et al. (1998), Italy	1992–96	M 437	≥25 vs < 25	1.1 (0.88–1.4)	NE	Age, education, physical activity, energy intake	Hospital-based
Colorectal adenoma, case–control studies							
Neugut et al. (1991), USA	1986–88	M 174 F 127	≥ 27.1 vs ≤23.1 (4) ≥ 33.5 vs ≤26.5 (4)	1.4 (0.8–2.5) 2.1 (1.1–4.0)	No Yes	Age	By colonoscopy
Shinchi et al. (1994), Japan	1991–92	M,F 228	>26.95 vs <22.5 (4)	1.9 (1.2–3.0)	No	Smoking, acohol, physical activity	By colonoscopy; age 49–55 years
Davidow et al. (1996), USA	1986–88	M 139	≥ 29.1 vs <24.4 (4)	1.9 (0.9–4.0)	No	Age, smoking, physical activity, energy intake	By colonoscopy
Bird et al. (1998), USA	1991–93	M,F 339 M,F 139	Highest vs lowest quartile	1.6 (0.9–2.6) 2.5 (1.1–5.4)	No Yes	Age, sex, smoking, NSAIDs, physical activity, energy intake, fibre	Small adenomas Large adenomas By colonoscopy
Kono et al. (1999), Japan	1995–96	M 189	≥ 26.9 vs < 22.45 (4)	2.4 (1.1–5.1)	No	Smoking, alcohol	By colonoscopy; age 47–55 years

* Either a significant test for trend or significant intermediate relative risks for intermediate exposure categories

1.4 (95% CI 0.86–2.4) for small adenomas.

Case–control studies

As seen in the cohort studies, the case–control studies of BMI and colon cancer risk show a pattern of association across most studies, with a stronger association for men than for women. Six case–control studies that used identical methods to study men and women found a stronger association between BMI and colorectal cancer among men (Graham et al., 1988; Gerhardsson de Verdier et al., 1990b; Kune et al., 1990; Le Marchand et al., 1997; Caan et al., 1998; Russo et al., 1998). Case–control studies also show an association between BMI and adenoma risk of a similar magnitude to that seen for colon cancer, though in the single study that reported separately for men and women (Neugut et al., 1991), the gender difference seen for colon cancer was not observed. The RR was higher for women.

The association between colorectal cancer risk and body weight is, in general, stronger and more consistently observed for cancers of the distal colon than for those of the proximal colon, among both men and women, especially in the very large studies (Dietz et al., 1995; Le Marchand et al., 1997; Caan et al., 1998; Russo et al., 1998). In contrast to the findings for colon cancer, studies of rectal cancer have generally shown little or no evidence for an association with BMI (Gerhardsson de Verdier et al., 1990b; Russo et al., 1998).

Weight change

Findings from studies that have examined the relationship between lifetime weight history and colon cancer risk are summarized in Table 24. These studies have reported colorectal cancer risks in relation to both BMI in early adulthood and BMI during later adult years, nearer the time of onset of cancer diagnosis. For only a few studies were direct estimates presented for the association

between weight gain per se and colon cancer risk (Dietz et al., 1995; Le Marchand et al., 1997; Kono et al., 1999; Russo et al., 1999).

Cohort studies

In general, cohort studies have not yielded evidence suggesting a stronger association between BMI earlier in life and colorectal neoplasia than for BMI later in life (Table 24). The studies by Lee & Paffenbarger (1992a) and Le Marchand et al. (1992) both showed similar relative risks for BMI in the late second and the third decades of life to those for BMIs in later adulthood (all in the range 1.4 to 1.6).

Case–control studies

Case–control studies do suggest that elevated BMI in the later adult years and weight gain between early adult ages and later adult ages increase risk for colon cancer (Dietz et al., 1995; Le Marchand et al., 1997), although this is less clear for adenomas (Bird et al., 1998; Kono et al., 1999). As in the cohort studies, there is no suggestion that body weight earlier in life is more important as a predictor of colon cancer risk than is body weight later in life.

Body fat distribution

Body fat distribution seems to be an additional predictor of chronic disease risk beyond the effect of overall obesity. Table 25 displays the evidence for an association between measures of body fat distribution and colon cancer risk. All studies expressed body fat distribution as the WHR, except for one which used the ratio of subscapular to triceps skinfold thickness (S/T ratio), another index of central adiposity (Ford, 1999).

Cohort studies

The relative risks or odds ratios for colorectal neoplasia associated with high versus low or normal levels of WHR are shown in Table 25. The ranges and distributions of WHR and of the S/T ratio

differ substantially across the various cohort studies, but as was observed with BMI, the WHR shows a pattern of a positive association with both colorectal cancer and colorectal adenoma risk. However, the single study using the S/T ratio did not find an association (Ford, 1999). In the studies reporting dose–response patterns, there was no specific threshold for this association except in the study of males by Giovannucci et al. (1995). As was seen for BMI, there is also an association between WHR and adenoma risk in cohort studies, which in one study was stronger for large adenomas.

Case–control studies

Like the cohort studies, case–control studies show an elevation of risk with higher WHR levels of a similar magnitude to the association with elevated BMI.

Discussion

High levels of body fat, as indicated by higher BMI during adult life and/or higher WHR, are associated with increased risk for colon cancer and for colon adenomas. This association is seen for both men and women, though the association with BMI is higher among men. The reason for this gender difference is unknown. If obesity was simply an indicator of energy imbalance, there should be no difference between the genders. On the other hand, there may be an offsetting beneficial effect of obesity among women. A factor such as the hyper-estrogenaemia that is associated with postmenopausal obesity could be responsible, as an estrogen benefit could serve to diminish the obesity-related risk in women. This hypothesis is further discussed later in this chapter.

The observation that BMI is more strongly associated with larger adenomas than with smaller adenomas suggests that obesity-related factors may act at a later stage in the development of cancer, perhaps by contributing to the

Table 24. Studies of weight change and risk of colorectal neoplasia

Author, date, study location	Study dates	No. of cases	BMI, Young adult ages BMI range contrasts (no. of categories)	RR (95% CI)	BMI near time of diagnosis BMI range contrasts (no. of categories)	RR (95% CI)	Adult weight change BMI range contrasts (no. of categories)	RR (95% CI)	Adjustment for confounding
Colon cancer, cohort studies									
Lee & Paffenbarger (1992a), USA	1962–88	M 266	>23.5 vs < 20 in college (5)	1.4 (0.99–2.0)	>26 vs <22.5 at age 47 (5)	1.5 (1.1–2.2)	NA	NA	Age, physical activity, family history
Le Marchand et al. (1992), USA	1942–86	M 203	Highest vs lowest tertile at age 15–29	1.6 (1.2–2.1)	Highest vs lowest tertiles at age 45–59	1.4 (1.1–1.8)	NA	NA	Age, socio-economic status
Rectal cancer, cohort studies									
Le Marchand et al. (1992), USA	1942–86	M 203	Highest vs lowest tertile at age 15–29	0.7 (0.6–1.4)	Highest vs lowest tertiles at age 45–59	0.8 (0.5–1.2)	Highest vs lowest tertiles, age 15–45 change	1.2 (0.8–1.8)	Age, socio-economic status
Colorectal adenoma, cohort studies									
Giovannucci et al. (1996), USA	1976–92	F 125	Highest vs lowest quintile at age 18	1.9 (1.1–3.5)	≥29 vs <21 (5)	2.21 (1.2–4.2)	NA	NA	Age, family history, screening, smoking, NSAIDs, four foods/ nutrients, alcohol; Large adenomas
Colon cancer, case–control studies									
Dietz et al. (1995), USA	1990–91	F 737			>72.6 kg vs <58.1 kg 5 y ago (4)	1.3 (1.0–1.7)	>23% gain vs <6% since age 18 (4)	1.3 (1.0–1.6)	Age, weight at 18 y, height, family history, screening
Le Marchand et al. (1997), USA	1987–91	M 698	>23 vs <20 at age 25 (4)	1.5 (1.0–2.2)	26 vs <22 5 y ago (4)	2.2 (1.5–3.2)	>14 kg gain vs <2 kg age 25 to 5 y ago (4)	1.6 (1.0–2.4)	Age, family history, alcohol, smoking, energy intake, three foods/nutrients, physical activity
		F 494	>22 vs <19 at age 25 (4)	1.5 (0.9–2.3)	>26 vs <21 5 y ago (4)	1.2 (0.8–1.9)	>11 kg gain vs <2 kg age 25 to 5 y ago (4)	0.8	

Table 24 (contd)

Author, date, study location	Study dates	No. of cases	BMI, Young adult ages — BMI range contrasts (no. of categories)	RR (95% CI)	BMI, near time of diagnosis — BMI range contrasts (no. of categories)	RR (95% CI)	Adult weight change — BMI range contrasts RR (no. of categories)	RR (95% CI)	Adjustment for confounding (95% CI)
Colorectal cancer, case–control studies									
Russo et al. (1998), Italy	1992–96	M 1124 F 819	>28.1 vs <22.5 at age 30 (5)	1.8 (1.3–2.4) 1.3 (0.97–1.7)	>28.7 vs <22.5 at age 50 (5)	1.7 (1.3–2.3) 0.92 (0.68–1.2)	Age 30–50 change (vs no change) Men – decrease Men – increase Women – decrease Women – increase	1.1 (0.88–1.4) 0.75 (0.63–0.88) 0.93 (0.71–1.2) 0.66 (0.54–0.80)	Age, education, physical activity, energy intake
Rectal cancer, case–control studies									
Dietz et al. (1995), USA	1990–91	F 234			>72.6 kg vs <58.1 kg 5 y ago (4)	1.1 (0.7–1.7)	>23% gain vs <6% since age 18 (4)	1.0 (0.7–1.5)	Age, weight at 18 y, height, family history, screening
Le Marchand et al. (1997), USA	1987–91	M 221 F 129	Highest vs lowest tertile at age 35	2.0 1.4	Highest vs lowest tertile 5 years ago	2.9 0.8			Age, family history, alcohol, smoking, energy intake, three foods/nutrients, physical activity
Colorectal adenoma, case–control studies									
Bird et al. (1998), USA	1991–92	483	Highest vs lowest quartile at age 18	1.1 (0.8–1.6)	Highest vs lowest quartile 5 years ago	1.3 (0.9–1.9)	Highest vs lowest quartile, weight gain or weight loss over last 10 years	1.8 (0.7–4.4)	Sex, age
Kono et al. (1999), Japan	1995–96	M 189	>26.5 vs <22.25 10 yrs ago	1.5 (0.7–3.1)	>26.9 vs <22.4 (4)	2.4 (1.1–5.1)	>6 kg gain vs ≤2 in past 10 yrs (4)	2.2 (1.0–4.8)	Smoking, alcohol

NA, not analysed

Table 25. Studies of body fat distribution and risk of colorectal neoplasia

Author, date, study location	Study dates	No. of cases	WHR range contrasts (no. of categories)	Relative risk (95% CI)	Trend*	Adjustment for confounding	Comments
Colon cancer, cohort studies							
Bostick et al. (1994), USA	1986–90	F 211	>0.91 vs <0.76 (5)	1.2 (0.83–1.9)	No	Age, energy intake, height, parity, two nutrients	Age 55–69 y
Giovannucci et al. (1995), USA	1986–92	M 117	> 0.99 vs <0.90 (5)	3.4 (1.5–7.7)	Yes	Age, screening, family history, smoking, physical activity, NSAIDs, five foods/nutrients, alcohol	Health professionals
Martinez et al. (1997), USA	1980–92	F 161	>0.83 vs <0.73 (5)	1.5 (0.88–2.5)	No	Age, smoking, family history, physical activity, hormone replacement therapy, NSAIDs, alcohol	Age 25–74 y
Ford (1999), USA	1971–92	M 102 F 117	Subscapular/triceps ratio >1.5 vs <0.6 (5)	0.81 (0.22–3.0) 0.88 (0.17–4.5)	No No	Age, race, education, smoking, cholesterol, physical activity, alcohol	Age 25–74 y
Colorectal adenoma, cohort studies							
Giovannucci et al. (1995), USA	1986–92	M 197 M 131	≥0.99 vs <0.90 (5)	0.77 (0.48–1.2) 3.4 (1.6–7.5)	No Yes	Age, screening, family history, smoking, physical activity, NSAIDs, five foods/nutrients, alcohol	Small adenomas Large adenomas
Giovannucci et al. (1996), USA	1976–92	F 125 F 330	Highest vs lowest quintile	1.2 (0.65–2.3) 1.4 (0.98–2.1)	No No	Age, family history, screening, smoking, NSAIDs, four foods/nutrients, alcohol, BMI	Large adenomas All adenomas
Colon cancer, case–control studies							
Caan et al. (1998), USA	1991–92	M 927 F 742	Highest vs lowest quintile	1.3 (0.98–1.7) 1.7 (1.2–2.4)	Yes Yes	Age, NSAIDs, energy intake, fibre, calcium, family history, physical activity	Population-based
Russo et al. (1998), Italy	1992–96	F 530	>0.90 vs <0.82 (3)	1.6 (1.1–2.1)	Yes	Age, education, physical activity, energy intake	Hospital-based

Table 25 (contd)

Author, date, study location	Study dates	No. of cases	WHR range contrasts (no. of categories)	Relative risk (95% CI)	Trend	Adjustment for confounding	Comments
Rectal cancer, case–control studies							
Russo et al. (1998), Italy	1992–96	F 289	≥ 0.9 vs <0.82 (3)	1.6 (1.1–2.4)	Yes	Age, education, physical activity, energy intake	Hospital-based
Colorectal adenoma, case–control studies							
Shinchi et al. (1994), Japan	1991–92	M,F 228 M,F 102	≥ 0.96 vs <0.88 (4)	1.5 (0.9–2.5) 2.9 (1.4–5.9)	No Yes	Smoking, alcohol, physical activity	All adenomas Large adenomas Age 49–55 years
Kono et al. (1999), Japan	1995–96	M 189	>0.96 vs <0.87 (4)	2.0 (0.9–4.2)	Yes	Smoking, aochol	Age 47–55 years

* Either a significant test for trend or significant intermediate relative risks for intermediate exposure categories

promotion and progression of adenomas towards cancer. Alternatively, this pattern could appear simply because many other factors can lead small adenomas not to progress, so that among people with small adenomas those other causes dilute the association of obesity with risk.

It is important to note that the strength of the association between colorectal neoplasia and WHR is no greater than the strength of the association with BMI. It is unlikely, therefore, that the association with BMI is simply a proxy for a body fat distribution phenotype such as that indicated by the WHR. BMI is strongly associated, however, with WHR, so it is difficult to be sure that, as measured, the independent effects of each are truly separable in epidemiological studies. In addition, it may be specifically the intra-abdominal fat stores that account for the associations with WHR, and that the crude measure of the total circumferences, which includes both intra-abdominal and subcutaneous fat depots, does not separate those two depots.

In most of the epidemiological studies, body weight (as a measure of obesity) has been obtained by self-reporting. Case–control studies use the weight before onset of symptoms leading to the diagnosis of cancer, as weight loss is a frequent consequence of undiagnosed colorectal cancer. In most of the case–control studies of adenomas, both the cases and controls came from screened populations, so these are truly cross-sectional studies by design. Nonetheless, because adenomas rarely cause weight loss, there should be no bias in the assessment of weight as a risk factor. In prospective studies, current weight at baseline is usually the measure, although some studies have also included retrospective recall of weight from earlier in life (e.g., Lee & Paffenbarger, 1992a; Le Marchand et al., 1992).

Latency can be inferred either by examining lifetime retrospective weight histories or from prospective studies by examining patterns of associations according to the length of follow-up. These analyses of differences in the association between BMI and cancer at different periods in life suggest that the observed association between adult obesity and colorectal neoplasia is probably not due simply to a residual effect from a stronger association earlier in life, nearer to the time of adenoma initiation. In view of the observation that the association with obesity is stronger for larger adenomas, the relationship between BMI-associated factors and cancer most likely follows the pathways of promotional effects on adenoma growth and progression.

In summary, both case–control and cohort studies have shown associations between various measures of adiposity and the risk of colorectal neoplasia. The association is not stronger for adenomas than for cancer, nor is it stronger earlier in life than later in life. The association is stronger, however, for larger adenomas than for smaller ones, and stronger for men than for women. These patterns suggest an effect of factors related to adiposity on the promotion of cancer and a possible counteracting effect on these factors by estrogens.

Breast cancer

The hypothesis that a chronic state of positive energy balance promotes tumour growth has been examined since the early 1930s in animal models as one rationale for the increasing incidence of female breast cancer in developing countries (Tannenbaum, 1945). Epidemiological studies in humans first demonstrated in the 1970s that heavier women were at increased risk of breast cancer (de Waard & Baanders-van Halewijn, 1974; Blitzer et al., 1976). The influence of various measures of body size has been most extensively explored for breast cancer, in part because of the inconsistency in observed associations. The most informative epidemiological studies are those that distinguish between pre- and postmenopausal breast cancer, examine the effect of weight, weight gain and central body fat at various ages and are designed to examine the possible differential effects of exogenous and endogenous estrogens. In view of intriguing evidence obtained in the late 1990s that insulin-related growth factors (IGF) may influence breast cancer risk (see section on Mechanisms later in this Chapter), recent studies have begun to explore possible effects of IGF and body weight (Yu & Rohan, 2000).

Over 100 studies have examined the association of three major anthropometric measures (weight or BMI at different ages, central fat distribution, adult weight gain) and female breast cancer incidence and prognosis, with most studies examining weight or BMI, often at different periods of life. Studies that have examined the association of weight or BMI with cancer at many different sites have limited information on breast cancer incidence, have generally not adjusted for confounding, and therefore are not included in this review. Because of the complexity of the association of the various anthropometric measures with breast cancer and the volume of the literature, only studies with at least 200 cases for either pre- or postmenopausal breast cancer are summarized in Tables 26–28. The information in these tables is organized by premenopausal and postmenopausal breast cancer incidence, with data on cohort and case–control studies summarized under each of these headings. Data are summarized in the table and text for three major anthropometric measures: (1) BMI or relative weight, (2) weight at different ages and adult weight change, and (3) body fat distribution. Findings on breast cancer prognosis and those relating to birth weight and the interaction of weight with age at menarche are briefly summarized in the text but not included in the tables. In general, the many studies conducted have found that taller women are at increased risk for breast cancer

Table 26. Studies of body mass index and risk of breast cancer

Author, date, study location	Study dates	No. of cases	BMI range contrasts (no. of categories)	Relative risk (95% CI)	Trend*	Adjustment for confounding	Comments
Premenopausal breast cancer							
Cohort studies							
Le Marchand et al. (1988a), USA	1972–83	289	Tertiles	Age 30–44: 0.78 (0.46–1.3) Age 45–49: 1.1 (0.63–1.8)	No	Age, age at first birth, socioeconomic status	< 50 years, Hawaii
Tretli (1989), Norway	1963–81	3305	RR given for 1 unit increase	0.84 (0.74–0.95)	Yes		< 50 years
Vatten & Kvinnsland (1992), Norway	1974–88	291	≥27 vs 22 (4)	0.78 (0.65–0.94)	Yes	Age, reproductive risk factors, occupation, country of residence	≤ 50 years
Törnberg & Carstensen (1994), Sweden	1963–87	373	≥ 28 vs <22 (5)	0.41	Yes	Age	< 55 years
Huang et al. (1997), USA	1976–92	1000	> 31.0 vs ≤20.0 (10)	0.62 (0.45–0.86)	Yes	Age, history of benign breast disease, family history, reproductive factors	Nurses, < 55 years
Case-control studies							
Paffenbarger et al. (1980), USA	1970–77	374	≥ 24.5 vs < 21.5 (3)	0.65	No	Age, ethnicity, parity	Hospital-based
Lubin et al. (1985), Israel	1975–78	363	Comparison of mean BMI	p not significant	NE	Age, ethnic origin	Hospital-based
Hislop et al. (1986), Canada	1980–82	306	≥ 27 vs ≤ 21 (4)	0.84 (0.52–1.4)	No	Age	Population-based
Hsieh et al. (1990), international	NS	3993 pre- and post	Normal BMI not defined; obese defined as + 4 kg/m²	1.0 (0.98–1.1)	No	Age, centre, reproductive factors	Hospital-based
Chu et al. (1991), USA	1980–82	2053	Sextiles – cutpoints not stated by menopausal status	1.3 (0.9–2.0)	Yes	Age, reproductive risk factors, family history, surgical biopsy for benign breast disease	Population-based

Table 26 (contd)

Author, date, study location	Study dates	No. of cases	BMI range contrasts (no. of categories)	Relative risk (95% CI)	Trend	Adjustment for confounding	Comments
Brinton & Swanson (1992), USA	1973–80	414	≥26 vs < 20 (5)	0.65 (0.4–1.0)	Yes	Age, age at menarche, education	Population-based, <50 years
Francheschi et al. (1996), Italy	1991–94	988	>28.8 vs <21.7 (5)	0.7 (0.5–0.9)	Yes	Age, centre, education, parity, total energy and alcohol intake	Hospital-based
Swanson et al. (1996), USA	1990–92	1588	>28.8 vs <22.0 (4)	0.65 (0.5–0.8)	Yes	Age, centre, ethnicity, reproductive factors, alcohol, oral contraceptive use	Population-based, <45 years
Yong et al. (1996), USA	1973–81	226	≥34.7 vs < 26.8 (5)	0.9 (0.6–1.4)	No	Age, education, reproductive risk factors, history of benign breast disease, family history	Population-based
Ziegler et al. (1996) Asia	1983–87	421	>31.3 vs <22.9 (6)	1.6 (0.87–2.9)	No	Age, ethnicity, centre, reproductive risk factors, history of benign breast disease, family history	Population-based
Chie et al. (1998), Taiwan	1993–94	334	≥25 vs <20 (4)	0.5 (0.2–1.2)	No	Age, education, family history, reproductive factors, oral contraceptive use	Hospital-based
Coates et al. (1999), USA	1990–92	1590	>30.4 vs <21.5 (5)	0.69 (0.54–0.88)	Yes	Age, centre, ethnicity, family history, history of breast biopsy, education, reproductive factors, history of mammograms, alcohol, height, oral contraceptive use	Population-based, <44 years
Peacock et al. (1999), USA	1983–90	845	≥27.1 vs ≤19.9 (5)	0.67 (0.49–0.91)	Yes	Age, age at menarche	Population-based, <45 years

Table 26 (contd)

Author, date, study location	Study dates	No. of cases	BMI range contrasts (no. of categories)	Relative risk (95% CI)	Trend	Adjustment for confounding	Comments
Enger et al. (2000), USA	1983–89	714	≥27.1 vs <21.7 (4)	ER+/PgR+: 1.1 (0.70–1.8) ER+/PgR–: 0.92 (0.34–2.5) ER–/PR–: 1.1 (0.56–1.7) Unknown: 0.80 (0.53–1.2)	No	Age, socioeconomic status, reproductive risk factors, family history, physical activity	Population-based
Hall et al. (2000b), USA	1993–96	389	>30.1 vs <24.6 (3)	Black: 0.89 (0.38–2.1) White: 0.46 (0.26–0.80)	No	Age, reproductive risk factors, education	Population-based
Postmenopausal breast cancer							
Cohort studies							
Le Marchand et al. (1988a), Hawaii, USA	1972–83	280	Tertiles	Age 50–54: 1.2 (0.70–2.0) Age 55–65: 1.2 (0.74–2.1)	No	Age, age at first birth, socioeconomic status	≥50 years
Tretli (1989), Norway	1963–81	5122	RR given for 1 unit increase	1.2 (1.1–1.2)	Yes		≥50 years
Sellers et al. (1992), USA	1986	469	≥30.7 vs ≤ 22.9	No family history : 1.5 (1.1–2.1) Family history: 2.2 (1.4–3.6)	Yes No	Age	≥ 55 years
Tornberg & Carstensen (1994), Sweden	1963–87	1093	≥28 vs <22 (5)	1.1	Yes	Age	≥55 years
Huang et al. (1997), USA	1976–92	1517	>31.0 vs ≤20.0 (10)	1.1 (0.87–1.5)	No	Age, history of benign breast disease, family history, reproductive factors	≥55 years
Case-control studies							
Paffenbarger et al. (1980), USA	1970–77	1029	≥24.5 vs <21.5 (3)	1.4	Yes	Age, ethnicity, parity	Hospital-based
Lubin et al. (1985), Israel	1975–78	664	≥27.1 vs ≤19 (4)	2.5	Yes	Age, ethnic origin, education, reproductive factors, history of benign breast disease, family history	Hospital-based

Table 26 (contd)

Author, date, study location	Study dates	No. of cases	BMI range contrasts (no. of categories)	Relative risk (95% CI)	Trend	Adjustment for confounding	Comments
Hislop *et al.* (1986), Canada	1980–82	517	≥27 vs ≤21 (4)	0.88 (0.59–1.3)	No	Age	Population-based
Kolonel *et al.* (1986) USA	1975–80	272	Weight: highest vs lowest quartile	Japanese: 1.6 (0.8–3.1) White: 1.7 (0.8–3.4)	No	Age, reproductive risk factors, history of benign breast disease, family history	Population-based; Hawaii
Bouchardy *et al.* (1990), France	NS	584	> 27 + vs <23 (3)	Age 55–64: 0.9 Age 65–92: 1.0	Yes	Socioeconomic status reproductive risk factors, prior breast biopsy, family history	Hospital-based, ≥ 55 years
Hsieh *et al.* (1990), Japan	NS	3993 pre- and post-	Normal BMI not defined; obese defined as + 4 kg/m^2	1.1 (1.1–1.2)	No	Age, centre, reproductive factors	Hospital-based
Chu *et al.* (1991), USA	1980–82	547	Sextiles – cutpoints not stated by meno-pausal status	2.7 (1.4–5.4)	Yes	Age, reproductive risk factors, family history, surgical biopsy for benign breast disease	Population-based
Brinton & Swanson (1992), USA	1973–80	1114	≥ 26 vs <20 (5)	0.98 (0.7–1.3)	No	Age, age at menarche, education	Population-based, ≥ 50 years
Harris *et al.* (1992), USA	1987–89	412	> 27 vs <22 (3)	1.5 (1.0–2.3)	Yes	Age, education, parity, family history	Hospital-based
Franceschi *et al.* (1996), Italy	1991–94	1574	>28.8 vs <21.7 (5)	1.4 (1.1–1.8)	Yes	Age, centre, education, parity, total energy and alcohol intake	Hospital-based
Yong *et al.* (1996), USA	1973–81	1198	≥34.7 vs 26.8 (5)	1.3 (1.1–1.6)	Yes	Age, education, reproductive risk factors, history of benign breast disease, family history	Population-based

Table 26 (contd)

Author, date, study location	Study dates	No. of cases	BMI range contrasts (no. of categories)	Relative risk (95% CI)	Trend	Adjustment for confounding	Comments
Chie et al. (1998), Taiwan	1993–94	216	≥25 vs < 20 (4)	1.9 (0.5–7.3)	No	Age, education, family history, reproductive factors, oral contraceptive use	Hospital-based
Galanis et al. (1998a), USA	1975–94	292	>26 + vs <19.6 (5)	1.5 (1.0–2.3)	Yes	Age, education, ethnicity and drinking status	Population-based, Hawaii, ≥50 years
Magnusson et al. (1998), Sweden	1993–95	2904	≥28.3 vs < 22.2 (5)	1.6 (1.4–2.0)	Yes	Age, reproductive factors, use of hormone replacement therapy	Population-based
Enger et al. (2000), USA	1987–89	1091	≥27.1 vs <21.7 (4)	ER+/PgR+: 2.4 (1.7–3.5) ER+/PgR–: 1.3 (0.78–2.2) ER–/PgR–: 1.2 (0.70–2.0) Unknown: 1.6 (1.1–2.2)	Yes No No Yes	Age, socioeconomic status, reproductive risk factors, family history, alcohol, physical activity	Population-based
Hall et al. (2000b), USA	1993–96	391	>30.1 vs <24.6 (3)	Black: 0.68 (0.33–1.4) White: 1.1 (0.58–2.0)	No	Age, reproductive risk factors, education	Population-based

NE, not estimated
ER, estrogen receptor
PgR, progesterone receptor
* Either a significant test for trend or significant intermediate relative risks for intermediate exposure categories

Table 27. Young adult, usual or recent BMI and adult weight change and risk of breast cancer

Author, date, study location	Study dates or date at diagnosis	No. of cases	BMI, Young adult (18–25 y)		BMI, usual or recent adult		Adult weight change		Adjustment for confounding
			BMI range contrasts (no. of categories)	RR (95% CI)	BMI range contrasts (no. of categories)	RR (95% CI)	BMI range contrasts (no. of categories)	RR (95% CI)	
Premenopausal breast cancer									
Cohort studies									
Le Marchand et al., (1988a), USA	1972–83	289	NA	NA	Tertiles	0.78 (0.46–1.3), age 30–44 y, 1.1 (0.63–1.8), age 45–49 y	Tertiles	0.67 (0.39–1.2), age 30–44 y 1.1(0.64–1.8), age 45–49 y	Age, age at first birth, socio-economic status
Huang et al. (1997), London et al. (1989), USA	1976–92	598	≥25 vs <20.0 (5)	0.6 (0.5–0.8), age 18	>31.0 vs ≤20.0 (10)	0.62 (0.45–0.86)	Gain >25 kg vs loss or gain ≤2.0 kg (6)	0.74 (0.54–1.0)	London: Age, height, history of benign breast disease, family history, reproductive factors, smoking Huang: Age, height, history of benign breast disease, family history, reproductive factors Weight gain data adjusted for BMI at age 18 y
Case–control studies									
Paffenbarger et al. (1980), USA	1970–77	372	≥22.0 vs <19.0 (3)	0.70, age 20 y	≥24.5 vs ≤21.5 (3)	0.65	NA	NA	Age, ethnicity, parity

Table 27 (contd)

Author, date, study location	Study dates or date at diagnosis	No. of cases	BMI, Young adult (18–25 y) BMI range contrasts (no. of categories)	RR (95% CI)	BMI, usual or recent adult BMI range contrasts (no. of categories)	RR (95% CI)	Adult weight change BMI range contrasts (no. of categories)	RR	Adjustment for confounding (95% CI)
Chu et al. (1991), USA	1980–82	2053	Sextiles – cutpoints not stated by menopausal status	0.6 (0.2–0.9), age 18 y	Sextiles – cutpoints not stated by menopausal status	1.3 (0.9–2.0)	NA	NA	Age, reproductive factors, family history, surgical biopsy for benign breast disease
Brinton & Swanson (1992), USA	1973–80	414	>25 vs <19 (5)	0.58 (0.3–1.1), age 20 y	>26+ vs < 20 (5)	0.65 (0.4–1.0)	Gain 6.0+ BMI vs no change (5)	0.47 (0.3–0.9)	Age, age at menarche, education
Coates et al. (1999), USA	1990–92	1590	>22.8 vs <18.5 (5)	0.75 (0.59–0.95), age 20	>30.4 vs <21.5 (5)	0.69 (0.54–0.88)	Gained ≥ 21 kg vs gained or lost ± 2 kg	0.72 (0.54–0.95)	Age, centre, ethnicity, family history, history of breast biopsy, education, reproductive factors, history of mammograms, alcohol, height, oral contraceptive use. Weight gain adjusted for BMI at age 20 y
Peacock et al. (1999), USA	1983–90	845	≥27.1 vs ≤19.9 (5)	0.71 (0.53–0.96), age 18 y	≥27.1 vs ≤19.9 (5)	0.67 (0.49–0.91)	Average annual BMI change of ≥0.25 units	0.70 (0.54–0.90)	Age at menarche

Postmenopausal breast cancer
Cohort studies

Author, date, study location	Study dates or date at diagnosis	No. of cases	BMI, Young adult (18–25 y) BMI range contrasts (no. of categories)	RR (95% CI)	BMI, usual or recent adult BMI range contrasts (no. of categories)	RR (95% CI)	Adult weight change BMI range contrasts (no. of categories)	RR	Adjustment for confounding (95% CI)
Le Marchand et al. (1988a), USA	1972–83	280	NA	NA	Tertiles	1.2 (0.70–2.0), age 50–54 y 1.2 (0.74–2.1), age 55–65 y	Tertiles Change in BMI	Age 50–54 y: 1.1 (0.66–1.8) Age 55–65 y: 2.3 (1.4–3.7)	Age, age at first birth, socioeconomic status

Table 27 (contd)

Author, date, study location	Study dates or date at diagnosis	No. of cases	BMI, Young adult ages (18–25 y) — BMI range contrasts (no. of categories)	RR (95% CI)	BMI, usual or recent adult — BMI range contrasts (no. of categories)	RR (no.(95% CI))	Adult weight change — BMI range contrasts (no. of categories)	RR	Adjustment for confounding (95% CI)
Folsom et al. (1990), Sellers et al. (1992), USA	1985–86	382	≥24.6 vs <20.0 (5), age 18	Family history –ve: 0.64 (0.45–0.91) Family history +ve: 0.88 (0.46–1.7)	≥30.7 vs ≤22.9 (5)	Family history –ve: 1.5 (1.1–2.1) Family history +ve: 2.2 (1.4–3.6)	Current–weight at age 18 y >17.3 vs <8.2 kg (3)	1.6 (1.1–2.3) (data on 225 women)	Age Weight gain data adjusted for BMI at age 18 y
Huang et al. (1997), London et al. (1989), USA	1976–92	384	≥25 vs <20.0 (5)	0.8 (0.6–1.2) age 18 y	> 31.0 vs ≤ 20.0 (10)	1.1 (0.87–1.5)	Gain > 25 kg vs loss or gain <2 kg (6)	1.4 (1.1–1.8)	London: Age, height, history of benign breast disease, family history, reproductive factors,smoking Huang: Age, height, history of benign breast disease, family history, reproductive factors Weight gain data adjusted for BMI at age 18
Case–control studies									
Paffenbarger et al. ethnicity, (1980), USA	1970–77	991	≥22.0 vs <19.0 (3) age 20 y		≥24.5 vs <21.5 (3)	1.0,	NA	1.4	Age, parity
Chu et al. (1991), USA	1980–82	547	Sextiles – cutpoints not stated by menopausal status	0.3 (0.03–2.2), age 18 y	Sextiles – cutpoints not stated by menopausal status	2.7 (1.4–5.4)	NA	NA	Age, reproductive factors, family history, surgical biopsy for benign breast disease

Table 27 (contd)

Author, date, study location	Study dates or date at diagnosis	No. of cases	BMI, Young adult (18–25 y) BMI range contrasts (no. of categories)	RR (95% CI)	BMI, usual or recent adult BMI range contrasts (no. of categories)	RR (95% CI)	Adult weight change BMI range contrasts (no. of categories)	RR (95% CI)	Adjustment for confounding
Brinton & Swanson (1992), USA	1973–80	1107	≥25 vs <19 (5), age 18 y	0.60 (0.4–0.9)	≥26 vs <20 (5)	0.98 (0.7–1.3)	BMI gain 6.0+ vs no change (5)	1.5 (1.1–2.2)	Age, age at menarche, education
Magnusson et al. (1998), Sweden	1993–95	2326	≥22.7 vs <18.7 (5) age 18 y	0.83 (0.69–1.0)	≥28.3 vs <22.2 (5)	1.6 (1.4–2.0)	≥30 kg vs <0 kg (5)	1.4 (1.1–1.9)	Age, reproductive factors, use of hormone replacement therapy
Enger et al. (2000), USA	1987–89	1091	≥27.1 vs <21.7 (4), age 18	ER+/PgR+: 0.75 (0.38–1.5) ER+/PgR−: 0.53 (0.16–1.8) ER−/PgR−: 0.79 (0.27–2.3) Unknown: 0.77 (0.38–1.6)	≥27.1 vs <21.7 (4)	ER+/PgR+: 2.4 (1.7–3.5) ER+/PgR−: 1.3 (0.78–2.2) ER−/PR−: 1.2 (0.70–2.0) Unknown: 1.6 (1.1–2.2)	% change age 18 to reference age, >29.2 vs ≤0 (4)	ER+/PgR+: 2.3 (1.6–3.4) ER+/PgR−: 0.99 (0.58–1.8) ER−/PR−: 1.8 (0.91–3.4) Unknown: 1.7 (1.2–2.5)	Age, socioeconomic status reproductive risk factors, family history, alcohol, physical activity

NA, not analysed
ER, estrogen receptor
PgR, progesterone receptor

Table 28. Studies of body fat distribution and risk of breast cancer

Author, date, study location	Study dates	No. of cases	WHR range contrasts (no. of categories)	Relative risk (95% CI)	Trend*	Adjustment for confounding	Comments
Premenopausal breast cancer							
Cohort studies							
Kaaks et al. (1998), Netherlands	1984–96	147	WHR: >0.80 vs ≤0.73 (4) Waist: >83.5 cm vs ≤71 cm (4)	WHR: 0.96 (0.60–1.5) Waist: 0.92 (0.57–1.5)	WHR: No Waist: No	Age, reproductive factors, height, weight	Breast cancer screening
Huang et al. (1999), USA	1976–94	197	WHR: ≥0.84 vs <0.73 (5) Waist: ≥36.0 vs <27.9 (5)	WHR: 1.4 (0.86–2.4) Waist: 1.7 (0.74–4.1)	WHR: No Waist: No	Age, BMI	Nurses
Case–control studies							
Franceschi et al. (1996), Italy	1991–94	947	> 0.88 vs < 0.78 (5)	0.7 (0.5–1.0)	No	Age, BMI, centre, education, parity, total energy and alcohol intake	Hospital-based
Swanson et al. (1996), USA	1990–92	1588	>0.858 vs 0.753 (4)	0.95 (0.8–1.2)	No	Age, BMI, centre, reproductive factors, oral contraceptive use, alcohol	Population-based, < 45 years
Hall et al. (2000b), USA	1993–96	370	> 0.86 vs <0.77 (3)	Black: 2.5 (1.1–5.7) White: 2.4 (1.2–5.1)	Yes	Age, BMI, reproductive factors, education	Population-based
Postmenopausal breast cancer							
Cohort studies							
Sellers et al. (1992), USA	1986	465	> 0.91 vs < 0.76 (5)	No family history 1.2 (0.87–1.7) Family history 3.2 (2.1–5.0)	No	Age	> 55 years
Huang et al. (1999), USA	1976–94	840	WHR: >0.84 vs <0.73 (5) Waist: >36.0 vs <27.9 (5)	WHR: 1.2 (0.96–1.6) Waist: 1.3 (0.88–1.8)	WHR: Yes Waist: No	Age, BMI	Nurses

Table 28 (contd)

Author, date, study location	Study dates	No. of cases	WHR range contrasts (no. of categories)	Relative risk (95% CI)	Trend	Adjustment for confounding	Comments
Case–control studies							
Franceschi *et al.* (1996), Italy	1991–94	1441	> 0.88 vs < 0.78 (5)	1.0 (0.8–1.3)	No	Age, BMI, centre, education, parity, total energy and alcohol intake	Hospital-based
Hall *et al.* (2000b) USA	1993–96	380	> 0.86 vs < 0.77 (3)	Black: 1.6 (0.70–3.8) White: 1.6 (0.88–3.1)	No	Age, BMI, reproductive risk factors, education	Population-based

* Either a significant test for trend or significant intermediate relative risks for intermediate exposure categories

WHR, waist/hip ratio

irrespective of menopausal status, while height has generally not been related to breast cancer prognosis, but data on height are not included in this review.

Premenopausal breast cancer
BMI or relative weight
Cohort studies
Cohort and nested case–control studies within cohorts are fairly few, but in general have found greater reductions in premenopausal breast cancer risk than case–control studies (Table 26). Estimates of 0.41 to 0.9 (Willett *et al.*, 1985; London *et al.*, 1989; Swanson *et al.*, 1989; Tretli, 1989; Vatten & Kvinnsland, 1992; Törnberg & Carstensen, 1994; Huang *et al.*, 1997) have been reported for recent or usual BMI greater than 27 to 28 kg/m². The studies of Willett, London, and Huang are all derived from the Nurses' Health Study and reflect longer periods of follow-up and more cancer cases in each subsequent study. Two early studies suggested that the protective effect among heavier women was limited to early-stage disease due to poorer detection of small tumours (Willett *et al.*, 1985; Swanson *et al.*, 1989). However, more recent studies including case–control (see below) and cohort studies presented in this chapter suggest that detection bias could not explain the increased risk for breast cancer observed among lean premenopausal women (London *et al.*, 1989; Brinton & Swanson, 1992). Some of the most precise estimates of risk derive from the Nurses' Health Study (Willett *et al.*, 1985; London *et al.*, 1989; Huang *et al.*, 1997). In an analysis from the 1992 follow-up of that cohort, the risk estimate for the top decile of recent BMI (>31.0 kg/m²) was 0.62. Relative risk estimates for the 2nd to 7th deciles were essentially null and then decreased to 0.86 and 0.80 for the 8th and 9th deciles, respectively, suggesting that the protective effect was limited to very high BMI. Questions have been raised about the selective nature of

the study population (all nurses) within the Nurses' Health Study. One other large, well designed population-based Norwegian cohort study provided risk estimates that are perhaps more generalizable to a population of white women (Tretli, 1989). In that cohort, relative risk estimates for stage I breast cancer for women in the top quintile compared with the bottom quintile of BMI were 0.80, 0.54, 0.54 and 0.63 for women aged 30–34, 35–39, 40–44 and 45–49 years. Relative risk estimates for stage II–IV breast cancer were 1.2, 1.2, 0.97 and 1.4, respectively, for the same five-year age groups. However, the only statistically significant relative risks were those for stage I breast cancer among women 35–49 years.

Case–control studies
Heavier women have been found to have a decreased risk of premenopausal breast cancer in most case–control studies (Paffenbarger *et al.*, 1980; Hislop *et al.*, 1986; Brinton & Swanson, 1992; Franceschi *et al.*, 1996, Swanson *et al.*, 1996; Chie *et al.*, 1998; Coates *et al.*, 1999; Peacock *et al.*, 1999). Risk estimates of 0.6 to 0.8 have generally been reported for the highest compared with the lowest BMI or weight groups. A limited number of case–control studies showed no association or a non-significant positive one (Hsieh *et al.*, 1990; Chu *et al.*, 1991; Ziegler *et al.*, 1996, Enger *et al.*, 2000; Hall *et al.*, 2000b). Two case–control studies have confirmed the findings in cohort studies that detection bias does not explain the increased risk for breast cancer observed among lean premenopausal women (Swanson *et al.*, 1996; Coates *et al.*, 1999). This risk may be modified by height. An informative large case–control study that allowed stratified analysis of the effects of both height and weight found that risk was increased about twofold among women who were tall and thin compared with women who were heavy and short (Swanson *et al.*, 1996).

Weight change and young adult weight
Data on weight change, young adult weight and premenopausal breast cancer are limited but generally show similar inverse associations irrespective of study design.

Cohort studies
Consistent with findings for recent BMI and premenopausal breast cancer, two cohort studies have reported that weight gain is associated with reduced risk of premenopausal breast cancer (Le Marchand *et al.*, 1988a; Huang *et al.*, 1997). As shown in Table 27, an analysis within the large Nurses' Health Study gave a risk estimate of 0.74 (95% CI 0.54–1.0) for the top sextile of weight gain (>25 kg) from age 18 years (Huang *et al.*, 1997). Heavier weight or BMI during young adulthood, generally reported for ages 18–20 years, was associated with a 25–40% decrease in breast cancer in the limited number of cohort studies in which it has been examined (Le Marchand *et al.*, 1988a; London *et al.*, 1989). In a large US cohort, the risk estimate for the 5th compared with the 1st quintile of BMI at age 18 years was identical to that for recent BMI (London *et al.*, 1989).

Case–control studies
In the limited number of case–control studies (Brinton & Swanson, 1992; Coates *et al.*, 1999; Peacock *et al.*, 1999), weight gain was associated with a 30% reduction in risk (Table 27). The largest case–control study that examined weight gain of 1590 women in the USA found a reduced relative risk of 0.72 (95% CI 0.54–0.95) with weight gain of 21 kg or greater. In case–control studies, heavier weight or BMI during young adulthood, generally reported as ages 18–20 years, was associated with a 25–40% decrease in breast cancer (Paffenbarger *et al.*, 1980; Chu *et al.*, 1991; Brinton & Swanson, 1992; Coates *et al.*, 1999; Peacock *et al.*, 1999). This

inverse association with young adult weight or weight gain was seen even in the absence of an inverse association between recent BMI and breast cancer (Chu et al., 1991).

Central adiposity

Data on central adiposity and premenopausal breast cancer risk are inconsistent but the most informative studies suggest that neither waist nor waist to hip ratio (WHR) is related to premenopausal breast cancer risk (Swanson et al., 1996; Kaaks et al., 1998).

Cohort studies

One study found no association between waist or WHR (Kaaks et al., 1998), one showed a modest non-significant increase in risk with WHR (Huang et al., 1999) and one reported a statistically significant increase in risk with WHR (Sonnenschein et al., 1999) (Table 28). A later follow-up, with more cases, of a cohort that first found a positive association (den Tonkelaar et al., 1995a) did not detect any association between WHR and breast cancer incidence (Kaaks et al., 1998).

Case–control studies

Two studies found no association between various measures of central adiposity (Petrek et al., 1993; Swanson et al., 1996), one found a non-significant decrease in risk (Franceschi et al., 1996), one found modest non-significantly increased risk (Hall et al., 2000b) and two reported statistically significant increases in risk with WHR (Männistö et al., 1996; Ng et al., 1997) (Table 28). A multi-centre population-based case–control study in the USA was particularly informative in terms of having a large number of premenopausal breast cancer cases and measured waist and hip circumferences (Swanson et al., 1996), and found no association of WHR with breast cancer risk.

Postmenopausal breast cancer
BMI or relative weight

In contrast to the evidence on premenopausal breast cancer, heavier women have been found to be at increased risk of postmenopausal breast cancer in most studies (Table 26).

Cohort studies

Findings from a number of prospective cohort studies indicate a modest increased risk associated with recent BMI (Le Marchand et al., 1988a; Tretli, 1989; Sellers et al., 1992; Törnberg & Carstensen, 1994; Huang et al., 1997). Other known risk factors that are likely to confound the association of weight with breast cancer include exogenous estrogen use and family history of breast cancer, and few studies have performed stratified analyses to explore the discrete effects of such factors. One of the largest cohort studies found no increase in risk (RR = 1.1; 95% CI 0.87–1.5) for all women (Huang et al., 1997). However, among women who had not used hormone replacement therapy, risk was increased to 1.6. In another large cohort, heavier women with a family history of breast cancer had a greater risk of developing breast cancer than heavier women without a family history (Sellers et al., 1992).

The Pooling Project included data from eight prospective cohorts (one each in Canada, the Netherlands and Sweden and five in the USA) comprising 337 819 women and 4385 incident invasive breast cancer cases. Risk of breast cancer increased above a BMI of 20 kg/m^2 up to a relative risk of 1.3 (95% CI 1.1–1.5) for women with BMI over 28 kg/m^2, and did not increase further. This analysis also found that the association between BMI and breast cancer was stronger and more significant among women who had never used postmenopausal hormone replacement therapy. In a subgroup analysis from the Oxford Pooling Project, which combined data on 50 cohorts primarily to examine the effect of estrogen replacement therapy (ERT) and breast cancer risk, among women who had recently used ERT for more than five years, the relative risk in those with a BMI over 25 kg/m^2 was 1.5 and was null among those with a BMI less than 25 kg/m^2 (Collaborative Group on Hormonal Factors in Breast Cancer, 1997). These risk estimates were not adjusted for duration of ERT. The results of these two analyses confirm the earlier finding of an significant interaction between body mass and hormone replacement therapy from the Nurses' Health Study (Huang et al., 1997). The stronger association among non-users of hormone replacement therapy provides strong support for the hypothesis that the mechanism for increased risk is largely due to increases in endogenous estrogen production among heavier women.

Case–control studies

Women with BMI above 27–28 kg/m^2 have been reported to be at 10–60% increased risk of breast cancer in many case–control studies (Paffenbarger et al., 1980; Kolonel et al., 1986; Hsieh et al., 1990; Harris et al., 1992; Franceschi et al., 1996; Yong et al., 1996; Galanis et al., 1998a; Magnusson et al., 1998), at a more than twofold increased risk in some others (Lubin et al., 1985; Chu et al., 1991; Chie et al., 1998; Enger et al., 2000) and at no increased risk in a few studies (Hislop et al., 1986, Bouchardy et al., 1990; Brinton & Swanson, 1992; Hall et al., 2000b). However, where examined, risk appeared to increase with age at diagnosis, from 1.1–1.3 among women younger than 60 years to 1.6–2.9 among women older than 65 or 70 years (Franceschi et al., 1996; Yong et al., 1996; La Vecchia et al., 1997a). Only one study has examined breast cancer incidence by estrogen (ER) or progesterone receptor (PgR) status of the tumour (Enger et al., 2000). Risk was 2.4 for a BMI over 27 kg/m^2 among women with ER- and PgR-positive tumours and was not increased among those with ER- or PgR-negative tumours or with ER-positive but PgR-negative tumours. In the same study, risk associated with BMI did not vary according to ER or PgR status among premenopausal women.

Weight change and young adult weight
At present, the most consistent body-size predictor of postmenopausal breast cancer risk is adult weight gain (Table 27).

Cohort studies
An association of postmenopausal breast cancer risk with adult weight gain has been found in cohort studies (Le Marchand *et al.*, 1988a; Ballard-Barbash *et al.*, 1990a; Folsom *et al.*, 1990; Huang *et al.*, 1997), including those that found no association between BMI at baseline and subsequent development of breast cancer and also adjusted weight gain for baseline BMI (Ballard-Barbash *et al.*, 1990a; Folsom *et al.*, 1990; Huang *et al.*, 1997). Findings from one of the largest cohort studies suggest that the doubling of risk associated with a weight gain of over 20 kg from age 18 years was limited to women who had never used post-menopausal hormone replacement therapy (Huang *et al.*, 1997). The data from this study can be examined to determine if there is a specific level of weight gain at which risk increases. A 20% increase in risk was observed for weight gains between 2 to 20 kg, although this was not statistically significant, while a statistically significant increase in risk of 40% was seen for weight gains of over 20 kg.

In two cohort studies, greater weight or BMI during young adulthood, generally reported for ages 18–20 years, was associated with a 20–30% decrease in breast cancer risk (London *et al.*, 1989; Sellers *et al.*, 1992).

Case–control studies
Weight gain is also a consistent predictor of increased risk in case–control studies

(Brinton & Swanson, 1992; Ziegler *et al.*, 1996; Magnusson *et al.*, 1998; Enger *et al.*, 2000). Two case–control studies also examined the effect of BMI or weight gain and hormone replacement therapy and reported similar results. In these studies, modest or no increase in breast cancer risk with increases in BMI was seen, but increases were larger among women not using hormone replacement therapy (Harris *et al.*, 1992; Magnusson *et al.*, 1998). In a large case–control study for which data were not presented in detail, it was noted that the association between weight gain and postmenopausal breast cancer risk was attenuated among current hormone users, although the test for interaction was not statistically significant (Trentham-Dietz *et al.*, 2000).

Greater weight or BMI during young adulthood, generally reported for ages 18–20 years, was associated with a 10–30% decrease in breast cancer risk in most case–control studies (Brinton & Swanson, 1992; Magnusson *et al.*, 1998; Enger *et al.*, 2000) but not in all (Paffenbarger *et al.*, 1980; Trentham-Dietz *et al.*, 2000). A few studies reported on a relative weight measure (Hislop *et al.*, 1986; Brinton & Swanson, 1992) and generally found that lower body weight or size relative to peers at young ages was associated with either no difference or a reduced risk of breast cancer. During the middle decades of life, the risk associated with BMI remains inverse for premenopausal breast cancer, though it shifts from a protective effect to null as women approach the menopause, and increases with age for postmenopausal breast cancer.

Central adiposity
Cohort studies
Increases in central adiposity have been associated with higher breast cancer risk among postmenopausal women in cohort studies (Ballard-Barbash *et al.*, 1990b; Folsom *et al.*, 1990; Sellers *et al.*,

1992; Kaaks *et al.*, 1998),(Table 28) particularly when possible differences in risk related to use of hormone replacement therapy were examined (Huang *et al.*, 1999). Some of these studies adjusted for baseline BMI and, therefore, the risk estimates suggest an independent effect of central adiposity. In the largest cohort study, risk increased from 1.2 among women overall to 1.9 among women who had never used postmenopausal hormone replacement therapy (Huang *et al.*, 1999). Family history of breast and ovarian cancer may modify the observed association in postmenopausal women. In a cohort of postmenopausal women, among women with elevated WHR, only those with a positive family history of breast cancer were at increased risk, while the combination of high WHR with a family history of breast and ovarian cancer was associated with a more than fourfold increase in risk of breast cancer (Sellers *et al.*, 1992). In another large US cohort, risk associated with waist circumference and WHR appeared to vary slightly with family history of breast cancer (Huang *et al.*, 1999). Among women having a family history of breast cancer, risk estimates for the 5th compared to the 1st quintile were 1.2 for waist and 0.73 for WHR. Conversely, amon women without a family history, risk estimates were 1.4 for waist and for WHR.

Case–control studies
Case–control studies have yielded less consistent results. Risk was significantly increased by about double in most studies (Bruning *et al.*, 1992a; Männistö *et al.*, 1996; Ng *et al.*, 1997), non-significantly increased by 60% in one (Hall *et al.*, 2000b) and not increased in some (Petrek *et al.*, 1993; Franceschi *et al.*, 1996). The majority of the studies finding a positive association adjusted for current BMI (Bruning *et al.*, 1992a; Männistö *et al.*, 1996; Ng *et al.*, 1997) and still found an independent effect of central adiposity. However, the largest case–control study found no increase in risk

with higher WHR after adjustment for recent BMI (Franceschi *et al.*, 1996).

Birth weight

Data on birth weight and breast cancer are sparse, somewhat inconsistent, but are accumulating rapidly and suggest a positive association for premenopausal breast cancer. However, most studies on birth weight and breast cancer risk are limited by a very small number of cases, with many having fewer than 100 cases and several less than 50 cases.

Cohort studies

One cohort study has suggested that the effect of birth weight may be modified by childhood height. Among premenopausal women, risk was not significantly increased (RR = 1.2; 95% CI 0.31–4.9) for a birth weight of 3500 g or greater and a height of less than 1.22 m at age seven years, compared with a much higher risk (RR = 5.9; 95% CI 2.0–17.4) for the same birth weight but height greater than 1.22 m at age seven years (De Stavola *et al.*, 2000).

Case–control studies

Two case–control studies found no association between birth weight and breast cancer (Le Marchand *et al.*, 1988b; Ekbom *et al.*, 1997); the 1997 report by Ekbom is an update of an earlier study with a more limited number of cases that did report a positive association (Ekbom *et al.*, 1992). However, more studies reported a positive association, with one case–control study of premenopausal cases under age 37 years showing an increased risk with birth weight over 4500 g (Innes *et al.*, 2000) and other studies finding an increase in risk with increasing birth weight for premenopausal but not postmenopausal breast cancer (Berstein, 1988; Michels *et al.*, 1996; Sanderson *et al.*, 1996) or stronger increases in risk for premenopausal than for postmenopausal breast cancer (De Stavola *et al.*, 2000; Kaijser *et al.*, 2001). Most of these

studies suggested that risk increased above a birth weight of 3500 g.

Weight and age at menarche

Age at menarche, an established risk factor for breast cancer, provides an indirect indicator of energy balance during childhood. Nutritional factors, in particular energy balance, appear to be the major determinants of age at menarche. In prospective studies among young girls, the major predictors of age at menarche were weight, height and body fatness (Meyer *et al.*, 1990; Maclure *et al.*, 1991; Merzenich *et al.*, 1993; Koprowski *et al.*, 1999). Early onset of menstrual cycles exposes the breast to ovarian hormones at a younger age and for a longer duration over a lifetime. The potential for energy balance to influence breast cancer risk through age at menarche is greater than might be appreciated by examining the distribution of this variable in developed countries. Although the average age at menarche in these countries is now 12–13 years, in rural China the typical age has been 17–18 years (Chen *et al.*, 1990), similar to that in the developed countries some 200 years ago.

Data from different ethnic populations

As is clear from Tables 26–28, the majority of studies on weight and breast cancer risk have been conducted in European and North American populations. With the exception of studies in Asian or Asian American women (Kolonel *et al.*, 1986; Tao *et al.*, 1988; Kyogoku *et al.*, 1990; Wang *et al.*, 1992; Chie *et al.*, 1996; Ziegler *et al.*, 1996; Ng *et al.*, 1997; Galanis *et al.*, 1998a; Tung *et al.*, 1999) and a single study including stratified results for African American women (Hall *et al.*, 2000b), data on specific non-white populations are limited. Generally, the results in these studies are similar to those reported for white women or from population-based studies that included women from diverse ethnic backgrounds

but did not report specific ethnic comparisons within their samples. For example, in a large case–control study (Hall *et al.*, 2000b), risk in African Americans was similar to that in white women for both premenopausal and postmenopausal women for both BMI and WHR. However, in this study, BMI was not related to risk for postmenopausal breast cancer (Table 26). Two smaller studies in China and Japan are not summarized in the tables, but the results were similar to those in other populations. In a small case–control study of 130 cases (menopausal status not stated) in Singapore, risk was markedly increased to 6.1 (95% CI 2.7–14.2) among women with a WHR greater than 0.86, while the risk associated with a BMI greater than 27.5 kg/m^2 was non-significantly elevated (1.2; 95% CI 0.7–2.3) (Ng *et al.*, 1997). In a case–control study of 190 premeno-pausal breast cancer cases and 186 postmenopausal breast cancer cases in Japan, BMI was not associated with premenopausal breast cancer (RR = 0.98; 95% CI 0.46–2.1, for BMI ≥25.1 kg/m^2) and was positively associated with postmenopausal breast cancer (RR = 1.9; 95% CI 1.1–3.2, for BMI ≥25.1 kg/m^2) (Tung *et al.*, 1999).

In a comparison of the effect of body size in various populations, seven countries were separated into those with low (Japan, Taiwan), moderate (Brazil, Greece, Yugoslavia) and high (USA, Wales) risk (Pathak & Whittemore, 1992). At a BMI of 24 kg/m^2, rates of breast cancer increased among postmenopausal women across all countries, with the greatest increases in risk at higher BMI among low- and moderate-risk countries, suggesting that increases in BMI now being observed in those countries (see Chapter 1) may be a major factor contributing to increases in breast cancer rates in countries that previously had low to moderates rates (Hodge *et al.*, 1995, 1996). Further, while risk ratios levelled off at higher BMIs in high-risk countries, this was not the case in low- to moderate-risk countries, where risk continued to increase exponentially across the full range of body weight.

Intentional weight control or loss

Data on an association between weight loss and breast cancer risk are limited. Four observational epidemiological studies that presented data on weight loss and breast cancer found no statistically significant association (Ballard-Barbash et al., 1990a; Brinton & Swanson, 1992; Ziegler et al., 1996; Huang et al., 1997). In three studies, weight loss occurring over a long interval was associated with a non-significant slight reduced risk (Ballard-Barbash et al., 1990a; Brinton & Swanson, 1992; Trentham-Dietz et al., 1997, 2000). In another, weight loss in the decade before diagnosis was associated with a non-significant decreased risk (Ziegler et al., 1996). One study of premenopausal women found a statistically significant decreased risk (RR = 0.64; 95% CI 0.42–0.98) with weight loss from age 20 years to interview (age 20–44 years) that was present only among cases with low-grade tumours (Coates et al., 1999). One study of postmenopausal women found a statistically significant decreased risk (OR = 0.76; 95% CI 0.61–0.96) with weight loss from age 18 years to interview (age 50–74 years) (Magnusson et al., 1998). These data suggest that weight loss may be beneficial, but are difficult to interpret as the cause of weight loss was not specified.

Breast cancer prognosis
BMI or relative weight

The association of BMI or weight with breast cancer prognosis has been examined in over 50 studies; all of which were cohort in design in terms of evaluating recurrence or death. Nearly all evaluated the effect of BMI at the time of diagnosis on breast cancer prognosis. Heavier women experienced poorer survival and increased likelihood of recurrence in most studies irrespective of menopausal status and after adjustment for stage and treatment (Greenberg et al., 1985; McNee et al., 1987; Hebert et al., 1988; Mohle-Boetani et al., 1988; Lees et al., 1989; Verreault et al., 1989; Coates et al., 1990; Kyogoku et al., 1990; Tretli et al., 1990; Vatten et al., 1991; Senie et al., 1992; Giuffrida et al., 1992; Bastarrachea et al., 1994; Zhang et al., 1995; den Tonkelaar et al., 1995b; Maehle & Tretli, 1996). In several studies, the association with prognosis was limited to or more pronounced among women with stage I and II disease (Verreault et al., 1989; Tretli et al., 1990), estrogen receptor (ER) and progesterone (PgR)-positive status (Coates et al., 1990; Giuffrida et al., 1992; Maehle & Tretli, 1996) and negative nodes (Mohle-Boetani et al., 1988; Newman et al., 1997). While many of the studies have used hospital-based samples of women, the most precise risk estimates are derived from large population-based cohorts of breast cancer cases. In the largest cohort of over 8000 women with breast cancer, risk varied by stage at diagnosis. Among women with stage I disease, women in the upper quintile of BMI had a 70% increased risk of dying from breast cancer; among women with stage II disease, women in the upper quintile had a 40% increased risk. BMI was not associated with risk among women with late stage III and stage IV disease (Tretli et al., 1990). In a subset of 1238 women of this cohort with unilateral breast cancer treated with modified radical mastectomy and followed for 15 years, the risk of dying from breast cancer relative to BMI varied markedly by hormone receptor status (Maehle & Tretli, 1996). Although women with ER- and PgR-positive tumours had nearly a 50% reduced risk of dying from breast cancer, the risk within hormone receptor-positive and -negative groups varied with BMI. Among women with hormone receptor-positive tumours, obese women had a risk of death three times higher than thin women. In contrast, among women with hormone receptor-negative tumours, thin women had a risk of death six times higher than obese women, even after adjustment for lymph node status, tumour diameter and mean nuclear area.

Weight gain

Weight gain is reported in the majority of women undergoing adjuvant therapy for breast cancer (Heasman et al., 1985; Goodwin et al., 1988; Camoriano et al., 1990; Demark-Wahnefried et al., 1993, 1997). Weight gain associated with treatment is lowest among women not receiving systemic therapy, intermediate among women receiving combination therapy and more pronounced among women receiving prednisone and ovarian ablation in addition to adjuvant chemotherapy. Recent research has begun to examine whether changes in energy intake and expenditure during treatment are associated with weight gain, in order to develop interventions to prevent weight gain during treatment (Demark-Wahnefried et al., 1993). Although data on the association of post-diagnosis weight gain and prognosis are limited, the largest study of 391 premenopausal women found that women who gained more than 5.9 kg were 1.5 times more likely to relapse and 1.6 times more likely to die than women who gained less weight (Camoriano et al., 1990).

Body fat distribution

Data on fat distribution and breast cancer prognosis are limited to one study of 119 postmenopausal women with breast cancer that found no association with two measures of skinfold thickness, subscapular and triceps (den Tonkelaar et al., 1995b). No study has examined prognosis in relation to waist or hip circumference.

Conclusion

In populations with a high incidence of breast cancer, the overall association of BMI with premenopausal breast cancer risk is inverse. This has been found in many cohort and case–control studies that carefully controlled for numerous reproductive and lifestyle factors. The reduction in risk of 0.6 to 0.7 is modest and does not appear to be observed below a BMI of 28 kg/m^2. In contrast to the consistency in the positive association of BMI for postmenopausal breast cancer in terms of both incidence and mortality or prognosis, mortality for premenopausal breast cancer is not lower among heavier women. This may relate to the observation that tumours have tended to be diagnosed at more advanced stages among overweight women. The results are largely from studies performed before mammographic screening was widespread, but are still relevant for young women, as mammographic screening does not begin until ages of 40 to 50 years in most countries. However, in moderate- and low-risk countries, risk of premenopausal breast cancer does not appear to decrease with increasing BMI, which may be due in part to a low prevalence of overweight in such populations.

More than 100 studies conducted during some 30 years in populations in many countries have established that higher body weight is associated with increased breast cancer risk among postmenopausal women. The large majority of cohort and case–control studies have seen positive associations, although the increase in risk with BMI has been somewhat modest. Nearly all of these studies have controlled for a wide variety of reproductive and lifestyle risk factors without altering this positive association. More recent studies have also adjusted for physical activity and still found an association. Risk appears to increase in a stepwise fashion with age.

Adult weight gain has been shown to be a strong and consistent predictor of postmenopausal breast cancer risk. Again, the association was particularly strong among women who were never users of hormone replacement therapy.

As with the studies on BMI and breast cancer, adjustment for many breast cancer risk factors, including physical activity, did not weaken these associations.

Endometrial cancer

There is convincing evidence from both cohort studies and case–control studies that adult obesity is associated with a two- to threefold increased risk of endo-metrial cancer (Table 29). Only studies with at least 100 cases are reviewed here, apart from some smaller studies conducted in less-studied populations.

Cohort studies
Cohort studies conducted in various developed countries, including the USA (Lew & Garfinkel, 1979; Le Marchand *et al.*, 1991a), Denmark (Ewertz *et al.*, 1984; Møller *et al.*, 1994), Norway (Tretli & Magnus, 1990) and Sweden (Törnberg & Carstensen, 1994; Terry *et al.*, 1999), have consistently found a direct association between endometrial cancer risk and adult weight or BMI. Only one of these studies adjusted risk estimates for reproductive risk factors (Le Marchand *et al.*, 1991a). In this study, in Hawaii, USA, using historically-recorded weight and height data, the association between adult weight and endometrial cancer was not explained by parity and age at first birth; the association was strongest in older women (over 60 years).

Case–control studies
Consistently with the cohort studies, the great majority of case–control studies have reported an increased risk of endometrial cancer with higher weight (Wynder *et al.*, 1966; Elwood *et al.*, 1977; Kelsey *et al.*, 1982; Henderson *et al.*, 1983; La Vecchia *et al.*, 1984, 1991; Lawrence *et al.*, 1987; Austin *et al.*, 1991; Shu *et al.*, 1991, 1992; Brinton *et al.*, 1992; Swanson *et al.*, 1993; Inoue *et al.*, 1994; Olson *et al.*, 1995; Goodman *et al.*, 1997; Shoff & Newcomb, 1998;

Weiderpass *et al.*, 2000). A particularly large and well conducted case–control study with 405 cases and 297 controls (Swanson *et al.*, 1993) reported a two-fold increase in endometrial cancer risk (95% CI 1.2–3.3) among women with BMI >30 kg/m^2 compared with those having BMI <23 kg/m^2. This association was observed in studies conducted in North America, northern Europe, southern Europe and China. Only two (Koumantaki *et al.*, 1989; Parslov *et al.*, 2000) out of 17 case–control studies (18 publications) found no association and none found an inverse association. In most studies, the association between body weight and endometrial cancer was independent of other known risk factors for the disease, such as age, parity, menopausal status, smoking, estrogen replacement therapy and socioeconomic status.

Discussion
A linear increase in risk with increasing weight or BMI has been observed in most studies (Elwood *et al.*, 1977; Kelsey *et al.*, 1982; Henderson *et al.*, 1983; Ewertz *et al.*, 1984; La Vecchia *et al.*, 1984, 1991; Lawrence *et al.*, 1987; Tretli & Magnus, 1990; Austin *et al.*, 1991; Le Marchand *et al.*, 1991a; Brinton *et al.*, 1992; Törnberg & Carstensen, 1994; Olson *et al.*, 1995; Goodman *et al.*, 1997; Terry *et al.*, 1999). However, in other studies, the increased risk was present only for the highest category of body mass (Shu *et al.*, 1991; Swanson *et al.*, 1993; Inoue *et al.*, 1994; Weiderpass *et al.*, 2000). Thus, it is unclear whether the risk of endometrial cancer is elevated only in overweight and obese women or whether the association is also present at lower levels of body weight. This inconsistency in the shape of the relationship across studies may be due to misclassification resulting from the use of weight or BMI as a measure of obesity (see below), to random variation or to true differences between populations.

Table 29. Studies of body mass index and risk of endometrial cancer

Author, date, study location	Study dates	No. of cases	BMI range contrasts (no. of categories)	Relative risk (95% CI)	Trend*	Adjustment for confounding	Comments
Cohort studies							
Lew & Garfinkel (1979), USA	1959–72	NR	40% > average weight	5.4	Yes	Age	Mortality study
Ewertz et al. (1984), Denmark	1943–77	115	> 31 vs < 22 (5)	2.3 (0.9–6.2)	Yes	Age	Cancer registry
Tretli & Magnus (1990), Norway	1963–81	2208	Highest vs lowest quartile	2.1 (1.9–2.5)	NE	Age	Tuberculosis screening programme
Le Marchand et al. (1991a), USA	1972	214	Weight: highest vs lowest tertile	2.3 (1.0–5.0)	Yes	Age, reproductive factors, socioeconomic status	Age > 60 years
Møller et al. (1994), Denmark	1977–87	114	Incidence relative to population	2.0 (1.6–2.4)	NE	Age, calendar period	Cohort of obese women
Törnberg & Carstensen (1994), Sweden	1963–87	412	≥ 28 vs < 22 (5)	2.6	Yes	Age, period of follow-up	Cancer registry
Terry et al. (1999), Sweden	1967–92	133	Weight: highest vs lowest quartile	2.4 (1.4–3.8)	Yes	Age	Twin registry
Case–control studies							
Wynder et al. (1966), USA	1959–63	112	Weight	Direct association	NE	Age	Hospital-based
Elwood et al. (1977), USA	1965–69	212	> 28 vs < 22 (4)	1.9	Yes	Age	Population-based
Kelsey et al. (1982), USA	1977–79	167	Weight ≥ 166 lb vs ≤ 125 lb (4)	2.3	Yes	Age, estrogen use, diabetes	Hospital-based
Henderson et al. (1983), USA	1972–79	110	Weight ≥ 190 lb vs ≤ 129 lb (5)	17.7	Yes	Age	Population-based
La Vecchia et al. (1984), Italy	1979–83	283	≥ 30 vs < 20 (4)	7.6 (4.2–14.0)	Yes	Age	Hospital-based
Lawrence et al. (1987), USA	1979–81	200	Weight ≥ 190 lb vs < 140 lb (4)	5.7	Yes	Age	Population-based Non-smokers

Table 29 (contd)

Author, date, study location	Study dates	No. of cases	BMI range contrasts (no. of categories)	Relative risk (95% CI)	Trend	Adjustment for confounding	Comments
Koumantaki *et al.* (1989), Greece	1984	83	Weight per 5 kg	1.0 (0.93–1.1)	NE	Age, reproductive factors estrogen use, smoking	Hospital-based
Austin *et al.* (1991), USA	1985–88	168	> 36.4 ≤ 28.4 (4)	2.3 (1.3–3.9)	Yes	Age, race, education	Hospital-based
La Vecchia *et al.* (1991), Italy	1983–88	562	Highest vs lowest quintile	3.4	Yes	Age, socioeconomic status, smoking, reproductive factors, estrogen use	Hospital-based
Shu *et al.* (1991, 1992), China	1988–90	268	≥ 31.9 vs ≤ 26.2 (4)	2.2 (1.3–3.8)	No	Age, parity	Population-based
Brinton *et al.* (1992) Swanson *et al.* (1993), USA	1987–90	405	≥ 32 vs < 23 (5) > 30 vs < 23 (4)	4.2 (2.5–6.8) 2.0 (1.2–3.3)	Yes No	Age, education, estrogen use, reproductive factors	Population-based
Inoue *et al.* (1994), Japan	1979–92	143	≥24.0 vs < 20 (3)	2.7 (1.6–4.7)	NE	Age	Hospital-based
Olson *et al.* (1995), USA	1986–91	232	≥26.63 vs < 22.61 (3)	3.2 (2.0–5.2)	Yes	Age, reproductive factors, hypertension, diabetes	Population-based
Goodman *et al.* (1997), USA	1985–93	332	≥27.3 vs <21.1 (4)	4.3	Yes	Age, race, reproductive factors, diabetes, total energy	Population-based
Shoff & Newcomb (1998), USA	1991–94	723	≥31.9 vs <29.1 (3)	3.9 (3.1–4.8)	NE	Age, education, diabetes, smoking, estrogen use, parity	Population-based
Parslov *et al.* (2000), Denmark	1987–94	237	≥30 vs < 20 (4)	No association	NE	Age, family history, reproductive factors, estrogen use	Population-based
Weiderpass *et al.* (2000), Sweden	1994–95	709	≥34 + vs <22.5 (6)	6.3 (4.2–9.5)	No	Age, reproductive factors, smoking, estrogen use, diabetes	Population-based

* Either a significant test for trend or significant intermediate relative risks for intermediate exposure categories

NR, not reported
NE, not estimated

Few studies have examined the association between weight and endometrial cancer separately for pre- and post-menopausal women or by age-group and the numbers of premenopausal women studied have been small. Most of these studies found increased risk in all groups, with somewhat greater risk estimates for older women (La Vecchia *et al.*, 1991; Le Marchand *et al.*, 1991a; Törnberg & Carstensen, 1994). However, in one study (Brinton *et al.*, 1992), the increase in risk was similar for younger and older women and in another study the association with obesity appeared stronger in premenopausal women (La Vecchia *et al.*, 1984). Studies that examined the relationship between body weight at an early age and endometrial cancer found either no association or a weaker association compared with the results for body weight in late adulthood (Henderson *et al.*, 1983; Le Marchand *et al.*, 1991a; Swanson *et al.*, 1993; Olson *et al.*, 1995; Terry *et al.*, 1999; Weiderpass *et al.*, 2000).

Weight gain during adulthood has generally been found to be associated with endometrial cancer risk independently of young adult obesity and in a dose-dependent manner (Le Marchand *et al.*, 1991a; Shu *et al.*, 1992; Swanson *et al.*, 1993; Olson *et al.*, 1995; Terry *et al.*, 1999). In four of the five studies that reported on this variable, the association with adult weight gain remained after adjustment for early-age weight (Le Marchand *et al.*, 1991a; Swanson *et al.*, 1993; Olson *et al.*, 1995; Terry *et al.*, 1999). Since, in most women, adult weight gain represents added fat tissue, it may be a better measure of adiposity than BMI, which reflects the weight of both fat and lean tissue. The linear dose–response relationship with weight gain suggests that any amount of adiposity contributes to endometrial cancer risk.

The distribution of body fat has been examined in relation to endometrial cancer risk using various measures, including WHR, waist-to-thigh ratio, subscapular skinfold and subscapular-to-thigh skinfold ratio. In a cohort study in Iowa, USA, WHR did not contribute additionally to BMI to the risk of endometrial cancer (Folsom *et al.*, 1989). Similarly, in a cohort study conducted in Sweden, WHR did not remain associated with endometrial cancer after adjustment for BMI (Lapidus *et al.*, 1988). Six case–control studies have examined the association of WHR with endometrial cancer. In three of these (Elliott *et al.*, 1990; Schapira *et al.*, 1991; Swanson *et al.*, 1993), WHR was independently associated with risk of the disease, whereas in the three other studies (Austin *et al.*, 1991; Shu *et al.*, 1992; Goodman *et al.*, 1997), this association did not remain statistically significant after adjustment for BMI. However, waist and hip circumferences may not be the most relevant measures of central obesity with regard to endometrial cancer risk. In a hospital-based case–control study in Alabama (Austin *et al.*, 1991) and a population-based case–control study in China (Shu *et al.*, 1992), measures based on subscapular skinfold were found to better predict endometrial cancer risk than WHR, with a threefold increase in risk across quartiles that remained unaffected by adjustment for BMI.

One study has examined the interaction between body weight and estrogen replacement therapy (La Vecchia *et al.*, 1982). Although the power of this study to detect an interaction was small, the effects of estrogen replacement therapy and of body weight on endometrial cancer appeared to be additive.

In conclusion, a direct association between body weight and endometrial cancer has been observed in all but three of 25 epidemiological studies, including in studies conducted in North America, Europe and Asia, and among pre- and postmenopausal women. Overweight women (BMI > 25 kg/m² or more) appear to be at a 2–3-fold increased risk of endometrial cancer.

Adult weight gain, which may be a better measure of middle-age obesity than BMI, has been found to be associated with risk in a linear dose-dependent fashion. There is evidence that fat distribution may also be important in endometrial cancer, with upper-body obesity particularly increasing risk.

Ovarian cancer

Since the relationship between obesity and ovarian cancer has been examined in only a relatively small number of cohort and case–control studies (Table 30), all but the smallest studies (less than 50 cases) were considered in this review. A potential methodological problem that may be particularly significant for ovarian cancer is the possibility of reverse causation, i.e., that a weight loss due to preclinical disease may confound an association with body weight.

Cohort studies
Lew and Garfinkel (1979) reported a statistically significant 1.63-fold increased risk of mortality from ovarian cancer in women with weight >40% above average compared with women of average weight in the American Cancer Society cohort study. However, Møller *et al.* (1994) found no increased risk of ovarian cancer in a cohort of obese women, compared with the Danish population. Similarly, a large cohort study of Swedish women (Törnberg & Carstensen, 1994) with 330 cases found no association with BMI (RR = 1.0; 95% CI 0.92–1.1). A report based on 97 cases and seven years of follow-up from the Iowa Women's Health Study (Mink *et al.*, 1996), which included information on possible confounders, also showed no association of BMI with ovarian cancer (RR = 1.1; 95% CI 0.64–1.9).

Case–control studies
The results of case–control studies have also been inconsistent (Table 30), with five studies finding a direct association (Casagrande *et al.*, 1979; CASH Study,

Table 30. Studies of body mass index and risk of ovarian cancer

Author, date, study location	Study dates	No. of cases	BMI range contrasts (no. of categories)	Relative risk (95% CI)	Trend*	Adjustment for confounding	Comments
Cohort studies							
Lew & Garfinkel (1979), USA	1959–72		40% > average weight	1.6	NE	Age	Mortality study
Møller et al. (1994), Denmark	1977–87	58	Incidence relative to population	1.1 (0.8–1.4)	NE	Age, calendar period	Cohort of obese women
Törnberg & Cartensen (1994), Sweden	1963–87	330	≥ 28 vs < 22 (5)	1.0 (0.92–1.1)	No	Age, period of follow-up	Cancer registry
Mink et al. (1996), USA	1985–92	97	>29.51 vs <23.45 (4)	1.1 (0.64–1.9)	No	Age	Age 55–69 yrs
Case–control studies							
Casagrande et al. (1979), USA	1973–76	150	20% > ideal weight	2.1	NE	Age, 'ovulatory age'	Population-based
Byers et al. (1983), USA	1957–65	274	> 30 vs < 21.5 (5)	0.74	No	Age	Hospital-based
CASH Study (1987), USA	1980–82	546	> 25.0 vs < 22.5 (3)	Direct association	NE	Age	Population-based
Mori et al. (1988), Japan	1980–86	110	> 20 vs ≤ 20	1.7 (0.9–3.3)	NE	Age	Hospital-based
Farrow et al. (1989), USA	1976–79	277	≥ 24.1 vs <19.8 (5)	1.7 (1.1–2.7)	Yes	Age, parity, estrogen use	Population-based
Hartge et al. (1989), USA	1978–81	296	Highest vs lowest quartile	1.1	No	Age, race	Hospital-based
Shu et al. (1989),	1984–86	172	≥ 22.32 vs ≤ 18.86 (4)	1.6 (0.8–3.3)	No	Age, education, animal fat intake	Population-China based
Purdie et al. (1995), Australia	1990–93	824	≥ 85th vs < 15th percentile	2.0 (1.4–2.8)	Yes	Age, reproductive factors, estrogen use	Population-based
Parazzini et al. (1997), Italy	1983–91	971	Severe overweight or obesity: yes vs no	0.66 (0.52–0.85)	NE	Age, education, reproductive factors	Hospital-based
Mori et al. (1998), Japan	1994–96	89	≥ 25.9 vs ≤ 21.9 (4)	1.6 (0.80–3.0)	No	Age, marital status	Hospital-based

* Either a significant test for trend or significant intermediate relative risks for intermediate exposure categories

1987; Farrow *et al.*, 1989; Purdie *et al.*, 1995; Mori *et al.*, 1998), four showing no association (Byers *et al.*, 1983; Mori *et al.*, 1988; Hartge *et al.*, 1989; Shu *et al.*, 1989) and one showing an inverse association (Parazzini *et al.*, 1997). The two largest case–control studies found clearly divergent results. The study by Purdie *et al.* (1995) conducted in Australia found a twofold increased risk of ovarian cancer (95% CI 1.4–2.8) for women with BMI above the 85th percentile whereas, in their study in Italy, Parazzini *et al.* (1997) reported a decreased risk (OR = 0.66; 95% CI 0.52–0.85) for women with "severe overweight".

Discussion

The evidence from the relatively few studies on body weight and ovarian cancer has been inconsistent and does not allow any conclusion to be drawn on a possible association.

In addition to BMI, measures of central obesity were examined in two cohort studies in relation to ovarian cancer risk. Lapidus *et al.* (1988) found no association between this cancer and WHR or subscapular skinfold in a small cohort of Swedish women after adjusting for BMI. In contrast, Mink *et al.* (1996) found a 2.3-fold increased risk of ovarian cancer (95% CI 1.2–4.5) for women in the fourth quartile of WHR compared with the lowest quartile in a cohort study in Iowa, USA. In this study, no association was found with BMI and the association with WHR was not attenuated by adjustment for other risk factors.

Prostate cancer

Although prostate cancer is a common cancer in many developed countries, very few risk factors have been identified for this disease. Because rates of the disease increase when migrants move from low-risk to high-risk areas, lifestyle and diet are thought to play major roles in its etiology. Much attention has been given to the possible importance of

nutrition, and in particular obesity and physical activity. Because latent or early-stage prostate tumours are often found at autopsy, the clinical significance of early-stage prostate cancer, as commonly detected by screening, is unclear. Also, it is possible that lifestyle characteristics that are associated with participation in screening may confound studies of other risk factors. Thus, analyses that focused on the more aggressive, high-grade tumours are particularly useful.

Cohort studies

Table 31 summarizes the prospective studies with at least 100 cases which have explored the relationship between anthropometric variables and prostate cancer. Most of these studies focused on adult weight and BMI. Four cohort studies found a direct association between weight or BMI and prostate cancer (Lew & Garfinkel, 1979; Chyou *et al.*, 1994; Andersson *et al.*, 1997; Putnam *et al.*, 2000). However, nine other cohort studies found no statistically significant association between body mass and prostate cancer (Greenwald *et al.*, 1974; Whittemore *et al.*, 1985a; Mills *et al.*, 1989; Thompson *et al.*, 1989; Le Marchand *et al.*, 1994; Giovannucci *et al.*, 1997; Lund Nilsen & Vatten, 1999; Schuurman *et al.*, 2000; Clarke & Whittemore, 2000). Although the majority of the significant associations with body mass were found in studies which focused on fatal or more aggressive tumours (Greenwald *et al.*, 1974; Andersson *et al.*, 1997; Putnam *et al.*, 2000), a clear pattern of a stronger association for the more clinically significant forms of the disease has not been consistently observed. Some studies having death from prostate cancer as the end-point did not find any association with BMI (Greenwald *et al.*, 1974; Whittemore *et al.*, 1985) and some large cohorts which conducted sub-group analyses on advanced prostate cancer did not clearly show a stronger effect for BMI in these

patients (Giovannucci *et al.*, 1997; Lund Nilsen & Vatten, 1999).

Three large, well conducted prospective studies illustrate the variation in the epidemiological findings on body weight and prostate cancer. In a retrospective cohort study, Andersson *et al.* (1997) studied 135 000 Swedish construction workers who participated in health check-ups between 1971 and 1975 and were followed through 1991. A total of 2368 incident prostate cancer cases and 708 deaths from this disease were observed. Height and weight were measured at baseline. Weak positive associations (13–17% increase in risk for the highest compared with the lowest quartile) were found for weight, height, BMI and estimated lean body mass. These associations were somewhat stronger (30–40% increase in risk) when prostate cancer death rather than incidence was used as the endpoint. Giovannucci *et al.* (1997) analysed data from the Health Professionals Follow-up Study, a cohort of 47 781 men who answered a mail questionnaire in 1986 and were followed until 1994. They identified 1369 cases of incident prostate cancer. Adult body mass was unrelated to the risk of total, advanced or metastatic prostate cancer. In contrast, higher BMI at age 21 years was associated with a significantly lower risk of advanced (RR = 0.53; 95% CI 0.33–0.86 for BMI ≥26 vs <20 kg/m^2 at age 21 years) and metastatic prostate cancer. Schuurman *et al.* (2000) used data from the Netherlands Cohort Study to investigate by a case–cohort approach the relationship of anthropometric variables with prostatic cancer. They studied 58 279 men aged 55–69 years who completed a self-administered questionnaire in 1986 and were followed until 1992. A total of 681 incident cases were identified. No association was found with baseline BMI, height or lean body mass for total, localized or advanced prostate cancer. However, a direct association was observed between BMI at age 20 years

Table 31. Studies of body mass index and risk of prostate cancer

Author, date, study location	Study dates	No. of cases	BMI range contrasts (no. of categories)	Relative risk (95% CI)	Trend	Adjustment for confounding	Comments
Cohort studies							
Greenwald et al. (1974), USA	1880–1916	268	Mean BMI	No association	NE	Age	Mortality study
Lew & Garfinkel (1979), USA	1959–72	NR	40% > average weight	1.3	No	Age	Mortality study
Whittemore et al. (1985), USA	1916–78	243	NR	No association	NE	Age	Mortality study
Mills et al. (1989), USA	1976–82	180	>25.9 vs ≤23.2 (3)	1.2 (0.79–1.7)	No	Age	7th day Adventists
Thompson et al. (1989a), USA	1972–87	100	BMI per 2.92 kg/m^2	1.2 (1.0–1.5)	NE	Age, diabetes, family history, systolic blood pressure, diet, smoking	Age 50–84 yrs
Chyou et al. (1994), USA	1965–92	306	Weight ≥ 70 + vs <57 kg (4)	1.5 (1.1–2.1)	Yes	Age	Hawaii Japanese
Le Marchand et al. (1994), USA	1975–89	198	> 26 vs < 22 (4)	0.7 (0.5–1.2)	No	Age, ethnicity, income	Hawaii residents
Giovannucci et al. (1997), USA	1986–94	1369	≥29 vs <23 (7)	0.90 (0.71–1.2)	No	Age, height	Health professionals
Andersson et al. (1997), Sweden	1971–91	2368	>26.2 vs <22.1 (4)	1.1 (0.99–1.3)	No	Age	Construction workers
Lund Nilsen & Vatten (1999), Norway	1984–97	642	≥28.3 vs ≤23.0 (5)	1.0 (0.8–1.3)	No	Age	Health screenees
Clarke & Whittemore (2000), USA	1971–92	201	Mean BMI	No association	No	Age, race	Caucasians (2000), African Americans
Putnam et al. (2000), USA	1986–95	101	> 26.6 vs <24.1 (3)	1.6 (0.9–2.8)	No	Age, diet, family history	Cancer registry
Schuurman et al.(2000), Netherlands	1986–92	681	≥28 vs <22 (5)	0.89 (0.58–1.4)	No	Age, family history, socioeconomic status	Age 55–69 yrs
Case–control studies							
Wynder et al. (1971), USA	1968–69	300	Relative weight	No association	NE	Age	Hospital-based

Table 31 (contd)

Author, date, study location	Study dates	No. of cases	BMI range contrasts (no. of categories)	Relative risk (95% CI)	Trend	Adjustment for confounding	Comments
Graham et al.(1983) (1983), USA	1957–65	311	BMI distribution	No association	NE	Age	Hospital-based
Talamini et al. (1986), Italy	1980–83	166	≥ 28 vs < 23 (3)	4.4 (1.9–9.9)	Yes	Age, marital status, occupation, diet	Hospital-based
Ross et al. (1987), USA	1977–80	142	Mean BMI	No association	NE	Age, ethnicity	Population-based
Kolonel et al. (1988), USA	1977–83	452	Mean BMI	No association	NE	Age, ethnicity	Population-based; Hawaii
West et al. (1991), USA	1984–85	358	Highest vs lowest quartile	No association	NE	Age	Population-based
Andersson et al. (1995, 1996), Sweden	1989–92	256	> 23.81 vs ≤20.83 (4) > 27.36 vs ≤ 23.84 (4)	1.0 (0.6–1.8) 1.2 (0.7–2.0)	No No	Age, region	Population-based
Whittemore et al. (1995), USA, Canada	1987–91	1655	Mean BMI	No association	NE	Age, race, ethnicity	Population-based
Grönberg et al. (1996), Sweden	1967–70	406	> 29 vs ≤23 (4)	1.8 (1.1–3.0)	Yes	Age, diet	Twin registry
Ilic et al. (1996), Yugoslavia	1990–94	101	≥ 28 vs < 22 (3)	No association	No	Age	Hospital-based
Key et al. (1997), United Kingdom	1989–92	328	Age 45 y, > 25.17 vs <22.75 (3)	1.4 (0.95–2.0)	No	Age	Population-based
Hsieh et al. (1999), Greece	1994–97	320	≥ 32 vs < 20 (8)	No association	No	Age, education	Hospital-based
Sung et al. (1999), Taiwan	1995–96	90	Age 40–45 y, >24.75 vs≤24.75	0.50 (0.26–0.95)	NE	Age, education, exercise, diet	Hospital-based
Villeneuve et al. (1999), Canada	1994–97	1623	≥ 30 vs < 20 (4)	0.9 (0.7–1.1)	No	Age, ethnicity, residence, smoking, diet, income	Population-based
Hsing et al. (2000), China	1993–95	238	≥24.03 vs <19.82 (4)	1.2 (0.73–1.8)	No	Age, education, marital status, total energy intake	Population-based

* Either a significant test for trend or significant intermediate relative risks for intermediate exposure categories
NR, not reported
NE, not estimated

and prostate cancer (RR = 1.3; 95% CI 0.81–2.2 for BMI ≥25 vs. <19 kg/m² at age 20 years). This association was limited to localized tumours and not observed for advanced tumours.

Case–control studies
Case–control studies of body mass and prostate cancer risk (Table 31) have been quite consistent in suggesting no association (Wynder *et al.*, 1971; Graham *et al.*, 1983; Ross *et al.*, 1987; Kolonel *et al.*, 1988; West *et al.*, 1991; Whittemore *et al.*, 1995; Andersson *et al.*, 1995, 1996; Ilic *et al.*, 1996; Key *et al.*, 1997; Hsieh *et al.*, 1999; Villeneuve *et al.*, 1999; Hsing *et al.*, 2000). Some of these studies were particularly large and informative. A population-based case–control study conducted by Whittemore *et al.* (1995) among 1655 cases and 1645 controls of African American, Asian or Caucasian origin, in California, Hawaii and Canada showed a clear lack of association with BMI. Similarly, the population-based case–control study conducted by Villeneuve *et al.* (1999) in eight Canadian provinces with 1623 cases and 1623 controls found an odds ratio of 0.9 (95% CI 0.7–1.1) for men with BMI >30 kg/m², compared with those having BMI <20 kg/m². Another population-based case–control study conducted in China reported an odds ratio of 1.2 (95% CI 0.73–1.8) for BMI >24.03 kg/m² compared with BMI ≤19.82 kg/m² (Hsing *et al.*, 2000).

Not all studies have been null, however. Two case–control studies conducted in Italy (Talamini *et al.*, 1986) and Sweden (Grönberg *et al.*, 1996) reported a direct association, and one in Taiwan (Sung *et al.*, 1999) reported an inverse association between BMI and prostate cancer.

Discussion
It is possible that adult weight and BMI do not well reflect the actual exposures most relevant to prostate cancer etiology. BMI reflects both lean body mass and adipose tissue, especially in men, and thus is not an ideal measure for studies of an androgen-dependent tumour, such as prostate cancer, since lean body mass is related to androgen levels. Only a few studies have investigated the body fat distribution patterns that may be more strongly related to the endocrine abnormalities typically associated with obesity. Giovannucci *et al.* (1997) failed to find an association between waist circumference or WHR and prostate cancer. However, they found a borderline statistically significant inverse association with hip circumference. No association with waist girth was found in a large case–control study conducted in California, Hawaii and Canada (Whittemore *et al.*, 1995). In contrast, a population-based cohort study conducted in China reported a direct dose-dependent association with WHR, with an OR of 2.7 (95% CI 1.7–4.4) for a WHR >0.92, compared with ≤0.86 (Hsing *et al.*, 2000).

It is also possible that body mass at a young age is more important than adult BMI. However, the results on body weight in young adulthood have also been inconsistent, with a large cohort study finding a weak direct association between BMI at age 20 years and prostate cancer (Schuurman *et al.*, 2000), one cohort study (Cerhan *et al.*, 1997) and two case–control studies (Andersson *et al.*, 1996; Key *et al.*, 1997) finding no association and another large cohort study finding an inverse association with advanced disease (Giovannucci *et al.*, 1997). A reduced risk was also associated in the latter study with obesity at ages 5 and 10 years, based on self-reported assessment using pictograms of body size and shape. Height, which partially reflects energy intake in childhood and androgen levels around the time of puberty, has been more intensively investigated. Four cohort studies (Le Marchand *et al.*, 1994; Andersson *et al.*, 1997; Giovannucci *et al.*, 1997; Hebert *et al.*, 1997) found a direct association between attained adult height and prostate cancer. However, six other cohort studies (Whittemore *et al.*, 1985; Severson *et al.*, 1988; Cerhan *et al.*, 1997; Veierod *et al.*, 1997; Lund Nilsen & Vatten, 1999; Clarke & Whittemore, 2000) and all but one case–control studies (Norrish *et al.*, 2000) that have reported on height failed to find an association.

High birth weight was found to be associated with increased risk of prostate cancer in a small cohort study in Sweden that used midwife records (Tibblin *et al.*, 1995). An attempt to reproduce this finding using self-reported birth weight in a large cohort study in the USA found no overall association with prostate cancer, although a weak association between birth weight and high-stage/grade tumours was suggested (Platz *et al.*, 1998). Thus, measures of body mass during childhood, adolescence or early adulthood have not been consistently associated with prostate cancer risk, mirroring the inconclusive results obtained for adult body mass.

In summary, a quite large number of studies have examined the association between body weight and prostate cancer in a variety of populations in North America, Europe and Asia, and have considered weight at different periods of life as well as body fat distribution. Some studies focused on the more aggressive forms of the disease which may be less subject to detection bias. No consistent pattern of association has emerged. The data suggest the absence of an important association between elevated body weight and the risk of prostate cancer.

Kidney cancer
Several studies worldwide have established BMI as a risk factor for renal-cell cancer (Bergström *et al.*, 2001) (Table 32) Additionally, diabetes and hypertension, which are both related to obesity, are established risk factors for renal-cell cancer. In contrast, no association between obesity and tumours of the renal

pelvis has been identified (McCredie & Stewart, 1992; Chow et al., 2000).

Cohort studies

Four studies based on at least 100 kidney cancer cases (Finkle et al., 1993; Hiatt et al., 1994; Heath et al., 1997; Chow et al., 2000) conducted in North America and Sweden have reported on the association between obesity and kidney cancer. Among women in the Kaiser Foundation Health Plan between 1980 to 1989, Finkle et al. (1993) identified 191 cases of histologically verified renal-cell cancer. The earliest recorded measure of weight/height was compared. Renal-cell cancer was associated with increasing relative weight, with a 2.6-fold increased risk in the highest quartile compared with the lowest and a significant trend ($p < 0.01$). In a similar study, Hiatt et al. (1994) identified 167 male and 90 female cases of renal-cell cancer that occurred between 1964 and 1988 among participants of the Kaiser Permanente Medical Care Program in northern California. Among neither men nor women was any increase in renal-cell cancer with BMI observed. Following 998 904 men and women for seven years (1982–89), Heath et al. (1997) identified 212 and 123 renal-cell cancer deaths among men and women, respectively. High BMI was associated with increased mortality from renal-cell cancer, in both men and women. In a study based on the health records of 363 992 Swedish male construction workers who underwent at least one physical examination between 1971 and 1992, Chow et al. (2000) identified 759 renal-cell cancer cases, as well as 136 cases of renal pelvis cancer. The risk of renal-cell cancer was significantly higher in those with a high BMI, with an approximate doubling of risk among those in the highest octile of the cohort compared with the lowest. A dose–response relationship was observed. No association was observed between BMI and cancer of the renal pelvis.

Case–control studies

Fifteen case–control studies covering populations in North America, northern and southern Europe, Asia and Australia have reported on the association between BMI and renal-cell cancer (Table 32). Four of these (McLaughlin et al., 1984; McCredie & Stewart, 1992; Lindblad et al., 1994; Mellemgaard et al., 1994) were included in a pooled analysis of 1050 male and 682 female renal-cell cancer cases, which provides the most accurate estimates of the relationship between BMI and renal-cell cancer (Mellemgaard et al., 1995). In this pooled analysis, including studies conducted in Australia, Denmark, Germany, Sweden and the USA, an increasing trend in renal-cell cancer with increasing BMI was observed for both men and women, with a 3.6-fold increased risk for women and a 1.6-fold increased risk for men in the fourth quartile of BMI compared with the first. In the remaining 11 case–control studies, an increasing risk of renal-cell cancer with BMI was observed either in men or women or in both in nine studies, an exception being a small hospital-based case–control study in northern Italy (Talamini et al., 1990). As well as the international pooled study which reported a greater effect of BMI among women than among men, four of the remaining studies provided evidence of a stronger association among women (McLaughlin et al., 1992; Benhamou et al., 1993; Kreiger et al., 1993; Chow et al., 1996), while one showed a greater effect among men (Asal et al., 1988).

Discussion

A consistently increased risk of renal-cell cancer with increasing BMI, with a dose–response relationship, was observed in most studies for both men and women. Furthermore, it was observed both in a large case–control study (Yuan et al., 1998) and in a cohort study (Chow et al., 2000) that obesity, independently of blood pressure, increased renal-cell cancer risk. This

may indicate that obesity and hypertension influence renal-cell cancer through different mechanisms.

BMI has been observed in some studies to increase renal-cell cancer risk more among women than men (McLaughlin et al., 1992; Mellemgaard et al., 1994). This suggests the importance of gender-specific fat distribution and hormonal levels. A high WHR has been observed in two studies to increase renal-cell cancer risk (Prineas et al., 1997; Bergström, 2001).

Weight change throughout life has been investigated in a population-based case–control study; subjects with a high BMI already at age 20 years who further gained 20 kg or more between ages 20 and 50 years had a 2.9-fold increased risk (95% CI 1.4–6.0) (Bergström, 2001). Those with a low BMI at age 20 years who gained weight up to age 50 years had a moderately increased risk of renal-cell cancer. Both weight cycling and weight loss have been observed to increase renal-cell cancer risk (Mellemgaard et al., 1995; Bergström, 2001). Losing weight was associated with increase in risk, especially among subjects with low BMI at age 20 years (RR = 2.6, 95% CI 1.4–4.7) (Bergström, 2001). These observations of increased risk of renal-cell cancer with weight loss may be explained by incomplete adjustment for preclinical disease.

In a recent meta-analysis including 11 studies, 6% and 7% increases in renal-cell cancer risk were observed for each unit increase in BMI in men and women, respectively. The estimated relative risks correspond to increases in risk of 36% for an overweight person (BMI >25.0 kg/m^2) and 84% for an obese person (BMI >30.0 kg/m^2) (Bergström et al., 2001).

In summary, all studies except for one of the 19 reviewed found a more than twofold increase in renal-cell cancer risk among obese men and women compared with those of normal weight. The studies, conducted in Australia, China, Europe and the USA, consistently found

Table 32. Studies of body mass index and risk of renal-cell cancer

Author, date, study location	Study dates	No. of cases	BMI range contrasts (no. of categories)	Relative risk (95% CI)	Trend	Adjustment for confounding	Comments
Cohort studies							
Finkle et al. (1993), USA	1980–89	F: 161	Weight/height F: ≥75 vs <25 (4)	2.6 (1.4–4.8)	Yes	Age	Medical care programme
Hiatt et al. (1994), USA	1964–88	M: 163 F: 88	M: ≥28.3 vs <24.6 (4) F: ≥27.8 vs ≤21.8 (4)	M: 0.9 (0.5–1.6) F: 1.2 (0.5–2.9)	M: No F: No	Age	Medical care programme
Heath et al. (1997), USA	1982–89	M: 208 F: 121	M: ≥31.1 vs ≤24.6 (4) F: ≥32.3 vs ≤21.9 (4)	M: 1.6 (0.9–2.7) F: 3.1 (1.5–6.4)	M: No F: Yes	Age	Mortality study
Chow et al. (2000), Sweden	1971–92	M: 759	≥27.8 vs ≤20.8 (8)	1.9 (1.3–2.7)	Yes	Age, smoking status, diastolic blood pressure	No association observed between BMI and renal pelvis cancer (N=136)
Case–control studies							
McLaughlin et al. (1984), USA	1974–79	M: 310 F: 178	M: >5.72 vs <4.83 lb/ft² F: >5.36 vs <4.42 lb/ft² (4)	M: 1.3 (0.8–1.8) F: 2.3 (1.3–4.1)	M: No F: Yes	Age, cigarette smoking	Population-based
Goodman et al. (1986), USA	1977–83	M: 173 F: 71	≥ 28 vs < 24 (3)	M: 2.7 (1.5–5.9) F: 2.4 (1.2–6.8)	M: Yes F: Yes	Age, saccharin additives, diet beverages, lifetime grams of artificial sweeteners, recreational and occupational activity, history of diabetes	Hospital-based
Asal et al. (1988), USA	1981–84	M: 209 F: 100	M: >6.02 vs <4.86 lb/ft² F: >6.16 vs <4.60 lb/ft² (4)	M: 3.3 (1.8–6.1) F: 1.2 (0.6–2.6)	M: Yes F: No	Age, education	Adjustment for smoking made little difference. Population-based
Maclure & Willett (1990), USA	1976–83	M: 135 F: 68	> 28 vs ≤22 (5)	M: 1.7 (1.1–2.8) F: 1.7 (0.9–3.2)	M: NE F: NE	Income, occupational status, education, history of cardiovascular disease	Population-based
Talamini et al. (1990), Italy	1986–89	M: 150 F: 90	>27 vs <24 (3)	0.74 (0.51–1.1)	No	Age, education, area of residence	Hospital-based

Table 32 (contd)

Author, date, study location	Study dates	No. of cases	BMI range contrasts (no. of categories)	Relative risk (95% CI)	Trend	Adjustment for confounding	Comments
McCredie & Stewart (1992), Australia	1989–90	M: 307 F: 173	M: >25.34 vs < 23.05 (3) F: >30.79 vs <27.21 (3)	M: 1.6 (1.1–2.5) F: 1.3 (0.8–2.1)	M: Yes F: No	Age, method of interview	Population-based
McLaughlin et al. (1992), China	1987–89	M: 76 F: 58	At age 50 y M: >23.3 vs ≤19.7 (4) F: >30.6 vs ≤24.4 (4)	M: 1.7 (0.5–5.7) F: 3.3 (0.7–15.1)	M: Yes F: No	Age, education, smoking Age, education	Population-based
Benhamou et al. (1993), France	1987–91	M: 138 F: 58	≥27 vs ≤20 (4)	M: 2.4 (1.0–5.9) F: 3.5 (1.0–11.8)	M: Yes F: Yes	Age, years at school, smoking	Hospital-based
Kreiger et al. (1993), Canada	1986–87	M: 282 F: 181	M: >25.1 vs ≤21.5 (4) F: >23.0 vs ≤19.7 (4)	M: 1.3 (0.8–2.2) F: 2.5 (1.4–4.6)	M: No F: Yes	Age, smoking status, BMI at age 25 y	Population-based
Lindblad et al. (1994), Sweden	1989–91	M: 207 F: 172	M: >25.8 vs <23.1 (4) F: >25.2 vs <21.3 (4)	M: 1.4 (0.78–2.4) F: 1.4 (0.71–2.9)	M: No F: No	Age, education, smoking, amphetamine use, weight cycling	Population-based
Mellemgaard et al. (1994), Denmark	1989–91	M: 225 F: 141	M: >26.4 vs <23.1 (4) F: >31.7 vs <27.2 (4)	M: 1.2 (0.7–2.0) F: 2.2 (1.1–4.2)	M: No F: No	Age, smoking, socio-economic status	Population-based
Muscat et al. (1995), USA	1977–93	M: 543 F: 245	Highest vs lowest quartile	M: 1.4 (1.1–1.9) F: 1.4 (0.9–2.1)	NE NE	Age, education, smoking	Hospital-based
Chow et al. (1996), USA	1988–90	M: 274 F: 163	Highest vs lowest quintile	M: 1.3 (0.7–2.3) F: 3.8 (1.7–8.4)	M: No F: Yes	Age, smoking, history of hypertension/hypertensive drug use	Population-based
Boeing et al. (1997), Germany	1989–91	259	>27 vs <25 (3)	2.2 (1.3–3.8)	Yes	Age, gender, smoking, alcohol, education	Population-based
Yuan et al. (1998), USA	1986–94	M: 781 F: 423	≥ 30 vs <22 (6)	M: 4.6 (2.9–7.5) F: 4.0 (2.3–7.0)	M: Yes F: Yes	Age, education	Population-based

* Either a significant test for trend or significant intermediate relative risks for intermediate exposure categories
NE, not estimated; 1 lb/ft^2 = 4.9 kg/m^2

the risk of renal-cell cancer to increase in a BMI-dependent manner in both men and women.

Lung cancer

A positive association between over-weight and cancer mortality has been well documented for both men and women (Lew & Garfinkel, 1979; Waaler, 1984; Møller et al., 1994; Calle et al., 1999) (Table 33). In contrast, there has been considerable debate as to whether lower body weight is associated with either higher total mortality (Lee et al., 1993) or lung cancer risk (Waaler, 1984; Goodman & Wilkens, 1993). Inclusion of individuals with pre-existing respiratory diseases and/or smoking-related weight loss may explain a U-shaped or a J-shaped relationship between body weight and cancer mortality rates observed in many studies (Singh & Lindsted 1998). Thus, the issue of whether body weight is related to increased risk of lung cancer remains controversial.

Cohort studies

Five cohort studies that investigated the association between weight and lung cancer risk were conducted in Finland (Knekt et al., 1991), the USA (Lee & Paffenbarger, 1992b; Chyou et al., 1994; Drinkard et al., 1995) and Israel (Kark et al., 1995). During 19 years of follow-up, 504 lung cancer cases were diagnosed among 25 994 Finnish men (Knekt et al., 1991). An inverse association between BMI and lung cancer risk was observed overall after adjustment for potential confounding factors including smoking and was even stronger among non-smokers. Lee and Paffenbarger (1992b), in a study of Harvard alumni including 286 lung cancer cases diagnosed between 1962/66 and 1988, observed a nearly twofold increase in lung cancer risk among those in the lowest tertile compared with the highest tertile of BMI, with a dose–response association in the first 11–15 years of follow-up. In a linkage study including 9975 male civil servants,

BMI was inversely related to lung cancer incidence in a dose-dependent manner, with a relative risk of 0.44 (95% CI 0.26–0.72) for the highest quintile of BMI compared with the lowest (Kark et al., 1995). Controlling for lung function did not change the association observed. In the study by Chyou et al. (1994), including 236 lung cancer cases, a clear inverse association between skinfold thickness and lung cancer risk was observed, but no association between BMI and lung cancer risk was seen after adjustment for smoking habits. In a prospective study of women in Iowa, USA (Drinkard et al., 1995), BMI was estimated through self-reporting at ages 18, 30, 40 and 50 years and at baseline. Among never-smokers, no association between BMI at baseline and lung cancer risk was observed among 233 lung cancer cases diagnosed during six years of follow-up.

Case–control studies

In a hospital-based case–control study including 3607 lung cancer cases, no significant association was observed in men who never smoked between the highest and lowest quartiles of BMI and lung cancer risk (RR = 1.1, 95% CI 0.5–2.5) (Kabat & Wynder, 1992). In contrast, in currently smoking men, after adjustment for smoking habits, a twofold decreased risk was observed (RR = 0.5; 0.4–0.7). However, a clear inverse dose–response relationship was observed between BMI and lung cancer risk in both currently smoking and never-smoking women. A population-based case–control study in Hawaii found an inverse association with BMI assessed only five years before diagnosis but not with BMI at ages 20 or 29 years, with an increased risk among the leanest men and women (Goodman & Wilkens, 1993). Information about preclinical disease was not available. A population-based case–control study in the USA included subjects who either had not smoked more than 100 cigarettes during their lifetime (never smokers) or had not

smoked during the past 10 years (former smokers) (Rauscher et al., 2000). Those in the highest octile of BMI (> 30.8 kg/m^2) had more than twice the odds of developing lung cancer compared with those in the lowest octile (BMI ≤ 21.3 kg/m^2).

Discussion

An inverse dose–response relationship between BMI and lung cancer was observed overall or in most subgroups in all studies except one (Rauscher et al., 2000) of those reviewed. However, several cohort studies suggested that an inverse association between BMI and lung cancer risk is limited to those who developed lung cancer in the first years of follow-up (Lee & Paffenbarger, 1992b; Drinkard et al., 1995). Thus, the inverse association observed between BMI and lung cancer may be explained by weight loss due to preclinical disease, i.e., latent undiagnosed lung cancer. This is supported by the observation that the inverse association between skinfold thickness and lung cancer did not persist as the time between examination and cancer diagnosis was lengthened (Chyou et al., 1994).

Since smoking is well established as the primary cause of lung cancer and is inversely associated with BMI, the inverse association between BMI and lung cancer may reflect incomplete adjustment for effects of smoking. This is supported by the observation that no significant association between BMI and lung cancer risk was observed among men who never smoked, while among currently smoking men, after adjustment for smoking habits, an increased lung cancer risk was observed with higher BMI. In the cohort study by Drinkard et al. (1995), multivariate analyses suggested that the inverse association of BMI with lung cancer could be explained by smoking status and that the positive association between WHR and lung cancer with lung cancer could be explained in terms of pack-years of smoking.

Table 33. Studies of body mass index and risk of lung cancer

Author, date, study location	Study dates	No. of cases	BMI range contrasts (no. of categories)	Relative risk (95% CI)	Trend*	Adjustment for confounding	Comments
Cohort studies							
Knekt et al. (1991), Finland	1966–84	M: 504	> 27.0 vs ≤ 22.5 (4)	0.55 (0.42–0.71)	Yes	Age, geographical area, social class, smoking, general health, number of stress symptoms, chest X-ray	Screening examination
Lee & Paffenbarger (1992b), USA	1962–88	M: 286	≥ 25.0 vs <22.0 (3)	Current smokers: 1962/66–77: 0.54 (0.30–0.99) 1978–88: 0.97 (0.57–1.7)	Yes No	Age, smoking, number of cigarettes per day, physical activity	Age 40–69 years
Chyou et al. (1994), USA	1965–92	M: 236	≥ 26.0 vs <22.0 (4)	0.69 (0.46–1.0)	No	Age, smoking	Hawaii Japanese
Drinkard et al. (1995), USA	1986–92	F: 233	Total population >29.7 vs <23.5 (4) Never smokers >28.4 vs <24.3 (4)	0.52 (0.36–0.74) 0.68 (0.31–1.5)	Yes No	Age, education, physical activity, alcohol, pack-years, years since last smoked	Effect not seen for non-smokers Age 55–69 years
Kark et al. (1995), Israel	1963–86	M: 153	≥22.9 vs < 20.2 (5)	0.44 (0.26–0.72)	Yes	Age, smoking, city of employment	Smokers included
Case–control studies							
Kabat & Wynder (1992), USA	1981–90	M: 69 F: 127	≥28 vs < 22 (4)	Never-smokers M: 1.1 (0.5–2.5) F: 0.34 (0.2–0.6)	M: No F: Yes	Age, education, race, hospital, history of chronic lung disease, alcohol	Hospital-based
Goodman & Wilkens (1993), USA	1979–85	M: 518 F: 230	M: >25.8 vs <21.9 (4) F: >25.5 vs <20.2 (4)	0.6 (0.4–0.8) 0.6 (0.4–1.0)	Yes Yes	Age, ethnicity, smoking	Population-based
Rauscher et al. (2000), USA	1982–85	M+F: 188	>30.8 vs ≤21.3 (8)	M: 2.6 (0.8–7.9) F: 2.1 (0.9–4.8)	NE	Age, years of smoking, number smoked per day, education	Population-based

* Either a significant test for trend or significant intermediate relative risks for intermediate exposure categories

Oesophageal cancer

During recent decades, the incidence of oesophageal and gastric cardia adeno-carcinoma has been increasing, while the incidence of oesophageal squamous cell carcinoma has remained relatively constant. Except for an association with Barrett's oesophagus, little is known about the etiology of these cancers. Certain epidemiological and molecular differences between oesophageal and gastric cardia carcinoma suggest that these cancers represent biologically different malignancies (Dolan *et al.*, 1999; Wijnhoven *et al.*, 1999).

Cohort studies

Data from the national Norwegian screening programme for tuberculosis (Tretli & Robsahm, 1999) were used in a study of 1 100 000 individuals aged 30–69 years at the time of examination who were followed until December 1989 (Table 34). High BMI was associated with increased risk of oesophageal ade-nocarcinoma, while the incidence of squamous cell carcinoma was linked to low BMI (men, RR = 2.4; 95% CI 1.3–4.4; women, RR = 1.6; 95% CI 0.5–4.8 for the highest quintiles).

Case–control studies

Out of eight reported case–control studies, six included more than 100 cases (Table 34). In a study of 173 male cases with adenocarcinoma of the distal oesophagus or cardia and 4544 controls, Kabat *et al.* (1993) found no association with reported BMI five years before diagnosis (BMI ≥28 vs <22 kg/m^2: OR = 0.8; 95% CI 0.4–1.7) for adenocarcinoma of the oesophagus or cardia. A smaller study by Zhang *et al.* (1996) also failed to find an association between BMI and oesophageal cancer. However, five case–control studies have observed positive associations with increasing BMI. In the US study of Brown *et al.* (1995), 162 male cases with oesophageal adenocarcinoma were compared with 685 controls. Risk was significantly elevated for subjects in the heaviest quartile compared to the lowest quartile of BMI, (OR = 3.1; 95% CI 1.8–5.3). Vaughan *et al.* (1995) studied 133 cases of adenocarcinoma of the oesophagus and 165 cases of cancer of the gastric cardia and found increased risks with higher BMI (OR = 2.5; 95% CI 1.2–5.0 and 1.6; 95% CI 0.8–3.0, respectively for the highest percentiles of BMI). Ji *et al.* (1997) reported ORs for adenocarcinoma of the cardia of 5.4 (95% CI 2.4–12.3) for men and 1.8 (95% CI 0.5–6.4) for BMI above 25 kg/m^2 in women in Shanghai, China. Chow *et al.* (1998) also found increasing risk associ-ated with BMI for both oesophageal adenocarcinoma and gastric cardia ade-nocarcinoma. The elevated risk was related mainly to excess weight *per se* and not to weight change over time. Men in the highest quartile of usual BMI had an OR of 3.0 (95% CI 1.7–5.0) and women OR 2.6 (95% CI 0.8–8.5) for oesophageal adenocarcinoma, while the ORs for cardia cancer were lower. The ORs for the highest versus lowest quar-tiles of usual BMI were 8.7 (95% CI 2.4–31.1) among non-smokers and 2.9 (95% CI 1.1–7.6) among current smokers, cigarette smoking being a significant effect modifier.

Lagergren *et al.* (1999a) studied 189 and 262 Swedish patients with oesophageal and cardia adenocarci-noma, respectively. Strong positive associations with oesophageal adeno-carcinoma were observed for BMI above 25.6 kg/m^2 for men or 24.2 kg/m^2 for women relative to the lowest quartile (OR = 7.6; 95% CI 3.8–15.2), and for obesity (BMI above 30 kg/m^2) relative to BMI less than 22 kg/m^2 (OR = 16.2; 95% CI 6.3–41.4).

Discussion

In six out of eight reported case–control studies, an increased risk was observed with higher BMI, notably at high BMI values. The risk is higher for oesophageal adenocarcinoma than for cardia adenocarcinoma. No association has been reported between squamous cell carcinoma and BMI. The association between BMI and adenocarcinoma of the oesophagus and cardia is strong and seems not to be explained by bias or confounding.

An increased incidence of gastric reflux has been proposed as the under-lying cause of the elevated risk of adenocarcinoma in persons with high BMI (Hagen *et al.*, 1987; Mercer *et al.*, 1987; Stene-Larsen *et al.*, 1988). Although the risk in one study (Lagergren *et al.*, 1999a) was indepen-dent of gastro-oesophageal reflux symp-toms, support for this hypothesis comes from the observation that medications that lower oesophageal sphincter pres-sure, thereby increasing reflux, have been associated with oesophageal ade-nocarcinoma (Lagergren *et al.*, 2000).

Pancreatic cancer

Due to its high fatality, pancreatic cancer is one of the leading causes of cancer death in developed countries. Most pan-creatic cancers derive from the exocrine component of the pancreas. Studies of migrants suggest that environmental factors influence the risk of pancreatic cancer; tobacco smoking is the single established cause (Ögren *et al.*, 1996). Studies of BMI and risk of pancreatic cancer with more than 100 cases are listed in Table 35.

Cohort studies

Only one cohort study out of four (Friedman & van den Eeden, 1993; Shibata *et al.*, 1994; Møller *et al.*, 1994; Ögren *et al.*, 1996) included more than 100 cases. In this exploratory nested case–control study in the San Francisco Bay area (Friedman & van den Eeden, 1993) within a large cohort of the Kaiser Permanente Medical Care Program, increased body weight measured at baseline was associated with somewhat higher pancreatic cancer risk (RR = 1.1; 95% CI 1.0–1.04). A unit increase in BMI

Table 34. Studies of body mass index and risk of adenocarcinoma of the oesophagus (AE) and of the gastric cardia (AC)

Author, date, study location	Study dates	No. of cases	BMI range contrasts (no. of categories)	Relative risk (95% CI)	Trend*	Adjustment for confounding	Comments
Cohort studies							
Tretli & Robsahm (1999), Norway	1963–89	M: 94, F: 25	Highest vs lowest (5)	AE: 2.4 (1.3–4.4), 1.6 (0.5–4.8)	No	Age, birth cohort, county of residence	Tuberculosis screening programme
Case–control studies							
Kabat et al. (1993), USA	1981–90	M:121 AE+AC	≥ 28 vs <22 (4)	0.8 (0.4–1.7)	No	Age, education, hospital, alcohol, smoking, dietary factors	Hospital-based
Brown et al. (1995), USA	1986–89	M:161 AE+AC	>26.6 vs <23.1 (4)	3.1 (1.8–5.3)	No	Age, area, liquor use, income, energy intake, smoking	Population-based
Vaughan et al. (1995), USA	1983–87	M+F: 131 AE, M+F: 164 AC	Percentiles 90–100% vs 10–49%	2.5 (1.2–5.0), 1.6 (0.8–3.0)	Yes, Yes	Age, gender, education, race, cigarette smoking, alcoho	Population-based
Zhang et al. (1996), USA	1992–94	M+F: 95 AE+AC	Not stated	AE+AC: 0.93 (0.83–1.03)	NE	Age, years of education, smoking, alcohol, total energy intake, sex, race, iron deficiency, stomach ulcers, hypertension, Barrett's oesophagus	Hospital-based
Ji et al. (1997), China	1988–89	M:148 AC, F: 37 AC	>22.2 vs <19.4 (4), >22.9 vs <19.5 (4)	3.0 (1.7–5.4), 1.4 (0.5–4.1)	Yes, Yes	Age, education, income, cigarette smoking, alcohol, total energy intake, chronic gastric diseases	Population-based
Chow et al. (1998), USA	1993–95	M: 244 AE, F: 48 AE, M: 223 AC, F: 38 AC	≥27.3 vs <23.1 (4), ≥27.4 vs <22.0 (4)	3.0 (1.7–5.0), 2.6 (0.8–8.5), 1.8 (1.1–2.9), 1.3 (0.4–4.2)	Yes, Yes, Yes, No	Age, cigarette smoking geographic location, race, sex	Population-based
Lagergren et al. (1999a), Sweden	1995–97	M+F: 189 AE, M+F: 262 AC	M: >25.6 vs <22.3 (4), F: >24.2 vs >21.1 (4) BMI 20 y before interview	AE+AC: 7.6 (3.8–15.2), AC: 2.3 (1.5–3.6)	Yes, Yes	Age, sex, tobacco smoking, socioeconomic status, reflux symptoms, energy intake, physical activity, fruit and vegetables	Population-based
Cheng et al. (2000), UK	1993–96	F: 68	BMI at age 20, ≥22.7 vs ≤19.5 (4)	AE: 6.0 (1.3–28.5)	Yes	Age, fruit consumption, breast-feeding, social class, no. of children	Population-based

* Either a significant test for trend or significant intermediate relative risks for intermediate exposure categories

Table 35. Studies of body mass index and risk of pancreas cancer

Author, date, study location	Study dates	No. of cases	BMI range contrasts (no. of categories)	Relative risk (95% CI)	Trend*	Adjustment for confounding	Comments
Cohort studies							
Friedman & van den Eeden (1993), USA	1964–88, follow-up 1 day–24.1 years	M+F: 450	BMI (per unit increase), measured at inclusion	1.02 (1.00–1.04)	No	Age, cigarette smoking, race	Exploratory study, testing 779 characteristics
Case–control studies							
Bueno de Mesquita et al. (1990), The Netherlands	1984–88	M: 89 F: 79	> 27.9 vs < 23.0 (5) > 28.7 vs <21.6 (5) two years before diagnosis	0.88 (0.40–1.9) 1.1 (0.46–2.8)	No	10-year age group, response status, total smoking	Population-based
			> 27.9 vs <23.0 (5) > 28.7 vs <21.6 (5), maximum BMI ever attained	0.72 (not given) 0.89 (not given)	No		
Ghadirian et al. (1991), Canada	1984–88	M+F: 179	> 26.5 vs <21.1 (4)	0.88 (0.42–1.8)	No	Age, sex, response status, cigarette smoking	Population-based
Ji et al. (1996), China	1990–93	M: 255 F: 183	> 22.5 vs < 19.4 (4) > 23.2 vs < 19.4 (4) usual BMI	1.4 (0.91–2.1) 1.5 (0.85–2.5)	Yes No	Age, income, smoking, physical activity, response status, diabetes, vitamin C, total energy	Population-based
Silverman et al. (1998), USA	1986–89	M: 218 F: 213	> 27.2 vs < 23.1 (4) > 34.4 vs < 27.5 (4) usual adult BMI	1.5 (1.0–2.3) 1.5 (0.9–2.5)	Yes No	Age, race, study area, diabetes, cholecystectomy, cigarette smoking, alcohol, income (men), marital status (women)	Population-based

* Either a significant test for trend or significant intermediate relative risks for intermediate exposure categories

was associated with an RR of 1.02 (95% CI 1.00–1.04). The studies of Ögren *et al.* (1996) and Møller *et al.* (1994), which included rather few cases, also found significant increased risk for pancreatic cancer in relation to high BMI.

Case–control studies

During 1984–88, a population-based case–control study of exocrine pancreas carcinoma was carried out in Utrecht, the Netherlands as part of the IARC SEARCH programme (Bueno de Mesquita *et al.*, 1990). The risk of pancreatic cancer in relation to high BMI suggested non-significant opposite effects for males and females, with reduced risk in men and increased risk in women for all quintiles of BMI two years before diagnosis, compared with the lowest quintile. In contrast, the highest BMI ever obtained was associated with non-significant reduced risks in both men and women.

Another participant in the SEARCH Collaborative Study Group carried out a case–control study in Montreal, Canada (Ghadirian *et al.*, 1991). No clear trend in risk of pancreatic cancer with increasing BMI was seen (OR = 0.88; 95% CI 0.42–1.8 for the highest versus lowest BMI quartiles).

In a case–control study in Shanghai, China (Ji *et al.*, 1996), interview data were obtained on weight during adulthood (usual weight) and at four different periods (ages 20–29, 30–44, 45–54 and ≥55 years). In both men and women, the highest quartile of usual BMI was associated with a non-significantly increased risk of pancreatic cancer, with the lowest quartile as reference category.

In a case–control study conducted in Atlanta, Detroit and New Jersey, USA, from 1986 to 1989, 436 patients and 2003 general population controls were interviewed (Silverman *et al.*, 1998). For both men and women, the highest quartile of BMI (≥27.2 and ≥34.4 kg/m^2, respectively) was associated with a 50% increase in risk of pancreatic cancer, compared with BMI 17.4–23.1 and BMI

20.5–27.5 kg/m^2, respectively. Blacks and whites experienced similar BMI-related risks.

Discussion

Only one exploratory cohort study and four case–control studies on the relationship between BMI and pancreatic cancer included 100 cases or more. Both lower and higher risks related to high BMI have been observed, with the studies finding an increased risk most often showing a dose–response effect. The highest risk was seen in the study in China, where the highest exposure category started at a rather low BMI compared with the other studies. All the case–control studies on pancreatic cancer were subject to bias because of a low participation rate among cases and use of information obtained from next-of-kin, due to the high mortality rate of this cancer.

Overall, the evidence is too limited to allow any firm conclusion to be drawn on the relationship between BMI and the risk of pancreatic cancer.

Cancer of the head and neck

Tobacco smoking and alcohol drinking account for over 90% of cancers of the oral cavity and pharynx in developed countries (IARC, 1986, 1988). Dietary factors (i.e., low consumption of fruit and vegetables and high intake of saturated fat (McLaughlin *et al.*, 1988) have also been related to risk. Several case–control studies on the association between weight and cancer of the head and neck have been reported, but no cohort studies (Table 36).

Case–control studies

An inverse association with weight and/or BMI was reported in four case–control studies on cancer of the oral cavity and pharynx in the USA (McLaughlin *et al.*, 1988; Marshall *et al.*, 1992; Day *et al.*, 1993; Kabat *et al.*, 1994), two in Italy (D'Avanzo *et al.*,1996a; Franceschi *et al.*, 2001), and one in China (Zheng *et al.*, 1993a). Two

case–control studies in the USA (Muscat & Wynder, 1992) and Italy (D'Avanzo *et al.*, 1996a) showed a similar, but somewhat weaker, inverse association between BMI and laryngeal cancer.

The risk pattern according to BMI seems to be similar in men and women, as well as in whites and blacks. Conversely, smoking and, possibly, heavy alcohol drinking seem to modify the apparent adverse effect of leanness. Three studies included an assessment of BMI according to smoking status, two of which found that BMI was not significantly related to oral cancer risk among never-smokers of either sex (Kabat *et al.*, 1994; Franceschi *et al.*, 2001). An association between oral and laryngeal cancers and BMI was found by D'Avanzo *et al.* (1996a) among never-smokers (OR = 0.5; 95% CI 0.3–0.7), but was weaker than among current smokers.

Weight at cancer diagnosis, but before disease-related weight changes, was generally considered in these studies. However, McLaughlin *et al.* (1988) reported that BMI at age 20 years was unrelated to oral cancer incidence. Franceschi *et al.* (2001) observed that male cases of oral cancer had significantly lower BMI than control subjects also at ages 30 and 50 years.

Discussion

A low BMI has emerged consistently as a marker, possibly a relatively early one, of increased risk of cancer of the head and neck in eight case–control studies in the USA, Europe and China. In the three studies where it was possible to restrict the analysis of BMI to never-smokers, however, the inverse association with BMI, if any, was weak.

Testicular cancer

Testicular cancer incidence has increased markedly in recent years among many populations worldwide, coincident with increases in obesity. Obesity often reflects altered levels of

Table 36. Case–control studies of body mass index and risk of cancer of the head and neck

Author, date, study location	Study dates	No. of cases	BMI range contrasts (no. of categories)	Relative risk (95% CI)	Trend*	Adjustment for confounding	Comments
Oral cavity and pharynx							
McLaughlin et al. (1988), USA	1984–85	871	Highest vs lowest quartile	M: 0.5 / F: 0.6	Yes / No	Age, sex, smoking, alcohol	Population-based
Marshall et al. (1992), USA	1975–83	290	≥ 28 vs ≤ 23 (4)	0.4 (0.2–0.6)	Yes	Age, sex, education, smoking, alcohol	Population-based
Day et al. (1993), USA	1984–85	1065 (194 Blacks)	F: Weight/height$^{1.5}$ M: weight/height^2 Highest vs lowest quartile	White: 0.6 / Black: 0.3	Yes / Yes	Age, sex, location, respondent, status, smoking, alcohol	Population-based
Zheng et al. (1993a), China	1989	404	≥26 vs ≤20 (4)	0.40 (0.23–0.69)	Yes	Age, sex, education, smoking, alcohol, inadequate dentition	Population-based
Kabat et al. (1994), USA	1977–90	M: 1097 F: 463	Highest vs lowest quartile	M: Current smokers: 0.3 (0.2–0.5) Never-smokers: 0.7 (0.3–1.7) F: Current smokers: 0.6 (0.3–1.1) Never-smokers: 0.6 (0.3–1.3)	Yes / No / No / No	Age, sex, education, race, smoking, alcohol	Hospital-based
D'Avanzo et al. (1996a), Italy	1985–91	M: 462	M: ≥26.8 vs ≤ 22.6 (4)	0.2 (0.2–0.3)	Yes	Age, sex, education, smoking, alcohol, β-carotene intake	Hospital-based
Franceschi et al. (2001), Italy and Switzerland	1992–97	M: 638 F: 116	≥ 28.5 vs < 22.7 (5) >26.9 ≤ 23.8 (3)	M: 0.3 (0.2–0.4) F: 0.5 (0.2–1.1) Non-smokers: 0.8 (0.4–1.7)	Yes / No / No	Age, centre, physical activity, alcohol, smoking, intake of energy, fruit and vegetables	Hospital-based
Larynx							
Muscat & Wynder (1992), USA	1985–90	M: 194	Highest vs lowest quartile	0.2 (0.02–0.6)	NE	Age, education, smoking, alcohol	Hospital-based
D'Avanzo et al. (1996a), Italy	1985–91	M: 369	M: ≥26.8 vs ≤22.6 (4)	0.5 (0.3–0.7)	Yes	Age, sex, education, smoking, alcohol, β-carotene intake	Hospital-based

* Either a significant test for trend or significant intermediate relative risks for intermediate exposure categories

estrogens and other sex hormones, which may be related to the risk of neoplasia of endocrine organs. Thus, obesity either early in life and/or later in life might affect testicular cancer risk. The five published studies are summarized in Table 37.

Cohort studies
In a large prospective study in Norway, a lower risk was observed among men with higher BMI as adults (RR = 0.70 for men with BMI of 20–25 kg/m² compared with below 20 kg/m²) (Akre *et al.*, 2000). A marginally reduced risk was seen for men who were obese (RR = 0.73 above BMI 30 kg/m² compared with below 20 kg/m²).

Case–control studies
Four case–control studies have focused on the association between weight and testicular cancer. A hospital-based case–control study including 259 cases (138 seminomas, 104 teratomas, 17 mixed histology) was conducted in England (Swerdlow *et al.*, 1989). Risk of testicular cancer was raised among men with a high BMI as adults, but not significantly, and there was no overall significant relationship. In a later population-based case–control study in England and Wales including 794 testicular cancer cases, no association with weight was observed (UK Testicular Cancer Study Group, 1994a). Similarly, a case–control study conducted in Canada including 510 men with testicular cancer aged 15–79 years found no association of BMI at age 21 years with increased risk (Gallagher *et al.*, 1995). In contrast, men with an adult BMI of 22–24 kg/m² were at lower risk (OR = 0.4; 95% CI 0.2–0.8) compared with those having BMI ≤ 21 kg/m² (Petridou *et al.*, 1997).

Discussion
Studies have reported either inverse associations between BMI and testicular cancer risk (Petridou *et al.*, 1997; Akre *et al.*, 2000) or no association (Swerdlow *et al.*, 1989; UK Testicular Cancer Study Group, 1994a; Gallagher *et al.*, 1995); no firm conclusion can be drawn on this relationship. Birth weight was not associated with increased testicular cancer risk in one case–control study (Sabroe & Olsen, 1998).

Cancer of the thyroid
Thyroid hormones are relevant to the growth and development of several body tissues, and weight is affected by hypo- and hyperthyroidism. An association between BMI (or weight gain) and thyroid cancer has been suggested by a number of case–control studies.

Case–control studies
Ron *et al.* (1987), in a study of thyroid cancer in Connecticut, USA, found an OR of 1.5 for women (but not men) in the highest BMI quartile at age 18 years and in adult life. Goodman *et al.* (1992), in a study from Hawaii, reported ORs of approximately 4.0 for men and 2.0 for women in the highest quartile of weight or BMI, and a significant direct association with weight and weight gain in women. In Shanghai, China, the ORs were 2.3 for the highest weight category and 2.0 for the highest level of weight gain; both estimates were significant (Preston-Martin *et al.*, 1993). In a study of 410 female cases and 574 control women in Washington State, USA, Rossing *et al.* (2000) reported an OR of 1.5 (95% CI 1.0–2.2) in women who weighed 185 pounds (84 kg) or more one year before diagnosis, compared with those who were lighter.

Dal Maso *et al.* (2000) carried out a pooled analysis of the relationship between anthropometric factors and thyroid cancer using individual data from 12 case–control studies (including those referred to above, except for Rossing *et al.*, 2000) conducted in the USA, Japan, China and Europe. A total of 2056 female and 417 male cases, 3358 female and 965 male controls were considered. Papillary carcinomas accounted for 78% of the thyroid cancers. ORs were derived by logistic regression, conditioning on age, A-bomb exposure (Japan) and study, and adjusting for radiotherapy.

Reported BMI at diagnosis was directly related to thyroid cancer risk for females in most studies, with a pooled OR of 1.2 (95% CI 1.0–1.4) for the highest tertile. The corresponding figure was 1.3 (95% CI 1.1–1.5) when the three Nordic studies were excluded. Similar to the finding for weight, no consistent association was observed in males (ORs 0.8 and 1.0 in subsequent tertiles). The pooled OR was 1.1 (95% CI 0.99–1.2). No consistent pattern of risk was observed for BMI between ages 17 and 20 years.

Discussion
A majority of the 13 case–control studies in the USA, China, Japan and Europe suggest a modest direct association between BMI and thyroid cancer risk in women. If such an association exists, it may be related to a potential association between thyroid tumours and steroid hormones or other endocrine factors. Overweight is related to increased estrogen levels in postmenopausal women (IARC, 1999) and exogenous estrogens are weakly related to increased thyroid cancer risk (La Vecchia *et al.*, 1999a; Negri *et al.*, 1999). In the pooled analysis, however, the influence of weight or BMI was of similar magnitude in older postmenopausal women and in younger ones. Some association with weight or BMI may be due to more frequent examination of the thyroid gland in overweight young women, particularly in the USA.

Gall-bladder cancer
Very few studies have investigated the relationship between weight or BMI and the risk of gall-bladder cancer. Descriptive studies have suggested that gallstones and obesity are risk factors for gall-bladder cancer. Of the cohort and case–control studies reported to date, only one included more than 100 cases.

Table 37. Studies of body mass index and risk of testicular cancer

Author, date, study location	Study dates	No. of cases	BMI range contrasts (no. of categories)	Relative risk (95% CI)	Trend*	Adjustment for confounding	Comments
Cohort studies							
Akre et al. (2000), Norway	1963–90	553	20.0–24.9 vs < 20.0 (5)	0.7 (0.5–0.9)	NE	Age	General population
Case–control studies							
Swerdlow et al. UK	1977–81	254	≥ 30 vs 20–24 (5)	2.0 (0.82–4.7)	No	Age, region of residence	Hospital-based
UK Testicular Cancer Study Group (1994a), UK	1984–86	790	Weight > 89 kg vs <60 kg (5)	1.1 (0.66–1.9)	No	Age, cryptorchidism, inguinal hernia	Population-based
Gallagher et al. (1995), Canada	1980–85	487	Age 21 y: ≥ 28 vs < 21 (5)	1.1 (0.7–1.7)	No	Age, ethnic origin, inguinal hernia, undescended testis	Population-based
Petridou et al. (1997), Greece	1993–94	97	22–24 vs ≤21 (5)	0.4 (0.2–0.8)	No	Age	Population-based

* Either a significant test for trend or significant intermediate relative risks for intermediate exposure categories

Cohort studies
In a cohort study on obese patients in Denmark, Møller et al. (1994) found a non-significant increased risk of gall-bladder cancer (RR = 1.4; 95% CI 0.9–2.1) in women.

Case–control studies
A study conducted in Mexico including 71 women and 13 men found a non-significant increased risk of gall-bladder cancer for higher BMI values (Strom et al., 1995). In a large case–control study conducted within the IARC SEARCH programme, including 196 cases (44 men and 152 women) of gall-bladder cancer from five centres in Australia, Canada, the Netherlands and Poland (Zatonski et al., 1997), higher BMI was associated with an elevated risk of gall-bladder cancer in females (OR = 2.1; 95% CI 1.2–3.8, for highest versus lowest quartiles), but not in males.

Discussion
Among the few reported studies, some have suggested a slight increased risk of gallbladder cancer related to a high BMI, especially for women. However, since only one study included more than 100 cases and this was the only one to control for potential risk factors such as age, alcohol drinking, tobacco smoking and socioeconomic status, the data remain inconclusive.

Malignant melanoma
Cohort studies
In one prospective study, BMI was associated with increased risk of malignant melanoma in men, while obese females were at lower risk compared with lean women (Thune et al., 1993).

Case–control studies
No association was observed between BMI and malignant melanoma in a case–control study of 361 patients conducted in Canada (Gallagher et al., 1985). This lack of association was supported in two other studies (Dubin et al.,

1986; Østerlind et al., 1988), but not in a study of men and women combined, where a positive association with BMI was found (Kirkpatrick et al., 1994).

Discussion
The results from the few studies conducted on malignant melanoma are inconsistent and do not allow any firm conclusion to be drawn on the relationship with BMI. BMI may influence sunbathing behaviour and hormonal factors, both of potential importance for development of skin cancer.

Cervical cancer
The international variation in cancer of the female reproductive system (breast, cervix uteri, corpus uteri and ovary) suggests certain common etiological factors. Overweight has been established as a risk factor for cancer of the corpus uteri (endometrial cancer; see above). However, few studies have focused on the association between cervical cancer and weight.

Cohort studies
The only cohort study identified included 271 cases of cervical cancer during 25 years of follow-up (Törnberg & Carstensen, 1994). No association with BMI was observed.

Case–control studies
Two small case–control studies have examined the association between weight and cervical cancer. A positive association with overweight was observed in a study including 39 cases in Italy (Parazzini et al., 1988), but no association with BMI was found in a study in Germany (Sönnichsen et al., 1990).

Discussion
Two case–control studies including less than 100 cases and one cohort study have been reported, and found either no association (Törnberg & Carstensen, 1994; Sönnichsen et al., 1990) or a positive relationship (Parazzini et al.,

1988; Guo et al., 1994) between cervical cancer and weight. Overall, the evidence is too limited to allow any conclusion on the relationship between BMI and risk of cervical cancer.

Other cancer sites
The Working Group was aware that certain other cancers (e.g., non-Hodgkin lymphoma, malignant myeloma, meningioma) have been studied in relation to weight. However, so few studies were identified for each cancer site that evaluation of the risks would be premature.

Population attributable risk
Overall, there is considerable evidence that overweight and obesity are associated with risk for some of the most common cancers. The proportion of any disease due to a risk factor in a population is determined by both the size of relative risk and the prevalence of the risk factor in the population. That proportion, often referred to as the population attributable risk (PAR), has been estimated by others for increased BMI in relation to many of the cancer sites reviewed here. Bergström et al. (2001) (Table 38) computed estimates of the PAR from overweight (BMI 25–29.9 kg/m^2) and obesity (BMI ≥30 kg/m^2) for selected cancers across countries of Europe, where about 50% of men and 35% of women are overweight, and 13% of men and 19% of women are obese. The risk estimates used in that analysis came from the authors' meta-analysis of the larger studies in the world literature, and are in line with those from the larger set of epidemiological studies included in the present review (see Tables 23–37). Because oesophageal cancer was not included in the analysis by Bergström et al. (2001), the PAR for oesophageal cancer due to overweight and obesity has been estimated here based on an RR of 2.0 for BMI over 25 kg/m^2 in Europe (see Table 34).

These PAR estimates are estimates that would apply to industrialized countries. However, the size of the PAR in any population will be dependent on the prevalence of elevated BMI in that population, which in some populations changes substantially over time. The prevalence of obesity continues to rise in many industrialized countries, and is also becoming a problem in many developing countries (see Chapter 2 and Popkin & Doak, 1998).

Physical activity

In view of the difficulty in measuring physical activity in a standardized manner, studies of the relationship between cancer and physical activity are described in some detail for the more important sites reviewed below.

Colorectal cancer

Occupational activity, leisure-time activities and participation in sports have been examined in a variety of populations to estimate the association between physical activity and colorectal cancer. Total activity and specific components of physical activity, such as level of intensity at which activities are performed, have been examined. Some studies have combined colon and rectal cancers (colo-rectal cancer), while others considered colon cancer separately and/or reported separate results for various subsites within the colorectal area. To clarify mechanisms and disease processes, some studies have looked at adenomas, the precursor lesion for most colorectal tumours. The results show that high levels of physical activity are consistently associated with reduced risk of colon cancer, although many of the studies that examined rectal tumours or colon and rectal cancers combined have yielded less consistent findings. However, this poorer consistency of associations for rectal cancers or colorectal cancer could stem in part from the less precise indicators of activity that were used.

The initial associations between physical activity and colon cancer were derived from observations that people involved in active occupations were less likely to develop colon cancer (Garabrant et al., 1984; Vena et al., 1987). Although physical activity was crudely categorized from occupational data in these studies, significant associations were detected and stimulated further examination of the associations, both for occupational activity and for other more comprehensive measures of total activity. Several studies have replicated the inverse association between job activity and colon or colorectal cancer (Fraser & Pearce, 1993; Hsing et al., 1998b; Levi et al., 1999a; Tavani et al., 1999), while others failed to detect differences between cases and controls on the basis of reported occupation (White et al., 1996; Le Marchand et al., 1997; Slattery et al., 1997a). Since occupational activity is tending to decrease for most people in developed societies, with leisure-time and recreational activities becoming a greater component of overall activity, it is likely that occupational activity is becoming a less sensitive discriminator of risk. For other populations where occupational activity remains more prevalent (Tavani et al., 1999), occupational activity is still associated with colon cancer.

The findings of the cohort and case–control studies (Table 39) are remarkably similar, suggesting that the associations are real and perhaps causal. Some of the larger, more rigorously conducted studies are described below, and details of all studies with more than 100 cases are presented in the table.

Cohort studies

Lee et al. (1991) evaluated long-term activity in a cohort of 17 148 Harvard alumni aged 30–79 years. Those who were active at several assessments had half the risk of developing colon cancer compared with those who were not (RR = 0.50; 95% CI 0.27–0.93). Similar associations were detected for those who were highly active and those who were moderately active. Physical activity as assessed at any single time period did not show a protective effect.

In the US Male Health Professionals Study cohort of 47 723 men (Giovannucci et al., 1995), there were 203 cases of colon cancer. Information was obtained by questionnaire on eight recreational activities and the amount of time spent per week on these activities. Physical activity was inversely associated with colon cancer after adjustment for age, BMI, diet and lifestyle factors (RR = 0.53; 95% CI 0.32–0.88, comparing high and low levels of activity).

A Norwegian cohort of 53 242 men and 28 274 women was followed for

Table 38. Estimates of population attributable risk due to overweight for selected cancer sites in developed countries (%)

	Attributable risk (%) for BMI > 25 vs <25 kg/m²
Colon cancer[a]	11
Postmenopausal breast cancer[a]	9
Endometrial cancer[a]	39
Kidney cancer[a]	25
Oesophageal cancer[b]	37

[a] From Bergstrom et al. (2001)
[b] Based on RR of 2.0 for BMI > 25 (see Table 34)

about 16 years, yielding 263 and 99 cases of colon cancer in men and women, respectively (Thune & Lund, 1996). Both occupation and recreational activity were considered. High levels of total physical activity were protective for women (RR = 0.63; 95% CI 0.39–1.0) but not for men (RR = 0.97; 95% CI 0.63–1.5).

Associations between physical activity and colon cancer were reported for the US Nurses' Health Study cohort of 52 875 women who completed a physical activity questionnaire in 1986 (Martinez et al., 1997). The questionnaire was the same as the one used in the Male Health Professionals Study and included questions on leisure and recreational activity only. In a multivariate analysis, physical activity was inversely associated with colon cancer (RR = 0.54; 95% CI 0.33–0.90) for those in the highest quintile of activity. Associations were slightly stronger for the distal colon (RR = 0.31; 95% CI 0.12–0.77) than for the proximal colon (RR = 0.77; 95% CI 0.38–1.6).

The Physicians' Health Study (Lee et al., 1997a) included 21 807 US physicians who were followed for an average of 10.9 years. A total of 217 cases of colon cancer were detected during the follow-up. This study was a randomized trial of low-dose aspirin and β-carotene, in which a crude indicator of physical activity was available. No association between physical activity and colon cancer was seen (RR = 1.1; 95% CI 0.7–1.6 for the highest versus lowest levels of activity). It is unclear whether the intervention had any effect on the results.

Case–control studies
In a study by Slattery et al. (1988), participants were asked to report activity performed at leisure and at work two years before diagnosis or interview as the number of hours spent in light, moderate and intense activity. The study consisted of 204 female and 180 male

controls and 119 female and 110 male colon cancer cases living in Utah, USA. Total physical activity was associated with a reduced risk of colon cancer for men; OR = 0.48; 95% CI 0.27–0.87 for women) after adjustment for diet, body size and age. Associations were present for intense activities (OR = 0.27; 95% CI 0.11–0.65) but not non-intense activities (OR = 1.2; 95% CI 0.68–2.3) among men. Both intense (OR = 0.55; 95% CI 0.23–1.3) and non-intense activities (OR = 0.53; 95% CI 0.29–0.95) were associated with colon cancer in women. However, since few women reported intense activities, estimates of association were imprecise. This study also showed significant interaction between dietary factors such as energy intake, protein and fat, and physical activity.

Three case–control studies reported in 1990 gave similar results to those of Slattery et al. (1988). Gerhardsson de Verdier et al. (1990a) assessed work and recreational activity among 452 colon cancer cases and 629 controls living in Stockholm, Sweden. People who reported being "very active" were at lower risk of developing colon cancer (OR = 0.6; 95% CI 0.3–1.0) relative to people who were sedentary, after adjustment for age, dietary factors, body size and gender. The associations were stronger for left colon cancer (OR = 0.32; 95% CI 0.14–0.71) than for right colon cancers (OR = 1.0; 95% CI 0.42–2.5).

Whittemore et al. (1990) examined associations between physical activity and colorectal cancer in Chinese living in North America and China. A total of 905 cases of colorectal cancer and 2488 controls were studied. Increased duration of exposure to a sedentary lifestyle was associated with increased risk of colorectal cancer. Inverse associations with colon cancer were detected for both job and lifestyle activities for men living in North America (OR = 0.4; 95% CI 0.2–0.9 for job activity; OR = 0.6; 95% CI 0.4–0.9 for lifestyle activity); women in North America reporting active

lifestyles had a reduced risk of colon cancer (OR = 0.5; 95% CI 0.3–0.8). In China, activity was not associated with reduced risk of colon cancer in men (OR = 1.2; 95% CI 0.5–2.6), although it was protective among women (OR = 0.4; 95% CI 0.2–1.0).

A study of 715 histologically confirmed cases of colorectal cancer and 727 age- and sex-matched controls in Melbourne, Australia, did not find any significant association with physical activity (Kune et al., 1990). People were classified as being totally inactive, not very active retired men and/or housewives or people in sedentary occupations; busy housewives; people on their feet most of the day doing moderate physical activity; or people performing strenuous activity such as manual labourers and athletes. This system of categorization may have led to misclassification.

Marcus et al. (1994) evaluated early adult physical activity in relation to colon cancer risk among women in Wisconsin, USA. The study population consisted of 536 cases and 2315 controls randomly selected from driver's license lists. Activity was reported for ages 14–22 years. After adjustment for age, family history of large bowel cancer, history of screening sigmoidoscopy and BMI, any strenuous physical activity during this time period was not associated with reduced risk of colon cancer (OR = 1.0; 95% CI 0.82–1.3).

A study by Longnecker et al. (1995) conducted in Los Angeles, California, USA, included data from 163 cases with right-sided colon cancer and 703 community controls. Questions about six specific leisure-time vigorous activities performed five years earlier were followed by an open-ended question about other forms of physical activity. People who reported two or more hours of vigorous activity per week were at reduced risk of colon cancer (OR = 0.57; 95% CI 0.33–0.97) after adjustment for smoking, income, race, family history of

Table 39. Studies of physical activity and risk of colorectal cancer

Author, date, study location	Study dates	No. of cases	Activity definition (no. of categories)	Relative risk (highest vs lowest categories) (95% CI)	Trend*	Adjustment for confounding	Comments
Colorectal cancer, cohort studies							
Colorectum							
Wu et al. (1987), USA	1981–82	M: 58 F: 68	Time spent per day in activities (3)	0.62 (0.45–0.87)	Yes	Age, alcohol, smoking, BMI	Retirement community residents
Albanes et al. (1989), USA	1971–84	M: 88 F: 53	Recreational exercise (3)	M: 0.6 (0.1–2.5) F: 0.8 (0.1–5.0)	NE	Age	Age 25–74 years
Ballard-Barbash et al. (1990c), USA	1954–82	M: 73 F: 79	Physical activity index (3)	M: 0.6 (0.3–1.0) F: 0.9 (0.6–1.7)	No	Age	Age 30–62 years
Steenland et al. (1995), USA	1971–87	M: 94 F: 82	Current non-recreational activity (3)	M: 1.0 (0.5–2.0) F: 1.1 (0.5–2.5)	NE	Age, BMI, smoking, alcohol, income, diabetes, recreational activity	NHANES 1 study
Thune & Lund (1996), Norway	1972–91	M: 236 F: 99	Moderate to intense activity per week in recreation and occupation (3)	Recreational M: 1.3 (0.90–2.0) F: 0.84 (0.43–1.6) Occupational M 0.82 (0.59–1.1) F 0.69 (0.34–1.4)	No	Age, BMI, geographic region	
Will et al. (1998), USA	1959–72	M: 2722 F: 2819	Usual level of activity at work or play (3)	M: 0.7 (0.6–0.9) F: 0.9 (0.8–1.1)	NE	Age, race, BMI, education, family history of colon cancer, diet, aspirin, smoking, parity (F), pipe/cigar smoking (M)	
Colon cancer, cohort studies							
Gerhardsson et al. (1986), Sweden	1961–79	5100	Occupational titles by census (2)	0.8 (0.7–0.8)	NE	Age, population density, social class	Age 20–64 years
Vena et al. (1987), USA	1974–79	M: 6459 F: 604	Occupational activity from death certificate (4 or 3)	PMR = M: 89 (p<0.1) F: 80 (p<0.01)	NE	Age	Mortality not incidence
Gerhardsson et al. (1988), Sweden	1969–82	M: 99 F: 92	Work and leisure activity by intensity (2)	0.3 (0.1–0.8)	NE	Age, gender	Age > 44 years
Marti & Minder (1989), Switzerland	1979–82	1995	Occupational data based on census (3)	SMR=0.8	NE	Age	Mortality

Table 39 (contd)

Author, date, study location	Study dates	No. of cases	Activity definition (no. of categories)	Relative risk (highest vs lowest categories) (95% CI)	Trend*	Adjustment for confounding	Comments
Severson et al. (1989), USA	1965–86	M: 191	24-h index of all activities plus time sleeping (3 or 2) home/leisure:	Total: 0.71 (0.51–0.99) Moderate /intense vs sitting: 0.66 (0.49–0.88)	No	Age, BMI	Hawaii Japanese
Lee et al. (1991), USA	1962–88	M: 225	Recreational activity, stair climbing, blocks walked (3)	Activity in 1962/66/77; 0.85 (0.64–1.1)	No	Age	College alumni
Thun et al. (1992), USA	1982–88	M: 611 F: 539	Current recreational and occupational activity (4)	M: 0.6 (0.3–1.3) F: 0.9 (0.4–2.0)	No	Age, familial history, fat, fruits, vegetables and grains, BMI, NSAIDs	Mortality study
Chow et al. (1993), China	1980–84	M: 302 F: 936	Occupational data census (3)	M: 0.9 (0.7–1.0) F: 0.8 (0.7–1.0)	Yes	Age	Age > 30 years
Bostick et al. (1994), USA	1986–90	F: 212	Two physical activity questions (3)	0.95 (0.68–1.4)	No	Age, energy intake, height, vitamin E intake, vitamin A supplements	Age 55–69 years
Chow et al. (1994), Sweden	1961–79	M: 13940 F: 4892	Occupational titles by census	SIR Professional: M: 1.2 (p < 0.01) F: 1.0 Agricultural: M: 0.8 (p < 0.01) F: 0.9	NE	Age, region	
Giovannucci et al. (1995), USA	1987–92	M: 203	Moderate and vigorous leisure activity (5)	0.53 (0.32–0.88)	Yes	Age, BMI, family history, endoscopic screening, smoking, aspirin, diet	Age 40–75 years
Lee et al. (1997a), USA	1982–94	M: 217	Frequency of vigorous activity (4)	1.1 (0.7–1.6)	No	Age, obesity, alcohol, treatment	Age 40–84 years

Table 39 (contd)

Author, date, study location	Study dates	No. of cases	Activity definition (no. of categories)	Relative risk (highest vs lowest categories) (95% CI)	Trend*	Adjustment for confounding	Comments
Martinez et al. (1997), USA	1976–92	F: 161	Time per week in walking and selected moderate and vigorous activities (5)	0.54 (0.33–0.90)	Yes	Age, cigarette smoking, family history of colorectal cancer, BMI, hormone replacement therapy, aspirin, red meat, alcohol	Age 30–55 years
Hsing et al. (1998b), 1966–86 USA		M: 120	Occupational history	Agricultural vs professional workers: M: 0.7 (0.3–1.4)	NE	Age, alcohol, physical activity	Mortality study
Rectal cancer, cohort studies							
Gerhardsson et al. (1986), Sweden	1961–79	4533	Occupational title by census (2)	0.9 (0.8–1.0)	NE	Age, population density, social class	Age 20–64 years
Thune & Lund (1996), Norway	1972–91	M: 170 F: 58	Recreational and occupational activity (3)	Recreational M: 0.98 (0.6–1.6) F: 1.5 (0.5–4.2) Occupational M: 1.0 (0.6–1.4) F: 0.88 (0.33–2.4)	NE	Age, BMI, geographic region	Age 40–75 years
Colorectal cancer, case–control studies							
Peters et al. (1989), 1975–82 USA		M: 147	Lifetime occupational titles (3)	1.1 (0.5–2.3)	No	Age, education	Population-based
Benito et al. (1990), 1984–88 Spain		M: 151 F: 135	Current occupational activity (4)	0.7	Yes	Age	Population-based
Kune et al. (1990), 1980–81 Australia		M: 388 F: 327	Recreational and occupational activity in previous 20 years (4)	M: 1.5 (0.8–2.7) F: 0.9 (0.3–2.8)	NE	Age, BMI, diet	Population-based
Le Marchand et al. (1997), USA	1987–91	M: 698 F: 494	Lifetime recreational activity and occupational activity (4)	Recreation M: 0.6 (0.4–0.8) F: 0.7 (0.5–1.1) Occupation M: 1.3 (0.9–1.9) F: 1.5 (0.9–2.3)	Yes No No No	Age, family history of colorectal cancer, alcohol, cigarettes, eggs, dietary fibre, calcium, energy, BMI	Population-based

Table 39 (contd)

Author, date, study location	Study dates	No. of cases	Activity definition (no. of categories)	Relative risk (highest vs lowest categories) (95% CI)	Trend*	Adjustment for confounding	Comments
Levi et al. (1999a), Switzerland	1992–97	M: 142 F: 81	Occupational and recreational activity at different ages (3)	Occupation 15–19: 0.63 (0.40–1.0) 30–39: 0.44 (0.26–0.73) 50–59: 0.63 (0.37–1.1) Leisure 15–19: 0.97 (0.62–1.5) 30–39: 0.53 (0.33–0.86) 50–59: 0.54 (0.30–0.96)	Yes	Age, sex, education, alcohol and energy intake	Hospital-based
Tang et al. (1999), Taiwan	1992	M: 90 F: 70	Current non-occupational activity (3)	M: 0.3 (0.1–0.8) F: 0.8 (0.3–1.9)	Yes	Age, energy intake, dietary fibre, vegetable, protein and water intake, smoking, alcohol	Hospital-based
Steindorf et al. (2000), Poland	1998–99	M+F: 180	Occupational activity (3) and three questions on recreational activity (3)	Occupational: 0.61 (0.29–1.3) Recreational: 0.45 (0.24–0.84)	NE	Age, energy intake, education	Hospital based
Colon cancer, case–control studies							
Garabrant et al. (1984), USA	1972–81	M: 2950	Occupational title (3)	0.55 (0.5–0.6)	Yes	Age	Population-based
Vena et al. (1987), USA	1957–65	M: 210	Lifetime occupation (4)	0.5 (p<0.001)	Yes	Age	Hospital-based
Slattery et al. (1988), USA	1979–83	M: 110 F: 119	Non-occupational and occupational activity by intensity (4)	Total M: 0.7 (0.4–1.3) F: 0.5 (0.3–0.9) Intense M: 0.3 (0.1–0.7) F: 0.6 (0.2–1.3)	Yes	Age, BMI, energy, fat, proteins	Population-based
Brownson et al. (1989), USA	1984–87	M: 1211	Occupational title from medical chart (3)	0.7 (0.5–1.0)	Yes	Age	Hospital-based
Fredriksson et al. (1989), Sweden	1980–83	M: 156 F: 156	Occupational history (5)	M: 0.8 (p<0.05) F: 0.7 (p<0.05)	NE	Age	Population-based

Table 39 (contd)

Author, date, study location	Study dates	No. of cases	Activity definition (no. of categories)	Relative risk (highest vs lowest categories) (95% CI)	Trend*	Adjustment for confounding	Comments
Gerhardsson de Verdier et al. (1990a), Sweden	1986–88	M+F: 352	Total work and leisure activity (3)	0.6 (0.3–1.0)	NE	Age, gender, BMI, energy, fat, protein, fibre, browning of meat	Population-based
Kato et al. (1990), Japan	1979–87	M: 756	Occupational codes (3)	0.6 (0.5–0.7)	Yes	Age	Hospital-based
Whittemore et al. (1990), Chinese in North America and China	1981–86	North America M: 179 F: 114 China M: 95 F: 78	Sedentary lifestyle (2)	North America M: 0.6 (0.4–0.9) F: 0.5 (0.3–0.8) China: M: 1.2 (0.5–2.6) F: 0.4 (0.2–1.0)	NE	Age	Population-based
Markowitz et al. (1992), USA	1985–90	M: 307	Occupational activity (3)	0.5 (0.3–0.8)	Yes	Age, race, geographical area, recreational activity at age 22–44 y	Hospital-based
Fraser & Pearce (1993), New Zealand	1972–80	M: 1651	Last occupation at registry (3)	0.8 (0.7–1.0)	NE	Age	Population-based
Marcus et al. (1994), USA	1990–91	F: 536	Participation in vigorous activity at ages 14–22 yrs (5)	≥ 7 times/wk: 0.46 (0.19–1.1) Any activity 1.0 (0.82–1.3)	No	Age, family history, screening, BMI	Population-based
Longnecker et al. (1995), USA	1986–88	M: 163	Occupational (3) and vigorous recreational activity (4)	Occupation 0.68 (0.31–1.5) Leisure 0.57 (0.33–0.97)	No Yes	BMI, family history, income race, smoking, alcohol, energy, fat, fibre, calcium	Population-based
White et al. (1996), USA	1985–89	M: 251 F: 193	Moderate/intense recreational activity (5); Occupational activity (3)	Total: M: 0.79 (0.48–1.3) F: 0.71 (0.39–1.3) Intense: M: 0.57 (0.35–0.92) F: 0.74 (0.43–1.3) Occupation: M: 0.84 (0.52–1.4) F: 0.89 (0.46–1.7)	No (M+F) Yes No No (M+F)	Age	Population-based

Table 39 (contd)

Author, date, study location	Study dates	No. of cases	Activity definition (no. of categories)	Relative risk (highest vs lowest categories) (95% CI)	Trend*	Adjustment for confounding	Comments
Slattery et al. (1997a,b), USA	1991–94	M: 1099 F: 894	Occupational (3), household and recreational activity 2 yrs before diagnosis, 10 and 20 yrs ago, by level of intensity (4 or 5)	Long-term vigorous: M: 0.61 (0.47–0.79) F: 0.63 (0.48–0.82) Total recent: M: 0.90 (0.70–1.2) F: 0.91 (0.67–1.2) Total recent vigorous: M: 0.71 (0.55–0.92) F: 0.88 (0.69–1.1) Occupation: M: 0.98 (0.77–1.2) F: 1.1 (0.87–1.4)	Yes	Age, BMI, energy, fibre, calcium, NSAIDs, family history of colorectal cancer	Population-based
Tavani et al. (1999), Italy	1991–96	M: 688 F: 537	Occupational activity at different ages (5)	15–19 yrs: M: 0.47 (0.31–0.71) F: 0.62 (0.44–0.89) 30–39 yrs: M: 0.64 (0.44–0.93) F: 0.49 (0.33–0.72) 50–59 yrs: M: 0.69 (0.45–1.0) F: 0.75 (0.47–1.2)	Yes	Age, energy, alcohol, education, centre	Hospital-based
Rectal cancer, case–control studies							
Garabrant et al. (1984), USA	1972–81	M: 1213	Occupational title (3)	1.0 (0.8–1.3)	No	Age	Population-based
Gerhardsson de Verdier et al. (1990a), Sweden	1986–88	M+F: 217	Total work and leisure activity (3)	1.0 (0.5–2.0)	NE	Age, BMI, calories, fat, protein fibre, browning of meat, gender	Population-based
Kato et al. (1990), Japan	1979–87	M: 753	Occupational codes (3)	0.8 (0.6–1.0)	Yes	Age	Hospital-based
Whittemore et al. (1990), Chinese in North America and China	1981–86	N: Amer. M: 105 F: 75 China M: 131 F: 128	Occupation and sedentary lifestyle (2)	North America: M: 0.67 (0.4–1.1) F: 0.53 (0.27–1.0) China: M: 1.4 (0.63–3.1) F: 1.4 (0.71–2.9)	NE	Age	Population-based

Table 39 (contd)

Author, date, study location	Study dates	No. of cases	Activity definition (no. of categories)	Relative risk (highest vs lowest categories) (95% CI)	Trend*	Adjustment for confounding	Comments
Markowitz et al. (1992), USA	1985–90	M: 133	Occupational activity (3)	0.6 (0.3–1.1)	No	Age, race, geographical area, recreational activity at age 22–44 y	Hospital-based
Fraser & Pearce (1993), New Zealand	1972–80	M: 1046	Last occupation at registry (3)	0.8 (0.7–1.0)	NE	Age	Population-based
Longnecker et al. (1995), USA	1986–88	M: 242	Occupational (3) and recreational activity (4)	Occupation: 0.99 (0.44–2.2) Leisure: 1.2 (0.70–2.0)	No	BMI, family history, income, race, smoking, alcohol energy, fat, fibre, calcium	Population-based
Le Marchand et al. (1997), USA	1987–91	M: 221 F: 129	Lifetime recreational activity and occupational activity (3)	Recreational M: 0.5, p = 0.07 F: 0.8, p = 0.97 Occupational: M: 0.8, p = 0.49 F: 1.1, p = 0.87	NE NE	Age, family history of colorectal cancer, alcohol, cigarettes, eggs, dietary fibre, calcium, energy, BMI	Population-based
Levi et al. (1999a), Switzerland	1992–97	M+F: 104	Occupational activity at 30–39 yrs (3)	0.49 (0.26–0.92)	No	Age, sex, education, alcohol and energy intake	Hospital-based
Tavani et al. (1999), Italy	1991–96	M: 435 F: 286	Occupational activity, at different ages (4)	Occupational 30–39 M: 1.3 (0.86–2.0) F: 0.88 (0.48–1.6)	No	Age, energy, alcohol, education, centre	Hospital-based

* Either a significant test for trend or significant intermediate relative risks for intermediate exposure categories

colorectal cancer, BMI, alcohol intake and diet.

A study conducted in the Seattle–Puget Sound area of Washington State, USA (White *et al.*, 1996) included 251 male and 193 female cases and 233 male and 194 female controls identified by random-digit dialling. Physical activity was assessed by questions on frequency and duration of types of recreational and occupational activities during the 10-year period ending two years before diagnosis. After adjustment for age, a reduced risk of colon cancer was observed for men and women who reported two or more sessions of moderate- or high-intensity activity per week (OR = 0.70; 95% CI 0.49–1.0) relative to those without any activity. Further adjustment for sex, BMI, dietary factors and other health-related behaviours did not significantly modify the risk estimates. Associations were slightly stronger for men aged less than 55 years at the time of diagnosis (OR = 0.29; 95% CI 0.12–0.69 for ≥14.5 hours per week of moderate activity versus none).

A US multi-centre study of 1099 male and 894 female cases of colon cancer and 1290 male and 1120 female controls was conducted in the Kaiser Permanente Medical Care Program of northern California, an eight-county area of Utah and the Twin Cities area of Minnesota (Slattery *et al.*, 1997b). A questionnaire was used to assess recreational and occupational activity; activities performed at moderate and intense levels; and activities performed for the referent period of two years before diagnosis as well as activities performed 10 and 20 years ago. Long-term intense activity was the best predictor of colon cancer risk (OR = 0.61; 95% CI 0.47–0.79 for men; OR = 0.63; 95% CI 0.48–0.82 for women). Adjustment for other dietary and lifestyle factors did not alter the risk estimates. Interaction between BMI and total energy intake was observed, with physical activity having its greatest impact among those who having high energy intake and those who had higher BMI. Occupational activity was not associated with reduced risk of colon cancer (Slattery *et al.*, 1997a).

In a study in Hawaii among Japanese, Caucasian, Filipino and Chinese participants, 698 male and 494 female cases of newly diagnosed histologically confirmed large bowel cancer were matched to population-based controls (Le Marchand *et al.*, 1997). Lifetime physical activity was evaluated for recreational and occupational activity that included duration and intensity of activities performed. Reduced risk of colorectal cancer was observed for both men and women (men, OR = 0.6; 95%CI 0.4–0.8; women, OR = 0.7; 95% CI 0.5–1.1) after adjustment for age, BMI and lifestyle factors. As in the study by Slattery *et al.* (1997b), there was significant interaction between physical activity and BMI and energy intake for men.

Adenomas
Fewer studies have focused on adenomas than on adenocarcinomas. Associations for adenomas are less consistent between subgroups of the population than those observed in most studies of cancer (Neugut *et al.*, 1996; Little *et al.*, 1993). In some studies, associations with physical activity appear to be strongest and most consistent for large adenomas (Giovannucci *et al.*, 1995, 1996). In several studies, a 40% reduction in risk of colorectal adenomas has been observed (Sandler *et al.*, 1995; Giovannucci *et al.*, 1995, 1996; Lubin *et al.*,1997).

Discussion
As shown in Table 39, most studies have shown a consistent reduction in risk of colon cancer with increasing levels of activity; studies of rectal cancer and of colon and rectal cancers combined have given less consistent results. Consistent associations have been shown across diverse populations in Europe, Asia and America, with use of different indicators of physical activity. The magnitude of the risk reduction is consistently around 40% for colon cancer. It has been estimated from the results of a large multi-centre study in the USA that 13–14% of colon cancer may be attributable to physical inactivity (Slattery *et al.*, 1997a).

Several studies have shown a trend of decreasing risk of colon cancer with increasing levels of activity. Such a trend has been seen both for increasing intensity of activities and for increasing amounts of intense activity. The greatest reductions in colorectal cancer risk appear to be associated with level of intensity of activities performed (Slattery *et al.*, 1988; Marcus *et al.*, 1994; Longnecker *et al.*, 1995; White *et al.*, 1996; Slattery *et al.*, 1997b; Giovannucci *et al.*, 1995; Thune & Lund, 1996; Martinez *et al.*, 1997), total activity (Gerhardsson *et al.*, 1988; Slattery *et al.*, 1988; Severson *et al.*, 1989; Gerhardsson de Verdier *et al.*, 1990a) and/or long-term involvement in physical activity (Lee *et al.*, 1991; Slattery *et al.*, 1997b; Le Marchand *et al.*, 1997). The amount of activity to reduce risk is not clear, given the variety of methods used to assess activity, but it has been estimated that 30–60 minutes of more intense types of activities are needed to see the greatest effect in risk reduction (Slattery *et al.*, 1997a; White *et al.*, 1996; Marcus *et al.*, 1994; Wu *et al.*, 1987; Thune & Lund, 1996).

Overall, it appears that intense activity may be more protective against colon cancer than moderate levels of activity. While it is possible that intense activity stimulates biological mechanisms that moderate levels of activity do not, it is also possible that intense activities are reported better than moderate activities. In fact, data support the better long-term recall of intense activities than of moderate activities (Slattery & Jacobs, 1995). Misclassification of moderate activities would decrease ability to detect real associations.

Long-term involvement in activity appears to be an important predictor of colorectal cancer risk. It is not clear if those who are more active over long periods of time report their activity more accurately, or if long-term involvement in activity increases protection over a long period of time. Results of studies that show inverse associations between physical activity and adenomas provide support for a long-term benefit of physical activity.

As shown in Table 39, the studies have differed in the number and types of adjustment factors used to assess associations. Studies that have attempted to adjust for factors associated with risk of colon cancer, such as body size, diet, age, cigarette smoking status, use of aspirin and sunshine exposure, have not reported that the associations were confounded (Ballard-Barbash et al., 1990c; Giovannucci et al., 1995; Le Marchand et al., 1997; Martinez et al., 1997; Slattery et al., 1997b). Also, given the consistency of the association between studies of colon cancer, it is likely that confounding contributes little to the observed associations. An evaluation of both cases and controls for reduced ability to exercise because of illness (Slattery et al. 1997a) suggests that cases do not report lower levels of past activities as a result of the tumour itself.

Studies to evaluate effect modification (Slattery et al., 1997b, c) have shown that physical activity may most importantly reduce risk of colon cancer in the presence of high levels of energy intake, a high glycaemic index or large body size.

Breast cancer

Results for cohort and case–control studies with more than 100 cases are summarized in Table 40. More detailed descriptions are provided in the text of studies that had relatively good measures of physical activity, used incident cases, had good follow-up (cohort studies) or

response rates (case–control studies) and adjusted for known and possible confounders of the association. No studies on physical activity in breast cancer among men have been reported.

Cohort studies

A few preliminary reports from cohort studies were not reviewed because the results were updated in a subsequent paper. This applies to the College Alumni Health Study (Paffenbarger et al., 1987, updated by Sesso et al., 1998), the National Health and Nutrition Examination I Survey (NHANES I) cohort (Albanes et al., 1989, updated by Steenland et al., 1995) and a Finnish cohort of teachers (Vihko et al., 1992, updated by Pukkala et al., 1993). The first report from the college graduates by Frisch et al. (1985) had only 69 cases, but in the later update by Wyshak and Frisch (2000) the size of the original cohort had decreased substantially, so that a 'healthy survivor' effect may have influenced the second follow-up results.

Of 14 separate cohort studies reviewed (Table 40), eight observed an inverse association between physical activity and breast cancer risk (Vena et al., 1987; Zheng et al., 1993b; Fraser & Shavlik, 1997; Thune et al., 1997; Sesso et al., 1998; Rockhill et al., 1999; Moradi et al., 1999; Wyshak & Frisch, 2000). The risk decreases ranged from 50–70% in the studies by Thune et al. (1997) and Sesso et al. (1998) to 20–30% in the studies by Vena et al. (1987), Zheng et al. (1993b), Fraser & Shavlik (1997), Rockhill et al. (1999) and Moradi et al. (1999). No association was found between physical activity in the follow-up study of the NHANES I cohort (Steenland et al., 1995), in the Nurses' Health Study II cohort that included premenopausal women only (Rockhill et al., 1998), in the Cancer Prevention II Study cohort (Calle et al., 1998a) and in the Iowa Women's cohort study (Moore et al., 2000a). Increased standardized incidence ratios for breast cancer were

observed in the Finnish teachers cohort study for physical education and language teachers compared with the total Finnish population (Pukkala et al., 1993). The follow-up of the Framingham Heart Study cohort also found an increased breast cancer risk among women who had the highest overall score on a physical activity index (Dorgan et al., 1994). However, both of these studies that observed an increased risk of breast cancer had limitations in the methods used for assessment of physical activity.

Thune et al. (1997) studied a cohort of 25 624 Norwegian women from three population-based surveys conducted in 1974–78 and 1977–83. The women were aged 20–54 years at baseline and 351 cases were identified during the follow-up to 1994, with 100% follow-up achieved. A self-administered questionnaire was used to measure current occupational and recreational activity. Risk was statistically significantly reduced with higher occupational and recreational activity and evidence was seen for a dose–response relationship. The multivariate relative risk for women who were consistently active versus those who were sedentary for recreational activity was 0.6 (95% CI 0.4–1.0). For regularly exercising women aged less than 45 years at baseline, the risk was 0.38 (95% CI 0.19–0.79) and for women who were in the lowest BMI tertile, the risk for recreational activity was 0.3 (95% CI 0.1–0.7). Risk reductions were found for both pre- and postmenopausal women, but the associations were stronger and statistically significant for premenopausal women.

Rockhill et al. (1998) analysed physical activity and breast cancer in the Nurses' Health Study II cohort of 116 671 nurses aged 25–42 years (mostly premenopausal) in 1989 at baseline, who were followed up for six years. No association with recreational activity performed during late adolescence or in the recent past was found.

Table 40. Studies of physical activity and risk of breast cancer

Author, date, study location	Study dates	No. of cases	Activity definition (no. of categories)	Relative risk (highest vs lowest categories) (95% CI)	Trend*	Adjustment for confounding	Comments
Cohort studies							
Vena et al. (1987), USA	1974–79	791	Usual lifetime occupational activity from death certificate (3)	PMR = 0.85, $p < 0.05$	NE	Age	Mortality study
Pukkala et al. (1993), Finland	1967–91	228	Current occupational title	SIR (vs general population) for: Physical activity teachers: 1.4 (1.0–1.9) Language teachers: 1.5 (1.3–1.7)	NE	Age	Based on national incidence figures
Zheng et al. (1993b), China	1980–84	2736	Current occupational activity from job title and index of sitting and energy expenditure (3)	SIR = 0.79, $p<0.01$	Yes	Age	Based on occupational data on census
Dorgan et al. (1994), USA	1954–88	117	Index of all types of physical activity performed in a day (4)	1.6 (0.9–2.9)	Yes	Age, age at FFTP, parity, menopausal status, alcohol intake, education, occupation	
Steenland et al. (1995), USA	1971–87	163	Current recreational and non-recreational activity (3)	1.1 (0.6–2.0)	NE	Age, BMI, smoking, alcohol, income, diabetes, menopausal status, recreational activity	NHANES I study
Fraser & Shavlik (1997), USA	1976–82	218	Current vigorous recreational and occupational activity (2)	0.7 (0.5–0.9)	NE	Age, age at FFTP, oral contraceptive and hormone replacement therapy use, family history, benign breast disease, energy and fat intake	Seventh-Day Adventists
Thune et al. (1997), Norway	1974–94	351	Current recreational (3) and occupational (4) activity	R: 0.6 (0.4–1.0) 0: 0.5 (0.3–0.9)	Yes	Age at entry, parity, BMI, height, county of residence	Age 20–54 years

Table 40 (contd)

Author, date, study location	Study dates	No. of cases	Activity definition (no. of categories)	Relative risk (highest vs lowest categories) (95% CI)	Trend*	Adjustment for confounding	Comments
Calle et al. (1998a), USA	1982–91	1780	Usual lifetime occupational activity	Housewives vs administratives: 1.1 (0.8–1.3)	NE	Age, age at menarche, age at FFTP, age at menopause, parity, BMI, benign breast disease, family history, oral contraceptive use, hormone replacement therapy use, smoking, alcohol, education, race, exercise	Mortality study
Rockhill et al. (1998), USA	1989–95	372	Recent recreational vigorous activity	1.1 (0.8–1.6)	No	Age, age at menarche, age at FFTP, parity, BMI, height, benign breast disease, family history, oral contraceptive use, alcohol consumption	Age 25–42 years
Sesso et al. (1998), USA	1962–93	109	Physical activity index composed of current recreational activity, blocks walked, stairs climbed (3)	0.7 (0.5–1.1)	Yes	Age, BMI	University alumnae
Moradi et al. (1999), Sweden	1960–89	51520	Current occupational titles classified by intensity (4)	0.9 (0.8–1.0)	No	Age in five-year intervals, place of residence, calendar year of follow-up, socio-economic status	Three overlapping cohorts from national census
Rockhill et al. (1999), USA	1976–92	3137	Current recreational activity (5)	0.8 (0.7–1.0)	Yes	Age, age at menarche, age at FFTP, parity, BMI at age 18, height menopausal status/ use of hormone replacement therapy, benign breast disease, family history, oral contraceptive use in premenopausal models	Age 30–55 years
Moore et al. (2000a), USA	1986–97	1362	Current recreational activity (4)	0.9 (0.8–1.0)	No	Age, age at menopause, age at FFTP, BMI at age 18 y, education, family history, estrogen use	Age 55–69 years
Wyshak & Frisch (2000), USA	1981–96	175	Recreational activity in college (2)	0.6 (0.4–0.8)	NE	Age, parity, oral contraceptive and hormone replacement therapy use, family history, current exercise, smoking, per cent body fat	College alumnae

Table 40 (contd)						
Author, date, study location	Study dates	No. of cases	Activity definition (no. of categories)	Relative risk (highest vs lowest categories) (95% CI)	Trend*	Adjustment for confounding	Comments
Case–control studies							
Dosemeci et al. (1993), Turkey	1979–84	241	Occupational titles to estimate average energy expenditure and sitting time over lifetime (2)	Energy: 0.7 (0.2–3.4) Sitting time: 1.0 (0.4–2.5)	No	Age, smoking and socio-economic status	Hospital-based
Bernstein et al. (1994), USA	1983–89	545	Lifetime recreational activity of at least 2h/wk (4)	Current activity 0.4 (0.3–0.6)	Yes	Age, age at menarche, age at FFTP, number of FFTPs, breastfeeding, oral contraceptive use, family history, BMI	Population-based age <40 years
Friedenreich & Rohan (1995), Australia	1982–84	444	Current recreational activity converted into kcal/wk expended (4)	0.7 (0.5–1.1)	No	Age, BMI and energy intake	Population-based
Hirose et al. (1995), Japan	1988–92	1063	Current recreational activity (3)	Premenopausal: 0.7 (0.6–1.0) Postmenopausal: 0.7 (0.5–1.0)	Yes	Age, age at menarche, age at FFTP, breastfeeding, BMI, height, smoking, alcohol intake, some dietary components (e.g., meats, vegetables)	Hospital-based
Mittendorf et al. (1995), USA	1988–91	6888	Strenuous recreational activity at ages 14–18 and 18–22 yrs (4)	0.5 (0.4–0.7)	Yes	Age, state, age at menarche, age at FFTP, parity, age at menopause, menopausal status, type of menopause, family history, benign breast disease, BMI, alcohol intake, interaction of BMI and menopausal status	Population-based
Taioli et al. (1995), USA	1987–90	617	Strenuous recreational activity at different ages (2)	15–21: 1.0 (0.6–1.8)	NE	Age, age at menarche, parity, education, BMI	Hospital-based controls

Table 40 (contd)

Author, date, study location	Study dates	No. of cases	Activity definition (no. of categories)	Relative risk (highest vs lowest categories) (95% CI)	Trend*	Adjustment for confounding	Comments
Coogan et al. (1996), USA	1988–91	6835	Usual lifetime occupational title	Administrative support occupation: 1.2 (1.1–1.2)	NE	Age, age at menarche, age at FFTP, parity, lactation, BMI, benign breast disease, family history, menopausal status, alcohol consumption, state education	Population-based All other occupation categories not associated with breast cancer Secondary analysis of Mittendorf et al. (1995)
D'Avanzo et al. (1996b), Italy	1991–94	2569	Occupational and recreational activity at different ages (5)	15–19 years: R: 1.0 (0.8–1.2) O: 0.8 (0.5–1.4) 30–39 years: R: 0.8 (0.6–1.1) O: 0.6 (0.4–1.0) 50–59 years: R: 0.7 0.4–1.1) O: 0.8 (0.4–1.5)	Yes	Age, age at menarche, age at FFTP, parity, age at menopause, menopausal status family history, benign breast disease, BMI, smoking, energy intake, education, centre	Hospital-based
McTiernan et al. (1996), USA	1988–90	537	Recreational activity 2 years before interview (3)	All women: 0.6 (0.4–1.0) Postmenopausal: 0.6 (0.3–0.9)	Yes	Age and education	Population-based
Chen et al. (1997), USA	1983–90	747	Recreational activity at ages 12–21 and 2 years before interview (5)	Two years before: 0.9 (0.7–1.2) 12–21 years: 1.1 (0.8–1.7)	No	Age	Population-based
Coogan et al. (1997), USA	1988–91	4863	Usual lifetime occupational activity (4)	0.8 (0.6–1.1)	Yes	Age, age at menarche, age at FFTP, menopausal status family history, benign breast disease, BMI, education, and alcohol intake, state, recreational activity at age 14–22 y	Population-based Secondary analysis of Mittendorf et al. (1995)
Hu et al. (1997), Japan	1989–93	157	Recreational activity in adolescence and in twenties (3)	Adolescence: Premenopausal: 0.7 (0.4–1.4)	No	Age	Population-based

Table 40 (contd)

Author, date, study location	Study dates	No. of cases	Activity definition (no. of categories)	Relative risk (highest vs lowest categories) (95% CI)	Trend*	Adjustment for confounding	Comments
Hu et al. (contd)				Postmenopausal: 1.4 (0.6–3.1) Twenties: Premenopausal: 1.0 (0.5–1.9) Postmenopausal: 0.5 (0.2–1.5)			
Gammon et al. (1998), USA	1990–92	1647	Recreational activity at ages 12–13, 20 and yr before interview (4)	12–13 years: 1.0 (0.8–1.2) 20 years: 1.1 (0.9–1.4) Year before interview: 1.1 (0.9–1.4)	No	Age, centre, age at menarche, age at FFTP, parity, lactation, abortions, miscarriages, menopausal status, marital status, education, family income race, BMI at age 20 y and adulthood, oral contraceptive and hormone replacement therapy use, alcohol, smoking, energy intake in past year, history of breast biopsy, family history	Population-based
Mezzetti et al. (1998), Italy	1991–94	2569	Occupational title at different ages (3)	30–39 years All women 0.7 (0.5–0.9) Premenopausal: 0.7 (0.5–1.1) Postmenopausal: 0.6 (0.4–0.9)	Yes	Age, centre, β-carotene, vitamin E, alcohol, BMI, energy intake, education, menopausal status	Hospital-based Re-analysis of D'Avanzo et al. (1996b)
Ueji et al. (1998), Japan	1990–97	139	Lifetime recreational activity (3) and most representative lifetime occupational activity (4)	Recreational activity: 0.4 (0.2–0.7) Occupational activity: 0.6 (0.3–1.1)	Yes No	Age, age at menarche, age at FFTP, menopausal status, parity, BMI, height, family history, education	Population-based
Carpenter et al., (1999), USA	1987–89	1123	Lifetime recreational activity of at least 2 h/wk (3)	0.6 (0.4–0.8)	Yes	Age, age at menarche, age at FFTP, age a menopause, BMI family history, interviewer	Population-based Age 55–64 yrs

Table 40 (contd)

Author, date, study location	Study dates	No. of cases	Activity definition (no. of categories)	Relative risk (highest vs lowest categories) (95% CI)	Trend*	Adjustment for confounding	Comments
Coogan & Aschengrau (1999), USA	1983–86	233	Lifetime occupational activity (3)	0.9 (0.4–1.9)	No	Age, vital status, education, total duration of work	Population-based
Levi et al. (1999b) Switzerland	1993–98	246	Recreational and occupational activity at different ages (3)	Recreational activity: 15–19 yrs: 0.4 (0.3–0.7) 30–39 yrs: 0.5 (0.3–0.8) 50–59 yrs: 0.4 (0.2–0.8) Occupational activity: 15–19 yrs: 0.6 (0.4–1.0) 30–39 yrs: 0.5 (0.3–1.0) 50–59 yrs: 0.7 (0.4–1.3)	Yes	Age, age at menarche, age at FFTP, age at menopause, parity, menopausal status, benign breast disease, family history, energy intake, education	Hospital-based
Marcus et al. (1999), USA	1993–96	527 white and 337 African-American	Recreational and household activity at age 12 converted into summary measure (5)	0.6 (0.3–1.1)	No	Age at diagnosis, race, sampling design	Population-based
Moradi et al. (2000a), Sweden	1993–95	2838	Childhood (< 18 yrs) and adult (18–30 yrs) and current recreational activity (4)	Childhood: 1.0 (0.9–1.3) 18–30 yrs: 0.9 (0.8–1.1) Recent: 0.8 (0.7–0.9)	No No Yes	Age, age at menarche, parity, age at FFTP, age at menopause, BMI, height, hormone replacement therapy use, oral contraceptive use	Population-based
Shoff et al. (2000), USA	1988–91	4614	Strenuous recreational activity at ages 14–18 and 18–22 yrs (4)	0.6 (0.4–0.8)	Yes	Age, age at menarche, age at FFTP, parity, age at menopause, BMI at age 18, family history, education	Population-based Secondary analysis of Mittendorf et al. (1995)
Verloop et al. (2000), Netherlands	1986–89	918	Lifetime recreational activity and title of longest job held (4)	0.6 (0.4–0.8)	NE	Age, education, family history	Population-based

Table 40 (contd)

Author, date, study location	Study dates	No. of cases	Activity definition (no. of categories)	Relative risk (highest vs lowest categories) (95% CI)	Trend*	Adjustment for confounding	Comments
Friedenreich et al. (2001a, b, c), Canada	1995–97	1233	Lifetime occupational, household, recreational activity (4)	Premenopausal women: 1.1 (0.7–1.6) Postmenopausal women: 0.7 (0.5–0.9)	No Yes	Age, hormone replacement therapy use, history of benign breast disease, family history, alcohol, smoking, waist/hip ratio, education	Population-based

PMR, proportional mortality ratio; OR, odds ratio; RR, relative risk; SIR, standardized incidence ratio; FFTP, first full-term pregnancy; BMI, body mass index; MET, metabolic equivalent
* Either a significant test for trend or significant intermediate relative risks for intermediate exposure categories

Rockhill *et al.* (1999) reported on the Nurses' Health Study I cohort of 121 701 women aged 30–55 years in 1976. Between 1980, when physical activity data were first collected and 1996, 3137 women were diagnosed with breast cancer, with 94% follow-up achieved. Breast cancer risks were slightly decreased among women who reported moderate or vigorous recreational activity levels compared with women who had low activity levels. The associations were nearly identical for pre- and post-menopausal women and there was no statistical interaction between menopausal status and cumulative average adult physical activity.

In the Iowa Women's Health Study, 37 105 postmenopausal study subjects aged 55–69 years at baseline in 1986 were followed to 1997, at which time 1380 women were diagnosed with breast cancer, with 79% follow-up (Moore *et al.,* 2000a). A self-administered questionnaire was used to measure current recreational activity at baseline and no follow-up assessments were made. No effect of physical activity on breast cancer risk was found.

Case–control studies
Several publications on different aspects of the certain case–control studies have been published. Thus, D'Avanzo *et al.* (1996b) first published results from a multi-centre case–control study in Italy, later extended by Mezzetti *et al.* (1998). Mittendorf *et al.* (1995) published the first results on recreational activity from a multi-centre case–control study conducted in four US states. Two subsequent publications from this study considered risk by occupation (Coogan *et al.*, 1996) and by occupational activity (Coogan *et al.*, 1997). The most recent publication from this study examined the effect of body size, weight change and early-life physical activity on risk of post-menopausal breast cancer (Shoff *et al.,* 2000). Bernstein *et al.* (1994) published data from a case–control study of

women up to age 40 years and Carpenter *et al.* (1999) published data from another case–control study in California of women aged 55–64 years. The data from these two case–control studies were combined into a subsequent analysis by Enger *et al.* (2000) that examined the influence of body size, physical activity and breast cancer hormone receptor status on breast cancer risk.

Of 19 separate case–control studies (Table 40) that have reported data on physical activity and breast cancer risk, 14 found an inverse association (Bernstein *et al.*, 1994; Friedenreich & Rohan, 1995; Hirose *et al.*, 1995; Mittendorf *et al.*, 1995; D'Avanzo *et al.*, 1996b; McTiernan *et al.*, 1996; Hu *et al.,* 1997; Ueji *et al.*, 1998; Carpenter *et al.*, 1999; Levi *et al.*, 1999b; Marcus *et al.*, 1999; Moradi *et al.*, 2000a; Verloop *et al.*, 2000; Friedenreich *et al.*, 2001a, b, c). The papers from two population-based case–control studies in California among premenopausal women (Bernstein *et al.,* 1994) and postmeno-pausal women (Carpenter *et al.*, 1999) and the further stratified analyses of these data by BMI and hormone receptor status (Enger *et al.*, 2000) all reported strong risk reductions ranging from 40 to 60%. The risk reductions were even greater among certain subgroups of the study populations; for example, parous premenopausal women had a risk of 0.3 (95% CI 0.2–0.5) (Bernstein *et al.*, 1994).

Equally strong risk reductions were reported by Mittendorf *et al.* (1995) for recreational activity during adolescence and early adulthood. The subsequent analyses of the occupational data from this study found either no association with occupational title (Coogan *et al.*, 1996) or a decreased risk for usual occu-pational activity performed over lifetime (Coogan *et al.*, 1997). A further stratified analysis of recreational activity in early life (Shoff *et al.*, 2000) on this data-set confirmed the initial findings by Mittendorf *et al.* (1995).

Similarly, strong breast cancer risk decreases were observed for occupa-tional and recreational activity performed during three time periods in life in the study by D'Avanzo *et al.* (1996b). These were confirmed in additional analyses of these data by Mezzetti *et al.* (1998), who presented only the occupational activity data for women at age 30–39 years, but provided more stratified analyses by menopausal status. McTiernan *et al.* (1996) observed strong risk reductions for recreational activity performed between adolescence and early adult-hood. Likewise, particularly strong risk decreases have been noted for lifetime recreational activity (Ueji *et al.,* 1998) and for recreational and occupational activity at different time periods of life (Levi *et al.,* 1999b). Strong risk reduc-tions were also found by Friedenreich *et al.* (2001a, b, c) for lifetime total physical activity, with the greatest reductions noted for occupational (0.59; 95% CI 0.44–0.81) and household activity (0.57; 95% CI 0.41–0.79) after menopause.

Bernstein *et al.* (1994) conducted a population-based case–control study among 545 cases and matched neigh-bourhood controls in California, USA. An interview-administered questionnaire was used to measure lifetime recre-ational activity in premenopausal women who were aged 40 years or less at the time of the interview. The initial study sample of 744 pairs was reduced to 545 pairs when the the method for recording physical activity was changed during the study. The response rate for the original sample of 744 cases was 78.4% and was not estimated for the controls because of the complex sampling strategy used to identify eligible controls. A statistically significant decrease in risk was found for women who performed 3.8 hours per week of recreational activity versus those who did none (OR = 0.4; 95% CI 0.3–0.6). The risk reduction was even stronger among physically active than among inactive parous women (OR = 0.28; 95% CI 0.16–0.50). Evidence of a dose–response effect was found. Adjustment for confounding and examination of effect modification were performed, but no data on dietary intake were available.

Carpenter et al. (1999) conducted a similar case–control study in California, USA, using the same recruitment and data collection methods as Bernstein et al. (1994). A total of 1579 cases (69% of eligible patients) and 1506 controls were interviewed; the analysis was restricted to 1123 cases and 904 controls who were postmenopausal. The subjects were 55–64 years old at the interview. The response rate for cases was 67% and for controls was not estimated. Significantly decreased risks of breast cancer were found for women who performed 17.6 MET-hours per week or more of recreational activity compared with those who did none (OR = 0.6; 95% CI 0.4–0.8), for women who exercised for four hours per week for at least 12 years (OR = 0.71; 95% CI 0.52–0.96) and for those who exercised vigorously during the most recent 10 years (OR = 0.71; 95% CI 0.48–1.1). Risk reductions were also stronger among women who had less than 17% change in body weight during adulthood. No adjustment for dietary intake was possible. A dose–response effect was seen.

Mittendorf et al. (1995) conducted a multi-centre population-based case–control study in the USA among women aged 17–74 years. A total of 6888 cases and 9539 controls were included. Response rates were 81% for cases and 84% for controls. A telephone interview was used to assess strenuous recreational activity at ages 14–18 and 18–22 years. A statistically significant decreased risk was associated with strenuous versus no strenuous recreational activity in the total study population (OR = 0.5; 95% CI 0.4–0.7). This risk reduction was greater among women over 40 years of age than those under 40 and no effect modification by parity or menopausal status was found. A dose–response

effect was seen. Full adjustment for confounding was made, although no data on dietary intake were available.

D'Avanzo et al. (1996b) conducted a multi-centre hospital-based case–control study in Italy in 1991–94 with women aged 23–74 years at interview. A total of 2569 cases and 2588 non-cancer controls were included and over 95% response rates were obtained. An interview-administered questionnaire was used to assess occupational and recreational activity at ages 15–19, 30–39 and 50–59 years. Non-significant decreased risks of breast cancer were found for activity performed at most of these time periods, except for occupational activity between ages 30–39 years, for which a risk of 0.6 (95% CI 0.4–1.0) was estimated. Evidence for a dose–response effect was found. Detailed adjustment for confounding was performed. Mezzetti et al. (1998) further analysed the data on occupational activity at age 30–39 years and found somewhat stronger risk reductions among postmenopausal women, for whom the risk was 0.6 (95% CI 0.4–0.9), but no effect modification on menopausal status was seen.

McTiernan et al. (1996) conducted a population-based case–control study in the state of Washington, USA, in 1988–90 among women aged 50–64 years at baseline. The study included 537 cases (81% of eligible) and 492 controls (73% of eligible). An interview-administered questionnaire was used to assess recreational activity performed between ages 12–21 years and two years before the interview. A borderline statistically significant decreased risk was found among women who performed high-intensity exercise during adulthood (OR = 0.6; 95% CI 0.4–1.0) compared with those who did no exercise. The effects were somewhat stronger for postmenopausal women (≥ 55 years of age only), for whom the risk was 0.6 (95% CI 0.3–0.9) among those who spent at least three hours weekly doing high-intensity exercise

compared with those who did none. Evidence for a dose–response effect was found and full adjustment was made for confounding.

A similar population-based case–control study conducted by Chen et al. (1997) in the state of Washington, USA, in 1983–90 used the same population sampling and data collection methods as were used by McTiernan et al. (1996). This study included premenopausal women aged 21–45 years at the time of the interview. No effect of physical activity was found; adjustment for age only was performed, although several other factors were considered with the exception of dietary intake. In the studies by Chen et al. (1997) and McTiernan et al. (1996) and the two cohort studies by Rockhill et al. (1998, 1999), the same study methods were used and all four found no effect of physical activity among premenopausal women but a risk reduction among postmenopausal study subjects.

Another multi-centre population-based case–control study conducted by Gammon et al. (1998) in the USA, with 1668 cases (86% of eligible) and 3173 controls (79% of eligible) and similar study methods to Chen et al. (1997), also found no effect of physical activity on breast cancer risk. The study subjects were premenopausal women under 45 years of age who reported the frequency of recreational activity at ages 12–13 and 20 years and in the preceding year. Detailed adjustment was made for all confounders.

A population-based case–control study by Marcus et al. (1999) in North Carolina, USA, included 527 white and 337 African American cases (77% of eligible) and 790 (68% of eligible) controls. An interview-administered questionnaire was used to assess recreational and household activity at age 12 years. Some evidence of risk reduction was found for the different summary measures of activity used, but no dose–response effect was detected. Control for confounding was made for most risk factors with the exception of dietary intake.

Verloop *et al.* (2000) conducted a population-based case–control study that included women aged 20–54 years in four regions of the Netherlands. A total of 918 case–control pairs were studied, with 60% and 72% response rates for cases and controls respectively. An interview-administered questionnaire was used to assess lifetime recreational activity and the title of the longest-held job. Several measures of physical activity were reported and most of these were associated with statistically significant risk reductions for breast cancer. For women who maintained recreational activity throughout their lifetime, the risk was 0.70 (95% CI 0.56–0.88) and when recreational and occupational activities were combined into one measure, women who were in the highest versus the lowest category had a risk of 0.58 (95% CI 0.42–0.82). Adjustment was made for risk factors except dietary intake. Effect modification by several other factors was explored and greater risk decreases were found among women who were parous, who ever had benign breast disease, who were leaner (lowest tertile of BMI) or who had a first-degree family history of breast cancer.

Moradi *et al.* (2000a) conducted a population-based case–control study in Sweden of women aged 50–74 years. The sample included 2838 cases (71% of original sample) and 3108 controls (76% of original sample). Recreational activity during childhood, early adulthood and current activity was assessed by questionnaire and occupational status in each decade between 1960 and 1990 was obtained from Swedish census data. A statistically significant risk reduction was observed for women who were the most active in combined recreational and occupational activities compared with the least active (OR = 0.32; 95% CI 0.13–0.76). When each type of activity was considered separately, slight

decreases in risk of breast cancer were observed among the highest activity categories. Effect modification by BMI, parity and hormone replacement therapy was found. Greater postmenopausal breast cancer risk reductions were observed in association with occupational activity for nulliparous women and for leaner women (lowest tertile of BMI) who never used hormone replacement therapy. There was also evidence for a dose–response effect and adjustment for all confounders, except dietary intake, was performed.

Friedenreich *et al.* (2001a, b, c) conducted a population-based case–control study of women aged up to 84 years in Canada. The sample included 1233 cases (78% of eligible) and 1237 (56% of eligible). An interview-administered questionnaire was used to obtain lifetime physical activity patterns including all types of physical activity (i.e., occupational, household and recreational activity) from childhood until the reference year and all parameters of activity (i.e., frequency, intensity and duration). A 30% decreased risk of breast cancer was found for high total lifetime activity and even greater risk reductions (OR = 0.6; 95% CI 0.4–0.8) were observed for both occupational and household activity after menopause. The risk decreases were observed for postmenopausal women only, with no associations found for premenopausal women. Risk reductions were also noted for non-drinkers, non-smokers and nulliparous women. The reductions were particularly strong for activity done after menopause. In terms of patterns of activity, the greatest reductions were observed for activity sustained throughout lifetime and for activity done between menopause and the reference year. There was no linear association between intensity of activity and breast cancer risk, with the most notable risk reductions occurring for moderate-intensity activity. This was the first study that examined all types of activity and all

parameters of activity throughout women's lifetimes.

Discussion

Results regarding the association between physical activity and breast cancer have been fairly consistent, since 22 of the 33 separate studies (eight of the 14 cohort studies and in 14 of 19 case–control studies) have found inverse associations among the most physically active participants compared with the least active. The decrease in risk of breast cancer was, on average, about 20–40%, with some studies observing up to 70% risk reductions. Evidence for a linear trend in decreasing risk of breast cancer with increasing activity was evident in the majority of the studies that examined the dose–response relationship. These associations were observed for both occupational and recreational activity, among pre- and post-menopausal women, for activity measured at different time periods in life and for different levels of intensity of activity. Although the relevant data are limited, it appears that physical activity has similar effects within different populations. An effect of physical activity on breast cancer risk is biologically plausible, since physical activity has direct effects on prevention of weight gain and on postmenopausal obesity, both established breast cancer risk factors. Physical activity has an independent effect on breast cancer risk, aside from those of weight and weight gain, as shown in these studies.

Neither occupational nor non-occupational activity is consistently clearly associated with breast cancer risk reduction. This lack of a clear pattern may be attributable to differences in the physical activity assessment methods and definitions used across studies. Seven of 11 studies of breast cancer that measured occupational activity found risk decreases among the most physically active, while for non-occupational activity, the most physically active subjects had decreased breast cancer risk in 15 of 22 studies. All five of the studies that measured total activity showed risk decreases (Fraser & Shavlik, 1997; Thune et al. 1997; Sesso et al., 1998; Verloop et al., 2000; Friedenreich et al., 2001a). Hence, it appears that total physical activity may be the most etiologically relevant parameter.

The most important time period(s) in life for breast cancer etiology are also unknown. Activity that is sustained throughout lifetime, or at a minimum performed after menopause, may be particularly beneficial in reducing breast cancer risk. Some studies have attempted to measure activity throughout lifetime (Bernstein et al., 1994; Carpenter et al., 1999; Verloop et al., 2000; Friedenreich et al., 2001b) or at specific age periods (Mittendorf et al., 1995; D'Avanzo et al., 1996b; McTiernan et al., 1996; Chen et al., 1997; Gammon et al. 1998; Levi et al., 1999b). In these studies, the strongest risk reductions were observed for activity that was sustained throughout lifetime (Verloop et al., 2000; Friedenreich et al., 2001b); however, substantial risk decreases were also observed in studies of activity performed earlier in life (e.g., < 40 years (Bernstein et al., 1994)).

The frequency, intensity, duration of activity that are most associated with risk decreases have also not been systematically examined in all studies. There is inconclusive evidence for a dose–response relationship between increasing intensity of activity and decreasing risk of breast cancer. Indeed, some investigations that measured intensity of activity found the greatest risk decreases for moderate-intensity activity rather than vigorous-intensity activity. Several possible explanations include the low prevalence of high-intensity activity among general female study populations and misclassification of intensity levels. There is more evidence for a trend of decreasing risk with increasing frequency and duration of physical activity.

The 'dose' of physical activity required for breast cancer risk reduction can be estimated from those studies that provided sufficient detail on the activity performed at which risk decreases were observed (Bernstein et al., 1994; Mittendorf et al., 1995; McTiernan et al., 1996; Thune et al., 1997; Carpenter et al., 1999; Rockhill et al., 1999; Moradi et al., 2000a; Verloop et al., 2000; Friedenreich et al., 2001a, b, c). A total of 30–60 minutes of moderate- to vigorous-intensity activity is needed for breast cancer risk reduction. In countries where women achieve higher intensities of activity through occupational and household activities, these activities will be sufficient for breast cancer risk reduction. In countries where women perform sedentary or light occupational and household activities, moderate and vigorous recreational activities are likely to be needed to attain the levels of activity needed for breast cancer risk reduction.

Some of the inconsistencies observed across these studies may be attributable to limitations in the methods used for assessment of physical activity, as the assessment methods used may not have captured the most appropriate parameters of activity in the etiologically relevant periods of life.

Endometrial cancer
Cohort studies
Cohort studies on the relationship of physical activity and endometrial cancer that have included at least 50 cases are presented in Table 41. A prospective study conducted in Sweden found a decreased risk in women who reported "light exercise", "regular exercise" or "hard physical training" compared with those who reported no physical activity during leisure (Terry et al., 1999). Occupational physical activity, as assessed from the job title, was also inversely associated with endometrial cancer risk in another large cohort study in Swedish women (Moradi et al., 1998).

Case–control studies
Seven case–control studies conducted in the USA, Europe and Japan (Table 41) examined the association of physical activity and endometrial cancer (Levi et al., 1993; Shu et al., 1993; Sturgeon et al., 1993; Hirose et al., 1996; Goodman et al., 1997; Olson et al., 1997; Moradi et al., 2000b). All found an inverse association with either occupational or recreational physical activity. The most informative was a large case–control study which included all 709 women aged 50–74 years who were diagnosed with endometrial cancer in Sweden in 1994–95 and 3368 population controls (Moradi et al., 2000b). Information on leisure-time physical activity during childhood, at age 18–30 years and before diagnosis was obtained through mailed questionnaire. Occupational physical activity was estimated from job titles obtained from census information in various calendar years. Risk estimates were adjusted for potential confounders. Women in the highest leisure-time activity category at age 18–30 years were at slightly decreased risk of endometrial cancer (OR = 0.8). A similar decreased risk was found for women in the highest category for recent leisure activity. Inverse associations were also found for occupational physical activity. These associations appeared to be independent of BMI.

Discussion
The results of the limited number of cohort and case–control studies on physical activity and endometrial cancer are consistent in suggesting a 20–40% decrease in risk for the highest levels of physical activity. Most of these studies have taken into consideration other known risk factors for this disease, including body mass, making it unlikely that the observed association was due to confounding. Two studies that reported age-specific results did not suggest any difference in the association by age (Shu et al., 1993; Moradi et al., 1998).

Table 41. Studies on physical activity and risk of endometrial cancer

Author, date, study location	Study dates	No. of cases	Activity definition (no. of categories)	Relative risk (highest vs lowest categories) (95% CI)	Trend*	Adjustment for confounding	Comments
Cohort studies							
Zheng et al. (1993b), China	1980–84	452	Current occupational activity (3)	SIR = 80	NE	Age	Based on occupational data on census
Moradi et al. (1998), Sweden	1967–98	213 / 708 / 729 / 299	Occupational activity at different ages (4)	< 50 yrs: 1.4 (0.67–2.7); 50–59 yrs: 0.62 (0.42–0.91); 60–69 yrs: 0.62 (0.43–0.91); 70+ yrs: 1.6 (0.80–3.1)	No / Yes / Yes / No	Age, residence, socioeconomic status, period of follow-up	Based on national census
Terry et al. (1999), USA	1967–92	112	Recreational activity (4)	0.1 (0.04–0.6)	Yes	Age, weight, parity	Swedish twin registry
Case-control studies							
Levi et al. (1993), Italy and Switzerland	1988–91	274	Occupational / Recreational / Household activity (4)	0.7 (0.5–1.0) / 0.5 (0.3–1.1) / 0.2 (0.1–0.4)	Yes	BMI, age, education, reproductive factors, oral contraceptive and estrogen replacement therapy use, energy intake, study centre	Hospital-based
Shu et al. (1993), China	1988–90	268	Occupational: (4) All / ≤ 55 yrs	1.1 (0.63–1.7) / 0.62 (0.26–1.4)	No / No	Age, parity, BMI, energy intake	Population-based
Sturgeon et al. (1993), USA	1987–90	405	Recent recreational and non-recreational activity (3)	0.83 (0.50–1.4) / 0.50 (0.32–0.77)	NE / NE	Age, BMI, parity, oral contraceptive and hormone replacement therapy use, smoking, education, study area, recreational or non-recreational activity	Population-based
Hirose et al. (1996), Japan	1988–93	145	Recreational activity (3)	0.6 (0.4–0.9)	Yes	Age, first visit year	Hospital-based
Goodman et al. (1997), USA	1985–93	332	Recreational / Non-recreational (4)	0.9 / 0.7	No / No	Age, parity, oral contraceptive and hormone replacement therapy use, diabetes, BMI, total energy	Population-based

Table 41 (contd)

Author, date, study location	Study dates	No. of cases	Activity definition (no. of categories)	Relative risk (highest vs lowest categories) (95% CI)	Trend*	Adjustment for confounding	Comments
Olson et al. (1997), USA	1986–91	232	Vigorous exercise Occupational (3)	0.67 (0.42–1.1) 1.2 (0.76–1.9)	No	Age, reproductive factors, BMI, estrogen replacement therapy use, diabetes, smoking education	Population-based
Moradi et al. (2000b), Sweden	1994–95	709	Recreational Occupational at different ages (4)	Recent years: 0.8 (0.6–1.0) 0.8 (0.5–1.1)	Yes Yes	Age, parity, reproductive factors, BMI, oral contraceptive use, hormone replacement therapy use, smoking	Population-based

* Either a significant test for trend or significant intermediate relative risks for intermediate exposure categories

Ovarian cancer

Cohort studies

A small number of studies have assessed the association of physical activity with ovarian cancer (Table 42). A Finnish retrospective cohort study comparing cancer risk found an elevated ovarian cancer risk among physical education and language teachers compared with the general population, with no difference between the two groups (Pukkala et al., 1993). A cohort study in Shanghai found that women with occupations entailing high physical activity had the same ovarian cancer risk as women in low-activity occupations (Zheng et al., 1993b). In an analysis of the Iowa Women's Health Study based on 97 cases and seven years of follow-up, Mink et al. (1996) found a two-fold increase in risk of ovarian cancer among the most active compared with the least active. In this study, women were asked how often they participated in moderate and vigorous leisure activity. Those who participated in vigorous physical activity two or more times per week and those who participated in moderate activity more than four times per week were considered to have a high physical activity level, regardless of the duration of the activity.

Case–control studies

In a detailed study of physical activity and ovarian cancer, Cottreau et al. (2000) interviewed 767 women with ovarian cancer and 1367 population controls about the frequency and duration of their leisure-time activities during each decade of life since adolescence. They found an odds ratio for ovarian cancer of 0.73 (95% CI 0.56–0.94) for women with the highest lifetime level of activity compared with those having the lowest level of activity. When the association was examined by decade of life, the corresponding odds ratios ranged from 0.64 to 0.78. In a hospital-based case–control study in Italy, Tavani et al. (2001) studied 1031 cases and 2411 controls, who char-

acterized their physical activity at work as "very heavy", "heavy", "average', "standing" or "mainly sitting". Physical activity during leisure time was assessed based on the number of hours per week spent in sports or household activities. After adjustment for other risk factors for ovarian cancer, the odds ratio for the highest versus lowest levels of occupational activity at age 50–59 years was 0.76 (95% CI 0.48–1.2). The corresponding OR for age 30–39 years was 0.67 (95% CI 0.47–0.98). No association was found with leisure-time activity.

Discussion

Only five studies have reported on physical activity and ovarian cancer and their findings have been inconsistent. The larger and more recent studies have included information on potential confounders. However, no firm conclusion on a possible association between physical activity and ovarian cancer can be drawn.

Prostate cancer

The great majority of the studies of the association between prostate cancer and physical activity have been conducted in developed countries, where participation in prostate cancer screening may differ between men who exercise and those with a more sedentary lifestyle. Thus, of particular interest are studies that focused on more advanced prostate tumours, the diagnosis of which is less dependent on participation in screening.

Cohort studies

Table 43 summarizes the prospective studies on physical activity and prostate cancer with at least 100 cases. Out of eight reports from cohort studies, six reported no association (Severson et al., 1989; Lee et al., 1992; Thune & Lund, 1994; Hartman et al., 1998; Giovannucci et al., 1998; Liu et al., 2000) and two observed a mostly weak protective effect (Clarke & Whittemore, 2000; Lund Nilsen et al., 2000). Some of the null studies observed an inverse association in sub-

group analyses (e.g., Thune & Lund, 1994; Hartman et al., 1998; Giovannucci et al.,1998), as described below.

Lee et al. (1992) found that Harvard alumni aged 70 years or older who expended more than 4000 kcal [16 800 kJ] per week in college or ten years later were at 50% decreased risk (95% CI 0.3–1.0) of developing prostate cancer, compared with those who expended less than 1000 kcal [4200 kJ] per week at either assessment. No association was found in younger subjects. Severson et al. (1989) reported no association between usual physical activity and prostate cancer in a cohort study of Japanese men in Hawaii. Similarly, in the Physicians' Health Study, a randomized trial of low-dose aspirin and β-carotene among 22 071 US men, physical activity (assessed as the frequency of exercise vigorous enough to work up a sweat) was unrelated to risk of prostate cancer (Liu et al., 2000). In the other cohort studies, physical activity was inversely associated with prostate cancer, overall or in subgroup analyses. One of these (Clarke & Whittemore, 2000) used the data from the NHANES I Epidemiological Follow-up Study. Participants were asked to rate their physical activity during a normal day and during their leisure activities as high, moderate or low. The most recent and detailed analysis of this cohort, based on 201 cases, showed that men who reported high levels of non-recreational physical activity had decreased prostate cancer risk compared with very sedentary men. This association was stronger for African Americans (RR = 0.27; 95% CI 0.12–0.60) than for Caucasians (RR = 0.60; 95% CI 0.44–1.3). Moderate levels of recreational activity were weakly associated with increased prostate cancer risk among African Americans but not among Caucasians, suggesting that only high physical activity levels were protective. A Norwegian study found that men who walked in their job and engaged in regular physical training

Table 42. Studies on physical activity and risk of ovarian cancer

Author, date, study location	Study dates	No. of cases	Activity definition (no. of categories)	Relative risk (highest vs lowest categories) (95% CI)	Trend*	Adjustment for confounding	Comments
Cohort studies							
Pukkala et al. (1993), Finland	1958–92	51	Current occupational title	SIR (vs general population) for: Physical activity teachers: 1.7 (0.8–3.2) Language teachers 1.6 (1.1–2.1)	NE	Age	Based on national incidence figures
Zheng et al. (1993b), China	1980–84	595	Current occupational activity (3)	SIR = 1.02	NE	Age	Based on occupational data on census
Mink et al., (1996), USA	1985–92	97	Recreational activity: Moderate (4) Vigorous (4) Overall index (3)	1.6 (0.87–2.9) 2.5 (1.0–6.3) 2.1 (1.2–3.5)	Yes Yes Yes	Age Age Age, smoking, education, parity, family history, waist/hip ratio	Post-menopausal women
Case–control studies							
Cottreau et al. (2000), USA	1994–98	767	Recreational index at different ages (3)	Lifetime 0.73 (0.56–0.94)	Yes	Ae, parity, estrogen use, family history, BMI, education, race, tubal ligation	Population-based
Tavani et al. (2001), Italy	1992–99	1031	Occupational Recreational at different ages (3)	30–39 years: 0.67 (0.47–0.98) 0.86 (0.65–1.1)	Yes No	Age, education, study centre, BMI, reproductive factors, family history, energy intake, estrogen use	Hospital-based

* Either a significant test for trend or significant relative risks for intermediate exposure categories

Table 43. Studies of physical activity and risk of prostate cancer

Author, date, study location	Study dates	No. of cases	Activity definition (no. of categories)	Relative risk (highest vs lowest categories) (95% CI)	Trend*	Adjustment for confounding	Comments
Cohort studies							
Severson et al. (1989), USA	1965–66	206	24 h index of all activities plus time sleeping (3)	1.0 (0.75–1.5)	No	Age, BMI	Hawaii Japanese
Lee et al. (1992) USA	1962–88	419	Recreational activity (3)	0.88 (0.64–1.2)	No	Age	College alumni
Thune & Lund (1994), Norway	1972–91	220	Occupational (4) Recreational (3)	0.81 (0.50–1.3) 0.87 (0.57–1.3)	NE NE	Age, region, BMI	Different counties in Norway
Giovannucci et al. (1998), USA	1986–94	200	Total Vigorous recreational activity (4)	0.72 (0.44–1.2) 0.46 (0.24–0.89)	No No	Age, height, vasectomy, diabetes smoking, diet	Metastatic tumours
Hartman et al. (1998), Finland	1985–94	317	Occupational (4) Leisure (2)	1.2 (0.74–2.0) 0.9 (0.73–1.1)	NE NE	Age, urban, smoking, history of benign prostate hypertrophy, intervention	ATBC trial
Clarke & Whittemore (2000), USA	1971–92	201	Non-recreational (3) or recreational (3) activity	0.58 (0.37–0.89) 0.85 (0.58–1.3)	Yes No	Age, education, family history	NHANES I
Liu et al. (2000) USA	1982–95	982	Vigorous exercise (4)	1.1 (0.91–1.4)	No	Age, height, intervention, smoking, alcohol, diabetes, plasma cholesterol, vitamins, hypertension, BMI	Physicians' Health Study
Lund Nilsen et al. (2000), Norway	1984–95	644	Recreational (3) or occupational (2) activity	0.80 (0.62–1.0) 1.0 (0.82–1.3)	No NE	Age	Health screenees
Case–control studies							
Brownson et al. (1991), USA	1984–89	2878	Occupational activity (3)	0.7 (0.6–0.8)	Yes	Age, smoking	Cancer registry data
Le Marchand et al. (1991b), USA	1977–83	214	Lifetime occupational activity (4)	2.0 (1.1–3.3)	Yes	Age, ethnicity, income, education	Population-based Age > 70 years
West et al. (1991) USA	1984–85	358	Total energy expended (2)	Aggressive tumours 2.0 (0.8–5.2)	NE	Age	Population-based controls

Table 43 (contd)

Author, date, study location	Study dates	No. of cases	Activity definition (no. of categories)	Relative risk (highest vs lowest categories) (95% CI)	Trend*	Adjustment for confounding	Comments
Hsing et al. (1994), China	1980–84	264	Occupational activity (3)	SIR = 0.92 (0.7–1.1)	No	Age	Population-based
Andersson et al. (1995), Sweden	1989–92	256	Adolescent physical activity (3)	0.7 (0.4–1.1)	No	Age, urban, farming	Population-based
Whittemore et al. (1995), USA, Canada	1987–91	1655	Time in light or vigorous activity	Means: no association	No	Age, ethnicity, region	Population-based
Ilic et al. (1996), Yugoslavia	1990–94	101	Occupational activity (2)	3.9 (2.1–7.2)	NE	Age, occupational exposure, nephrolithiasis no. of brothers, no. of sexual partners	Hospital-based
Sung et al. (1999), Taiwan	1995–96	90	Recreational exercise	2.2 (1.2–4.0)	NE	Age, education, BMI, diet	Hospital-based
Villeneuve et al. (1999), Canada	1994–97	1133	Leisure (strenuous) activity (5)	0.7 (0.4–1.4)	No	Age, province, race, smoking, BMI, diet, income, family history	Population-based

* Either a significant test for trend or significant relative risks for intermediate exposure categories

during leisure time had significantly lower risk of prostate cancer (RR = 0.45; 95% CI 0.20–1.0) compared with sedentary men (Thune & Lund, 1994). In the Alpha-Tocopherol, Beta-Carotene (ATBC) Cancer Prevention Study, a chemoprevention trial among smokers in Finland, no association between occupational activity and prostate cancer was found (Hartman et al., 1998). However, among working men, there was an inverse association with leisure-time physical activity. Participants who ranked their exercise level as "heavy" had a relative risk of 0.7 (95% CI 0.5–0.9) compared with those who described themselves as sedentary during leisure. Giovannucci et al. (1998) analysed the data from the Health Professionals Follow-up Study, the largest and most informative study of lifestyle and prostate cancer published to date. Subjects reported in a self-administered questionnaire the average time spent on a variety of non-occupational activities. No relationship was found with total or advanced prostate cancer for total, vigorous or non-vigorous physical activity. For metastatic prostate cancer, no linear trend was found for these activities, but a significantly lower risk was observed in the highest category of vigorous physical activity (RR = 0.46; 95% CI 0.24–0.89). Finally, in a large cohort study in Norway in which men self-characterized their leisure-time and occupational physical activity as low, medium or high, a weak inverse association was found with recreational exercise, whereas occupational physical activity was unrelated to risk (Lund Nilsen et al., 2000).

Case–control studies
Case–control studies that included at least 100 cases are summarized in Table 43; the results have been inconsistent. Among the five studies reporting on occupational physical activity, two observed an increased risk with high activity (Le Marchand et al., 1991b; Ilic et al., 1996), one showed no association

(Hsing et al., 1994) and two reported decreased risks (Brownson et al., 1991; Villeneuve et al., 1999). Among the case–control studies that reported on usual or leisure-time physical activity, two found no association (West et al., 1991; Whittemore et al., 1995) and one found an increased risk (Sung et al., 1999). In a case–control study in Utah, USA, West et al. (1991) found that men aged 45–67 years who were in the highest quartile of total energy expenditure were at slightly increased risk of 'aggressive' prostate tumours (a group including localized undifferentiated and advanced tumours). No association was found for older men. Two case–control studies reported on physical activity at an early age in relation to prostate cancer risk. In a subset of their Canadian subjects, Villeneuve et al. (1999) inquired about participation in strenuous and moderate leisure-time activity and assessed occupational physical activity at different periods of life (mid-teens or early 20s, early 30s, early 40s and two years before diagnosis). They found no association with prostate cancer, except for a protective effect of strenuous occupational physical activity performed in the mid-teens or early 20s (OR = 0.6; 95% CI 0.4–0.9 for strenuous activities compared with sitting activities). In a population-based case–control study in Sweden, Andersson et al. (1995) found that subjects who reported being more physically active than their classmates around the time of puberty were at somewhat lower risk of prostate cancer (OR = 0.7; 95% CI 0.4–1.1) compared with those who said that they exercised less than their classmates. Thus, the data are inconsistent with regard to the period of life at which physical activity may be most relevant.

Discussion
Less than twenty epidemiological studies were available to assess the relationship of physical activity to prostate cancer. As for other cancer sites, these studies are

difficult to evaluate due to the differences in the methods used to assess physical activity. Questionnaires have focused either on usual physical activity (i.e., amount of time spent at various levels of physical activity during a usual day) or on leisure-time activities and the questions have ranged from those covering details of the frequency and duration of various activities to simple questions asking the subjects to rate themselves as sedentary, moderately active or very active. Studies of occupational exercise have typically assumed that a man in a particular job has performed the level of physical activity that has been estimated as the average level for his job category and this for the duration of his employment in this job. However, despite these methodological differences, a majority of studies have suggested a protective effect; the relationships have tended to be of moderate strength and sometimes were observed only in subgroups. The findings in well conducted cohort studies of an inverse association with metastatic disease and in groups of low socioeconomic status (e.g., African Americans) suggest that the observed effects may not be due to detection bias.

Overall, the available evidence suggests that physical activity may protect against prostate cancer.

Kidney cancer
Cohort studies
In a Swedish study, occupational physical activity was inversely associated with renal-cell cancer risk among men but not in women (Lindblad et al., 1994). No association was found in the Harvard Health Alumni study (Paffenbarger et al., 1987).

Case–control studies
One case–control study reported a protective effect of occupational activity on renal-cell cancer risk among men (Bergström et al., 1999). Three others, however, found no association with physical activity (Goodman et al., 1986;

Mellemgaard *et al.*, 1994, 1995). One of these studies was a multi-centre population-based case–control study conducted in Australia, Denmark, Germany, Sweden and the USA that included 1732 cases (Mellemgaard *et al.*, 1995).

Discussion
The results from the few published studies regarding the association between physical activity and renal-cell cancer are inconsistent for both occupational and recreational physical activity and do not permit an adequate assessment to be made.

Lung cancer
Five cohort studies (Paffenbarger *et al.,* 1987; Severson *et al.*, 1989; Steenland *et al.*, 1995; Thune & Lund, 1997; Lee *et al.*, 1999a) and two case–control studies (Brownson *et al.,* 1991; Dosemeci *et al.*, 1993) on physical activity and lung cancer have been reported (Table 44). Earlier publications from the NHANES I study (Albanes *et al.* 1989) and the Harvard Health Alumni study (Lee & Paffenbarger, 1994) were excluded because the subsequent follow-ups from the same cohorts updated the results.

Cohort studies
A lower risk of lung cancer was associated with physical activity in all of the cohort studies. The largest studies were the Harvard Health Alumni Study (Lee *et al.*, 1999a) and a population-based cohort in Norway (Thune & Lund, 1997). The Norwegian cohort study measured both recreational and occupational activity and found a 30% decreased risk when these activities were combined into a total activity variable for the male study subjects (Thune & Lund, 1997), but no comparable risk decrease was observed for females. In the Harvard Health Alumni study (Lee *et al.*, 1999a), even stronger risk decreases were associated with total energy expended, with 40% decreases observed among men who

expended the greatest amount of energy. Overall, the risk decreases in these studies ranged from 20–60% for both non-occupational and occupational physical activity, with an inverse dose–response relationship.

Case–control studies
The two case–control studies of occupational physical activity do not support a decrease in risk of lung cancer; one observed an increased risk (Brownson *et al.*, 1991) and the other found no effect (Dosemeci *et al.*, 1993). Given the fact that these two studies were both hospital-based case–control studies and used only occupational title to assess physical activity, it is difficult to draw firm conclusions from these results.

Discussion
Five of the seven studies reviewed demonstrated a decreased risk of lung cancer among the most physically active subjects. The risk decreases ranged from 20 to 60% and evidence for a dose–response relationship was observed. This effect could be confounded by smoking which, although it was appropriately controlled for in these studies, could have been associated with other lung diseases (e.g., chronic obstructive lung disease) among the study participants. Given the uncertainty of the association and the limited amount of data available, the evidence for an association remains inconclusive.

The level of activity that appears to confer a protective effect on lung cancer can be estimated from the two largest studies. These studies indicate that four hours per week of hard leisure-time activity (Thune & Lund, 1997) and participation in activities of at least moderate activity (> 4.5 MET), but not light activity (< 4.5 MET) (Lee *et al.*, 1999), reduced lung cancer risk independently after adjustment for smoking and other possible risk factors. Different effects of physical activity on various histological types of lung cancer have

also been reported (Thune & Lund, 1997). Physical activity may reduce the concentration of carcinogenic agents in the airways, the duration of agent–airway interaction and the amount of particle deposition through increased ventilation and perfusion.

Testicular cancer
Two cohort studies (Paffenbarger *et al.*, 1992; Thune & Lund, 1994) and five case–control studies (Brownson *et al.*, 1991; Dosemeci *et al.*, 1993; UK Testicular Cancer Study Group, 1994b; Gallagher *et al.*, 1995; Srivastava & Kreiger, 2000) have been conducted on the association between physical activity and testicular cancer (Table 45). The two cohort studies both had sample sizes of less than 100 cases and have been excluded from the table but are mentioned briefly below.

Cohort studies
No effect of physical activity on testicular cancer risk was found in either of the two cohort studies (Paffenbarger *et al.*, 1992; Thune & Lund, 1994).

Case–control studies
A large case–control study conducted in the United Kingdom found a decreased risk of testicular cancer for recreational activity performed either early in life or during the reference year (UK Testicular Cancer Study Group, 1994b). These results were corroborated by a subsequent population-based case–control study conducted in Canada that found risk decreases for recreational activity performed at age 21 years and five years before diagnosis (Gallagher *et al.*, 1995). The results from these two studies and two earlier case–control studies that found either no effect (Dosemeci *et al.*, 1993) or a decreased risk with occupational activity (Brownson *et al.*, 1991) are in contrast to those of the most recent study, that observed an increased risk among physically active men (Srivastava & Kreiger, 2000). In this

Table 44. Studies of physical activity and risk of lung cancer

Author, date, study location	Study dates	No. of cases	Activity definition (no. of categories)	Relative risk (highest vs lowest categories) (95% CI)	Trend*	Adjustment for confounding	Comments
Cohort studies							
Paffenbarger et al. (1987), USA	1951–72	M+F: 112	Occupational titles (4)	0.4	NE	Age	Mortality study
Severson et al. (1989), USA	1965–86	M: 192	24-hour physical activity index as sum of time in all activities plus sleeping (3)	0.7 (0.5–1.0)	Yes	Age, BMI, smoking	Hawaii Japanese
Steenland et al. (1995), USA	1971–87	M: 151 F: 59	Current non-recreational activity (3)	M: 0.8 (0.5–1.4) F: 0.7 (0.3–1.7)	NE	Age, BMI, smoking, alcohol, income, recreational activity	NHANES 1 study Longer follow-up of cohort reported in Albanes et al. (1989)
Thune & Lund (1997), Norway	1972–91	M: 413 F: 51	Recreational and occupational activity (2, 3 or 4)	Occupational activity M: 1.0 (0.7–1.4) F: 0.8 (0.3–2.1) Recreational activity: M: 0.7 (0.5–1.0) F: 1.0 (0.4–2.8) Total activity: M: 0.7 (0.5–1.0) F: 0.9 (0.2–3.6)	No (M+F) Yes No NE	Age, geographical area, smoking habits, BMI	Age 20–49 years
Lee et al. (1999a), USA	1962–88	M: 245	Current walking, stair climbing and recreational activity at baseline (4)	Energy expended: 0.6 (0.4–0.9) Distance walked 0.7 (0.5–0.9) Stairs climbed: 0.7 (0.5–1.0) Moderate recreational activities: 1.0 (0.7–1.5) Vigorous recreational activities: 0.6 (0.4–1.0)	Yes Yes No No Yes	Age, smoking habits, BMI and other three components of physical activity	College alumni Update of Lee & Paffenbarger (1994)

Table 44 (contd)

Author, date, study location	Study dates	No. of cases	Activity definition (no. of categories)	Relative risk (highest vs lowest categories) (95% CI)	Trend*	Adjustment for confounding	Comments
Case–control studies							
Brownson et al. (1991), USA	1984–89	M: 4700	Occupational titles (3)	1.3 (1.1–1.7)	Yes	Age, smoking	Cancer registry data
Dosemeci et al. (1993), Turkey	1979–84	M: 1148	Occupational titles to estimate energy expenditure over lifetime (3)	1.0 (0.8–1.3)	No	Age, smoking, socioeconomic status	Hospital-based

RR, relative risk; OR, odds ratio; SIR, standardized incidence ratio; BMI, body mass index.
* Either a significant test for trend or significant intermediate relative risks for intermediate exposure categories

Table 45. Studies of physical activity and risk of testicular cancer

Author, date, study location	Study dates	No. of cases	Activity definition (no. of categories)	Relative risk (highest vs lowest categories) (95% CI)	Trend*	Adjustment for confounding	Comments
Case–control studies							
Brownson *et al.* (1991), USA	1984–89	252	Occupational titles (3)	0.5 (0.3–0.8)	Yes	Age, smoking	Cancer registry data
Dosemeci *et al.* (1993), Turkey	1979–84	191	Occupational titles to estimate energy expenditure over lifetime (3)	1.0 (0.5–1.8)	No	Age, smoking, socioeconomic status	Hospital-based
UK Testicular Cancer Study Group, (1994b), UK	1984–87	793	Recreational activity at age 20 and at reference age (6)	Age 20: 0.6 (0.4–0.9) Reference age: 0.5 (0.3–0.9)	Yes	Age, undescended testis, inguinal hernia before age 15 y	Population-based
Gallagher *et al.* (1995), Canada	1980–85	510	Lifetime occupational and recreational activity (4)	Recreational activity: 0.7 (0.5–0.9) Occupational activity: 0.9 (0.6–1.3)	Yes No	Age, ethnic origin, undescended testis, inguinal hernia	Population-based
Srivastava & Kreiger (2000), Canada	1995–96	212	Frequency of moderate recreational activity at different ages (4 or 5) Intensity of occupational activity by life period (4)	Recreational Teens: 2.4 (1.2–4.6) Early 30s: 1.7 (0.7–4.4) 2 yrs before: 1.4 (0.6–3.3) Cumulative lifetime: 1.0 (0.4–1.7) Occupational Early 20s: 1.7 (0.9–3.0) Early 30s: 1.3 (0.6–2.8) 2 yrs before: 0.9 (0.5–1.9) Cumulative lifetime: 0.8 (0.3–1.7)	NE	Age, BMI, education, smoking, marital status	Population-based

RR, relative risk; OR, odds ratio; SIR, standardized incidence ratio; BMI, body mass index
* Either a significant test for trend or significant relative risks for intermediate exposure categories

Canadian study, a 2.4-fold increase in risk was observed among subjects who participated in strenuous leisure-time activity more than five times per week during adolescence as compared with those who performed strenuous leisure-time activity less than once a month. At later ages and for cumulative lifetime exposure, the risks associated with recreational activity for the highest versus lowest quartiles were not elevated nor statistically significant. Likewise, increased risks were not statistically significant for occupational activity. Hence, it appears that in this study, only activity performed during adolescence was associated with increased testicular cancer risk.

Discussion

Three of the seven studies have found decreased testicular cancer risks among the most physically active participants. The risk decreases were fairly modest and since one study noted an increased risk and three a null effect, the results remain inconsistent and weak regarding this putative association. Little evidence exists for a dose–response relationship. The studies also suffered from weak exposure data and limited control for confounding. Overall, there is insufficient evidence to draw any conclusion on the nature of the relationship between physical activity and testicular cancer.

Population attributable risk

In summary, there is considerable evidence that physical inactivity is associated with some of the most common cancers. The proportion of any disease due to a risk factor in a population is determined by both the size of relative risk and the prevalence of the risk factor in the population. That proportion, often referred to as the population attributable risk (PAR), has not been estimated for most of the cancer sites reviewed here. Slattery et al. (1997a) estimated, from the results of a large US study, that the PAR for physical inactivity (20–25% of the population reported no activity) was 13% for colon cancer. This is similar to the PAR of 14% for colon cancer estimated by La Vecchia et al. (1999b) in an Italian study. Mezzetti et al. (1998) estimated that 11% of breast cancer might be attributable to physical inactivity. Although the measures of physical activity vary widely between the studies reviewed here, it is likely that in many industrialized countries the PARs for colon and breast cancers are at least this large. Random measurement error will result in underestimation of the size of relative risks. These PAR values for physical inactivity may therefore be substantially underestimated, perhaps by a factor of two. It is also important to point out that physical activity and weight control are clearly interrelated, as physical activity is an important factor in lifetime weight maintenance. Therefore, all the attributable risks for elevated BMI for colon, breast and endometrial cancers could also be interpreted as risks that are attributable, in part, to physical inactivity.

Intervention studies of intermediate markers of cancer

Studies of effects on cancer incidence or mortality of interventions to lose weight or to increase physical activity would require very large numbers (usually tens of thousands) of participants followed up for long periods of time. Such endeavours entail considerable difficulties in recruiting and retaining participants and in funding. Small randomized clinical trials of effects of exercise on biomarkers for cancer can provide insights into the biological effects of weight loss or physical activity interventions. In this section, the term 'intervention study' refers to a study in which a behavioural, medical or other intervention is prescribed to a group of study participants. 'Randomized controlled clinical trial' refers to a study in which participants are recruited, screened for eligibility and interest, randomly assigned to one or more interventions or to one or more control groups, and followed forward in time for the development of end-points. These end-points can be disease-specific morbidity and mortality or can be biomarkers of disease or health.

Clinical trials can focus on one or two specific interventions, so that the effect of a given level of exercise for a defined period of time can be assessed. The specific physiological aspects of physical activity can be studied. Many of the difficulties associated with measuring exercise exposure in observational studies can be avoided, because direct observation of study participants exercising can be made and physiological measures of fitness can be used. Properly designed and executed randomization can minimize bias from potential confounding variables. Homogeneity of exercise exposure can be avoided, because the trial design can include one or more groups with defined exercise prescriptions and, usually, a control condition. Measuring change in exercise exposure is difficult in observational settings because most people do not significantly change their exercise habits, and because recall of changes in physical activity can be difficult. Clinical trials can be designed so that change in physical activity is prescribed and maximized to allow assessment of effect. Randomized trials can focus on specific populations such as high-risk individuals, who may be highly motivated to make changes in exercise behaviour. The clinical trial design allows assessment of effects of physical activity on intermediate end-points and biomarkers, which is difficult to do in observational studies. Synergistic or antagonistic effects with other behaviours or with treatments can be studied in clinical trials, especially with factorial designs with two or more interventions. Finally, several end-points can be efficiently measured in a single trial. There are some limitations in randomized clinical trials. Volunteers for such studies are a selected group and may not represent the general population of overweight, obese or sedentary persons. The range of exercise or dietary exposure is normally limited to the type of intervention and individual adherence.

There have been a small number of intervention studies of weight loss or physical activity effect on intermediate markers of cancer. In addition, intervention studies without randomization or without a control group have been reported. Because of the potential for biased results in uncontrolled intervention studies, the optimal design for intervention studies is the randomized controlled trial. In several instances, trials have been conducted to assess intermediate markers of coronary or other diseases. The results of these studies are applicable to cancer in so far as the intermediate markers and biomarkers are shared.

Weight reduction
Hormones

Observational data suggest links between diet, overweight and risk of certain cancers, as well as between certain metabolic hormones and cancers. A full discussion of how diet and weight loss might affect sex and metabolic hormones and the proteins to which they bind in blood is included in Chapter 4. There have been many intervention studies, but few well powered randomized controlled trials, assessing the effect of weight loss on endogenous hormones. The studies in subjects with normal weight were not planned as such; weight loss occurred rather as a secondary effect of a change in dietary intake (of, for example, lowered fat, increased fibre or increased vegetables and fruits). Overall, there is clear evidence of reduction in circulating insulin levels with either type of weight loss. Consistent evidence from controlled and uncontrolled clinical trials shows that weight loss leads to

increased levels of SHBG. There is no convincing evidence from intervention studies that weight loss can reduce circulating estrogen levels in premenopausal women. However, some types of dietary change, such as increased fibre and decreased fat, may cause decreases in estrogen levels. A smaller body of data suggests that weight loss can affect IGF and IGFBP levels. Hormonal effects vary with the length of intervention and follow-up.

Mammographic densities

There is considerable evidence that women with extensive areas of mammographic densities are 4–6 times more likely to develop breast cancer than those with little or no density on their mammogram. High-risk mammographic patterns may be used as a surrogate end-point for breast cancer in etiological research as well as in prevention studies. In a randomized dietary intervention study, Boyd et al. (1997) examined the effect of a two-year low-fat, high-carbohydrate diet on breast radiological densities. Women with radiological densities ($n = 817$) in more than 50% of the breast area on mammography were recruited and randomly allocated to an intervention group taught to reduce their dietary intake of fat (mean, 21% of energy) and increase their complex carbohydrate intake (mean, 61% of energy) or to a control group (mean, 32% from fat and 50% from carbohydrates). Mean body weight was similar at baseline (62.3 and 62.7 kg in the intervention and control groups, respectively, $p = 0.47$), decreased 0.3 kg in the intervention group, and increased 0.9 kg in the control group ($p = 0.0003$). After two years, the area of density was reduced by 374 mm^2 (6.1%) in the intervention group compared with an average of 128 mm^2 (2.1%) in the control group ($p = 0.01$). The effect of the intervention on breast densities, however, was only marginally significant after weight change and change in

menopausal status were taken into account, suggesting that part of the dietary effect may have been mediated by weight loss.

Colorectal polyps

The Polyp Prevention Trial has provided data on effects of diet on colorectal polyp recurrence (Schatzkin et al., 2000) This trial was conducted in 2079 men and women aged 35 years or older who had one or more incident colorectal adenomatous polyps removed. Participants were randomized to either a low-fat (20% of energy), high-fibre (18 g/1000 kcal [4.3 g/1000 kJ]), and high fruits and vegetables (3.5 servings per 1000 kcal [0.8 servings per 1000 kJ]). Although the intervention was not focused on weight loss, the intervention participants lost a mean of 1.4 lb [0.64 kg], while controls gained an average of 1.0 lb [0.45 kg] during the course of the study. After four years of follow-up, there was no difference in the rate of polyp recurrence between the groups. The overall weight loss observed in this trial was too small to be informative.

Physical activity
Hormones

As for weight control, exercise causes significant reductions in circulating insulin levels in normal, hyperinsulinaemic and diabetic persons. Observations of amenorrhoea and other menstrual abnormalities in trained female athletes have led to closer scrutiny of the effects of exercise on hormonal patterns in girls and young women. There have been several uncontrolled trials of exercise effect on hormones, as discussed in Chapter 4. Overall, there is moderately strong evidence that vigorous exercise lowers endogenous estrogen levels in premenopausal women. There are no published data from intervention studies in postmenopausal women. In men and women of all ages, exercise raises SHBG levels. Effects of exercise on IGF levels have been tested in few intervention studies, with variable results.

Immune function

Interest in effects of exercise on immune function stems from observations of impaired immunity in highly trained athletes. While immune status has not been clearly linked to cancer etiology, it is biologically plausible that immune function is important in the development and growth of cancers. Many small uncontrolled trials have assessed effects on immune function of training-level and moderate-intensity exercise, with varying results depending on baseline fitness level, age and the type of immune parameter studied. Overall, moderate-intensity exercise appears to improve immune function, as discussed more fully in Chapter 4.

Summary

There have been many intervention studies of the effects of weight loss and physical activity on insulin, but fewer on sex hormones and immune function. Nevertheless, there are indications that various sex and metabolic hormones, immune function and other biomarkers of cancer are affected by weight loss and exercise.

Experimental systems

Animal experiments are classified as studies of energy restriction, diet restriction or exercise. These categories should be viewed as experimental approaches by which prevention of weight gain in animals is achieved. The majority of studies of restriction or physical activity in experimental animal models of carcinogenesis do not involve weight loss; instead, the animals are in a state of positive energy balance but achieve a smaller mass with a lower percentage of body fat than animals allowed free access to diet or sedentary animals. This situation directly parallels

and models conditions in humans associated with different levels of cancer risk. Thus the experimental carcinogenesis studies reviewed below do not involve extreme underweight (starvation), as exemplified by anorexia nervosa, nor do they model obesity.

It is not at present known, and may never be known, to what extent healthy individuals in modern societies restrict their dietary intake. The range of restrictions or physical activity used in animal experiments can be viewed as an approach to preventing adult body weight gain in these animals and is intended to resemble the range of energy balances that occur in healthy people. However, healthy rodents differ from healthy humans in that they experience adult linear growth.

Design issues in diet, exercise and experimental carcinogenesis

Selection of model

Experimental animal models must be selected that mimic as closely as possible the human disease. Characteristics that should be considered in choosing a model include the similarity of tumour morphology and biological traits such as (hormonal) responsiveness to those seen in humans. Such models are available for many organ sites. For example, in rat models for breast cancer, not only are tumours morphologically similar to their human counterparts, but the majority are ovarian steroid-responsive and factors such as full-term pregnancy protect against disease occurrence. *N*-Nitrosobis-2-(oxopropyl)amine (BOP)-induced ductular pancreatic cancer in the Syrian hamster is a model that has been useful in studying aspects of human pancreatic cancer that cannot be addressed with humans (Pour *et al.*, 1993), whereas other induced pancreatic tumours are acinar cell carcinomas, which are not a common pancreatic lesion in humans. Furthermore, it is best to minimize the time of treatment with a chemical carcinogen, unless the chemi-

cal carcinogen is one to which humans are chronically exposed. A short-term carcinogen treatment will allow the investigator to feed the experimental diet or provide the physical activity intervention of interest at times when the chemical carcinogen is not being administered. The impact of diet or exercise on the metabolism of a chemical carcinogen to which people are not exposed may be of scientific interest, but the observations may have limited relevance to the prevention of human cancer.

Selection of diet

Both cereal-based and semi-purified diets have been used in studies of dietary impact on carcinogenesis. It is of the utmost importance that the control diet in either case be adequate in all nutrients, not excessive in any component, and that it be free of potentially toxic components. Cereal-based diets have the advantage that they are designed using whole food ingredients. However, the food ingredients are not commonly used in the same manner in human diets and the complexity of their composition makes it difficult to attribute observations to a particular nutrient or constituent. This issue is addressed below for studies of dietary restriction with cereal-based diets. Semi-purified diets have the advantage that each component can be modulated independently of other constituents in a highly controlled fashion, but since these diets do not use common human foods, extrapolation to such foods must be made with caution.

Design of intervention protocol

Dietary or exercise interventions should be provided separately from the chemical carcinogen in studies where the cancer-causing stimulus is not a cancer-causing agent for human disease. With such models, it is common to apply the dietary or activity intervention after exposure to the carcinogenic stimulus, in order to obtain information on the development of the disease process. In cases where the cancer-causing stimuli do represent conditions that may induce human cancer, it is important to assess the impact of the intervention strategy both on the cancer-induction phase (preceding and at the time of carcinogen treatment) and on the promotion/progression (development) of the cancer (following treatment with the carcinogen). Models involving a short induction phase provide the possibility of assessing the impact of diet on early or late stages of promotion. If tumours are allowed to develop before the intervention, it is possible to assess the impact of the intervention on the regression or progression of the lesions. Finally, recently developed genetically modified animal models of human cancers allow scientists to determine if interventions of interest can prevent the development of cancer that is driven by genes known to be mutated in human cancer. Such studies should provide information on how diet or physical activity may be useful in the prevention of cancer in people with particular genetic predisposition.

Weight control

Weight control involves balancing energy intake with energy expenditure to maintain a targeted body weight and presumably body composition. In general, energy restriction has been shown to be associated with cancer prevention, while an excess intake of energy is associated with an increased risk for cancer. While some evidence implies a role of body fat in these effects, other results suggest that the effects are not due to body fat *per se*. Thus, in assessing the cancer-preventive effects of weight control, predominant attention is given here to the role of energy restriction. In the literature, energy restriction is also referred to as calorie restriction, dietary restriction or food restriction. These terms are not synonyms. Energy restriction is used in this volume to characterize studies in

which the energy intake was selectively reduced while all micronutrients were fed at the same level as in the control group. The terms food restriction and diet restriction are used to refer to underfeeding of a complete diet such that less of all nutrients and dietary factors is ingested; this approach can lead to an intake of micronutrients and/or macrocomponents that is incompatible with optimal health. The term dietary restriction is used for such protocols in this review. Dietary restriction, which does not allow the investigator to detect effects due specifically to a limitation in dietary energy, was frequently used in early studies of restriction. With the cereal-based diets used until the 1940s, dietary restriction was the most expedient approach and is still sometimes used. Such studies can provide valuable insights, but their results must be interpreted with caution. The earliest experimental studies of dietary restriction assessed the growth of transplanted tumours. Owing to the limited relevance of transplantable tumour model systems to primary cancer prevention, these studies (see reviews by Tannenbaum & Silverstone, 1953; Birt, 1987; Weindruch *et al.*, 1991; Kritchevsky, 1992, 1999) are not considered in detail below. Examples of studies with dietary restriction are included in this report only if they provide information not available with energy restriction protocols in which energy intake was selectively reduced. Calorie restriction and energy restriction are the terms generally applied to experimental approaches in which diets are formulated so that, when animals are fed different numbers of calories, they still receive the same levels of other nutrients, such that the only variable is energy intake.

The present review of energy restriction and dietary restriction approaches to prevent excessive adult body weight gain as cancer-preventive strategies covers dietary restriction studies only if similar energy restriction studies have

yielded comparable results. The aim was to ensure that the body weight maintenance resulting from the dietary restriction was likely to be the cause of the cancer prevention, and the parallel energy restriction protocol would provide this evidence. Dietary restriction protocols without parallel energy restriction studies must be viewed with caution, since a multitude of dietary constituents that may not affect body weight but are known to influence cancer rates are also reduced in these diets.

Studies described below are summarized in Table 46.

Colon

Chemically induced rodent colon tumours can be considered to model those in humans for the following reasons. They are induced more frequently in the distal part of the colon, which is the preferential site of the human lesions. The developmental sequence from preneoplastic lesions, aberrant crypt foci, to adenoma and carcinoma is well established. Furthermore, a similar incidence of K-*ras* mutations has been observed in adenocarcinomas in rats, mice and humans.

Reddy *et al.* (1987) reported the inhibition of azoxymethane (AOM)-induced colon carcinogenesis in rats by continuous energy restriction starting four days after AOM treatment. Colon carcinogenesis in rats was not inhibited when dietary restriction was initiated at day 63 after treatment with methylazoxymethanol (MAM) or when animals were fed *ad libitum* or fasted every other day from day 8 or 31 after MAM treatment (Pollard *et al.*, 1984). Newberne *et al.* (1990) studied the preventive effects of pre- and postnatal energy restriction against colon cancer in rats treated with dimethylhydrazine (DMH). After birth, rat litters were adjusted to four or eight rats per litter. The rats in litters of four and fed *ad libitum* became heaviest and developed the greatest number of tumours. Rats in litters of four, but pair-fed the

Table 46. Studies of prevention of spontaneous and carcinogen-induced tumours by dietary restriction in experimental animals

Organ site, species, strain (sex)	Age at beginning of study (wk)	No. of animals per group	Carcinogen/ dose/route	Dietary restriction/ amount, type	Timing of restriction	Prevention effect	Summarized effect	Reference
Colon								
Rat								
Lobund Sprague-Dawley (M)	Weanling	7–10	30 mg/kg bw MAM, s.c., killed 20 weeks after MAM	Dietary restriction: Natural ingredient diet fed 25% less of diet	DR day 10–140; DR day 63–140; AL/fasted alternate days for 8 days; AL/fasted alternate days for 31 days	Av. no. of tumours/rat[4]: AL throughout, 1.4–2.7[b]; 25% DR day 10–140, 0.4[a]; 25% DR day 63–140, 0.4[a]; 25% DR day 63–140, 2.2; AL/fasted alternate days 8 d, 1.1; AL/fasted alternate days 31 d, 2.0	DR throughout inhibited tumours	Pollard et al. (1984)
Fischer 344 (M)	Weaning	30	15 mg/kg bw AOM, s.c. x 2, at 7 and 8 wks. Killed at 32 weeks after AOM	Semipurified diet, HF and 30% ER	4 days after AOM until the end of experiment	Colon cancer incidence[4]: HF AL, 9%[b]; ER, 0%[a]	ER of HF inhibited tumours	Reddy et al. (1987)
Charles River Sprague-Dawley (dams M/F offspring)	Birth	25–40 females and litters and 25–40 offspring	10 mg/kg bw DMH, s.c., 2 x wk for 10 wk, beginning 1 mo post weaning, killed 20 wks after last DMH	Semipurified diet, litter size adjusted to 4 or 8 pups/litter	Before and after DMH	% colon tumours:[4] 8 pups/litter – M, 48%[a] and F, 42%[a], 4 pups/litter – M, 85%[b] and F, 60%[b], 4 pups/litter, birth–weaning, 76%[b], pair-fed to 8 pups/litter after weaning, 52%	Reducing litter size enhanced tumours	Newberne et al. (1990)
Zucker (fa/fa), (Fa/Fa) and (Fa/fa) (M)	8	9–10	15 mg/kg bw AOM, s.c. at 10 and 11 wks killed at 12 wks after last AOM	Crude natural ingredient diet, LF, 10% calories from fat; HF, 40% calories from fat	Throughout	Tumour incidence[4]: fa/fa (obese) LF, 89%[b], Fa/Fa (lean) HF, 0%[a], Fa/fa, LF, 0%[a], Fa/fa HF, 0%[a]	Obesity phenotype increased tumours	Weber et al. (2000)

Table 46 (contd)

Organ site, species, strain (sex)	Age at beginning of study (wk)	No. of animals per group	Carcinogen/ dose/route	Dietary restriction/ amount, type	Timing of restriction	Prevention effect	Summarized effect	Reference
Mammary gland								
Mouse								
Pure bred (M/F)	Weanling	48–50	Spontaneous, killed at 100 wks of age	Cereal based (fox chow diluted with cornstarch, removed cornstarch for restriction): control 10–12 kcal/day; intermediate 8.2 kcal/day; low energy 7.1 kcal/day	Throughout	Tumour incidence: 10–12 kcal/day, 54% 8.2 kcal/day, 12%, 7.1% kcal/day, 0%	ER inhibited	Tannenbaum (1945)
C3H/HeOu (F)	4	24	Spontaneous, killed at 60 wks	Energy restriction: 0 (control) and 40% restriction; energy restricted by reducing calories from protein and carbohydrate	From 5 up to 40%: control ER, 60 wks ER, wks 4–12 of age	% mammary tumour-free[3]: 17%[c] 87%[b] 50%[a]	ER late in promotion inhibited	Engelman et al. (1994)
B6C3F1 (F)	4	55	Spontaneous, longevity study	40% DR with vitamin supplementation	From 16 weeks throughout	Tumour (benign and malignant) incidence: Control 13%; DR 2% Control, 15%; DR, 0% Control, 5%; DR, 0%	DR decreased tumours	Sheldon et al. (1996)
B6D2F1 (F)	4	56						
C57BL/6 (F)	4	37						
Rat								
Sprague-Dawley (F)	50 days	17–18	5 mg DMBA, i.v. at 57 days of age, killed at 26 wks	Cereal-based diet, 50% diet restriction	Diet restricted 7 d before and 30 d after DMBA treatment	Mammary tumour incidence:[4] Control, 76%[b] DR, 29%[a]	DR around DMBA inhibited tumours	Sylvester et al. (1981)
Sprague-Dawley (F)	50 days	[18–21]	5 mg DMBA, i.v. at 57 days of age, killed at 21 wks	Cereal-based diet, 50% diet restriction	Diet restricted 1 wk before and 1 wk after DMBA treatment, or for 2 wks starting 1, 3 wks after after DMBA, or for 4 wks starting 5 wks after DMBA	Mammary tumour incidence:[4] Control, 81%[b], diet restricted 1 wk after DMBA treatment, 28%[a] or for 2 wks starting 1, 76%, 3, 75% after DMBA, or for 4 wks starting 5 wks,	Only ER 1 wk before and 1 wk after DMBA inhibited tumours	Sylvester et al. (1982)

Table 46 (contd)

Organ site, species, strain (sex)	Age at beginning of study (wk)	No. of animals per group	Carcinogen/dose/route	Dietary restriction/amount, type	Timing of restriction	Prevention effect	Summarized effect	Reference
Fischer 344 (F)	52 days	14–15	65 mg/kg bw DMBA by gavage, killed at 24 wks after DMBA	Control semi-purified (5% fat), HF (30% fat), HF restricted to the net energy value consumed by the control group (HFR)	Beginning one day after DMBA	Cumulative adenocarcinoma incidence: Control, 40% HF, 73% HFR, 8%	Restriction of HF diet inhibited tumours	Boissonneault et al. (1986)
Sprague-Dawley (F)	50 days	20	5 mg DMBA by gavage, killed at 20 wks	Energy restriction: 0 (control), 10, 20, 30, and 40% restriction	Throughout	Tumour incidence[4]: Control, 60%[b]; 10% ER, 60%; 20% ER, 40%[a]; 30% ER, 35%[a]; 40% ER, 5%[a]	Dose–response inhibition with ER	Klurfeld et al. (1989a)
Sprague-Dawley (F)	50 days	20	5 mg DMBA by gavage, killed at 20 wks	Energy restriction: 0 (control) and 25% restriction	Beginning one week after DMBA: control ER, 4 mo ER, 1 mo/C, 3 mo ER, 2 mo/C, 2 mo C, 1 mo/ER, 2 mo/C, 1 mo C, 2mo/ER 2 mo	Cumulative incidence of palpable tumours: 50% 20% 60% 40% 45% 30%	ER late in promotion inhibited tumours	Kritchevsky et al. (1989)
Sprague-Dawley (F)	50 days	10–80	5 mg DMBA by gavage, killed at 20 wks after feeding regimens	Energy restriction: 0 (control) 25 and 40% restriction	Beginning one week following DMBA	Tumour incidence[5]: Control, 90%[*]; 25% ER, 61%[*]; 40% ER, 20%[*]	Dose–response inhibition with ER	Ruggeri et al. (1989)
LA/N phenotypically lean or obese (F)	65 days	15 pairs obese and 19 pairs lean	5 mg DMBA by gavage, killed at 16 wks	Energy restriction: 0 (control) and 40% restriction	Beginning one week after DMBA: control, obese ER, obese Control, lean	Cumulative incidence of palpable tumours 100% 27% 21%	ER of obese inhibited tumours	Klurfeld et al. (1991)

Table 46 (contd)

Organ site, species strain (sex)	Age at beginning of study (wk)	No. of animals	Carcinogen/ dose/route	Dietary restriction/ amount type	Timing of restriction	Prevention effect	Summarized effect	Reference
Sprague-Dawley (F)	50 days	20	25 mg/kg bw MNU, i.v., killed at 20 wks	Energy restriction: 0 (control) and 30% restriction	Beginning one day after MNU: all rats fed 50 kcal/day/45% fat diet (control/HF) until tumours were 1 cm³, then some were fed for 10±2 weeks on this diet: 35 kcal/day/45% fat (ER/HF), 50 kcal/day/25% fat (control/LF), 35 kcal/day/25% fat (ER/LF)	Tumour/body weight (%): ER/HF, 2.2; Control/LF, 2.5; ER/LF, 1.3	ER of LF or HF inhibited tumours	Zhu et al. (1991)
Fischer 344 (F)	4	54–180	Spontaneous longevity study	40% DR with vitamin supplementation	From 16 weeks throughout	Adenocarcinoma incidence: Control, 6%; DR, 1%	DR decreased tumours	Thurman et al. (1994)
Fischer 344 (F)	50 days	30–32	50 mg/kg bw MNU, i.p., x 2, 50 and 57 d, killed at 20.5 wks after MNU	Meal-fed control semi-purified diet and 20% ER	Beginning at 64 d of age, with or without exercise (progressively up to running 20 m/min at 15% grade for 30 min, 5 days/wk)	Cumulative adeno-carcinoma incidence:[4] Control, sedentary, 23%[b]; ER, sedentary, 7%[a], control, exercise, 28%[b]; ER, exercise, 34%[b]	ER or sedentary inhibited tumours	Gillette et al. (1997)
Sprague-Dawley (F)	21 days	24	50 mg/kg bw MNU, i.p., killed at 35 days after MNU	Energy restriction: 0 (control) 10, 20 and 40% restriction	Following carcinogen treatment to end of study	Proportion of carcinoma[5]: Control, 4.55%*; 10% ER, 2.72%*; 20% ER, 1.76%*; 40% ER, 0.29%*	Dose-response inhibition of tumours	Zhu et al. (1997)

Table 46 (contd)

Organ site, species, strain (sex)	Age at beginning of study (wk)	No. of animals per group	Carcinogen/ dose/route	Dietary restriction/ amount, type	Timing of restriction	Prevention effect	Summarized effect	Reference
ACI	7	21	17β-Estradiol (E2) in silastic tubing implants from 8.5 wks, killed when tumours were 1.5–2.0 cm diameter or at 220 days of E2	Energy restriction: 0 (control) and 40% ER from fat and carbohydrate	Throughout	Mammary cancer incidence at end of study in E2-treated groups:[4] Control, 100[b] ER, 60%[a]	ER inhibited tumours	Harvell et al. (2001a)
Prostate								
Rat								
Lobund Wistar germ-free and conventional (M)	Weanling	100	Spontaneous, killed at 6, 18, 30 or 30+ months	Cereal-based diet; diet restricted 30%	Throughout	Prostate adeno-carcinoma: Control-conventional, 26%; DR-conventional, 6%; control-germ-free, 5%; DR-germ-free, 10%	DR inhibited tumours in conventional rats	Pollard et al. (1989)
Pancreas								
Rat								
Lewis (M)	2	22–24	30 mg/kg bw azaserine × 1 i.p. at suckling, killed at 14 mo after azaserine	Meal fed: AL 5–6 h day	For the first two months after initiation, for the second two months after initiation or for 4 months after initiation	Carcinoma incidence:[2] control, 65%[c]; MF/C, 26%[b]; C/MF, 21%[b]; MF/MF, 0%[a]	Meal feeding for 4 months inhibited more than meal feeding during 2 months in early or late promotion	Roebuck et al. (1993)
Hamster								
Syrian golden (M)	8	25–35	20 mg/kg bw BOP × 1, s.c., killed at 94 wks	AL (av, 29–35 kcal /day); 'control fed' (av, 27 kcal/day); with control diet (4.3% fat) or high fat (20.5% fat)	1 week after initiation	Ductular carcinoma incidence:[3] AL/ control, 8%[a]; AL/HF, 30%[b]; control fed/control, 13%[c]; control fed/ HF, 52%[d]	HF diet increased tumours	Birt et al. (1989)

Table 46 (contd)

Organ site, species, strain (sex)	Age at beginning of study (wk)	No. of animals per group	Carcinogen/ dose/route	Dietary restriction/ amount, type	Timing of restriction	Prevention effect	Summarized effect	Reference
Syrian golden (M) (M)	8	33–38	20 mg/kg bw BOP weekly, x 3 s.c., killed at 42–44 wks after last BOP	Control, 20 and 40% ER from fat and carbohydrate	After initiation	No. of carcinomas/ effective animals[4]: control, 0.9[a]; 20% restricted, 1.2; 40% 1.7[b]	40% ER increased multiplicity	Birt et al. (1997)
Skin *Mouse* Rockland (F)	8–12	48	Benzo[a]pyrene; 60 µg 2 x wk, 38 weeks, terminate at 38 week, topical	50% ER, removal of carbohydrate	Throughout	Tumour incidence: control, 82%; 50% restriction, 16%	ER reduced tumours	Boutwell et al. (1949)
Sencar (F)	9	23–30	10 nmol DMBA x 1 + 3.2 nmol TPA, 2 x wk, 20 weeks, topical, killed at 50 wk	40% restriction, removal of fat and carbohydrate (ER) or feeding less diet (DR)	Restriction only before DMBA or only after DMBA	Carcinoma incidence[4]: control, 71%[b], ER before, 69%; DR before, 58%; ER after, 28%[a]; DR after, 41%	ER inhibited more than DR	Birt et al. (1991)
Sencar (F)	9	45	10 nmol DMBA x 1 + 3.2 nmol TPA, 2 x wk, 20 weeks, topical, killed at 59 wks after DMBA	35% ER, removal of fat or carbohydrate	Restriction during and after TPA	Carcinoma incidence[4]: control 70%[b]; removal of fat, 45%[a], removal of carbohydrate, 45%[a]	ER from fat or from carbohydrate inhibited	Birt et al. (1993)
Sencar (F)	9	31–48	10 nmol DMBA x 1 + 3.2 nmol TPA, 2 x wk, 2 weeks, then 10 nmol Mezerein 2 x wk, 16 weeks, topical, killed at 62 wk after DMBA	40% energy restriction from fat and carbohydrate	Restriction during TPA, or during Mezerein or during both exposure periods	Carcinoma incidence[1]: control, 29%[f]; ER during TPA, 33%[f]; ER during Mezerein, 15%[e]; ER during both, 10%[e]	ER during late promotion or throughout inhibited	Birt et al. (1994a)

Table 46 (contd)

Organ site, species, strain (sex)	Age at beginning of study (wk)	No. of animals per group	Carcinogen, dose/route	Dietary restriction/ amount, type	Timing of restriction	Prevention effect	Summarized effect	Reference
Sencar (F)	9	35	10 nmol DMBA x 1 + 3.2 nmol TPA, 2 x wk, 18 weeks topical, killed at 45 wk after DMBA	20 and 40% ER from fat and carbohydrate from LF (10% fat) or HF (42% fat) diets	Restriction during and after TPA	Carcinoma incidence[1]: Control, 40%[d]; 20% restriction from LF, 40% restriction from LF, 15%[c]; HF, 35%[b], 20% restriction from HF, 35%; 40% restriction from HF, 0%[a]	LF diets: 20% ER and 40% ER inhibited; HF diets: only 40% ER inhibited	Birt et al. (1996)
Liver								
Mouse								
Swiss OF1 (M/F)	Weanling	14–17	0.4 µmol/g bw DEN, i.p. killed at 48 wk	Cereal-based diet, 30% DR	Ad libitum thoughout DR thoughout AL-36 wk/DR-12 wk DR-36 wk/AL-12 wk	Incidence of hepatocellular adenoma or carcinoma AL throughout 14%[b] DR throughout 10%[a] AL-36 wk/DR-12 wk 14% DR-36 wk/AL-12 wk 13%	DR throughout inhibited	Lagopoulos et al. (1991)
B6C3F₁ (M)	4	56	Spontaneous, longevity study	40% DR with vitamin supplementation	From 16 weeks throughout	Tumour (benign and malignant) incidence Control, 39%; DR, 9%;	DR decreased tumours	Sheldon et al. (1996)
(F)		56				Control, 11%; DR, 11%		
B6D2F₁ (M)	4	56				Control, 24%; DR, 2%		
(F)		56				Control, 13%; DR, 4%		
C57BL/6 (M)	4	50				Control, 12%; DR, 0%		
(F)		37				Control, 3%; DR, 0%		
Pituitary gland								
Mouse								
B6C3F₁ (F)	4	55	Spontaneous, longevity study	40% DR with vitamin supplementation	From 16 weeks throughout	Adenoma incidence: Control, 30%, DR, 0% tumours	DR decreased	Sheldon et al. (1996)

Table 46 (contd)

Organ site, species strain (sex)	Age at beginning of study (wk)	No. of animals per group	Carcinogen/ dose/route	Dietary restriction/ amount, type	Timing of restriction	Prevention effect	Summarized effect	Reference
B6D2F$_1$ (F)	4	56				Control, 17%; DR 0%		
C57BL/6 (F)	4	37				Control, 57%; DR, 2%		
Rat								
Fischer 344 (M)	4	54–180	Spontaneous longevity study	40% DR with vitamin supplementation	From 16 weeks throughout	Tumour incidence; Control, 72%; DR 36%	DR decreased tumours	Thurman et al. (1994)
Fischer 344 (F)	4					Tumour incidence: Control, 74%; DR, 44%		
Fischer 344			17β-Estradiol in silastic tubing implants for 12 wks	40% energy restriction from fat and carbohydrate	Throughout	Fold induction of pituitary weight by E2 compared with untreated rats:[4] Control, 5x[b], 40% ER, 2 x[a]	ER reduced adenoma	Harvell et al. (2001b)
Copenhagen			17β-Estradiol in silastic tubing implants for 12 wks	40% energy restriction from fat and carbohydrate	Throughout	Fold induction of pituitary weight by E2 compared with untreated rats:[4] Control, 2.5x[b], 40% ER, 1.5x[a]	ER reduced adenoma	Harvell et al. (2001b)
ACI			17β-Estradiol in silastic tubing implants for 12 wks	40% energy restriction from fat and carbohydrate	Throughout	Fold induction of pituitary weight by E2 compared with untreated rats:[4] Control, 3.5 [a], 40% ER, 4.5x[b]	No effect of ER	Harvell et al. (2001b)

Table 46 (contd)

Lymphoma

Mouse

Organ site, species, strain (sex)	Age at beginning of study (wk)	No. of animals per group	Carcinogen/ dose/route	Dietary restriction/ amount, type	Timing of restriction	Prevention effect	Summarized effect	Reference
B10C3F₁ (M)	45–50	67–68	Spontaneous, killed when moribund	Semipurified diet DR with supplementation: Control (160 kcal/wk) DR (90 kcal/wk)	Diet initiated at 12–13 mo of age	Tumour incidence[4]: Control, 47%[b]; DR, 31%[a]	DR inhibited	Weindruch & Walford (1982)
C57BL/6 (M)	45	60–72	Spontaneous, killed at 25 mo of age	ER, 25%	Diet initiated at 12 mo of age	Tumour incidence[4]: Control, 19%[b]; DR, 5%	DR inhibited	Volk et al. (1994)
B6C3F₁ (M) (F)	4	56 56	Spontaneous, longevity study	40% DR with vitamin supplementation	From 16 wks throughout	Tumour incidence: Control, 41%; DR, 11%; Control, 61%; DR, 29%	DR decreased tumours	Sheldon et al. (1996)
B6D2F₁ (M) (F)	4	56 56				Control, 38%; DR, 29% Control, 36%; DR, 21%		
C57BL/6 (M) (F)	4	50 37				Control, 8%; DR, 7% Control, 30%; DR, 9%		
C57BL/6 & 129/Sv p53⁻ᐟ⁻ p53⁺ᐟ⁺	Weanling	28–30	Spontaneous, genetically engineered mouse p53⁻ᐟ⁻, killed when moribund	Semi-purified energy restricted by 40% reduction from carbohydrate	Throughout	Time to death (tumour mortality) p53⁻ᐟ⁻/control, 110 days p53⁻ᐟ⁻/ER, 162 days p53⁻ᐟ⁻/control, 384 days; p53⁻ᐟ⁻/ER, 643 days	ER increased time to death	Hursting et al. (1997)

AL, *ad libitum*; AOM, azoxymethane; BOP, *N*-nitrosobis-(2-oxopropyl)amine; C, carcinogen; DMBA, 7,12-dimethylbenz[a]anthracene; i.m., intramuscular; i.p., intraperitoneal; i.v., intravenous; DMH, 1,2-dimethylhydrazine; DR, dietary restriction; ER, energy restriction; HF, high fat; LF, low fat; MAM, methylazoxymethanol; MF, meal fed; MNU, *N*-methyl-*N*-nitrosourea; s.c., subcutaneous; TPA, 12-*O*-tetradecanoylphorbol 13-acetate

[1]Statistically significant differences: pooled e < pooled f
[2]Statistically significant differences: a < b < c
[3]Statistically significant differences: a < b; c < d
[4]Statistically significant differences: a < b
* Significant trend

intake of the animals in the group with eight per litter, had intermediate cancer rates. The rats in litters of eight had the lowest rates. In a recent study on the relationship of obesity and high-fat diet to colon cancer, AOM induced large colon cancers in 8 out of 9 genetically obese Zucker rats (*fa/fa*) fed a low-fat diet, while parallel groups consisting of their genetically lean genotypes (*Fa/Fa* and *Fa/fa*) developed no gross lesions (Weber *et al.,* 2000). Furthermore, more colon aberrant crypts were observed in the obese Zucker rats fed low-fat diet than in the lean counterparts fed low- or high-fat diet.

Mammary gland

The most extensively studied organ system for cancer-preventive effects of dietary energy restriction is the mammary gland. Mammary carcinogenesis induced by viruses in mice or by chemical carcinogens such as 7,12-dimethylbenz[*a*]anthracene (DMBA), *N*-methyl-*N*-nitrosourea (MNU) and benzo[*a*]pyrene (BP) in mice and rats is inhibited by energy restriction (Freedman *et al.,* 1990; Decarli *et al.,* 1997; Kritchevsky, 1997). In general, mammary carcinomas induced in mice are alveolar in origin and are not dependent on ovarian steroids for their development and growth. For this reason, the majority of studies reviewed in this section were selected because they used one of two chemical carcinogens which induce mammary cancers that have many characteristics similar to the human counterparts. These characteristics include: ductal origin, ovarian hormone dependence and morphology.

Recent studies to assess the effect of energy restriction on mammary carcinogenesis have differed in strategy in various ways: restricting diet to different extents, feeding during different phases of cancer development, comparing the sources of energy or assessing the relation of body fatness to cancer prevention. Two related strategies that are covered elsewhere are comparing the effects of reduced calorie availability by dietary or energy restriction with those of increased energy use through an exercise regimen (covered in the next section of this chapter) and cyclic feeding, which results in a reduction in or loss of the protection due to restriction and is therefore covered in Chapter 7. Furthermore, several investigations have attempted to link changes in body composition with underfeeding and cancer prevention.

Tannenbaum (1945) investigated the influence of the level of energy restriction on spontaneous mammary cancer in mice. He noted that a reduction in daily energy intake from 12 to 7 calories [from 50 to 29 J] completely eliminated spontaneous mammary tumours, while the mean age at death of the non-tumour-bearing mice increased from 76 ± 5.1 weeks to 83 ± 2.8 weeks. Klurfeld *et al.* (1989a) compared rats subjected to 10, 20, 30 or 40% energy-restriction with freely fed controls and found a slight reduction in DMBA-induced mammary cancer incidence and multiplicity with 20% restriction and significant inhibition with 30 or 40% energy restriction. Reduced body weight and body fat were correlated with the reduction in tumour weight. Similar results were obtained by Ruggeri *et al.* (1989), but while inhibition of mammary carcinogenesis with 40% energy restriction was significantly correlated with reduced levels of circulating insulin, a reduction in carcinogenesis with 25% energy restriction was not paralleled by a significant reduction in circulating insulin (discussed further in the section on mechanisms later in this chapter). In a longevity study on Fischer 344 rats, 40% energy restriction also decreased the incidence of spontaneous adenoma and adenocarcinomas (Thurman *et al.,* 1994). Zhu *et al.* (1997) observed dose-related inhibition of mammary carcinogenesis, in terms of both incidence and multiplicity, in rats treated with 50 mg/kg bw MNU followed by an observation period of 35 days. Dramatic inhibition by 10, 20 or 40% energy restriction was seen in this rapid mammary tumorigenesis model, in comparison with freely fed controls, and the inhibition correlated with elevated excretion of corticosterone. Indeed, corticosterone excretion could serve as an independent predictor of the animal's cancer response in this study (Zhu *et al.,* 1997).

The impact of dietary or energy restriction during different stages of mammary carcinogenesis has also been assessed (Sylvester *et al.,* 1981, 1982; Kritchevsky *et al.,* 1989; Engelman *et al.,* 1994). Sylvester *et al.* (1981) studied the effect of short-term dietary restriction (50%) on DMBA-induced mammary carcinogenesis. They found that restriction for seven days before and for 30 days after treatment with the carcinogen resulted in a significant reduction in the average number of carcinomas by the end of a 26-week experiment. Short-duration under-feeding one week before and one week after DMBA treatment decreased tumour incidence, but underfeeding for two weeks beginning one or three weeks after treatment or for four weeks starting five weeks after treatment failed to inhibit the carcinogenic response as assessed 21 weeks later (Sylvester *et al.,* 1982). Kritchevsky *et al.* (1989) treated rats with DMBA and restricted their energy intake by 25% at different times during the next four months. The animals were placed on restricted energy during all the four months, during the first one or two months of this period, during the middle two months or during the last two months. Energy restriction reduced mammary cancer rates when applied throughout the four months or when initiated late in the process, but was not effective when administered early followed by *ad libitum* feeding (Kritchevsky *et al.,* 1989). These results showed that inhibition of the carcinogenic process was dependent on the time-frame over which energy restriction was imposed, the duration of energy restriction and the proximity of the energy restriction to the termination of the study. Engelman *et al.* (1994) examined the effect of the time of energy restriction (5–40% restriction) on spontaneous mammary cancer in C3H/HeOu mice. Mice were subjected to energy restriction from four weeks until the end of the study at 60 weeks of age or from weeks 4 to 12 followed by *ad libitum* feeding. The reduction in cancer was greatest with energy restriction throughout the study (about 90% of mice tumour-free at 60 weeks), intermediate with energy restriction from weeks 4–12 (about 50% of mice tumour-free at 60 weeks of age) and least in controls (17% of mice tumour-free at 60 weeks of age) (Engelman *et al.*, 1994). These observations were paralleled by reduction of numerous indices of mammary gland development by energy restriction. Reduction of tumour incidence by 40% dietary restriction was also observed in several strains of mice by Sheldon *et al.* (1996).

From a review of the literature and by comparing the effects of reductions in dietary fat with those of reductions in dietary energy intake, Freedman *et al.* (1990) concluded that both high-energy and high-fat diets increased mammary tumour incidence, with the magnitude of the effect of fat being two thirds that of energy. They further summarized data showing that the enhancement by dietary fat of mammary tumorigenesis was not simply due to elevations in body weight, but that there was a "specific enhancing effect of dietary fat" on mammary carcinogenesis. Ip (1990) observed the greatest reduction in mammary cancer when both fat and energy were reduced. Boissonneault *et al.* (1986) studied the influence of fat and energy intake on mammary carcinogenesis in DMBA-treated Fischer 344 rats. They calculated relative net energy values and restricted the intake of a high-fat diet (30%) to the net energy intake of the low-fat group (5%). Carcass energy was highest in the high-fat group, intermedi-

ate in the high-fat restricted (HFR) group and lowest in the low-fat group, while the mammary cancer incidence was lowest in the HFR group. It was concluded that mammary cancer development was related to a complex interaction of energy intake, energy retention and body size rather than to the percentage of fat in the diet. Zhu *et al.* (1991) assessed the effects of dietary fat and dietary energy on the growth of established mammary tumours in Sprague-Dawley rats. Mammary cancers were induced with 25 mg/kg MNU at 50 days of age and when tumours reached 1 cm^3, the rats were fed diets containing 25% or 45% dietary fat either *ad libitum* or with 30% energy restriction. Tumour growth was lowest in the low-fat 30% energy-restricted group. Reductions in fat intake did not significantly inhibit tumour growth.

The importance of body fat for mammary carcinogenesis has been evaluated. Studies with reduced energy intake after DMBA treatment comparing genetically obese LA/N-cp female rats with phenotypically lean littermates suggested that body fatness *per se* was not directly related to the risk of mammary carcinogenesis (Klurfeld *et al.*, 1991). In fact, energy restriction of the obese rats reduced lean body mass more than body fatness. Gillette *et al.* (1997) subjected rats treated with MNU (50 mg/kg at 50 and 57 days of age) to a treadmill-exercise regimen (20 m/min at a 15% grade for 30 min on five days per week) with or without energy restriction (20% reduction). Body weight gain, carcass fat and carcass energy were reduced in the exercised and energy-restricted groups, but mammary carcinogenesis was inhibited only in the sedentary energy-restricted rats. This finding is consistent with that of Klurfeld *et al.* (1991), indicating that carcass fat *per se* was not directly associated with cancer risk.

Recent studies of 17β-estradiol-induced mammary cancer in the ACI rat have demonstrated marked inhibition by

dietary energy restriction of mammary cancers but no prevention of 17β-estradiol-induced focal regions of atypical hyperplasia and no alteration in circulating estradiol (Harvell *et al.*, 2001a). This suggests that energy restriction may inhibit tumour development by blocking the progression of hyperplasia to mammary cancers.

Prostate

Pollard *et al.* (1989) examined spontaneous tumours in the prostate, liver and adrenal glands of conventional and germ-free Lobund-Wistar rats. A 30% reduction in dietary intake reduced prostate tumours from 25.7% to 6.3% and extended latency from 26.6 months to 36.7 months in conventional rats. The spontaneous prostate tumours were squamous-cell carcinomas, unlike the prostate adenocarcinomas observed in humans. In this study, although spontaneous liver adenomas were inhibited by reduced dietary intake, adrenal adenomas were not.

Pancreas

The effect of modifying energy intake has been assessed using two models of pancreatic cancer, azaserine-induced acinar carcinogenesis and BOP-induced ductular carcinogenesis. Azaserine induces acinar-cell acidophilic foci acinar carcinomas. Although such lesions are seen in human pancreas, acinar carcinomas account for a minor fraction of human pancreatic cancer. In contrast, BOP-induced pancreatic ductular carcinoma is highly representative of the human disease (Pour *et al.*, 1993). Using the azaserine model, Roebuck *et al.* (1993) demonstrated that meal feeding of rats for 5–6 h/day (matching a 10–15% energy restriction) resulted in an approximately 40% reduction in carcinoma incidence. Birt *et al.* (1989, 1997) fed restricted intakes to Syrian golden hamsters as part of a study of the impact of dietary fat on carcinogenesis. A delay of about eight weeks was observed in the induction of ductular pancreatic cancer by BOP in the 'control-fed' high-fat group compared with the *ad-libitum*-fed high-fat group. The reduction in dietary intake in the 'control-fed' high-fat hamsters compared with the *ad-libitum*-fed high-fat hamsters was about 23% (Birt *et al.*, 1989). Since this suggested that energy restriction delayed pancreatic carcinogenesis, the second study assessed the impact of 10, 20 and 40% dietary energy restriction on pancreatic carcinogenesis by BOP (Birt *et al.*, 1997); no inhibition of ductular pancreatic carcinogenesis was detected, and in contrast, a nearly twofold increase was seen in the multiplicity of pancreatic ductular carcinogenesis in the 40% dietary energy-restricted hamsters (see section on mechanisms later in this chapter).

Skin

The two-stage model of skin carcinogenesis has been particularly useful in assessing the inhibition of carcinogenesis by dietary energy restriction because of the ability to separate effects on initiating events from those on promoting events and because of the wealth of information available on the biochemical processes and the gene mutations that are important in carcinogenesis in this model. While chemically induced skin cancers are a good model of epithelial carcinogenesis, they do not well resemble human skin cancers, which are induced primarily by ultraviolet light. Boutwell *et al.* (1949) demonstrated that enhancement of BP-induced skin carcinogenesis by high levels of dietary fat was dependent upon the higher energy intake of the mice. More recent studies by Birt and colleagues have been reviewed (Birt *et al.*, 1995). Energy restriction was effective in protecting against skin carcinogenesis induced by DMBA and promoted by 12-*O*-tetradecanoylphorbol 13-acetate (TPA) when restriction was implemented during promotion, but was not effective when

given for a short time before and during the initiation phase (Birt *et al.*, 1991). Restriction either of fat plus carbohydrate energy or of all dietary constituents during skin tumour promotion resulted in fewer papillomas and carcinomas, but selective restriction of fat and carbohydrate energy gave greater inhibition of papilloma growth, papilloma number and carcinoma incidence than diet restriction (Birt *et al.*, 1991). Furthermore, while high dietary fat intake did increase skin carcinogenesis, reductions in energy intake were much more potent in inhibiting carcinogenesis (Birt *et al.*, 1993). In particular, restricting carbohydrate energy was more effective than restricting fat energy in the prevention of skin papillomas, although these two dietary restriction protocols were equally effective in preventing development of DMBA-initiated, TPA-promoted squamous cell carcinomas in Sencar mice. Restricting mice to either 20 or 40% of the energy intake of freely fed controls reduced the incidence of skin carcinomas by more than 50% in mice on a control fat (10% of energy) diet, while 40% energy restriction, but not 20% energy restriction, was effective in preventing skin cancer in mice fed high-fat (42% of energy) diets (Birt *et al.*, 1996). Studies with a two-stage promotion model using TPA as an early-stage promoter (two weeks) or mezerein as a late-stage promoter (16 weeks) showed that energy restriction was most effective in inhibiting late-stage promotion (Birt *et al.*, 1994a).

Liver

Chemically induced and spontaneous liver tumours in rodents are considered to model those occurring in humans because of their close similarity in morphological appearance (Scarpelli, 1988). Furthermore, rodent liver tumours often metastasize to the lung, as occurs in humans. Dietary energy restriction for prevention of liver carcinogenesis has been studied in animal models. For

example, Lagopoulos *et al.* (1991) examined liver tumours induced in mice by diethylnitrosamine (DEN) and demonstrated reductions in numbers of basophilic foci, adenomas and hepatocellular carcinoma after dietary restriction. *Ad libitum* feeding after long-term restriction resulted in the resumption of hepatic carcinogenesis and restriction was most effective when administered early in life. However, the mice fed restricted diets for 12 or 24 weeks followed by *ad libitum* feeding developed fewer hepatic lesions than the fully fed positive control group.

Liver tumours are often induced in chronic toxicity studies. Dietary restriction, used to achieve body weight control, reduced the incidence of both spontaneous liver tumour incidence and salicylazosulfapyridine-induced liver tumours (Iatropoulos *et al.*, 1997). Moreover, the incidences of liver tumours of unknown etiology (spontaneous) in rodents are also correlated with resultant body weight. In an analysis of over 100 chronic bioassays conducted by the US National Toxicology Program, from 75 to 90% (depending on study type) of the variance in control tumour (adenoma plus carcinoma) incidences (which ranged from 20 to 90%) was accounted for by variations in average body weight at approximately 14 months of age (Turturro *et al.*, 1996). Individual animal body weight at the same age was directly related, in an approximately quadratic relationship, to the probability of developing a tumour (liver, mammary, etc.) by the end of a toxicity test (Seilkop, 1995). [The Working Group noted that the potential role of genetic factors in accounting for these relationships was not considered.]

Direct modification of dietary intake, e.g., by dietary restriction, also inhibited spontaneous liver tumour incidences. A 40% dietary restriction (with supplementation) resulted in a reduction of tumour incidence in several mouse strains (Sheldon *et al.*, 1996). Changes in liver physiology occur as a result of dietary restriction. In histological sections from animals sacrificed during the course of this study, the incidence of apoptosis in liver parenchymal cells was elevated and the estimated cellular proliferation rate decreased throughout the lifespan, compared with *ad libitum*-fed controls (Muskhelishvili *et al.*, 1995).

Pituitary gland

Dietary restriction has long been known to reduce the incidence of these usually benign but commonly fatal tumours in Sprague–Dawley rats (Everitt *et al.*, 1980). The tumours show many of the same characteristics as human tumours, with similar cell types affected. Dietary restriction also lowers the incidence of these lesions in Fischer 344 rats (Shimokawa *et al.*, 1991; Thurman *et al.*, 1994) and mice (Sheldon *et al.*, 1996).

The correlation of early dietary restriction and pituitary tumour incidence accounted for approximately half the variance in the wide range of pituitary tumour incidences (10–60%) in National Toxicology Program studies (Turturro *et al.*, 1998), while there was a direct relationship between individual animal body weight and the probability of developing a pituitary tumour in long-term chronic studies (Seilkop, 1995).

Estrogen-induced prolactin-producing pituitary tumours that are observed in rats are markedly enlarged benign masses that display diffuse lactotroph hyperplasia and hypertrophy. They are highly vascularized but generally lack adenomatous foci (Spady *et al.*, 1999). In humans, the majority of pituitary tumours are microadenomas, usually composed of a single secretory cell type. Prolactin-producing pituitary tumours, referred to as prolactinomas, are the most frequently occurring neoplasm in the human pituitary. Several case reports suggest that estrogens act as a causative factor in the development of prolactinomas in humans. Similarities in the manner in which pituitary cells of the prolactin-producing cell type respond to estrogen in rats and humans suggest that estrogen is a risk factor for pituitary tumour development in both species.

The effect of 40% energy restriction on estrogen-induced pituitary adenomas was assessed in three rat strains: Fischer 344, Copenhagen and ACI (Harvell *et al.*, 2001b). Pituitary wet weight, commonly used as an indicator of pituitary tumorigenesis, was increased by estrogen in all strains and energy restriction reduced this increase in Fischer 344 and Copenhagen rats but not in ACI rats. Therefore, genetic background may be an important determinant in prevention of pituitary tumours by energy restriction.

Lymphomas

A series of investigations of tumours of unknown etiology (spontaneous) determined that dietary restriction beginning during mid-life was effective in preventing spontaneous lymphomas in B10C3F$_1$ mice (Weindruch & Walford, 1982). Lymphomas were significantly reduced in number and delayed in occurrence, although hepatomas were equally prevalent in the underfed and control-fed groups. Similarly, fewer lymphomas were found in energy-restricted C57BL/6 mice and this was paralleled by inhibition of age-associated interleukin-6 (IL-6) dysregulation, including prevention of the increasing serum level of IL-6 observed in control mice (Volk *et al.*, 1994). Reduction of spontaneous lymphomas by 40% dietary restriction in mice has also been demonstrated (Sheldon *et al.*, 1996).

Other tumours

Inhibition due to dietary restriction (with vitamin supplementation) has been observed for a number of other tumours in rodents. These include: thyroid follicular tumours in mice, which are similar to the follicular form seen as the minority of human thyroid cancers (which are mostly of the papillary type) (Sheldon *et al.*, 1996; Hill *et al.*, 1998); interstitial cell tumours of the testes in rats, which are similar to human Leydig cell tumours, both morphologically and in overall hormonal sensitivity (Thurman *et al.*, 1994; Cook *et al.*, 1999); preputial and clitoral gland tumours in rats, which are sebaceous gland tumours that appear to be most similar to skin and urogenital tumours in humans (Raso *et al.*, 1992); thyroid C-cell and adrenal phaeochromocytomas in rats, which can be good models for multiple endocrine neoplasia type 2 in humans (Schulz *et al.*, 1992; Thurman *et al.*, 1994) and affect cells that are smaller than the usual chromaffin cells seen in humans but are otherwise similar (Tischler *et al.*, 1996); and lung tumours in male B6C3F$_1$ and B6D2F$_1$ mice, which are excellent models of human tumours in both morphology and oncogene features (Malkinson, 1992; Sheldon *et al.*, 1996). A comprehensive, though dated, review of the effects of dietary restriction on tumour development is available (Weindruch & Walford, 1988).

Genetically engineered mouse models

New genetically engineered animal models have been developed to study the misregulation of specific genes singly and in combination during the carcinogenic process. Both transgenic and knock-out models can be used. In one such model, both allelic copies of the wild-type *p53* tumour-suppressor gene are deleted (knocked out). This model is considered to have relevance to human cancer in general because mutations of the *p53* gene are the most commonly observed mutation in human cancer (Mowat, 1998). The *p53*-deficient mice are extremely susceptible to spontaneous occurrence of tumours. Using this model, Hursting *et al.* (1997) studied the effect of energy restriction on genetically induced lymphoma. The fact that energy restriction inhibits cancer development in p53 knock-out mice (*p53*$^{-/-}$) and that inhibition of genetically induced carcinogenesis was similar in p53 wild-type ($p53^{+/+}$) and in $p53^{-/-}$ mice demonstrates that cancer prevention by energy restriction is independent of the functional status of *p53*. The use of genetically engineered animals raises the possibility of looking at the effects of energy restriction on incidence of tumours that are normally rare but are increased in such animals.

Physical activity

Laboratory experiments in which animal models are used to investigate the relationship between physical activity and cancer prevention have the potential: (1) to identify the characteristics of physical activity or exercise that are most likely to be critical to cancer prevention in humans; (2) to define mechanisms and markers of those mechanisms that would allow monitoring of disease progression in human populations over a short time frame; (3) to identify physical activity or fitness-related biomarkers of the 'cancer-protected state', and (4) to identify potentially confounding variables, for example dietary factors, that might mask the protective effects of physical activity if their existence were unrecognized (see review by Thompson, 1997).

Physical activity model (voluntary)

In the context of experimental studies, physical activity can be defined as any voluntary movement of an animal in which the skeletal muscles contract resulting in a quantifiable expenditure of energy. This definition does not require that the physical activity be designed to improve fitness, nor does the activity need to be done in a regular, structured or repetitive manner. Physical activity can be distinguished from exercise in that efforts to increase physical activity do not require an intent to improve physical fitness (Caspersen *et al.*, 1985). Providing animals with free access to an activity wheel provides an excellent model for studying the effects of increased levels of physical activity. Because animals choose when to run in the wheel and this behaviour has been demonstrated to vary between animals, there is nothing planned or structured about the physical activity associated with free access to the running wheel. Thus free use of an activity wheel, because it is voluntary, meets the definition of physical activity, but not exercise, and this is consistent with the way investigators studying carcinogenesis have designed experiments involving wheel-running. The amount of wheel-running activity has been quantified in terms of distance run or energy expended, without any attempt to set fitness goals and/or to assess training effects. Providing animals with free access to activity wheels appears well suited to answering questions about physical activity and cancer, particularly the question of whether total cumulative physical activity is predictive of risk for cancer. Apart from the expense of obtaining a sufficient number of properly engineered activity wheels for conducting a carcinogenesis experiment, issues that need to be considered if this model is used are the general decline in activity observed in experiments of several months duration, and the behaviour of some animals that turn their wheels without actually running in them.

Exercise models (involuntary)

Exercise can be defined as planned, structured and repetitive activity with the intent to develop and/or maintain some defined attribute of physical fitness. Of the animal models which are most frequently used, running on a treadmill, motorized drum or wheel has the potential to satisfy this definition. If animals are to be exercised, the activity will inevitably be involuntary and will usually require some type of reinforcement, depending on the intensity and duration of the exercise. Concern has been expressed that reinforcement of exercise behaviour to maintain compliance is likely to be stressful. While this is clearly a possibility, it must also be recognized that all exercise involves the imposition of a stress on muscles in order to improve fitness. Thus stress is an inherent component of studying exercise; a greater difficulty lies in defining the chemical basis of the various components of stress induced when animals are exercised to achieve and maintain defined fitness goals.

There are three primary components of exercise that can be varied and that may have different effects relative to carcinogenesis. They are the intensity (work-rate), the duration (length per activity bout) and the frequency (times per week) of the activity performed.

The most widely used animal model of exercise is the running of rodents on a variable-speed, incline-adjustable treadmill. The use of such a treadmill permits great flexibility in studying the effects of exercise intensity, since both the incline and the belt speed can be altered to achieve a particular work rate. Use of a warm-up and a warm-down period in the training protocol can reduce physiological stress and avoid injury to the animals. Metabolic treadmills are available that permit the measurement of aerobic capacity throughout an experiment. This procedure requires minimal alteration of an animal's routine so that the process of assessment can guide the training programme without independently affecting study results. When a treadmill is used, the animals need to be continuously monitored to minimize the risk of injury and ensure adherence to the exercise training protocol.

Physical activity and exercise control conditions

Two important issues must be considered in determining what constitutes an appropriate control for animal experiments in which either physical activity or exercise is studied. The first relates to the use of 'sham' conditions for physical activity or exercise. When access to wheel-running is used as the model, the general approach has been to house control animals in the same type of activity cage as the experimental animals, but to lock the wheel so that it does not rotate. For the treadmill model, handling and placing animals in a stationary or slowly moving treadmill has been successfully used as a sham control. The key point is to expose the sham control animals to a set of stimuli similar to those faced by the experimental group. A second critical element of control in such experiments is the exposure of all animals to the same overall levels of environmental activity, including that of research technicians conducting the work, related to the implementation of the physical activity or exercise protocol. Such factors can significantly influence the carcinogenic response in some target organs such as the mammary gland. The control of this situation is straightforward. All animals in such studies should be housed in the same room in which the physical activity or exercise is performed. While this approach can require review by an institution's animal care and use committee for an exception to standard operating procedures, it is essential that this aspect of methodology be considered in order to preserve the integrity of the experiment.

The body of experimental information regarding the influence of physical exercise on development of premalignant and malignant lesions in animal models is very limited. The following review is organized with reference to organs and tissues (Table 47). The growth of transplantable tumours in experimental animals is not considered, since these studies have limited relevance to the primary prevention of cancer (see Rusch & Kline, 1944; Hoffman et al., 1962; Good & Fernandez, 1981).

Colorectum

In a study of the influence of physical activity on DMH-induced colon carcinogenesis in the rat, Andrianapoulos et al. (1987) found that animals that were allowed running-wheel activity showed a significant reduction in the incidence of colon tumours (exercise group, 54.5%; non-exercise group, 90%).

Reddy et al. (1988) assessed the effects of voluntary exercise on AOM-induced colon carcinogenesis in male Fischer 344 rats. At five weeks of age, animals were divided into two groups (sedentary and exercise) and fed AIN-76A semi-purified diet ad libitum. They received a subcutaneous injection of 15 mg/kg bw AOM at seven weeks of age and another one week later. Those in the exercise group were then placed in individual wheel-cage units while the sedentary group were housed in normal plastic cages. At 38 weeks after AOM treatment, body weights of the exercise and sedentary groups were similar. The incidence and multiplicity of colon adenocarcinomas, but not of adenomas, were significantly reduced by the exercise. Incidences of small intestinal carcinomas and of liver foci were also reduced.

Colbert et al. (2000a) examined the effect of exercise training on polyp development in a mutant mouse strain predisposed to multiple intestinal neoplasia (Min mouse). Three-week-old male and female heterozygotes were randomly assigned to control (10 males, six females) or exercise (11 males, 11 females) groups. In the first week, exercised mice were acclimatized to treadmill running at 10–18 m/min for 15–60 min per day on five days per week. From four to 10 weeks of age, mice ran at 18–21 m/min for 60 min. Control mice sat in Plexiglas lanes suspended above the treadmill for the same time periods. At 10 weeks of age, the mice were killed. There were no significant effects of exercise on the multiplicity of small intestine, colon or total intestinal polyps in the males and females combined ($p > 0.05$). Among the males, when analysed separately, there were fewer colon and total polyps in the exercised than in the control mice, although the difference was not statistically significant ($p = 0.06$).

Mammary gland

Thompson and co-workers (Thompson et al., 1988, 1989b, 1995; Gillette et al., 1997) studied the effects of exercise and its interaction with dietary factors on mammary carcinogenesis in the rat. In the first two studies, low-intensity and short-duration exercise was shown to enhance cancer incidence. These studies are reviewed in Chapter 7.

Female Fischer 344 rats were given intraperitoneal injections of 50 mg/kg bw MNU at 50 and 57 days of age and subjected to sham exercise or 35% and 70% maximal treadmill running intensity for 20 or 40 min per day on five days per week. Mammary cancer incidence and multiplicity was lower in all exercise groups compared with the sham controls. As the degree of protection was proportional to the exercise intensity, rather than its duration, the authors concluded that intensity may be the more important factor determining protective activity (Thompson et al., 1995).

Gillette et al. (1997) concentrated on energy availability and mammary carcinogenesis, looking at effects of both energy restriction and exercise. Female Fischer 344 rats were given intraperitoneal injections of MNU (50 mg/kg bw at 50 and 57 days of age) and then randomized into four groups: (i) unrestricted, sedentary; (ii) energy-restricted, sedentary; (iii) unrestricted, exercised; (iv) energy-restricted, exercised. The mammary carcinoma incidence was significantly lower in the energy-restricted sedentary group than in all other groups. No effect of exercise was seen, despite significant reductions in carcass fat and carcass energy.

Cohen et al. (1988, 1991, 1993) reported on the influence of dietary fat, energy restriction and voluntary physical activity on MNU- and DMBA-induced mammary carcinogenesis in rats.

Table 47. Studies of prevention of spontaneous and carcinogen-induced tumours by physical activity and exercise in experimental animals

Organ site species/ strain (sex)	Age at beginning of the study (wk)	Study type	No. per group	Carcinogen exposure	Type of exercise	Results	Reference
Colon and small intestine							
Rat							
Sprague-Dawley (M)	5	Pre-/post-initiation	11–21	20 mg/kg bw DMH, 1 x wk, 6 weeks, i.p., killed 20 weeks after final DMH	Voluntary – wheel cage	Decrease	Andriana-poulos et al. (1987)
Fischer 344 (M)	7	Post-initiation	12–27	15 mg/kg bw AOM, 1 x wk, 2 weeks, s.c., killed 38 weeks after carcinogen	Voluntary – wheel cage	Decrease of adenocarcinomas	Reddy et al. (1988)
Mouse							
C57BL/6Min (M+F)	Weaning	Spontaneous	6–11	Killed at 10 weeks of age	Treadmill	No effect	Colbert et al. (2000a)
Mammary gland							
Mouse							
BALB/cMed (F)	8	Post-initiation	29–48	1 mg DMBA, 1 x wk, 6 weeks, p.o. killed at 44 weeks of age	Treadmill – rotating drum	Decrease with diet restriction and high fat	Lane et al. (1991)
Rat							
Fischer 344 (F)	7	Post-initiation	30–36	37.5 mg/mg bw MNU i.v., killed 20 weeks after carcinogen	Voluntary – wheel cage	Decrease	Cohen et al. (1988, 1991)
Fischer 344 (F)	8	Post-initiation	30	5–10 mg/kg bw DMBA, p.o., killed at 77 or 133 days after carcinogen	Voluntary – wheel cage	No effect	Cohen et al. (1993)
Fischer 344 (F)	7	Post-initiation	28–30	50 mg/kg bw MNU, 1 x wk, 2 weeks, i.p., killed 3 months after carcinogen	Treadmill	Decrease	Thompson et al. (1995)

Table 47 (contd)

Organ site/ species/ strain (sex)	Age at beginning of the study (wk)	Study type	No. per group	Carcinogen exposure	Type of exercise	Results	Reference
Sprague-Dawley (F)	3	Pre-initiation	26–29	50 mg/kg bw MNU, at 50 days i.p., killed 24 weeks after carcinogen	Treadmill	Decrease	Whittal & Parkhouse (1996)
Fischer 344 (F)	7	Post-initiation	30–32	50 mg/kg bw MNU, 1 x wk, 2 weeks, i.p., killed 20.5 weeks after carcinogen	Treadmill[a]	No effect	Gillette et al. (1997)
Sprague-Dawley (F)	3	Pre-initiation	40	37.5 mg/kg bw MNU, at 50 days, i.p., killed 22 weeks after carcinogen	Treadmill	No effect	Whittal-Strange et al. (1998)
Pancreas *Hamster* Syrian hamster (F)	4	Pre-/post-initiation	25–28	20 mg/kg bw BOP, 1 x wk, 2 weeks, s.c., killed 44 weeks after last BOP	Voluntary – wheel cage	No effect	Kazakoff et al. (1996)
Liver *Rat* Jc1:Wistar (M)	10	Concurrent	17–19	0.0177 g/kg bw/day 3'-Me-4-DAB diet starting at 27 weeks, killed at 62 weeks of age	Voluntary – wheel cage	Decrease	Ikuyama et al. (1993)

AOM, azoxymethane; BOP, *N*-nitrosobis(2-oxopropyl)amine; DMBA, 7,12-dimethylbenz[a]anthracene; DMH, 1,2-dimethylhydrazine; i.p., intraperitoneal; i.v., intravenous; 3'-Me-4-DAB, 3'-methyl-4-dimethylaminoazobenzene; MNU, *N*-methyl-*N*-nitrosourea; p.o., orally

Voluntary activity during the post-initiation stage reduced tumour yields and extended the latency period. Cohen et al. (1992) reported a U-shaped relationship between cumulative distance run in an activity wheel and the magnitude of the carcinogenic response, the greatest response being observed at intermediate distances.

Whittal and Parkhouse (1996) reported the effects of exercise on mammary gland development, proliferation and MNU-induced tumorigenesis. Female Sprague-Dawley rats were divided into two groups, sedentary and exercised from 21 to 50 days of age (progressive treadmill training programme with a final workload of 18 m/min at 15% incline for 60 min per day). At 50 days of age, 24 hours after exercise, animals were given an intraperitoneal injection of MNU at 50 mg/kg bw. At the termination of the experiment at 24 weeks after carcinogen treatment, the total number of tumours was reduced by exercise (from 58 to 33 carcinomas, $p < 0.05$, 1.3 ± 0.24 tumours per animal versus 2.0 ± 3.5 in the sedentary group). The latency period was not affected and the tumour incidences were similar (68.9% and 61.5%) in sedentary and exercised rats. The results were not associated with any change in the degree of mammary gland development or proliferation status at the time of MNU administration.

Whittal-Strange et al. (1998) further described effects of exercise on MNU-induced mammary tumorigenesis. Female Sprague-Dawley rats, divided into two groups, sedentary and exercised from 21 to 50 days of age (progressive treadmill training programme with a final workload of 18 m/min at 15% incline for 60 min per day), were given an intraperitoneal injection of MNU at 35 mg/kg bw at 50 days of age. At the termination of the experiment 22 weeks after carcinogen treatment, the tumour incidence, multiplicity and latency did not show any difference between the groups, but the tumour growth rate and the final tumour weight

were significantly higher in the exercised animals.

In BALB/c mice treated with DMBA, tumour incidence was not affected by treadmill exercise in animals fed a standard diet, but was significantly reduced in exercised mice fed a restricted or a high-fat diet (Lane et al., 1991).

Pancreas

Kazakoff et al. (1996) determined the effects of voluntary physical activity on high-fat diet-promoted pancreatic carcinogenesis in hamsters. Groups of female Syrian hamsters were fed a high-fat diet (24.6% w/w corn oil) or low-fat diet (4.5% w/w corn oil). Each group was subdivided into an exercise and a sedentary group. All hamsters were fed their diets for four weeks, then given two injections of 20 mg/kg bw BOP with a one-week interval. Diets were continued until week 44 after the BOP treatment. No significant difference in incidence of carcinomas in situ or pancreatic ductal/ductular adenocarcinomas was observed between the exercise and sedentary groups.

Liver

The effects of voluntary physical activity on induction of hepatomas by 3′-methyl-4-dimethylaminoazobenzene were investigated in male Jc1:Wistar rats, divided into sedentary and exercise groups and maintained in individual cages (Ikuyama et al., 1993). Food intake and wheel-running were automatically controlled in the cages of the exercise group. From 27 weeks to the termination of the study at week 62, the animals were fed the carcinogen in the diet at 0.0177 g/day/kg body weight. The incidence of hepatomas [histology not specified] was significantly lower in the exercise group (0% versus 65% in the sedentary group).

Intermediate biomarkers – weight control

Intermediate end-point biomarkers are cellular, biochemical and/or molecular

determinants of the risk for subsequent development of cancer. These markers may represent intermediate stages in the development of cancer or be causally involved in the etiology of cancer, and/or reflect changes in cellular processes that occur in parallel to the initiation, promotion and/or progression stage(s) of carcinogenesis. Intermediate markers discussed in this section can be grouped under one of these categories. Some of these markers are also discussed in the section on mechanisms later in this chapter, since mechanistic studies frequently identify candidate intermediate biomarkers.

The number of animal experiments in which the effects of energy restriction on intermediate end-point biomarkers for cancer have been investigated is limited (Table 48).

Colon

The effects of 20–30% energy restriction on the rate of colonic cell proliferation, stated by the authors to be an intermediate biomarker for colon cancer risk, was investigated in male Fischer 344 rats treated with AOM as a colon-specific carcinogen (Steinbach et al., 1993). Energy restriction was shown to inhibit tumour formation. Both the DNA labelling index, determined by [3H]thymidine incorporation, and the number of labelled cells per crypt column were reduced by energy restriction in both carcinogen-treated and control rats in normal-appearing mucosa. The effect was seen after as little as 10 and 20 weeks of energy restriction and persisted at 34 weeks. These findings are indicative of a reduced risk for cancer. Lasko and co-workers also studied the effects of 20% energy restriction on a different intermediate biomarker for colon cancer, aberrant crypt foci (ACF), in rats treated with AOM (Lasko & Bird 1995; Lasko et al., 1999). A moderate level of energy restriction (20%) reduced the total number of ACF regardless of the level of fat, but retarded the appearance of

Table 48. Modulation by energy restriction of intermediate biomarkers in animal models

Organ site/ species/strain (sex)	Magnitude of restriction	Duration of feeding	Genotoxic agent (dose and schedule)	Investigated effect	Result[a]	Reference
Colon						
Rat						
Fischer 344 (M)	20 or 30%	10, 20, 21, 34 wks	AOM, 15 mg/kg bw, 1 x wk, 2 weeks, s.c.	Colon cell proliferation ([^{3}H]thymidine incorporation)	Decreased	Steinbach et al. (1993)
Fischer 344 (M)	20%	Restriction delayed for 11 wks and imposed for 12 wks	AOM, 15 mg/kg bw, 1 x wk, 2 weeks, s.c.	Aberrant crypt foci	Decreased	Lasko & Bird (1995)
Fischer 344 (M)	20%	Restriction delayed for 16 wks and imposed for 6 wks	AOM, 15 mg/kg bw, 1 x wk, 3 weeks, s.c.	Aberrant crypt foci	Decreased	Lasko et al. (1999)
Mammary gland						
Mouse						
C3H/HeOu (F)	19%	6, 8, 10 and 12 wks	Spontaneous	EGF mRNA or protein at 12 weeks: Submandibular gland; Mammary gland; Serum EGF protein	Decreased; Decreased; No change	Engelman et al. (1995)
Pancreas						
Rat						
Lewis (M)	10–30%	16 wk	Azaserine, 30 mg/kg, once	Acidophilic pancreatic foci	Dose-dependent decrease	Roebuck et al. (1993)
Liver						
Mouse						
B6C3F$_1$	40%	Continuous, multiple age groups	Spontaneous model	Pi-class glutathione S-transferase (GST-II) hepatic foci	Decreased	Muskhelishvili et al. (1996)
Rat						
Fischer 344 (M)	30%	32 wks	AOM, 15 mg/kg bw, 1 x wk, 2 weeks, s.c.	GST-P (placental form)-positive hepatic foci	Decreased	Sugie et al. (1993)
Fischer 344 (M)	40%	6 wks	Aflatoxin B$_1$ 0.1 mg 1,6 or 15 times, p.o. Benzo[a]pyrene (BP) 1 mmol/ml/kg bw, 1 or 3 times, i.p.	Aflatoxin B$_1$-DNA; BP-DNA adducts	Decreased; Increased	Chou et al. (1993a)

AOM, azoxymethane; BP, benzo[a]pyrene; i.p., intraperitoneal; p.o., oral; s.c., subcutaneous
[a] Statistically significant, $p < 0.05$

advanced ACF only when dietary fat was low (5% w/w) but not high (23% w/w). This effect, which was consistently observed only in animals fed the low-fat diet, was seen when energy restriction was initiated either 11 or 16 weeks after AOM treatment, times at which advanced ACF were present in the colon.

Mammary gland

Insulin-like growth factor metabolism has been proposed as a candidate intermediate marker for cancer at several sites including the mammary gland. The effects of energy restriction on this intermediate end-point are considered in the section on mechanisms later in this chapter. The effect of energy restriction (19%) on the expression of epidermal growth factor (EGF, mRNA and protein levels) was investigated in the submandibular gland, mammary gland and serum (protein only) of female C3H/HeOu mice that develop mammary tumours in response to mouse mammary tumour virus (MMTV) (Engelman et al., 1995). Effects were evaluated at 6, 8, 10 and 12 weeks. Levels of EGF mRNA and protein in tissue were lower in energy-restricted animals than in ad libitum-fed controls at the later time points, but no differences were observed in serum concentrations of EGF. The authors suggested that reduced levels of EGF in tumour tissue might contribute to the antiproliferative effects of energy restriction and reduced incidence of carcinomas in this mammary tumour model.

Pancreas

The effect of several levels of energy restriction (10, 15, 20 and 30%) on azaserine-induced pancreatic carcinogenesis in the rat has been studied (Roebuck et al., 1993). A progressive reduction in the occurrence of acidophilic pancreatic foci, an intermediate biomarker for pancreatic carcinomas, was observed with increasing degree of energy restriction.

Liver

Energy restriction has been reported to inhibit the occurrence of glutathione-S-transferase (GST)-positive hepatic foci, an intermediate biomarker for the development of hepatocellular carcinomas. Muskhelishvili et al. (1996) studied the effects of dietary restriction on the spontaneous occurrence of GST-II (pi-class)-positive foci in male B6C3F1 mice that are tumour-prone. [The Working Group noted that GST-pi-positive foci have not been shown to be precursor lesions for hepatocellular carcinoma in mice.] Dietary restriction diminished GST-II expression with a marked reduction in the incidence of liver tumours. Sugie et al. (1993) examined the effect of energy restriction (30%) on the induction of GST-P (placental form)-positive foci in rat liver following administration of AOM, which is usually considered a colon-specific carcinogen. The density and size of GST-P-positive foci were significantly lower in AOM-treated, energy-restricted animals, but the incidence of foci was unaffected in AOM-treated energy-restricted rats relative to the AOM-treated control group. Energy restriction (40%) has been reported to modulate the formation of carcinogen–DNA adducts in the liver. Whereas the formation of aflatoxin B_1–DNA adducts was reduced in parallel with a reduction in CYP2C11, which is involved in aflatoxin B_1 activation, BP–DNA adducts were increased (Chou et al., 1993a). The increase correlated with an increase in BP-metabolizing enzymes. The implications of these findings are discussed in the section on mechanisms later in this chapter.

Oncogene expression

Effects of energy restriction (30–40%) on oncogene expression have been reported (Nakamura et al., 1989; Baik et al., 1992; Himeno et al., 1992; Fernandes et al., 1995). Three of these experiments were not designed specifically to investigate the cancer-preventive activity of

energy restriction and in one (Fernandes et al., 1995), oncogene expression was studied in tumours that occurred despite energy restriction. Therefore, the results must be interpreted with caution, since the changes in oncogene expression observed may have little relevance to cancer prevention per se. Nonetheless, the data suggest that energy restriction leads to down-regulation of expression of c-Ha-ras and c-fos mRNA in mammary tissue (30% restriction) but not in liver (Baik et al., 1992). Hepatic c-myc proto-oncogene expression was reduced in chronically restricted (40%) C57B16 × C3HF1 hybrid mice (Nakamura et al., 1989). The authors speculated that c-myc expression may be linked to metabolic activity and to lower rates of hepatic cell proliferation in energy-restricted mice. Oncogene expression during liver regeneration was also studied (Himeno et al., 1992). Energy restriction (40%) preserved inducible cellular responses in response to partial hepatectomy, i.e., [^{3}H]thymidine incorporation, but lowered the elevated oncogene expression observed in response to partial hepatectomy relative to the response observed in ad libitum-fed controls.

Fernandes et al. (1995) studied the correlation of oncogene and tumour-suppressor gene changes with the cancer-preventive activity of energy restriction in an MMTV/v-Ha-ras model. In mammary tumours that occurred despite 40% energy restriction, the restriction led to lower expression and mRNA levels of v-Ha-ras and neu, and increased wild-type p53 expression. The authors speculated that these changes reflected molecular alterations involved in the inhibition of mammary carcinoma induction in this model.

Intermediate biomarkers – physical activity

Few animal experiments have investigated the effects of physical activity on intermediate end-point biomarkers for cancer (Table 49).

Table 49. Modulation by physical activity of intermediate biomarkers in animal models

Organ site/species/strain (sex)	Type of physical activity	Duration and intensity of physical activity	Genotoxic agent (dose and schedule)	Investigated effect	Result	Reference
Liver Rat Fischer 344 (M)	Wheel-running for 38 weeks, initiated 4 days after last AOM injection	Voluntary Peak: wk 6 Distance run diminished over time	AOM, 15 mg/kg bw, 1 × wk, 2 weeks, s.c.	GST-P hepatic foci Density Size Incidence	Decreased* Decreased* No effect	Sugie et al. (1992)
Pancreas Rat Lewis (M) Fischer 344 (F)	Wheel-running for up to 18 weeks, started after azaserine injection	Voluntary Peak: 6–12 week depending on gender Distance run diminished over time	Azaserine males: 30 mg/kg bw once, i.p. Females: 30 mg/kg bw × 3 times, i.p.	Volume% 4 months after initiation Acidophilic acinar-cell foci Basophilic acinar-cell foci Labelling index: [³H]thymidine incorporation	Reduced in males* and females – NS No effect in males; reduced in females* Reduced – NS	Roebuck et al. (1990)
Lewis (M)	Treadmill running	Progressive training programme, final work-load of 16 m/min, 7.5° incline, 5 days/week, 7 wk training, 18 wk exercise	Azaserine, 30 mg/kg bw once, i.p.	Acidophilic pancreatic foci: Volume%	Increased – NS	Craven-Giles et al. (1994)
Mammary gland Rat Sprague-Dawley (F)	Treadmill running with air jet reinforcement	Progressive training programme: final workload of 18 m/min on a 15% incline for 60 min, 5 days per week from 21 to 50 days of age	MNU, 50 mg/kg bw, i.p. at 50 days of age	Continuous labelling with BrdU for 4 days at 46 days of age (mammary gland) Developmental score for the mammary gland	No difference No difference	Whittal & Parkhouse (1996)

*Reported effect was statistically significant, $p < 0.05$; NS, not statistically significant
AOM, azoxymethane; BrdU, bromodeoxyuridine; GST, glutathione-S-transferase; i.p., intraperitoneal; MNU, N-methyl-N-nitrosourea; NS, not significant; s.c., subcutaneous

Liver

The effect of voluntary physical activity (wheel-running) on carcinogen-induced GST-P (placental form)-positive (enzyme-altered) foci in liver was studied by Sugie et al. (1992). Voluntary access to an activity wheel was initiated following carcinogen administration (AOM, subcutaneous injection, 5 mg/kg bw × 2). The density and size of GST-P hepatic foci were reduced significantly in active versus sedentary animals; the incidence of altered foci was unaffected. These results were interpreted by the authors to indicate that activity may inhibit chemically induced hepatocarcinogenesis. [The Working Group noted that activity was not uniform throughout the experiment, peaking at week 6 after carcinogen treatment and declining thereafter].

Pancreas

Roebuck et al. (1990) studied the effect of wheel-running on intermediate biomarkers for pancreatic cancer, namely formation of acidophilic and basophilic pancreatic foci and [3H]thymidine incorporation as a measure of cell proliferation within foci. Variable effects on these markers in response to exercise were observed and frequently differences between the active and sedentary groups did not reach the level of statistical significance. The authors concluded that male and female rats with free access to running wheels had significantly smaller foci and lower rates of thymidine incorporation into foci four months after initiation. These effects occurred late in the post-initiation phase and were not directly related to the extent of running activity early in the post-initiation phase. [The Working Group noted the reduction of running activity over time during this study. Also, the responses were not consistent with gender, and/or were not statistically significant.]

In a second series of studies, Craven-Giles et al. (1994) investigated modulation of pancreatic foci by treadmill running. Male Lewis rats were treated with azaserine at two weeks of age and weaned to experimental protocols at three weeks of age. Two experiments were undertaken: treadmill exercise began at six weeks of age (Experiment 1) or at 13 weeks of age (Experiment 2). Rats were exercised for 15–20 min/day and for three to five days per week. Treadmill speed and angle of incline were adjusted to afford a range of exercise intensities. The development of pancreatic acinar foci was evaluated by quantitative stereological analysis using light microscopy. In Experiment 1, exercise resulted in a known paradoxical reduction in food intake by about 15% of the intake of the sedentary group fed ad libitum. The burden of azaserine-induced foci was decreased by approximately 37%, and this was attributed to the known effects of reduced energy intake in these young, rapidly growing rats. In Experiment 2, the higher-intensity treadmill exercise group had an increased focal burden compared with their sedentary pair-fed controls despite a reduction in food intake and body fat stores. These experiments demonstrate that exercise may reduce or enhance the occurrence of acinar foci, depending upon the intensity of the exercise and the stage in the life cycle of the animal at which exercise is imposed. This enhancement of focal burden represents a potential adverse effect of physical activity, as noted in Chapter 7.

Mammary gland

Whittal and Parkhouse (1996) studied the effects of treadmill exercise for four weeks on both the developmental stage and level of proliferation in the mammary gland at the time of carcinogenic initiation. Both factors have been reported to be associated with risk for carcinogenic transformation. Neither parameter was affected by treadmill exercise. Cancer end-points were also assessed in additional groups of animals that received identical treatment. Exercise reduced the multiplicity of mammary carcinomas but not their incidence (see above).

Enzymes

Since activities of phase II enzymes have been inversely associated with cancer risk, their activities may have value as intermediate biomarkers. Duncan et al. (1997) examined whether a progressive treadmill training programme for seven weeks would modulate constitutive levels of phase II or antioxidant enzymes in liver or lung. While response to exercise varied with the tissue and the enzymes assayed, in general the activities of superoxide dismutase, catalase, UDP-glucuronosyl transferase and GST were increased by exercise. The authors interpreted their data as being consistent with the hypothesis that exercise would prevent liver and lung cancer. [The Working Group noted that no data were presented to show that the exercise training programme investigated would actually affect the occurrence of either liver or lung cancer in an animal model system.]

Mechanisms of cancer prevention

The observations that weight, weight change and physical activity are associated with cancer occurrence are supported by evidence of biological plausibility for these associations. In Chapter 3, the relationships between physical activity and BMI, and in particular the possible contribution of physical activity to preventing or reducing weight excess, have been discussed. As reviewed in Chapter 4, body mass, fat distribution and physical activity can have profound effects on many physiological factors that may be important in cancer etiology. These reviews show that the effects of physical activity on metabolic factors are mediated only in part by improved weight control.

This section reviews the human and animal evidence for the role of physiological and metabolic factors in cancer development. These factors include mainly endogenous hormones, particularly those hormones (sex steroids, insulin, insulin-like growth factor-I (IGF-I)) for which epidemiological studies have shown at least some direct or indirect evidence for involvement in cancer development. Other mechanisms briefly discussed relate to gastro-oesophageal reflux in relation to oesophageal adenomas, intestinal transit time and bile acid metabolism in relation to colorectal cancer, and immune function.

Human studies
Endogenous hormones and cancer risk
Sex steroids
One major class of mechanisms that may form a physiological and causal link between energy balance and cancer risk comprises alterations of endogenous hormone metabolism. Much attention has been focused on endogenous sex steroids as possible determinants of tumours of, in particular, the breast, endometrium, ovary and prostate. The role of sex steroids in regulating the balance between cellular differentiation, mitosis and apoptosis is well established, and it has been postulated that alterations in the endocrine environment may favour the selective growth of pre-neoplastic and neoplastic cells (Henderson et al., 1988; Dickson et al., 1990).

The risks of cancers of the breast, endometrium and ovary are related to factors such as early menarche, late menopause, age at first full-term pregnancy and parity. With increasing age, age-specific incidence rates of cancers of the breast and endometrium rise faster before than after menopause, when the ovaries stop producing estrogens and progesterone. Together, these observations provide indirect evidence for the role of ovarian activity and sex

steroids as modulators of the risk of these cancers. This hypothesis is supported by observations that risk of cancers of the breast, endometrium and ovary can be increased or decreased by use of exogenous estrogens or progestogens (or combinations of these) for contraception or postmenopausal therapy.

The predominant theory relating the risk of endometrial cancer to endogenous sex steroids is the 'unopposed estrogen' hypothesis. This proposes that risk is increased among women who have normal or elevated plasma levels of bioavailable estrogens but low levels of progesterone, so that biological effects of estrogens are insufficiently counterbalanced by those of progesterone (Key & Pike, 1988; Grady & Ernster, 1996). This hypothesis is supported by observations that use of exogenous hormones for contraception or postmenopausal replacement therapy is associated with an increase in endometrial cancer risk when the hormone preparations contain only estrogens, whereas combinations of estrogens plus progestogens confer a relative protection (van Leeuwen & Rookus, 1989; Grady & Ernster, 1996; IARC, 1999; Weiderpass et al., 1999a, b). Studies in vitro have shown that estrogens stimulate the proliferation of normal endometrial tissue as well as of endometrial tumour cells, and that at least part of this effect may be mediated by an increase in local IGF-I concentrations (Rutanen, 1998). The opposing effects of progestogens, on the other hand, appear to be due largely to progesterone's capacity to increase levels of IGF-binding protein-1 (IGFBP-1) in endometrium (Rutanen, 1998).

Case–control studies have shown an increase in endometrial cancer risk in women who have low levels of plasma sex-hormone-binding globulin (SHBG), elevated levels of androgens (Δ4-androstenedione, testosterone) and, particularly after menopause, elevated levels of total and bioavailable estrogens (estradiol, estrone) (Austin et al., 1991;

Möllerström et al., 1993; Nyholm et al., 1993; Grady & Ernster, 1996; Potischman et al., 1996). Before menopause, endometrial cancer risk may be related more to the lack of progesterone than to an excess of total or bioavailable estrogens (Key & Pike, 1988; Grady & Ernster, 1996; Potischman et al., 1996). Ovarian hyperandrogenism appears to be an important risk factor for endometrial cancer in premenopausal women, as suggested by a large number of case reports of polycystic ovary syndrome (PCOS) in young cancer patients (Grady & Ernster, 1996) and by case–control (Dahlgren et al., 1991; Shu et al., 1991; Niwa et al., 2000) and cohort (Coulam et al., 1983) studies showing an increased risk of endometrial cancer among women who have PCOS. PCOS is generally associated with chronic anovulation, and hence with low production of progesterone.

Taken together, these observations, along with those discussed above on relationships with insulin and IGFBP-1, strongly support the hypothesis that, in premenopausal women, obesity and chronic hyperinsulinaemia may increase endometrial cancer risk by inducing ovarian hyperandrogenism, chronic anovulation and insufficient ovarian progesterone production. The lack of progesterone plus elevated plasma insulin level causes a drop in endometrial IGFBP-1 levels, while normal or moderately elevated estrogen levels increase local IGF-I concentrations. The ensuing increase in local IGF-I activity, plus other effects of estrogens and progesterone on endometrial tissue, may favour tumour development. After meno-pause, when progesterone production has ceased altogether, chronic hyperinsulinaemia may also increase endometrial cancer risk because of elevated insulin levels, decreased endometrial IGFBP-1 concentrations and increases in total and bioavailable plasma estrogen concentrations.

With respect to breast cancer, there is strong evidence that risk is increased in women with elevated plasma and tissue levels of estrogens ('estrogen excess' hypothesis) (Bernstein & Ross, 1993). This is supported by observations from prospective cohort studies showing increased breast cancer incidence in postmenopausal women who have low levels of SHBG and elevated levels of total and bioavailable androgens and estrogens (Thomas *et al.,* 1997; Hankinson *et al.,* 1998a; Kabuto *et al.,* 2000). Since obesity and the associated chronic hyperinsulinaemia decrease levels of SHBG and, in postmenopausal women, increase levels of androgens plus estrogens, the estrogen excess theory can also explain the increased breast cancer risk in postmenopausal women who are overweight or obese.

A second, more extensive theory is that, beyond the effect of exposure to estrogens alone, breast cancer risk is increased further when women are exposed to a combination of estrogens and progestogens ('estrogen-plus-progestogen' hypothesis). This hypothesis is supported by recent results showing that women using combined estrogen-plus-progestogen preparations for postmenopausal replacement therapy have a greater increase in risk than women using preparations containing only estrogens (IARC, 1999; Magnusson *et al.,* 1999; Ross *et al.,* 2000b; Schairer *et al.,* 2000). In addition, since in premenopausal women obesity may lead to chronic anovulation and decreased progesterone levels (especially in women with a predisposition towards ovarian hyperandrogenism), this second theory could also explain why on average obesity appears to be inversely related to breast cancer risk in premenopausal women.

Reducing cumulative exposure to ovarian hormones by delaying menarche and/or by reducing the number of ovulatory cycles (Bernstein *et al.,* 1987; Keizer & Rogol, 1990; Loucks, 1990;

Meyer *et al.,* 1990; Moisan *et al.,* 1991; Greene, 1993; Merzenich *et al.,* 1993; Petridou *et al.,* 1996) may decrease the risk of cancers of breast. Anovulatory cycles are associated with marked changes in endogenous estrogens and progesterone, which may lower risk for breast cancer (Pike *et al.,* 1983).

Further theories propose that specific metabolites of estradiol and estrone that may be formed locally within breast tissue increase risk. One such theory is that an increased ratio of 16-hydroxy- to 2-hydroxy-estrogens increases risk (Bradlow *et al.,* 1986). This hypothesis is supported by some recent findings (Kabat *et al.,* 1997; Meilahn *et al.,* 1998; Muti *et al.,* 2000) but not by others (Ursin *et al.,* 1999). The ratio of 16-hydroxy- to 2-hydroxy-metabolites has been found to be increased in obese subjects and low in women with anorexia nervosa (Fishman *et al.,* 1975). Exercise, on the other hand, has been reported to reduce 2-hydroxy-estrogen levels (de Crée *et al.,* 1997c).

The etiopathogenesis of ovarian cancer is still poorly understood. One hypothesis is that many years of uninterrupted ovulatory cycles increase risk by enhancing entrapment of ovarian epithelium in inclusion cysts and/or by repeated damage of the surface epithelium during ovulation ('incessant ovulation' hypothesis) (Fathalla, 1971; Cramer & Welch 1983; Cramer *et al.,* 1983). This hypothesis is based almost entirely on indirect epidemiological evidence, which shows that high parity and regular use of oral contraceptives are protective factors. A second complementary hypothesis, based largely on evidence from animal experiments, is that tumour development is promoted by elevated ovarian exposure to luteinizing hormone (LH) ('gonadotropin' hypothesis) (Weiss *et al.,* 1996; Blaakaer, 1997). Both the incessant ovulation hypothesis and the gonadotropin hypothesis find some indirect support in observations that oral contraceptives decrease

ovarian cancer risk (Whittemore, 1993; Weiss *et al.,* 1996; Blaakaer, 1997). Exercise might prevent ovarian cancer by reducing the number of lifetime ovulatory cycles, since it has been shown to be associated with delayed menarche, amenorrhoea and anovulatory cycles (Frisch *et al.,* 1981; Russell *et al.,* 1984; Bernstein *et al.,* 1987; Moisan *et al.,* 1991; Whittemore, 1993). However, regular strenuous exercise seems to be needed to produce these effects.

Elevated pituitary secretion of LH is also a characteristic of women who have PCOS, and in one prospective study, PCOS was found to be associated with increased ovarian cancer risk (Schildkraut *et al.,* 1996). In another prospective study, 13 premenopausal women and 18 postmenopausal women who eventually developed ovarian cancer had higher prediagnostic serum levels of Δ4-androstenedione than age-matched control subjects from the same cohort (Helzlsouer *et al.,* 1995). These and other observations led to an extension of the gonadotropin hypothesis, which proposes that ovarian tumour development may be enhanced by excess ovarian production of androgens (Risch, 1998). Ovarian hyperandrogenism might also provide a link between a positive energy balance and ovarian cancer risk, since in women with a predisposition towards ovarian hyperandrogenism, adiposity and chronic hyperinsulinaemia might exacerbate the ovarian androgen excess. However, in hyperandrogenic women, obesity and chronic hyperinsulinaemia also cause more frequent anovulation; thus, following the incessant ovulation hypothesis, one could equally well expect that obesity or chronic hyperinsulinaemia would reduce risk. There is currently insufficient evidence to evaluate whether only milder forms of ovarian androgen excess, without chronic anovulation, constitute a risk factor for ovarian cancer. As reviewed earlier in this chapter, there is also insufficient evidence to conclude whether or not ovarian cancer risk is related to obesity.

Overall, the observation that, depending on cancer site and type of preparation used, exogenous hormones can either increase or decrease risk of cancers of the breast, endometrium or ovary shows that hormones can affect the development of these cancers at a relatively late stage during adulthood. Combined with the fact that weight loss can favourably change endogenous hormone profiles in initially obese women, this strongly suggests that weight loss may also have cancer-preventive effects even if initiated relatively late in life.

In men, a strong indication for the implication of sex steroids in prostate tumour progression is that surgical or medical castration can dramatically improve the clinical course of prostate cancer patients. Extensive animal research has also indicated the involvement of endogenous sex steroids in the development of such tumours. Nevertheless, the etiopathogenesis of prostate cancer remains poorly understood, although a role for androgens and/or estrogens appears likely (Bosland, 2000; Kaaks et al., 2000a). The predominant hypothesis is that risk is increased in men who have elevated intraprostatic concentrations of dihydrotestosterone (DHT). DHT is formed from testosterone within the prostate by the enzyme 5-reductase type II (SRD5A). Interindividual differences in SRD5A activity, due to polymorphic variations in the SRD5A gene (Ross et al., 1998) or to differences in physiological regulation, may cause variations in amounts of DHT formed and thus in prostate cancer risk (Bosland, 2000).

Another possible determinant of levels of intraprostatic DHT formation is the level of bioavailable testosterone in the circulation. One large prospective cohort study found a strong trend of increasing prostate cancer risk with increasing levels of plasma testosterone adjusting for SHBG, whereas risk was inversely related to levels of SHBG after adjustment for testosterone (Gann et al., 1996). However, these results have not been confirmed by other prospective cohort studies (Bosland, 2000; Kaaks et al., 2000a) and in a formal meta-analysis of all reported prospective studies, risk was found to be unassociated with levels of either total or bioavailable testosterone (Eaton et al., 1999). It remains possible, however, that difficulties in accurately measuring levels of bioavailable hormones obscured the presence of a relatively weak association with prostate cancer risk (Kaaks et al., 2000a). Besides androgens, estrogens have also been proposed to either enhance or inhibit prostate cancer development (Farnsworth, 1996; Chang & Prins, 1999; Bosland, 2000), but the lack of any association of prostate cancer risk with plasma estrogen levels supports neither of these hypotheses (Eaton et al., 1999; Bosland, 2000).

In summary, it remains unclear whether variations in bioavailable androgens (and possibly other sex steroids) are entirely unrelated to prostate cancer risk, or whether weak associations exist that may have been obscured by, for example, inaccuracies in hormone measurements. Even if prostate cancer risk were related to bioavailable androgen levels, however, the lack of any direct relationship of plasma bioavailable androgens with anthropometric measures of adiposity or physical activity levels would be consistent with the absence of an association between either obesity or physical activity and prostate cancer risk, as reviewed earlier in this chapter.

There is indirect evidence that sex steroids may also influence the development of colorectal cancer. Incidence rates are higher in men than in women, especially for the more distal colon, and use of postmenopausal estrogen supplements by women is associated with decreased risk of colorectal cancer (Calle et al., 1995; Kampman et al., 1997; Crandall, 1999) and colorectal adenomas (Potter et al., 1996). The mechanisms for this association are not well understood, but estrogen receptors are expressed by colonocytes. It has been proposed that the weaker association between BMI and colon cancer for women than for men might also be related to differences in estrogen metabolism between men and women. Women who are overweight after the menopause have higher circulating estrogen levels due to the conversion of estrogen precursors to estrogen in adipose tissues. If estrogens do, indeed, reduce colorectal cancer risk, this could account for the gender difference in the strength of the association with obesity. A counterargument, however, is that obesity is related to increased plasma estrogen levels also in men and that plasma estrogen concentrations in men and postmenopausal women are approximately identical.

Insulin, IGFBP-1 and IGFBP-2

Insulin, IGF-I and IGF-binding proteins are receiving increasing attention from molecular biologists, pathologists and epidemiologists (Giovannucci, 1995, 1999; Kaaks et al., 2000a; Khandwala et al., 2000; Pollak, 2000; Kaaks & Lukanova, 2001). Insulin and IGF-I stimulate the proliferation (mitosis) and inhibit the programmed death (apoptosis) of both normal and neoplastic cells of many types (Werner & LeRoith, 1996; Khandwala et al., 2000). Both hormones also have effects on cellular (de-) differentiation (Benito et al., 1996; Stewart & Rotwein, 1996; Werner & LeRoith, 1996; Yu & Berkel, 1999; Khandwala et al., 2000) and angiogenesis (Grant et al., 1993; Kluge et al., 1995) and have been reported to favour neoplastic transformation. Insulin and IGF-I exert these trophic effects on a wide variety of tissue types including cells from the breast (Foekens et al., 1989; Yee et al., 1989), endometrium (Rutanen, 1998; Wang & Chard, 1999), ovary (Wang & Chard, 1999;

Poretsky et al., 1999), colon (Singh & Rubin, 1993; Kim, 1998; Burroughs et al., 1999; Rosen, 1999), prostate (Pollak et al., 1998; Wong & Wang, 2000) and kidney (Hammerman, 1999). In some tissue types (e.g., breast, endometrium and prostate), these effects of IGF-I have been proven to be synergistic with those of other growth factors and steroids (Dickson et al., 1990; Westley & May 1994; Westley et al., 1998; Yee & Lee, 2000).

As reviewed in the first part of this chapter, epidemiological studies have shown that excess body weight and obesity are positively associated with risk of cancers of the endometrium (in pre- and postmenopausal women), breast (only for tumours diagnosed several years after menopause) colon, oesophagus (adenocarcinoma) and kidney (renal cell cancer). The risk of breast cancer before menopause, by contrast, appears to be slightly decreased by obesity. As discussed in Chapter 4, one major metabolic consequence of obesity is insulin resistance, an increase in fasting plasma glucose and insulin concentrations, and decreases in IGFBP-1 and IGFBP-2 levels (down-regulated by insulin). The relationship of colon cancer risk with obesity, as well as with other dietary and lifestyle factors thought to be related to insulin resistance (e.g., low intake of n–3 polyunsaturated fatty acids, dietary fibre and fruits and vegetables; high intake of sucrose and other carbohydrates of high glycaemic index; low levels of physical activity), led to the hypothesis that chronically elevated insulin levels may be a direct risk factor for colon cancer (McKeown-Eyssen, 1994; Giovannucci, 1995; Kim, 1998). Similar hypotheses have been formulated for cancers of the breast (Kaaks, 1996; Stoll, 1999), pancreas (Weiderpass et al., 1998) and endometrium (Rutanen et al., 1993; Rutanen, 1998). The tumour-enhancing effects might be due either to insulin itself or to an increase in IGF-I bioactivity that may result from insulin-induced

reductions in IGFBP-1 and -2. One physiological mechanism through which regular physical exercise may decrease cancer risk, and actually oppose the metabolic effects of obesity, is reduced insulin resistance, chronic hyperinsulinaemia and increased IGFBP-1 (see Chapter 4).

The hypothesis that chronic hyperinsulinaemia may enhance the development of these various forms of cancer finds indirect support in observations that the risk of cancers of the colon (or colorectum) (McKeown-Eyssen, 1994; Giovannucci, 1995; La Vecchia et al., 1997b; LeMarchand et al., 1997; Weiderpass et al., 1997; Will et al., 1998; Hu et al., 1999a), endometrium (Adami et al., 1991; Moseson et al., 1993; O'Mara et al., 1985; Parazzini et al., 1999; Niwa et al., 2000; Weiderpass et al., 2000), pancreas (Everhart & Wright, 1995; Wideroff et al., 1997; Calle et al., 1998b; Weiderpass et al., 1998; Silverman et al., 1999) and kidney (O'Mara et al., 1985; Coughlin et al., 1997; Wideroff et al., 1997; Lindblad et al., 1999) is increased in diabetics. A limitation of many of these studies is that they lacked detail as to whether diabetes was of early onset (type I) or adult onset (type II) and whether or not the subjects depended on insulin injections. However, within the general population, the majority (>80%) of diabetes is of adult onset and non-insulin-dependent. This type of diabetes is usually associated with pancreatic hypersecretion and increased plasma levels of insulin, even though the high insulin levels are insufficient to maintain normal plasma glucose levels because of insulin resistance. Case–control and prospective cohort studies have shown no consistent evidence for any association of diabetes with risk of breast cancer (Kaaks, 1996) or prostate cancer (Kaaks et al., 2000a).

In addition to studies relating cancer risk to diabetes, a few recent studies have directly related cancer risk to plasma levels of insulin, C-peptide (a

marker of pancreatic insulin secretion), or IGFBPs -1 and -2.

A recent cohort study showed an increase in colorectal cancer risk in men and women who had elevated fasting plasma glucose levels and higher plasma levels of glucose and insulin two hours after a standard dose of oral glucose (Schoen et al., 1999). The association of colorectal cancer risk with fasting glucose levels confirmed results from some previous studies, reviewed by McKeown-Eyssen (1994) and by Giovannucci (1995). Another prospective study, in New York women, showed an approximately fourfold increase in colorectal cancer risk between subjects in the highest and lowest quartiles of (non-fasting) serum C-peptide levels (Kaaks et al., 2000b). The association with C-peptide remained unaltered after adjustment for BMI. Furthermore, colorectal cancer risk was inversely associated with levels of IGFBP-1 and IGFBP-2.

For endometrial cancer, one large case–control study showed an increase in risk in postmenopausal women with elevated serum levels of C-peptide (Troisi et al., 1997), which did not however persist after adjustment for BMI. The effect of hyperinsulinaemia on endometrial cancer risk may be mediated by a decrease in IGFBP-1, and hence an increase in IGF-I bioactivity. In endometrial tissue, IGFBP-1 is the most abundantly expressed IGF-binding protein and strongly inhibits the mitogenic action of IGF-I (Rutanen, 1998). A small study of 23 endometrial cancer patients and 27 healthy control women in Japan found lower IGFBP-I levels in the cases (Ayabe et al., 1997) Another small study in Finland also showed higher fasting plasma insulin levels and lower expression of the IGFBP-1 gene in endometrial tissue samples from endometrial cancer patients than in those from healthy controls (Rutanen et al., 1994).

Two case–control studies have shown an association of both premenopausal (Bruning *et al.*, 1992b; Del Giudice *et al.*, 1998) and postmenopausal (Bruning *et al.*, 1992) breast cancer with measurements of insulin or C-peptide, but this was not confirmed in a prospective study with measurements of (non-fasting) C-peptide (Toniolo *et al.*, 2000).

As reviewed in the first part of this chapter, prostate cancer risk appears to be independent of BMI, and there is also no clear evidence that a more central body fat distribution is a risk factor. These conclusions seem to be confirmed by the findings of one prospective cohort study, in which prostate cancer risk showed no clear relationship with plasma levels of (fasting) insulin, IGFBP-1, and IGFBP-2—peptides that are usually correlated with indices of adiposity (Stattin *et al.*, 2000).

For pancreas cancer, no studies have examined associations with plasma insulin or C-peptide. However, one recent prospective study showed an increase in risk of pancreas cancer in men and women who had elevated plasma glucose levels two hours after a standard oral glucose dose (Gapstur *et al.*, 2000). Elevated plasma glucose levels are indicative of insulin resistance and hence of chronically elevated pancreatic insulin production (DeFronzo, 1988).

For lung cancer, one prospective cohort study found a borderline significant association of risk with serum insulin concentration, which persisted after adjustment for BMI and for current and previous smoking (Lukanova *et al.*, 2001).

IGF-I and IGFBP-3
As reviewed in Chapter 4, growth hormone (GH) provides the key stimulus for the synthesis of IGF-I and IGFBP-3, and absolute levels of IGF-I and IGFBP-3 in the circulation are regulated largely along the GH/IGF-I axis. However, dietary intake and body reserves of energy and protein (essential amino acids) modulate these stimulatory effects

of GH on the synthesis of IGF-I and IGFBP-3. Chronic energy restriction strongly reduces circulating IGF-I and IGFBP-3 levels. Paradoxically, however, obese subjects also have mildly reduced absolute IGF-I concentrations, compared with well nourished but non-obese subjects. Possible mechanisms of these paradoxical observations are discussed briefly in Chapter 4. Taken together, the data suggest that, within the low range of 18 to about 24 kg/m^2, BMI may be positively associated with IGF-I concentrations, whereas BMI values above 25 kg/m^2 may be inversely related, but this still requires confirmation.

Two case–control studies (Peyrat *et al.*, 1993; Bruning *et al.*, 1995) and two prospective cohort studies (Hankinson *et al.*, 1998b; Toniolo *et al.*, 2000) have shown an increased risk of premenopausal breast cancer in women with elevated levels of IGF-I in plasma or serum, but no association of IGF-I with postmenopausal breast cancer. A possible explanation for these findings is that IGF-I enhances breast tumour development only in the presence of, and in interaction with, elevated concentrations of estrogens. In several of these studies, the association of IGF-I with risk was stronger after adjustment for levels of IGFBP-3 (Hankinson *et al.*, 1998b) or when IGF-I levels were expressed as molar ratios to IGFBP-3 (Bruning *et al.*, 1995). Two other case–control studies, however, did not show any association between IGF-I and pre- or postmenopausal breast cancer risk (Del Giudice *et al.*, 1998; Ng *et al.*, 1998).

For colorectal cancer, three prospective cohort studies showed very small, statistically non-significant increases in risk with increasing absolute levels of IGF-I (Ma *et al.*, 1999; Giovannucci *et al.*, 2000; Kaaks *et al.*, 2000b). However, in two of these studies, the association of colorectal cancer risk with IGF-I levels became stronger, and statistically significant, after adjustment for levels of IGFBP-3 (Ma *et al.*, 1999; Giovannucci

et al., 2000). Furthermore, in two case–control studies, colorectal cancer risk also related directly to levels of IGF-I (Manousos *et al.*, 1999; Renehan *et al.*, 2000a) and inversely to IGFBP-3 (Manousos *et al.*, 1999). The prevalence of colorectal adenomas has long been known to be higher in patients with acromegaly, a pathology due to GH excess and associated with elevated IGF-I levels (Giovannucci, 1995). Furthermore, in one case–control study (Giovannucci *et al.*, 2000), but not another (Renehan *et al.*, 2000b), the presence of large, but not small, colorectal adenomas was found to be associated with more elevated IGF-I levels, compared with adenoma-free controls. Taken together, these observations suggest that elevated IGF-I levels may favour the progression of small to large adenomas, and possibly to carcinomas.

With regard to prostate cancer, two case–control (Mantzoros *et al.*, 1997; Wolk *et al.*, 1998) and three prospective cohort (Chan *et al.*, 1998; Harman *et al.*, 2000; Stattin *et al.*, 2000) studies have all shown an increase in prostate cancer risk in men with elevated absolute levels of IGF-I and one found an increase with elevated levels of IGF-I for given levels of IGFBP-3 (Chan *et al.*, 1998).

One case–control study showed an increase in lung cancer risk in subjects with elevated levels of IGF-I (Yu *et al.*, 1999). This association became more pronounced after adjustment for IGFBP-3 level, and after adjustment for IGF-I, risk was inversely related to IGFBP-3 levels. This study also showed a synergism between elevated IGF-I and measures of mutagen sensitivity, assessed by quantitating bleomycin- and benzo[*a*]-pyrene-induced chromatid breaks in peripheral blood lymphocyte cultures (Wu *et al.*, 2000). Another study, however, showed significantly lower IGF-I levels in lung cancer cases than in controls (Lee *et al.*, 1999b). One prospective cohort study showed no significant association of lung cancer risk with circulating IGF-I or IGFBP-3 (Lukanova et al., 2001).

Overall, these epidemiological studies show associations of risk of various forms of cancer with elevated levels of IGF-I, either as absolute concentrations or relative to levels of IGFBP-3. The increased strength of these associations, in some studies, after adjustment for IGFBP-3 may reflect increased bioavailability or bioactivity of IGF-I when IGFBP-3 levels are low. Irrespective of whether risk is associated with total IGF-I, with IGF-I adjusted for IGFBP-3, or both, these observations suggest a possible relationship of cancer risk with elevated pituitary GH secretion. Conditions of elevated GH levels, such as during the pubertal growth spurt or, at extreme levels, in acromegaly, are associated with increased levels not only of absolute IGF-I, but also of the IGF-I/IGFBP-3 ratio (Juul et al., 1994; Jasper et al., 1999). As discussed above, however, the relationships of absolute IGF-I levels or of IGF-I relative to IGFBP-3 with BMI are not straightforward. Further studies are required to elucidate the degree to which body fat stores and/or physical (in)activity may result in the relative increase in IGF-I (or IGF-I relative to IGFBP-3) observed in subjects who subsequently develop cancer.

It is unclear why hyperinsulinaemia and related decreases in IGFBP-1 and IGFBP-2 appear to increase the risk of some forms of cancer (e.g., colon, endometrium) but not of others (e.g., prostate cancer), for which risk is unrelated to obesity. One possible explanation for these contrasting observations is that, depending on tissue type, a decrease in IGFBP-1 or IGFBP-2 does not have the same effect on overall IGF-I bioactivity, cell proliferation and apoptosis. Paradoxically, however, those forms of cancer (e.g., of the prostate, or of the breast in premenopausal women) do show an association with absolute plasma IGF-I concentrations, or with

levels of IGF-I relative to IGFBP-3. As mentioned in Chapter 4, the relationships between between circulating levels of IGF-I and IGFBPs and the concentrations of these peptides in different types of tissue remain unclear, and it is also not fully understood which specific effects each of the IGFBPs may have, in combination with IGF-I, on cellular growth, differentiation and apoptosis.

Other hormones, growth factors and non-hormonal factors

Several studies have examined the association of leptin, a hormone that reflects total fat mass, with cancer risk. Premenopausal breast cancer patients were found to have a non-significantly lower level of leptin than controls (Mantzoros et al., 1999; Petridou et al., 2000). This finding is consistent with the inverse association between BMI and premenopausal breast cancer. For prostate cancer, one case–control study (Lagiou et al., 1998) showed no association with risk of prostate cancer or benign prostatic hyperplasia. However, the results from one prospective study suggested a possibly non-linear relationship of prostate cancer with plasma leptin concentration, with an increased risk only for moderately elevated leptin levels but not for the highest levels (Stattin et al., 2001).

Platelet-derived growth factor (PDGF) is a potent mitogen for a variety of cells, and may be associated with cancer occurrence (Ross et al., 1993). PDGF can also potentiate the action of growth factors such as IGF-I. Initiation of an exercise programme has been observed to cause eventual decrease in platelet responsiveness and aggregation (Rauramaa et al., 1986; Sinzinger & Virgolini, 1988; Davis et al., 1990). However, there have been no direct observations on a possible relationship between PDGF and cancer risk.

Prostaglandins have been associated with tumour growth in animal studies (Tutton & Barkla, 1980). Prostaglandin

F_2 alpha inhibits tumour growth in the colon and increases gut motility; prostaglandin E_2 decreases colonic motility and increases the rate of colonic cell proliferation, especially in cancer cells (Bennett et al., 1977; Tutton & Barkla, 1980). Strenuous physical activity appears to increase levels of prostaglandin F2 alpha and inhibit synthesis of prostaglandin E_2 (Demers et al., 1981; Rauramaa et al., 1984). In a cross-sectional analysis, Martinez et al. (1999b) observed that changes in both BMI and physical activity were associated with prostaglandin E_2 in rectal mucosa. An increase in BMI from 24.2 to 28.8 kg/m^2 was associated with a 27% increase in prostaglandin E_2 and an increase in activity level from 5.2 to 27.7 MET-hours per week was associated with a 28% decrease in prostaglandin E_2. The association of mucosal prostaglandin levels with cancer risk has not been studied directly, however.

Other mechanisms

There are several other hypothesized mechanisms of cancer occurrence that could explain associations of energy balance and physical activity with cancer occurrence. Except for a strong relationship between gastro-oesophageal reflux and oesophageal adenoma, however, the associations of these factors with cancer etiology are still largely unsubstantiated by direct observations in humans. Nevertheless, they are presented as potential explanations of etiological pathways and as areas for future research.

Gastro-oesophageal reflux

A number of epidemiological studies have shown a strong association between frequent gastro-oesophageal reflux and risk of Barrett's oesophagus and oesophageal adenoma. Relative risk estimates for usual BMI values ranged from 5.5 to 43.5 (Chow et al., 1995; Lagergren et al., 1999b; Farrow et al., 2000). The use of medications that relax the lower oesophageal sphincter has also been also found to increase the risk of oesophageal adenoma (Lagergren *et al.*, 2000). As described earlier in this chapter, gastro-oesophageal reflux disease is also strongly associated with BMI, and these observations provide evidence for gastro-oesophageal reflux as a mechanism relating obesity to oesophageal adenoma risk.

Intestinal transit time

A mechanism that might mediate the protective effects of physical activity against colorectal cancer is a reduction of gastrointestinal transit time (Holdstock *et al.*, 1970). Physical activity may shorten the faecal transit time through increased vagal tone and thus increased peristalsis. Reduced transit time would reduce the period of contact between carcinogens and colonic mucosal cells. Moderate-level activities such as walking or a training programme lead to a decreased transit time, resulting in increased propulsion of colonic contents through the colon (Cordain *et al.*, 1986; Koffler *et al.*, 1992). However, not all studies have found that physical activity reduces bowel transit time (Coenen *et al.*, 1992).

Immune function

Evidence for the potential of the immune system to destroy tumour cells and prevent tumour growth is compelling (Hoffman-Goetz, 1998; Nieman & Pedersen, 1999; Woods *et al.*, 1999). The immune surveillance theory hypothesizes that malignant cells survive in part because of impaired immune attack, due to either absence of immunogenicity (e.g., lack of tumour antigen expression) in the tumour cells or depressed immune response in the host system (Burnet, 1970). Immune-compromised individuals tend to show an excess of lymphomas, skin cancers and some other cancers (Penn, 1994; Schulz *et al.*, 1996; Schenkein & Schwartz, 1997), but the role of immune function in those cancers

for which risk is associated with excess body weight and physical inactivity is not established.

There is little epidemiological data linking immune function and cancer in the general population. One recent cohort study of 3625 Japanese persons aged 40 years and older found that individuals with lower natural cytotoxic activity of blood lymphocytes had increased risk of cancer (all sites combined) compared with individuals having high activity (Imai *et al.*, 2000). The assays were performed at study entry and follow-up amounted to 11 years.

Bile acid metabolism

Physical activity and weight control may also induce favourable effects on bile acid levels in humans. A decrease in the ratio of secondary to primary bile acids has been observed in obese patients after treatment with subcaloric diet and graded physical activity (Kadyrova & Shakieva, 1986). Bile acids have been observed to influence the growth and proliferation of colonic cells (Bernstein *et al.*, 1999).

Summary

In conclusion, several effects of weight, weight control and physical activity have been linked with cancer risk in epidemiological studies. Findings on the association of metabolic and sex hormones and etiology of several cancers are intriguing. Data on links between immune function and the cancers most strongly related to weight and physical activity are not available and other potential mechanisms have not yet been supported by observational data.

Experimental studies

Experiments using animal models can provide information relevant to the mechanisms in human subjects in ways that are not otherwise possible. In identifying studies for review here, it was considered essential that mechanisms were evaluated within the context of experi-

ments in which a cancer end-point was also studied. This approach has the advantage of increasing the likelihood of establishing causality, while being accompanied by the disadvantage of excluding some potentially relevant studies.

Weight control

Mechanistic considerations will be focused on following topics: carcinogen metabolism, DNA damage and repair, tissue size homeostasis which includes consideration of cell proliferation and apoptosis as well as the regulation of the relevant cellular machinery that carries out these processes, angiogenesis, modulation of immune function, and other mechanisms. Within these broad categories, the effects of energy restriction (or dietary restriction, as noted) on hormones and growth factors are reviewed. It should be emphasized that the operational division of carcinogenesis into stages is a useful tool for the investigation of this disease process, although the distinction between stages is in many respects arbitrary. Mechanisms generally considered to operate during initiation are likely to also affect post-initiation events and similarly, mechanisms that are described as post-initiation events clearly affect the process of initiation.

Effects on the initiation phase of carcinogenesis

Energy restriction has been reported to inhibit the initiation phase of the carcinogenic process, but a lack of effect on tumorigenesis has been noted in some model systems. Energy restriction (30–40%) before exposure of C3H/He male mice to 3 Gy of whole body X-radiation reduced the subsequent occurrence of myeloid leukaemia (Yoshida *et al.*, 1997). Energy restriction (50%) also reduced, to a limited extent, DMBA-induced mammary carcinogenesis when the restriction was imposed before and for a short time after carcinogen administration (Sylvester *et al.*, 1982) and energy restriction (25%) has been reported to inhibit colon tumorigenesis induced by a carcinogen requiring metabolic activation, methylazoxymethanol acetate, but not by the direct-acting carcinogen MNU (Pollard & Luckert, 1985). However, energy restriction has been reported to have no effect on the initiation phase of skin tumorigenesis in Sencar mice following a single application of DMBA (Birt *et al.*, 1991) or in NMRI mice after chronic dermal application of DMBA (Fischer & Lutz, 1994). Effects of energy restriction on phase I and II metabolism and on DNA damage and repair mechanisms could account, at least in part, for the variable responses to carcinogenic insult when animals are energy-restricted during cacinogenic initiation.

Modulation of phase I drug-metabolism systems – cytochrome P450 enzymes

Energy and/or dietary restriction alters the activities of drug-metabolizing enzymes in a number of tissues, including liver, lung, kidney and testis, and it modulates the formation of carcinogen–DNA adducts in carcinogen-treated animals (see section on intermediate biomarkers in this chapter). Restriction has been observed to reduce the metabolic activation of aflatoxin B_1 in liver, but to increase the activation of benzo[*a*]-pyrene in both rats and mice (Chen *et al.*, 1996; Chou *et al.*, 1993a,b, 1997). In these studies, both increases and decreases in the activities of specific CYP enzymes have been noted (see Table 50), and in general changes in enzyme activity have correlated with changes in detected levels of adducts as predicted by the CYP activity profile. There are species, strain and gender differences that appear to modulate the effect of dietary restriction on CYP activities and adduct formation (Manjgaladze *et al.*, 1993). However, a moderate level of dietary restriction also

has been reported not to affect the activity of either phase I or phase II drug-metabolizing enzymes (Keenan *et al.*, 1996). Collectively, these data indicate that dietary restriction has the potential to modulate DNA-adduct formation following carcinogenic insult, but it is not possible to make generalizable predictions about the potential for these effects to be beneficial against carcinogenic initiation due to the complexity of the systems involved.

Modulation of phase II drug-metabolism systems – conjugating enzymes

The effects of energy restriction on the activities of phase II conjugating enzymes have not been extensively studied, and contradictory results have been obtained (Chen *et al.*, 1995; Keenan *et al.*, 1996; Leakey *et al.*, 1989), as summarized in Table 50. Consequently, it is not possible to make generalizable statements about effects that these changes are likely to have on the initiation stage of the carcinogenic process.

Decreased oxidative DNA damage and increased DNA repair/antioxidant enzymes

Damage to DNA that leads to mutations and/or chromosomal alterations in specific genes, e.g., proto-oncogenes and tumour-suppressor genes, is causally involved in the genesis of cancer. Agents that can induce DNA damage come from both exogenous and endogenous sources. Effects of energy restriction on the metabolism of potential DNA-damaging agents of exogenous origin have been discussed in the preceding paragraphs. The present section focuses on agents that are endogenously produced and more specifically on reactive oxygen species. Oxidative damage to DNA can be decreased by reducing the formation of reactive species, increasing the scavenging of reactive species by low-molecular-weight compounds such as glutathione and/or by

antioxidant enzymes, and by increasing the rate of DNA repair and the fidelity of repair. Numerous studies have reported that dietary restriction affects these processes at levels of restriction that have been demonstrated to prevent tumour development in an array of experimental model systems. However, such information must be recognized to be indirect. No studies in experimental models have demonstrated a direct relationship between energy restriction, reduction of oxidative DNA damage, decreased mutations, and the prevention of cancer. Moreover, there is limited evidence to indicate that reactive oxygen species are essential for the promotion and progression of carcinogenesis in the model systems in which energy restriction has been shown to prevent cancer. Hence, while a reduction in DNA damage as a mechanism for cancer prevention is clearly biologically plausible, evidence that energy restriction prevents cancer by decreasing DNA oxidation is inferential.

Energy restriction has been shown to decrease the accumulation of oxidized bases in DNA. It also reduces oxidative damage to proteins and lipids (Youngman *et al.*, 1992; Shigenaga *et al.*, 1994). With respect to DNA damage, energy restriction has been shown to reduce levels of 8-hydroxydeoxyguanosine by 20–25% in rat liver DNA isolated from nuclei or mitochondria (Chung *et al.*, 1992) and in five different tissues of mice, namely skeletal muscle, brain, heart, liver and kidney (Sohal *et al.*, 1994a). The effects of energy restriction on another oxidized base, 5-hydroxymethyluracil, in DNA isolated from liver or mammary gland was also investigated in rats; dietary restriction (40%) resulted in statistically significant reductions (approximately 40%) of this base in both tissues (Djuric *et al.*, 1992). Evidence exists that implicates a reduction in the formation of reactive oxygen species (Sohal *et al.* 1994b) via the inhibition, by energy restriction, of mitochondrial state

Table 50. Effect of energy restriction on the activities of phase I and phase II drug-metabolizing enzymes

Species/strain (sex)	Tissue	Enzymes	Effect of energy restriction on activity	Reference
		Phase I		
Rat				
Fischer 344 (M)	Testis	CYP2A1	Decrease	Seng *et al.* (1996)
Fischer 344 (M)	Liver	CYP2C11	Decrease	Manjgaladze *et al.* (1993)
Fischer 344 (M) (late in life)	Liver	CYP2E1-selective 4-nitrophenol hydroxylase	Increase	Manjgaladze *et al.* (1993)
Mouse				
B6C3F$_1$(M)	Lung	CYP1A1	Increase	Chen *et al.* (1996)
DBA/2J or C57BL/6N	Liver	AHH CYP1A1-dependent EROD, CYP2B-dependent PROD	Increase	Cou *et al.* (1993b)
		Phase II		
Rat				
Fischer 344 (M)	Liver	GST towards 1,2-dichloro-4-nitrobenzene	Decrease	Leakey *et al.* (1989)
Fischer 344 (M)	Liver	UDP-glucuronyltransferase and sulfotransferase towards hydroxysteroids	No effect	Leakey *et al.* (1989)
Fischer 344 (M)	Liver	UDP-glucuronyltransferase towards bilirubin Gamma-glutamyltranspeptidase	Increase	Leakey *et al.* (1989)
Fischer 344 (M)	Liver	GST towards aflatoxin B$_1$-8-9-epoxide	Increase	Chen *et al.* (1995)

AHH, aryl hydrocarbon hydroxylase; EROD, ethoxyresorufin-*O*-deethylase; GST, glutathione-*S*-transferase; PROD, pentoxyresorufin-*O*-dealkylase

4 respiration, the state primarily responsible for the generation of superoxide. Besides effects on the production of reactive species, lower levels of oxidized DNA could result from increased scavenging of reactive oxygen species, but contradictory findings have been reported, showing increases or no clear-cut patterns of the effect of energy restriction on activity of the antioxidant enzymes superoxide dismutase (SOD), catalase and glutathione peroxidase (Rao *et al.*, 1990; Sohal *et al.*, 1994b).

Enhancement of DNA repair mechanisms has been reported in response to 40% dietary restriction with or without supplementation. Ultraviolet-induced unscheduled DNA synthesis was found to be increased (Weraarchakul *et al.*, 1989) and O^6-methylguanine DNA-methyltransferase activity to be elevated (73%) by restriction (40%) (Lipman *et al.*, 1989). However, effects of restriction on the activities of enzymes that repair specific oxidized bases have not been reported. Finally, one study has shown that the fidelity of DNA repair by certain polymerases purified from liver is increased in dietary-restricted (40%) mice (Srivastava *et al.*, 1991).

Effects on the post-initiation (promotion/progression) stage of carcinogenesis

Most studies on effects of energy restriction in the prevention of cancer using experimental models have found inhibition of the post-initiation stage of the disease process; this stage is also referred to as promotion or pro-gression.

Tissue size homeostasis

The processes of clonal expansion and selection of transformed foci of cells in a tissue can occur only if a dysequilibrium exists between the rates of cell prolifera-tion and cell death by apoptosis such that abnormal cells can accumulate in excess of their non-transformed neigh-bours (Thompson et al., 1992). Several laboratories have reported that dietary restriction (20%) decreases the rate of cell proliferation and increases the rate of apoptosis (Grasl-Kraupp et al., 1994; James & Muskhelishvili, 1994; Dunn et al., 1997; Hikita et al., 1997; Zhu et al., 1999a). The directions of both effects are considered beneficial in terms of cancer prevention. By inducing levels of apopto-sis, which can occur independently of wild-type p53 activity (Dunn et al., 1997), the potential for deletion of damaged and pre-malignant cells from a tissue is enhanced. Data relating to the effects of energy restriction on each of these processes is presented in the following sections.

Inhibition of cell proliferation: Since most *in-vivo* assessments consider synthesis of DNA as synonymous with cell prolifer-ation, they are here considered as one. Three general statements can be made about the effects of energy restriction on cell proliferation. First, in the many tis-sues and organs examined in energy-restricted animals, a reduction in the absolute number of cells present in a given tissue is uniformly observed. In some tissues, the reduction in cell num-ber is directly proportional to body weight such that the cell number in an organ or tissue per 100 g body weight is essen-tially the same in dietary-restricted and *ad-libitum*-fed mice or rats (James & Muskhelishvili, 1994; Zhu et al., 1999a). Second, the inhibitory effect of energy restriction on cell proliferation is constitu-tively expressed, i.e., it is non-specific and the magnitude of suppression is

directly proportional to the degree of energy restriction (Lok et al., 1990). Both normal and transformed or premalignant cell populations are affected (Grasl-Kraupp et al., 1994; Dunn et al., 1997; Zhu et al., 1999a). Third, the inhibitory effect of energy restriction has been seen in most tissues that have been evaluated, although some investigators have not observed an effect (Merry & Holehan, 1985; Lok et al., 1990). In the colon, energy restriction has been reported to reduce the activity of ornithine decarboxylase and mucosal protein tyrosine kinase activity, which would be consistent with decreasing the potential of cells to transit the cell cycle (Kumar et al., 1990).

Cell cycle regulation: The evidence pre-sented in the previous paragraph implies that energy restriction arrests the pas-sage of cells through the cell cycle. The cells are likely to be arrested in the G1 phase of the cell cycle (Lu et al., 1991). Female rats with 40% restricted energy intake had increased activity of the cyclin-dependent kinase inhibitor, P27, a member of the Cip/Kip family of kinase inhibitors (Zhu et al., 1999b). High levels of P27 have been associated with arrest of cells in the G0/G1 phase of the cell cycle, at least in part via the inhibitory effect of P27 on the activity of the cdk2–cyclin E complex. Additionally, a lower percentage of mammary epithelial cells from energy-restricted animals stained positive for cyclin D1; this also is consistent with arrest of cells in the G0/G1 phase of the cycle as a result of a reduced capacity to initiate phosphoryla-tion of the retinoblastoma protein (Rb), which is required for cells to traverse the G1/S transition in the cell cycle (Sherr, 2000). An associated issue is whether the effects on cell-cycle regulatory mole-cules are direct or are mediated by events upstream of cell cycle machinery. No data were available concerning direct effects of energy restriction on these cell-cycle molecules. However, three reports

indicate inhibitory effects of energy restriction on protein kinase C isozymes α and ζ in epidermal and pancreatic cells (Birt et al., 1994b, 1996; Nair et al., 1995); these could be involved in signal transduction events that modulate cell proliferation. Moreover, energy restric-tion (40%) has also been reported to inhibit signalling down the mitogen-acti-vated protein kinase (MAPK) pathway (Liu et al., 2001). In particular, tumour promoter induction of the specific MAPK extracellular response kinase (ERK 1,2) was selectively inhibited in the epidermis of energy-restricted mice, while JNK and p38 kinase were not influenced. This inhibition may be particularly relevant to the prevention of skin tumours by energy restriction because ERK 1,2 induction directly activates the c-fos gene and indi-rectly activates the c-jun gene. These two genes are constituents of the tran-scription factor AP-1, induction of which by tumour promoters is fundamental to carcinogenesis.

Induction of apoptosis: Apoptosis is a means of deleting cells from a tissue in the absence of a significant inflammatory response. Apoptosis is induced in response to physiological, pharmacolog-ical and toxic stimuli. Either chronic energy restriction or acute fasting can induce apoptosis. Three laboratories have reported the induction of apoptosis in liver by either fasting or energy restric-tion (Grasl-Kraupp et al., 1994; James & Muskhelishvili, 1994; Muskhelishvili et al., 1995; Hikita et al., 1997, 1999). It appears that constitutive rates of apopto-sis are elevated but that preneoplastic hepatic cell populations are more sensi-tive to the apoptotic stimulus than are non-transformed hepatocytes. Whereas fasting was associated with a transient reduction in the number and volume of altered hepatic foci (Hikita et al., 1999), chronic energy restriction was reported to cause a permanent reduction in the number of hepatic adenomas and carci-nomas induced in comparison to controls fed *ad libitum*, due to deletion of initiated hepatocytes (Grasl-Kraupp *et al.*, 1994). Energy restriction has also been reported to enhance rates of apoptosis in focal hyperplasia in the bladder (Dunn *et al.*, 1997) and in premalignant lesions in the mammary gland (Zhu *et al.*, 1999a). Induction of apoptosis has been noted to account for the decreased cellularity of the thymus and spleen in energy-restricted mice (Poetschke *et al.*, 2000), and under these circumstances the T-cell subsets had higher levels of plasma membrane Fas receptor and Fas ligand, and increased annexin-V positivity (Reddy Avula *et al.*, 1999). The authors suggested that these conditions reflect an increased potential for apoptosis.

Cell death machinery: While several studies have determined that energy restriction induces apoptosis, there have been no reports of which initiator caspases are activated by energy restriction, or of the signalling events that result in caspase activation. Nonetheless, the work cited above indicates that a death receptor pathway may be involved (Reddy Avula *et al.*, 1999).

Angiogenesis : The process of vascularization is intimately involved in regulating tissue size homeostasis. In order to support new growth, it is essential for neo-vascularization to occur, a process referred to as angiogenesis. Many findings indicate that energy restriction is likely to have an effect on this process. One report shows that energy restriction inhibits the progression of a transplantable prostate cell line. Inhibition of angiogenesis accompanied by reduced levels of vascular endothelial growth factor (VEGF) was one of the responses observed in energy-restricted animals that were inoculated with prostatic tumour cells (Mukherjee *et al.*, 1999). The authors suggested that the inhibition of angiogenesis by energy restriction protected animals against tumour development in this model system.

Hormones and growth factors

Modulation of insulin and insulin-like growth factors (IGFs): As described earlier in this chapter, energy-restriction in rodents prevents DMBA-induced mammary tumorigenesis in proportion to the degree of restriction imposed. In the same studies, energy restriction also resulted in a reduction in plasma insulin levels that was proportional to the degree of restriction imposed (Klurfeld *et al.*, 1989a, b). The development of DMBA-induced mammary tumours is also inhibited by alloxan-induced diabetes and alloxan- or streptozotocin-induced diabetes in rats causes a regression of 60–90% of DMBA-induced mammary tumours (Heuson & Legros, 1972; Cohen & Hilf, 1974; Hilf *et al.*, 1978; Gibson & Hilf, 1980). Tumour growth was restored and tumour latency reduced upon insulin administration to diabetic rats.

Energy restriction has also been reported to prevent the development of DMBA-induced mammary tumours in genetically obese LA/N-cp female rats. In both the obese animals and their genetically normal lean controls, energy restriction led to low plasma insulin levels. The authors speculated that insulin might be mediating the effect of energy restriction on tumour occurrence in this model system (Klurfeld *et al.*, 1991).

The effects on IGF metabolism of levels of energy restriction that inhibited tumour development have been investigated in four studies. Ruggeri *et al.* (1989) reported that a level of energy restriction that inhibited DMBA-induced mammary tumorigenesis reduced circulating levels of insulin and IGF-I, but not those of IGF-II. Initially, levels of both insulin and IGF-I were reduced, but only the effect of energy restriction on insulin persisted. Two studies found that energy restriction inhibited the development of either leukaemias or bladder cancer (Hursting *et al.*, 1993; Dunn *et al.*, 1997). The inhibitory effects on tumour development were accompanied by reductions in circulating levels of IGF-I. Both studies found rates of cell proliferation to be reduced in restricted animals, and in the bladder cancer model, the rate of apoptosis was markedly elevated in focal hyperplasias in energy-restricted animals. Administration of IGF-I to restricted animals restored the rates of proliferation and apoptosis to those observed in animals fed *ad libitum* (Hursting *et al.*, 1993; Dunn *et al.*, 1997). It was proposed that the effects of dietary restriction are mediated via changes in the availability of IGF-I, which modulates tissue size homeostasis by increasing cell proliferation and decreasing the rate of apoptosis. This hypothesis has significant biological plausibility given the role of IGF-I as a potent mitogen and as a survival factor (Kari *et al.*, 1999).

Modulation of adrenal cortical steroids: As early as 1948, a role was hypothesized for the adrenal gland in mediating the tumour-preventive effects of energy restriction (Boutwell *et al.*, 1948). In mice, adrenalectomy has been shown to abolish the protective activity of dietary restriction against chemically induced tumorigenesis in the skin and lung (Pashko & Schwartz, 1992, 1996). Elevated levels of corticosterone also accompanied dietary restriction in animals with an intact adrenal gland. The hyperplastic response normally observed during the carcinogenic initiation–promotion protocol was inhibited by energy restriction, but this inhibitory effect was abolished by adrenalectomy (Pashko & Schwartz, 1992). In rats, energy restriction leads to increased urinary excretion of corticosterone, and urinary corticosterone concentration was inversely associated with tumour multiplicity (Zhu *et al.*, 1997). In these studies, the authors hypothesized a causal role for adrenal cortical steroids in accounting for the cancer-preventive activity of energy restriction. Consistent with this observation, the inhibition of mouse skin carcinogenesis in the DMBA-initiation/-TPA-promoted Sencar mouse model by energy restriction was paralleled by reductions in protein kinase C α and ζ (Birt *et al.*, 1994b, 1996). Subsequently, mice were administered corticosterone in the drinking-water in a manner that elevated circulating corticosterone levels to an extent similar to that observed with energy restriction (Birt *et al.*, 2001). The pattern of reduced epidermal expression of protein kinase C isozymes α and ζ and elevation of isozyme η was strikingly similar to the alterations observed in the epidermis of dietary energy-restricted mice.

The role of glucocorticoid hormone in the prevention of rodent carcinogenesis has been studied (Yaktine *et al.*, 1998; Birt *et al.*, 1999); elevated glucocorticoid hormone levels have been reported to be associated with prevention of carcinogenesis and an intact adrenal gland is claimed to be essential for prevention of cancer by dietary restriction (Pashko & Schwartz, 1992, 1996). In contrast to findings in rats (Morimoto *et al.*, 1977; Armario *et al.*, 1987) and humans (Chiappelli *et al.*, 1991; Kennedy *et al.*, 1991), underfeeding hamsters did not result in elevated levels of glucocorticoid hormones. This hormonal response of hamsters may have been a factor in the inability of energy restriction to prevent ductular pancreatic carcinogenesis in the hamster model (Birt *et al.*, 1997).

Modulation of sex steroids: The hypothesis that energy restriction might act as a pseudohypophysectomy has its origins in early work in the field (Boutwell *et al.*, 1948). The relevance of the sex steroids estrogen and progesterone to the development of cancer has been covered in Chapter 4 and earlier sections of this chapter. The number of studies that have examined the effects of energy restriction on sex hormone function in parallel with its effects on the development of experimentally induced breast cancer is fairly limited. Sylvester *et al.* (1981) and Sarkar *et al.*, 1982) both observed sup-

pression of estrogen and prolactin secretion under conditions of energy restriction that inhibited mammary tumour development, but Sinha *et al.* (1988) failed to find differences in plasma estradiol levels at different stages of the estrous cycle or disruption of estrous cycling in rats subject to energy restriction. While such effects are not anticipated from the human findings reviewed in this volume, they imply that other mechanisms are likely to be involved. Conditions of energy restriction can be defined that inhibit mammary carcinogenesis with or without an effect on the hypophyseal–pituitary–ovarian axis. This finding is supported by the work of Harvell *et al.* (2001a), who found no effect of energy restriction on circulating 17β-estradiol in a rat model of estradiol-induced mammary carcinogenesis.

In reviewing the literature on this topic, the Working Group noted a lack of discussion on which experimental tumour systems model postmenopausal breast cancer. Therefore, although the mammary carcinogenesis model systems that have been studied show sensitivity to ovarian steroids, ovariectomy and anti-estrogen therapy, it is not clear how these observations relate to the epidemiological findings on the role of weight control and physical activity in postmenopausal breast cancer reviewed in the first part of this chapter. It appears possible to amplify the cancer-preventive effects of energy restriction on hormone-sensitive target organs by modulating the activity of the hypophyseal–pituitary–ovarian axis, but effects on these hormones do not appear to be obligatory in accounting for the cancer-preventive activity of energy restriction in such model systems.

Other mechanisms

Alterations of energy metabolism: Energy restriction produces an effect on intermediary metabolism in the liver that favours the role of glucagon in regulation of glycolysis and glucose synthesis,

while limiting the role of insulin. This results in higher glucose synthesis and lower glucose catabolism (Feuers *et al.*, 1989). The former effect was interpreted as providing for the efficient support of peripheral tissues and the latter a level of energy production necessary for self-maintenance. Using c-DNA array technology to characterize patterns of change in gene expression with ageing and the effects of energy restriction in a post-mitotic tissue (mouse muscle), Lee *et al.* (1999c) showed that energy restriction alters the expression of a number of genes involved in energy metabolism.

The potential interaction between effects of energy restriction on energy metabolism, changes in energy metabolism that occur in target cells following carcinogenic insult, and the inhibition of cancer by energy restriction has received limited attention. However, there is evidence that biologically plausible relationships exist that may underline, at least in part, the protective activity of energy restriction against cancer. Zhang *et al.* (1998) studied energy metabolism during AOM-induced colon carcinogenesis in male Sprague Dawley rats. They concluded that colonocyte energy metabolism differs between AOM-treated rats and saline controls and that it changes during tumorigenesis. A positive relationship between intracellular energy status and patterns of cell proliferation was observed. Using a yeast model for energy restriction, Lin *et al.* (2000) found that limiting the availability of glucose led to activation of a gene-silencing pathway by NAD+. The existence of homologues of these genes in mammalian cells remains to be established. It is still unclear whether effects of energy restriction on the availability of high-energy molecules (ATP, NADH and NADPH) play either a direct role in inhibiting the development of cancer by silencing genes involved in tumour initiation, promotion or progression, or an indirect role by regulating cell proliferation, apoptosis and/or angiogenesis.

Prevention of obesity: Data from experimental studies indicate that prevention of obesity is likely to affect endocrine function, i.e., insulin sensitivity and circulating levels of hormones such as estrogen. It could also affect levels of DNA damage by exogenous as well as endogenous agents. These topics have been reviewed above and will not be further discussed.

Modulation of immune function: The effects of energy restriction on immune function have been investigated most extensively in studies of the ageing process. In general, energy restriction has been reported to improve cell-mediated immune function by preventing age-related declines in activity (Cheney *et al.*, 1983; Weindruch *et al.*, 1986; Fernandes *et al.*, 1997; Frame *et al.*, 1998). Specific effects on CD4+ and CD8+ T cells and on natural killer cell activity have been reported as well as on T-lymphocyte proliferation. While experiments investigating the effects of dietary restriction on ageing-related changes in immune function have also noted the effects on spontaneous tumour occurrence, little effort has been made to determine if modulation of immune function is involved in the cancer-preventive activity of energy restriction. Most studies have used models in which tumour cells were inoculated and effects of energy restriction on tumour metastasis and immune function were measured. In three reports, effects of energy restriction on cell-mediated immunity were noted (Ershler *et al.*, 1986; Hodgson *et al.*, 1996, 1997), but in one of these (Hodgson *et al.*, 1996), energy restriction was associated with an increase in metastasis. Thus, while it is biologically plausible that effects of energy restriction on immune function could, at least in part, account for its cancer-preventive activity, experimental data remain limited and inconclusive.

Physical activity

There are a number of plausible mechanisms by which physical activity may prevent the development of cancer, but data in support of these mechanisms remain limited. In experimental tumour models, most work has focused on inhibition of the post-initiation (promotion and progression) stages of carcinogenesis by physical activity. However, it appears that physical activity can also affect the process of initiation (see the section on experimental studies of physical activity earlier in this chapter).

Immune status and function

Considerable attention has been directed to the hypothesis that physical activity prevents cancer in humans by enhancing immune function. Studies of this hypothesis in experimental tumour models have been limited to investigating the effects of physical activity in transplantable tumour systems. Thus, exercise-mediated effects on the immune system during either the initiation or the promotion phase of experimentally induced carcinogenesis have not been investigated.

The immune mechanisms most likely to be involved in protection against cancer include exercise- or training-induced increases in the number and/or activity of lymphokine-activated killer cells, tumour-infiltrating macrophages and/or activated natural killer cells. Since most of the immediate immune responses to exercise are relatively short-lived, susceptibility to cancer is more likely to be affected by training-induced changes in resting function of the immune system than by the immediate responses to a bout of exercise (Shephard & Shek, 1995). Many investigators have reported effects of various exercise regimes and/or training programmes on components of the immune system, but only a few studies have combined these measurements with data on the effects of the physical activity regime on a tumour outcome. Hoffman-Goetz *et al.* (1992) exercised

C3H mice on a treadmill and inoculated them with CIRAS 3 tumour cells at four weeks into the training protocol. At eight weeks of training, exercise was significantly associated with increased natural killer (NK) cytotoxicity against tumour targets *in vitro*, but this effect was observed only in animals without visible lung tumours. Consequently, the authors were doubtful about the physiological significance of exercise-induced changes in immune function on tumour progression. Hoffman-Goetz *et al.* (1994) also compared the effects of exercise on an activity wheel with those due to treadmill exercise on the occurrence of pulmonary metastases in female BALB/c mice inoculated intravenously with the MMT 66 tumour cell line. In general, exercise tended to increase NK activity and lymphokine-activated killer (LAK)-mediated cytotoxicity; however, no effect of exercise on lung metastasis was observed. Thus, although exercise training influences natural immune cytotoxic mechanisms *in vitro*, this may not translate into clinically significant changes in tumour burden (Hoffman-Goetz *et al.*, 1994). Woods *et al.* (1994) studied the effects of treadmill exercise on phagocytic capacity of intratumoural phagocytes in C3H/He male mice inoculated subcutaneously with SCA-1 mammary adenocarcinoma cells. While moderate exercise increased phagocytic capacity, no effect of exercise on tumour incidence or tumour size was observed. Jäpel *et al.* (1992) also reported enhanced phagocytosis of macrophages in tumour-bearing animals trained on a treadmill; this effect strongly depended on the duration and onset of the training programme.

Sex hormones

Data from human studies suggest that physical activity could prevent cancer by an endocrine route through an effect on sex steroids. Cohen *et al.* (1993) examined this possibility in carcinogenesis studies in female

Sprague-Dawley rats given access to activity wheels. Using DMBA to induce mammary tumours, access to exercise was associated with lower tumour occurrence; the nature of the protective activity depended on the dose of carcinogen. No difference in cytosolic estrogen receptor levels in the induced tumours was noted between animals that were sedentary and those that were exercised. The authors considered these data to cast doubt on the idea that physical activity selects, via an endocrine effect, for estrogen-non-responsive tumours. Cohen *et al.* (1991) observed that voluntary exercise on activity wheels reduced yields of MNU-induced mammary tumours and delayed time of tumour appearance (see page 185). They found no effect of wheel-running on circulating bioactive or immunoreactive prolactin and deduced that this cast doubt on mediation of the cancer-preventive effect of exercise by prolactin.

Insulin/glucose

Effects of exercise on insulin and/or IGF-I have been reported in two experimental tumour systems. Kazakoff *et al.* (1996) studied the effect of access to an activity wheel on induction of pancreatic cancer in female Syrian hamsters given an injection of BOP. They found exercise to have no effect on tumorigenesis, despite the fact that animals with access to exercise had significantly lower levels of circulating insulin, though unchanged plasma IGF-1 levels. The authors concluded that since exercise did not modulate tumour incidence, the effects of exercise on insulin probably do not mediate its effect on tumour development. While using a model not directly applicable to cancer prevention, Daneryd *et al.* (1990) studied the effects of access to an activity wheel in female Wistar Furth rats implanted with a transplantable tumour. Tumour-bearing exercised animals had higher insulin sensitivity and the exercised animals had a smaller tumour mass, the magnitude of reduction depending on the type of tumour implanted.

Other mechanisms

Various other plausible mechanisms could account for the cancer-preventive effects of physical activity (Cohen *et al.*, 1992). However, no experimental data were available to the Working Group for any exercise protocol known to prevent cancer in relation to the following mechanisms: stimulation of colonic peristalsis, altered prostaglandin production, increased endorphin production, altered adiposity/fat distribution (obesity), enhanced free-radical/antioxidant functions.

What counts as moderate physical activity ?

- **Raking leaves**
- **Digging in the garden**
- **Walking the dog**
- **Mowing the lawn**
- **Climbing stairs**
- **Dancing**
- **Cleaning windows**
- **Household chores**
- **Swimming**
- **Hiking**
- **Shovelling snow**
- **Riding a bike**

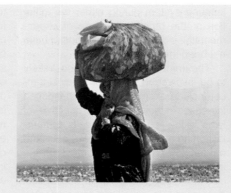
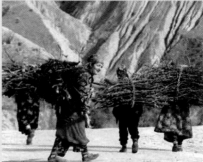
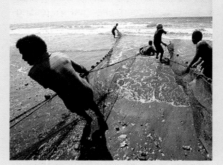
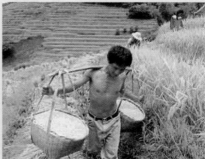

Chapter 6
Other beneficial effects

Weight control

Many prospective observational studies have investigated the impact of relative weight, measured as BMI, on risk of mortality and disease endpoints. Other prospective observational studies have looked at the effect of change in body weight that often occurred later in life. Relative weight has also been studied in relation to biological markers of disease and quality of life in observational and experimental settings. The results of experimental weight loss trials have often provided further evidence on effects of weight control on health.

Some major reports have summarized current evidence on the role of obesity and weight control with respect to risk for non-cancer diseases and all-cause mortality (WHO Expert Committee, 1995; National Task Force on the Prevention and Treatment of Obesity, 2000); these reports have provided the scientific background for major public health initiatives on weight control.

All-cause mortality
Weight status

The earliest data on the importance of relative weight for mortality and disease occurrence came from studies that prospectively related existing BMI to risk. This concept is straightforward because there is in general considerable variation in BMI between individuals within a study population which persists with nearly unchanged ranking for long time periods.

All-cause mortality increases with both higher and lower BMI in the general population. The association between relative weight and mortality was first demonstrated in a study of life insurance policy holders (Build and Blood Pressure Study, 1959) and the non-linearity of this association was confirmed in a later study of volunteers in the American Cancer Society Study (Lew & Garfinkel, 1979). Most subsequent studies have documented U-, reversed J-, and J-shaped associations between BMI and mortality in men and women; see for example Waaler (1988).

The increase in risk among subjects with the lowest BMI values has attracted particular attention in recent years (Seidell et al., 1999). The low BMI values in such studies were usually in the range defined as normal. Smoking was long believed to account for the excess mortality among lean individuals, and it has also been speculated that pre-existing disease is another factor. The exclusion of subjects who die during the first years of follow-up has therefore been recommended to avoid confounding. However a meta-analysis of studies specifically conducted on the relation between BMI and all-cause mortality revealed that the effect of excluding early death from the analysis was significant but of minor magnitude (Allison et al., 1999a).

Some more recent prospective studies have analysed the relationship between BMI and mortality particularly among non-smokers, excluding subjects with pre-existing diseases, and ignoring mortality in the first years of follow-up. Attempts were made to adjust for direct consequences of obesity such as diabetes and hypertension and to exclude subjects with a large loss of weight. Some studies with proper control of confounding demonstrated no significant increase in risk of all-cause mortality among subjects in the lower end of the BMI range (Wannamethee & Shaper, 1989; Lee et al., 1993; Sorkin et al., 1994; Manson et al., 1995; Stevens et al., 1998; Baik et al., 2000). Baik et al. (2000) found evidence that lean men particularly suffer from death due to respiratory diseases and that risk of mortality is particularly high among inactive lean subjects. Allison et al. (1997, 1999b) demonstrated that the higher mortality risk among lean subjects can be attributed to low lean body mass, whereas a low fat mass decreases mortality risk.

It appears that gender is a major modifier of the shape of the BMI–mortality association in the general population. For instance, Waaler (1988) found a U-shaped association in middle-aged men, while a reversed J-shaped association was observed in females, with the highest mortality rates among lean women. In a study of slightly younger adults in the Netherlands, a U-shaped association was seen in men but not in women (Seidell et al., 1996). It has been suggested that the gender difference in obesity-related mortality can be explained in part by a greater tendency for males to develop abdominal obesity (Larsson et al., 1992).

Stevens et al. (1998) conducted the largest recent study on a non-smoking population and showed in general a direct relationship between BMI in young age and all-cause mortality. This cohort study of the American Cancer Society also strongly indicated that age is a modifier of the effect of weight on all-cause mortality (and cardiovascular diseases). In this cohort of 62 116 men and 262 019 women, the increased relative risk of mortality with higher BMI decreased with age. The trend was similar in men and women. The modifying effect of age was further evaluated by Stevens (2000), taking previous research into account. Baik et al. (2000) also recently highlighted this issue and provided further evidence that in older subjects BMI may be less important compared with direct measurements of fatness such as waist circumference. Comparative analyses of different measures of fatness in the same study population are rare, but have shown that other measures of fatness than BMI are also related to risk and add further information on the relationship between fatness and mortality (Folsom et al., 2000). Seidell and Visscher (2000) considered five possible explanations for the observed modifying effect of age: (1) BMI is not a good indicator; (2) there is selective survival of only the fittest obese subjects; (3) a ceiling effect occurs because most study participants in old age groups die during follow-up; (4) cohort effects arise because of different experience in terms of development of obesity and morbidity/mortality across birth cohorts; (5) excess fat is less detrimental in older than in younger age groups. They also presented empirical data showing that ageing is associated with a change in body composition, with an increase in fat mass at the expense of lean body mass.

In a prospective study in the USA of the relationship of BMI and fitness to risk of all-cause mortality, 21 925 men, aged 30–83 years, had a body composition assessment and a maximal treadmill exercise test. The 428 deaths over the eight-year follow-up period (on average) were linked to obesity and cardiorespiratory fitness. Compared with lean fit subjects, obese fit subjects (% body fat ≥ 25) experienced a similar relative risk for all-cause mortality (RR = 0.92; 95% CI 0.65–1.3) which was lower than the relative risk of unfit subjects with normal weight (RR = 1.6; 95% CI 1.2–2.3) after adjustment for age, year of examination, smoking habits, alcohol intake and parental history of ischaemic heart disease (Lee et al., 1999d). The highest

relative risk compared with lean fit subjects was found for the unfit lean subjects (RR = 2.1; 95% CI 1.2–3.7) taking the lean fit subjects as reference. However this study population was highly selective and cardiorespiratory fitness is not identical with physical activity (see Chapter 1).

Methodological issues still dominate the debate about the relation between BMI and mortality. However, the data from studies with proper control of confounding clearly indicate that risk of all-cause mortality is lower at BMI < 25 kg/m^2 (Wannamethee & Shaper, 1989; Lee et al., 1993; Sorkin et al., 1994; Manson et al., 1995; Stevens et al., 1998; Baik et al., 2000). Ethnic differences probably exist for optimal BMI; there is evidence that the optimal BMI is higher for blacks, while in Pima Indian women no relationship between BMI and mortality was found (National Task Force on the Prevention and Treatment of Obesity, 2000).

Weight change

Weight change in the adult population is a common phenomenon often recorded in the prospective cohort studies that form the basis for the evaluation of long-term effects of weight on risk for all-cause mortality. In some studies, in addition to repeated measurements of weight and other anthropometric variables, weight histories were obtained. Subjects can also be asked about dieting behaviour, their intention to lose weight and how they lost weight. Thus it is possible to follow the development of weight over time in subjects and to compare groups with different patterns of weight development in terms of subsequent risk. In theory, data on the effect of weight change on risk in adult life may be much more relevant to weight reduction programmes focusing on change of weight in adult life than studies based on BMI at a given point in time.

The design of studies on weight change is more complex than that of

studies on BMI status. In most recent prospective studies, weight change was first measured and then the risk associated with such changes was assessed over the subsequent follow-up period. Only a few studies have incorporated data on weight changes during follow-up until end-point occurrence in their analysis (e.g., Deeg et al., 1990). The effect of weight change on risk was usually controlled for initial BMI. Thus, these studies allow simultaneous investigation of both weight and weight change, and have often led to the conclusion that these two aspects act independently of each other (Mikkelsen et al., 1999).

However, these studies have severe limitations. Whereas it is relative easy to record weight change over time, it is very hard to obtain information about the reason for changes. It is known that weight change in itself affects further weight development (Colditz et al., 1990). For example, weight reduction is a good predictor of subsequent increase in weight. Background information relating to weight change may be less important for weight gain but is very important in the case of weight loss. Weight loss is often related to underlying chronic diseases in an early stage, not yet verified by a physician. In some studies, specific enquiry was made about reasons for weight loss. Two studies have found that among weight losers, the percentages of intentional and unintentional loss of weight were about 50 and 50% (French et al., 1995) in women and about 40 and 60% in men (Wannamethee et al., 2000). However, even if a person has intentionally reduced weight, the various ways of doing so may affect disease risk differently: reduction of energy intake, increase of physical activity, change of dietary pattern, use of drugs etc. A recent large study of 4713 British men shed some light on the characteristics of those who indicated that they intentionally or unintentionally lost weight as they aged (Wannamethee et al., 2000). Intentional weight loss was associated with higher BMI than in those with unintentional loss and the latter group felt more unhealthy. However, both groups clearly differed from those with stable weight in having poorer health. A group of weight cyclers comprising only 82 of the men in this study showed the highest BMI and the poorest health. In conclusion, it seems very difficult to identify subjects in a cohort who reduced their weight for preventive reasons only with no relation to acute or chronic illness. Weight loss due to health impairment, even if considered as intentional, might therefore be particularly subject to the phenomenon of reverse causation, so that available data may be misleading.

It is nevertheless worthwhile to examine the results of prospective observational cohort studies that have analysed effects of weight change on risk of all-cause mortality in more detail. In such studies, stable weight is usually the reference category. For the determination of weight variability (cycling), at least three measurement points over time per subject are needed. In most of the studies that investigated this aspect, weight variability was defined as standard deviation of the subject-specific measurements or as the variation of the measurement points along a regression line (Lissner et al., 1990). The latter was considered particular useful because weight variability could be separated from weight development over time, allowing differentiation between the two aspects of weight change.

Only a few of the studies analysing the effect of weight change on all-cause mortality investigated all aspects of weight change, including the effect of stable weight, simultaneously in one study population. It is more usual to find studies within the same cohort but looking at different time periods, specific aspects of weight change and different disease outcomes. In addition, it is nearly impossible to standardize the results of the different studies. Wide variation exists across studies in terms of the age range of the population, the time period at which weight change was measured and the follow-up period used, as well as in the categories of weight change used. The study-specific definition of weight change has often mixed various aspects depending on the study design and the information available. For example, weight variability might be specifically measured in a study population or included in the weight change measure.

Studies of the effect of weight change on mortality were reviewed by Lee and Paffenbarger (1996) and a meta-analysis was performed by Andres et al. (1993). The earliest study was that of Dublin (1953), which used data from a life insurance company, and was followed by a similar study published in 1959 (Build and Blood Pressure Study), based on about five million subjects. Subsequent studies were those conducted by the American Cancer Society (Hammond & Garfinkel, 1969) and a second Build and Blood Pressure Study (1980) of members of a health insurance scheme. The first studies indicated a reduction of mortality with weight loss in both men and women. However, the detailed analysis by Hammond and Garfinkel (1969) revealed that weight loss might not only have beneficial effects by reducing the risk of mortality but also increase risk particularly for cardiovascular death in some strata. Table 51 summarizes the results of most of the subsequent studies, as far as they directly reported relative risk estimates. The relative risk estimates presented in this table refer in general to the highest or lowest weight change category if there was a linear trend. In addition to the studies reporting relative risk in Table 51, Deeg et al. (1990) found increased risk with increase and decrease of weight in a national sample of 604 Dutch subjects aged 65 to 99 years, particularly among males. Rhoads and Kagan (1983) reported increased risk with decreased weight and a slight increase in risk with increased weight among Honolulu Japanese men aged 45 to 68 years.

Overall, the studies indicate excess mortality associated with both weight loss and weight gain. Significantly increased risks were often seen for weight loss and studies that investigated weight cycling usually found consistently elevated risks for all-cause mortality. In most studies, weight gain was associated with only slightly increased risk compared with stable weight, often in a non-significant manner. However, many of the studies were conducted in older age groups. Effect modification by age similar to that seen for BMI should be considered. The same applies to modifying effects of initial BMI. Data from some studies suggest that weight loss and weight cycling in obese subjects are less strongly associated with risk than in subjects of normal weight (Blair et al., 1993; Pamuk et al., 1993) and some studies of obese subjects have not revealed increased risk associated with weight reduction (Williamson et al., 1995, 1999).

Studies that have separately investigated intentional and unintentional weight loss have failed to show reduced all-cause mortality for intentional weight loss compared with stable weight (Williamson et al., 1995, 1999; French et al., 1999b). However, two of these studies (Williamson et al., 1995; French et al., 1999b) found that the excess mortality associated with weight loss seemed to be attributable to unintentional loss. Intentional weight loss was associated with decreased premature mortality among obese women with obesity-related co-morbidities but not those without co-morbidities (Williamson et al., 1995).

In conclusion, methodological problems remain serious in the area of research into weight change and all-cause mortality. The current data do not indicate that weight loss lowers the risk of all-cause mortality.

Table 51. Studies of total mortality in relation to weight gain or loss

Reference	No. of total outcome	Total number of participants	Study population	Time-scale	Effect of intentional (I) or unintentional (U) weight change on risk			Remarks
					Increase	Decrease	Cycling	
Harris et al. (1988)	528	1723	USA, Framingham Study, men and women, 65 y	Weight change period: 10 y / Follow up period: 1 to 23 y	M: 1.5 (0.9–2.4) F: 1.1 (0.8–1.7)	M: 1.9 (1.1–3.2) F: 1.8 (1.2–1.6)		Non-smoking
Hamm et al. (1989)	736	1959	USA, Western Electric Study, men, 40–56 y	Weight change period: since age 20 y / Follow-up period: 25 y	1.4 (1.0–2.1)		1.5 (1.0–2.3)	
Lissner et al. (1991)	942	3130	USA, Framingham Study, men and women, 30–62 y	Weight change period: since age 2 y / Follow-up period: 32 y			M: 1.6 (1.3–2.1) F: 1.3 (1.0–1.6)	
Pamuk et al. (1992)	1496	4690	NHANES I Study, men and women, 45–74 y	Weight change period: maximum change / Follow-up period: 10 y		2.0 (1.5–2.8)		BMI $\geq$ 29 kg/m^2
Lee & Paffenbarger (1992c)	1441	11 703	USA, Harvard University alumni, men, 45–84 y	Weight change period: 11 to 15 y / Follow-up period: 11 y	1.4 (first 5 y) 1.3 (second 2 y)	1.8 (first 5 y) 1.5 (second 6 y)		
Blair et al. (1993)	228	10 529	USA, Multiple Risk Factor Intervention Trial, men, 35–57 y	Weight change period: 6–7 y / Follow-up period: 4 y	1.2 (0.86–1.7)	1.6 (1.2–2.2)	1.6 (1.2–2.2)	Effect of weight cycling only in normal weight men
Higgins et al. (1993)	Not reported	2500	USA, Framingham Study, men and women, 35–54 y	Weight change period: 10 y / Follow-up period: 20 y	M: 0.78 (0.60–1.0) F: 1.2 (0.87–1.6)	M: 1.3 (1.1–1.7) F: 1.3 (0.98–1.7)		
Paffenbarger et al. (1993)	476	10 269	USA, Harvard College alumni, men, 45–84 y	Weight change period: 11–15 y / Follow-up period: 8 y	1.4 (non-sign.)	1.3 (non-sign.)		Recalculated: BMI <26 kg/m^2 in both periods as basis
Ho et al. (1994)	35	374	Hong Kong women (> 70 y)	Weight change period: 2 y / Follow-up period: 2 y	1.3 (0.2–7.1)	4.8 (1.3–18.4)		

Table 51 (contd)

Reference	No. of total outcome	Total number of participants	Study population	Time-scale	Effect of intentional (I) or unintentional (U) weight change on risk			Remarks
					Increase	Decrease	Cycling	
Iribarren et al. (1995)	1217	6537	Japanese American men, 45–68 y	Weight change period: 6 y / Follow-up period: 15 y	0.99 (0.79–1.3)	1.2 (1.0–1.4)	1.2 (1.0–1.5)	
Losonczy et al. (1995)	2650	6387	USA, whites over 70 y	Weight change period: ≥20 y / Follow-up period: 3 and 6 y	M: 0.91 (0.76–1.1) F: 0.90 (0.90–1.1)	M: 1.7 (1.4–2.0) F: 1.6 (1.4–1.9)		Old subjects, increased risk disappeared after controlling for chronic conditions
Manson et al. (1995)	1059	115 195	USA, nurses, women, 30–55 y	Weight change period: since age 18 y / Follow-up period: 16 y	1.6 (1.3–1.9)	0.7 (0.4–1.4)		
Peters et al. (1995)	1845	6441	EU, Seven Countries Study men, 40–59 y	Weight change period: 10 y / Follow-up period: up to 15 y	1.0 (0.92–1.2)	1.3 (1.2–1.5)	1.2 (1.0–1.4)	
Williamson et al., (1995)	1819	28 388	USA, Cancer Prevention Study, overweight men, 40–64 y	Weight change period: 22 to 46 y / Follow-up period: 13 y	0.99 (0.74–1.3)	I: 0.98 (0.82–1.2) U: 1.2 (0.93–1.6)		Subjects with no preexisting illness, non-smoking
Folsom et al. (1996)	1068	33 760	Iowa Health Study, women, 55–69 y	Weight change period: 44 y / Follow-up period: 6 y	1.20 (0.8–1.8)	2.0 (1.3–3.1)	1.8 (1.2–2.8)	
Yaari & Goldbourt (1998)	2983	9228	Israel, Ischaemic Heart Disease Study, men, 40–65 y	Weight change period: 5 y / Follow-up period: 18 y	0.91 (0.80–1.0)	1.2 (1.1–1.4)		
Allison et al. (1999b)	321	1890	USA, Tecumseh Study, men and women	Weight change period: 4 y / Follow-up period: 16 y		1.3 (1.1–1.5)		Risk per 4.6 kg weight loss, fat loss was protective
	507	2731	USA, Framingham Study, men and women	Weight change period: 14 y / Follow-up period: 8 y		1.4 (1.2–1.5)		Risk per 6.7 kg weight loss, fat loss was protective

Table 51 (contd)

Reference	No. of total outcome	Total number of participants	Study population	Time-scale	Effect of intentional (I) or unintentional (U) weight change on risk			Remarks
					Increase	Decrease	Cycling	
French *et al.* (1999b)	1038	25 897	Iowa Health Study, women, 55–69 y	Weight change period: 25 y Follow-up period: 3 y		I: 1.2 (0.94–1.5) U: 1.3 (1.1–1.6)		
Mikkelsen *et al.* (1999)	3160	15 113	Denmark, men and women, 20–93 y	Weight change period: 5 to 25 y Follow-up period: 10 y	1.2 (0.94–1.4)	1.6 (1.3–1.9)		Compared at initial BMI 22–24 kg/m²
Reynolds *et al.* (1999)	106	648	Baltimore, women, 65+ y	Weight change period: 2 y Follow-up period: 6 y		3.8 (2.1–6.9)		
Williamson *et al.* (1999)	3726	36 280	USA, Cancer Prevention Study, overweight men, 40–64 y	Weight change period: 22–46 y Follow-up period: 13 y	1.1 (0.92–1.3)	I: 1.1 (0.98–1.2) U: 1.0 (0.91–1.2)		Subjects with no reported health conditions
Dyer *et al.* (2000)	686	1281	USA, Western Electric Company Study, men, 40–56 y	Weight change period: 8 y Follow-up period: 25 y			1.1 (1.0–1.2)	

Cardiovascular disease

Excess body weight has been demonstrated in many studies to increase the risk for mortality from cardiovascular disease in subjects of both genders (Pi-Sunyer, 1999). Also studies on weight change have analysed, in addition to all-cause mortality, coronary heart or cardiovascular disease mortality or morbidity (e.g., Lissner *et al.*, 1991; Lee & Paffenbarger, 1992d; Blair *et al.*, 1993; Higgins *et al.*, 1993; Iribarren *et al.*, 1995; Rimm *et al.*, 1995; Willett *et al.*, 1995; Folsom *et al.*, 1996; Fulton & Shekelle, 1997; French *et al.*, 1997; Yaari & Goldbourt, 1998; Galanis *et al.*, 1998b; French *et al.,* 1999b; Dyer *et al.*, 2000). In general, weight gain seems to be more tightly linked to an increase of risk for coronary heart diseases than for all-cause mortality, while the risk in connection with weight loss was on average less elevated for coronary heart diseases than for all-cause mortality and only slightly higher compared with stable weight. The three studies that addressed the question of intentional or unintentional weight loss (Williamson *et al.*, 1995, 1999; French *et al.*, 1999b) showed similar risk associated with intentional weight loss and with stable weight, while among women, unintentional loss of weight was associated with increased risk. However, the limitations of the current studies on weight loss discussed above also apply in relation to cardiovascular diseases and therefore the evidence for an effect of weight loss on cardiovascular diseases can be considered as limited.

This conclusion has to be weighed against the benefits seen in intervention studies among high-risk subjects (see following sections). Weight reduction improved cardiovascular disease clinical measurements and symptoms (Ornish *et al.*, 1990) and decreased mortality in a secondary prevention trial (Singh *et al.*, 1992). The National Task Force on the Prevention and Treatment of Obesity (2000) pointed out that most of the effects of weight on coronary heart diseases presumably act throught its impact on other risk factors including hypertension, impaired glucose tolerance, type II diabetes mellitus and dyslipidaemia.

Hypertension

Both systolic and diastolic blood pressure increase with increasing BMI (Stamler *et al.*, 1978; Van Itallie, 1985). Observational studies on risk of hypertension in relation to weight change suggest that an increase in weight increases the risk of hypertension (e.g., Curtis *et al.*, 1998; Huang *et al.*, 1998; Field *et al.*, 1999). Weight reduction seems to decrease the risk of hypertension (Huang *et al.,* 1998). Little information is available on the effect of weight cycling on risk of hypertension and no firm conclusion can currently be drawn. However, a recent small case–control study in Italy with a group of 103 hypertensive obese women aged 25–64 years and 155 controls revealed an increased risk associated with weight cycling (Guagnano *et al.*, 2000). It was concluded that weight cycling leads to increased weight and to a larger waist-to-hip ratio, both of which are associated with increased risk for hypertension.

Prevention of hypertension in overweight normotensive individuals

Stevens *et al.* (2001) randomized 1191 overweight subjects with non-medicated diastolic blood pressure of 83 to 89 mm Hg and systolic blood pressure less than 140 mm Hg to two groups. The intervention group lost weight through a three-year programme including dietary changes, physical activity and social support. After three years, the mean weight loss in the intervention group was 0.2 kg, while the control group had gained a mean of 1.8 kg. The risk ratio for hypertension in the intervention group was 0.81 (95% CI 0.70–0.95) at three years. Subjects who had lost at least 4.5 kg at six months and maintained this weight loss up to three years had the lowest risk ratio for hypertension, of 0.35 (95% CI 0.20–0.59).

Established hypertension

A systematic review of 18 randomized trials (Mulrow *et al.*, 2000) evaluated whether weight-loss diets are more effective than other antihypertensive therapies in controlling blood pressure in hypertensive subjects. The trials included 2611 hypertensive participants. Most studies excluded subjects with normal weight. Intervention periods with a weight-loss diet ranged from two weeks to three years. In general, participants assigned to weight-reduction groups lost weight compared with the control groups. Six trials involving 361 participants assessed a low-energy diet versus a normal diet. A 4–8% weight loss was associated with a decrease in blood pressure in the range of 3 mm Hg systolic and diastolic. The review included three trials that assessed a weight-loss diet versus treatment with antihypertensive medications and suggested that a stepped-care approach with antihypertensive medications produced greater decreases in blood pressure (6 and 5 mm Hg systolic and diastolic, respectively) than did a weight-loss diet. However, the review suggested that patients on a weight-reducing diet required less intensive antihypertensive drug therapy.

Type II diabetes

The development of type II diabetes is characterized by obesity, early insulin resistance and progressive deterioration of glucose homeostasis over several years from hyperinsulinaemia with normal fasting glucose to impaired fasting glucose ('impaired glucose tolerance') and ultimately to fasting hyperglycaemia accompanied by a cluster of other metabolic abnormalities predisposing to vascular disease (Laakso & Lehto,1997). Excess weight, particularly abdominal obesity, has a deleterious effect on all phases of this process. An increasing risk of diabetes with greater initial BMI and weight gain has been amply documented in prospective studies from various parts of the world (Maggio & Pi-Sunyer, 1997). The risk increases almost linearly, being 2.1 and 3.5 for BMI 22–22.9 and 23–23.9 kg/m^2, respectively, compared with BMI < 22 kg/m^2 in US women aged 30–55 years who were followed for eight years (Colditz et al., 1990). The positive effects of sustained weight loss on glycaemic control and associated metabolic complications in obese type II diabetes patients can be expected to have a favourable effect on mortality and morbidity among these patients. However, some studies have reported no association or an increased risk of mortality in obese diabetic patients with weight loss (Knatterud et al., 1982; Chaturvedi & Fuller, 1995; Hanson et al., 1995); these studies were not able to differentiate between in tentional and unintentional weight loss. Some studies suggest that weight cycling increases the risk of type II diabetes (French et al., 1997; Moore et al., 2000b), but this issue needs further research. In a recent re-analysis of the American Cancer Society Study (Williamson et al., 2000), overweight people with type II diabetes who reported intentional weight loss had lower total mortality (RR = 0.75; 95% CI 0.67–0.84) and cardiovascular disease and diabetes mortality (RR = 0.72; 95% CI 0.63–0.82) than those not reporting such weight loss. Weight loss of 20–29 lb [9–13 kg] was associated with the greatest reductions in mortality (0.67; 95% CI 0.58–0.77).

Prevention of diabetes in non-diabetic individuals

Short-term studies have shown a significant correlation between improved insulin sensitivity and percentage decrease in fat mass, especially in visceral adiposity (Goodpaster et al., 1999). Weight loss produced by a low-energy diet reduces blood glucose and insulin levels in obese individuals (National Institutes of Health and National Heart, Lung and Blood Institute, 1998). It also reduces the risk of developing type II diabetes, but the weight loss achieved by dietary interventions is usually not maintained and the benefit is short-lived. However, the protective effect is maintained if weight loss is maintained. After a two-year programme of diet and exercise in obese (30–100% overweight) persons with a family history of diabetes (Wing et al., 1998), no overall difference in weight loss between the intervention and control groups was found at the end of the trial, despite impressive results in the first six months. However, among the participants maintaining a weight loss of 4–5 kg or more, regardless of study group, the risk of developing diabetes was reduced by 30%. The protective effect of a small maintained weight loss is also illustrated by a pooled analysis of randomized placebo-controlled weight loss trials (Heymsfield et al., 2000). In this study, 10.8% of the obese subjects receiving diet only (mean weight loss 3.7 kg) developed impaired glucose tolerance and 1.2% developed diabetes in two years, whereas in the group on diet plus orlistat (a gastro-intestinal lipase inhibitor) (mean weight loss 6.7 kg), impaired glucose tolerance developed in 6.6% and none developed diabetes. The benefits of a modest amount of sustained weight loss is preserved for extended periods of time. In a long-term follow-up of the Framingham cohort (Moore et al., 2000b), weight loss of 3.5 kg or more maintained for eight years substantially lowered the risk of diabetes (RR = 0.38; 95% CI 0.18–0.81) in subjects with BMI ≥ 29 kg/m^2, whereas those who regained the weight they had lost had no reduction in diabetes risk. The most impressive protective effect is seen in subjects who lose a large amount of weight by obesity surgery (Long et al., 1994; Sjöström et al., 1999). In the Swedish Obese Subjects (SOS) Study, the eight-year incidence of diabetes among surgically treated morbidly obese subjects (maintained weight loss about 20 kg) was greatly reduced compared with matched controls (no weight change), with an odds ratio of 0.16 (95% CI 0.07–0.36) (Sjöström et al., 2000).

Prevention of diabetes in subjects with impaired glucose tolerance (IGT)

Several studies have demonstrated the potential of modest weight loss achieved by lifestyle modification to reduce the risk of diabetes in persons with IGT (e.g., Pan et al., 1997; Heymsfield et al., 2000; Tuomilehto et al., 2001). In Chinese subjects with IGT followed for six years after an intervention of diet or exercise or both, the conversion rate to diabetes at six years was reduced by 31% in the diet intervention group achieving permanent weight loss of 1–3 kg (Pan et al., 1997b). In a pooled analysis of two-year randomized placebo-controlled weight reduction trials comparing orlistat plus diet (mean weight loss 6.7 kg) versus diet alone (3.8 kg), half as many subjects with IGT progressed to diabetic status in the orlistat group (3.0%) as those with placebo (7.6%). In a randomized trial in Finland (Tuomilehto et al., 2001), a weight loss of about 3.5 kg resulting from lifestyle intervention (versus 0.9 kg in controls) reduced the incidence of diabetes by more than 50% during the first four years of follow-up.

Greater sustained weight loss appears to almost completely reverse the risk of diabetes in subjects with IGT. A randomized controlled trial by Long et al. (1994) examined the progression of IGT to type II diabetes in 109 morbidly obese individuals with gastric bypass and in 27 non-surgical controls. Maintenance of the weight loss, corresponding to about 50% of the excess weight in the surgery group, was associated with a more than 30-fold decrease in the risk of developing diabetes over six years.

Established type II diabetes

The health benefits of weight loss in obese patients with type II diabetes are well documented (Maggio & Pi-Sunyer, 1997; National Institutes of Health and National Heart, Lung and Blood Institute, 1998, Williamson et al., 2000). Negative energy balance results in rapid improvement of hyperglycaemia, independent of weight loss, which is followed by a more enduring improvement in glycaemic control and other metabolic risk factors with loss of (abdominal) fat (Markovic et al., 1998). Several studies have reported improved metabolic control with modest short-term weight loss (Liu et al., 1985; Wing et al., 1987; Goldstein, 1992). A meta-analysis of 89 short-term intervention studies using diet or a behavioural approach to induce negative energy balance concluded that a low-energy diet alone (often denoting a period of very low-energy diet) had a significant impact on weight (loss of about 9 kg), glycaemic control (−2.7% in glycosylated haemoglobin) and lipids and blood pressure, whereas the effects were smaller for behavioural therapies alone (about 2.9 kg and −1.5%) and for exercise alone (1.7 kg and −0.8%) (Brown et al., 1996).

The short-term reduction in fasting hyperglycaemia is usually greatest in patients who lose the most weight (UKPDS Group, 1990), but in most trials a modest weight loss of 5–15% body weight has been associated with distinct improvements in glycaemic control (e.g., Heller et al., 1988; UKPDS Group, 1990; Franz et al., 1995; Manning et al., 1995). For instance, in the randomized controlled trial by Heller et al. (1988), a median weight loss of 7 kg through dietary education (versus 2 kg in controls) resulted in a significant improvement in glycaemic control (median haemoglobin A1 7.5% versus 9.5%) at six months. However, glucose control

does not always improve with weight loss (Watts et al., 1990). The benefits may also depend on the type of diet, e.g., total energy content and fat and carbohydrate composition (Heilbronn et al., 1999).

Unfortunately, most of the benefit of weight loss seen in the early months of an intervention is lost with the weight regain that almost invariably later occurs, especially in diabetics (Guare et al., 1995). The improvement in metabolic control is sustained if weight loss is maintained, as in a 12-month trial comparing the efficacy of orlistat plus diet versus diet only in drug-treated diabetics (Hollander et al., 1998). A mean weight loss of 6 kg was seen in the orlistat group versus 4 kg with placebo at 12 months, in addition to decreased haemoglobin A1c and reductions in the use of sulfo-nylurea medication and in serum lipids. One of the few reports of successful long-term weight loss with diet comes from the Diabetes Treatment Study (Hadden et al., 1986), an uncontrolled prospective trial of 223 patients with recently diagnosed diabetes who were seen for up to 72 months. Average weight loss at six months was 9 kg, and this was maintained for the six years of the study. At the end, about 80% of the patients could still be managed by diet alone. Prospective studies of patients with surgically treated obesity convincingly demonstrate the benefits of sustained weight loss (Pories et al., 1995; Long et al., 1994; Sjöström et al., 1999). Over 80% of the 146 morbidly obese diabetics followed for 14 years after a gastric bypass operation had attained normoglycaemia, although they still were considerably overweight after a sustained weight loss of about 40 kg (Pories et al., 1995).

Taken together, these data indicate that maintained major weight loss results in dramatic improvement of metabolic control or even in cure of obese type II diabetics. Although successful weight

loss due to diet and lifestyle modification is difficult to achieve and even more difficult to maintain, even modest maintained weight loss offers considerable benefits. The unexplained variability of the metabolic response of type II diabetics to moderate weight loss may be due to the heterogeneity of the disease.

Other morbidity

Obesity is also associated with increased risk of gallbladder disease, liver disease, reproductive problems, sleep apnoea, poor pulmonary function and degenerative joint disease (Pi-Sunyer, 1999; National Task Force on the Prevention and Treatment of Obesity, 2000). BMI and weight gain are associated with risk of adult-onset asthma (Camargo et al., 1999). Weight loss decreases symptoms of these diseases, except for gallbladder disease. Significant improvement in both symptoms and objective findings of obstructive sleep apnoea syndrome after weight loss have been demonstrated (Lojander et al., 1998). In a randomized trial, weight reduction in obese patients with asthma improved their lung function, symptoms and health status (Stenius-Aarniala et al., 2000). In the Framingham study (Felson et al., 1992), a decrease of 2 BMI units or more during a 10-year period decreased the odds of developing knee osteoarthritis by more than 50%, while weight gain was associated with a slight increase in risk.

Effects on surrogate markers

Effects of weight on insulin resistance, IGF, sex steroids, other hormones and immune function are covered in Chapter 4. Notably, associations between obesity and blood pressure, type II diabetes, dyslipidaemia and cardiovascular disease risk differ between racial and ethnic groups (Fujimoto, 1996; Cappuccio, 1997; Zoratti, 1998; Brown et al., 2000)

Visceral adipose tissue

Hormonal and metabolic disturbances observed in abdominal obesity affect cardiovascular disease risk (Després et al., 1990). A weight-loss diet promotes the loss of visceral adipose tissue (VAT). A review (Smith & Zachwieja, 1999) covered only studies measuring VAT with computed tomography or magnetic resonance imaging. The 16 eligible studies comprised 399 subjects. The duration of the studies ranged from 7 days to 16 months. Reductions in body weight ranged from 3.9% to 19.8% and in VAT from 9.4% to 49.3%. Diet intervention led to a greater loss of VAT than total fat loss. Individuals with greater visceral fat mass appear to lose more visceral fat, when adjustment is made for loss of body fat.

Dyslipidaemia

A higher BMI is associated with higher plasma triglyceride levels and lower high-density lipoprotein (HDL) cholesterol level, but the association with low-density lipoprotein (LDL) cholesterol levels is inconsistent (Després et al., 1990). A meta-analysis (Yu-Poth et al., 1999) evaluated the effects of the National Cholesterol Education Program's Step I and Step II dietary interventions on blood lipids. The 37 eligible randomized trials included 9276 subjects in intervention groups and 2310 subjects in control groups. The duration of intervention ranged from three weeks to four years. There was no restriction as to baseline obesity. Mean baseline total and LDL cholesterol concentrations were 6.04±0.53 mmol/L and 4.01±0.46 mmol/L, respectively. Mean baseline HDL cholesterol concentration was 1.24±0.23 mmol/L and triacylglycerol concentration was 1.67±0.46 mmol/L. Reductions in dietary fat and saturated fatty acids had beneficial effects on blood lipids. Plasma total cholesterol, LDL cholesterol, and triacylglycerol concentrations and the ratio of total cholesterol to HDL cholesterol significantly

decreased after both Step I (by 10%, 12%, 8% and 10%, respectively) and Step II (by 13%, 16%, 8% and 7%, respectively) dietary interventions. In many of the studies, the subjects lost weight (mean 3.38 kg). The changes in body weight significantly affected plasma HDL cholesterol and triacylglycerol concentrations; for every 1 kg decrease in body weight, plasma triacylglycerol concentrations decreased by 0.011–0.012 mmol/L (0.77–0.87%), whereas HDL cholesterol concentrations increased by 0.011 mmol/L ($\cong$1%). The correlations between body weight reduction and changes in total cholesterol and LDL cholesterol were significant only when the analyses were weighted by the number of subjects in each study. Another meta-analysis found that during active weight loss, HDL cholesterol levels tend to decrease, but when reduced weight stabilizes, HDL cholesterol levels increase to above the level before weight loss (Dattilo & Kris-Etherton, 1992).

Psychosocial aspects and quality of life

There are probably ethnic and cultural differences in reactions and attitudes to overweight and obese individuals. There is an inverse association between weight and socioeconomic status, especially among women (Sobal & Stunkard, 1989). Low socioeconomic status of origin is predictive of weight gain during adulthood (Lahmann et al., 2000). Obese individuals may be prone to discrimination and negative attitudes in the areas of marital, employment and educational opportunities (Wadden & Stunkard, 1993). Most of the psychological disturbances (poor mental well-being, anxiety and depressive symptoms) associated with morbid obesity are believed to be consequences rather than causes of obesity. Decreasing psychological and behavioural symptoms after weight loss support this direction of causality (Wing et al., 1984; Karlsson et al., 1998).

Some studies have found that overweight (measured either as BMI or waist circumference) leads to poorer physical functioning (Le Pen et al., 1998; Lean et al., 1998). However, mental and social dimensions of quality of life (QOL) seem to remain unchanged with overweight. Only the additional burden of other chronic conditions compromises the mental and social dimensions of QOL in persons suffering from obesity (Doll et al., 2000). Compared with the general population, obese patients seeking treatment suffer impairment in all dimensions of quality of life (Fontaine et al., 2000).

Most of the studies assessing the effects of weight loss on QOL (functioning and well-being) have been conducted on surgically treated morbidly obese patients. The marked weight loss achieved by surgical techniques has been shown to improve deteriorated QOL in all of its dimensions (Karlsson et al., 1998; Choban et al., 1999). Positive changes in QOL have been related to the magnitude of weight loss and the duration of follow-up, with some tendency for QOL scores to return to baseline levels in subjects with less than 20 kg weight loss at long term (Karlsson et al., 1998). As regards non-surgical methods of weight loss, one randomized controlled trial showed that a 7-kg difference between groups in weight outcome achieved by increased physical activity, low-energy diet and group support led to improved QOL in the intervention group (Rippe et al., 1998). The duration of this study was only 12 weeks; the long-term effects of non-surgical weight loss interventions on QOL remain largely unknown.

Physical activity

A large body of evidence shows that physical inactivity increases mortality and morbidity (US Department of Health and Social Services, 1996). In the following review, priority has been given to health outcomes where the effects of physical activity have been demonstrated consistently in different populations, to studies with sound measures of physical activity or physical fitness, and—because of their relevance to developing public health recommendations for physical activity—to studies providing information on dose–response issues. The evidence discussed is derived for the most part from studies in Caucasian populations.

Total mortality

Physical activity is inversely associated with all-cause mortality rates in middle-aged and older ($\geq$ 60 years) men and women (Table 52). The relationship with volume of physical activity (estimated energy expenditure or a proxy for this) is linear, at least up to a level of about 14.7 MJ (3500 kcal) per week (Lee *et al.*, 1995), but approaches an asymptote at higher levels. Information on independent effects of the components of volume of physical activity (intensity, duration, frequency of sessions) is sparse. Some reports suggest a benefit only from vigorous activities ($\geq$ 6 METs) (Lee *et al.*, 1995; Lee & Paffenbarger, 2000) and others a benefit from moderately vigorous activity ($\geq$ 4.5 METs) (Paffenbarger *et al.*, 1993). Simple, non-sporting activities such as walking and stair climbing have been associated with lower risk. Distance walked and storeys climbed were predictive of longevity, independently of other components of physical activity, among male graduates of Harvard (Lee & Paffenbarger, 2000). Bicycling to work was associated with a 40% lower risk of mortality among Danish men and women, after multivariate adjustment which included leisure-time physical activity (Andersen *et al.*, 2000). Among retired men aged 61–81 years at the start of a 12-year follow-up period, the mortality rate among those who walked less than 1.6 km per day was nearly twice the rate in those who walked more than 3.2 km per day (Hakim *et al.*, 1998).

Inverse gradients for mortality exist across categories of increasing fitness (Sandvik *et al.*, 1993; Blair *et al.*, 1996); adjusted relative risks for medium and/or high fitness vs low fitness of 0.66 (95% CI 0.55–0.78) (Blair *et al.,* 1996) and 0.54 (95% CI 0.32–0.89) (Sandvik *et al.,* 1993) for men and 0.48 (95% CI, 0.31–0.74) for women (Blair *et al.*, 1996) have been reported. The available data suggest that a fitness level (assessed as maximal oxygen uptake) below 8–9 METs in middle-aged men is associated with a significant increase in risk (Whaley & Blair, 1995). Too few data are available for women to make a comparable estimate.

Low fitness is an important determinant of mortality risk. Among North American men, individuals with none of the established risk factors for coronary heart disease (smoking, high total cholesterol, hypertension) but who were in the lowest quintile for fitness had higher death rates than men who had two or three of these factors but were in the top quintile for fitness (Blair *et al.*, 1996).

Differences in mortality associated with physical activity levels are not explained by familial factors, as shown by comparison of death rates during follow-up in physically active twins with those of their less active siblings (Kujala *et al.*, 1998). Controlling for known confounders, including BMI, had relatively little impact on the relative risks of inactivity (Lee *et al.*, 1995) or low fitness (Sandvik *et al.*, 1993; Blair *et al.*, 1996). The effect of low fitness *per se* is evident from the report that unfit (bottom quintile of population studied) but lean men had significantly higher all-cause mortality than men who were fit (top quintile) but who had a BMI > 30 kg/m^2 (Lee *et al.*, 1999d). The importance of physical activity, as opposed to constitutional factors, is clear from reports that men and women who take up moderately vigorous activity or who increase their fitness level between two observations separated by some years

experience substantially lower all-cause mortality rates than their peers who remain inactive or unfit (Paffen-barger *et al.*, 1993; Blair *et al.*, 1995).

Cardiovascular disease

Physical inactivity is linked to increased risk of mortality and morbidity from coronary heart disease (CHD). A meta-analysis of the findings from studies of 27 cohorts showed that the protective effect probably lies in prevention of occurrence of major events, rather than in the reduction in the severity of events which do occur (Berlin & Colditz, 1990). The relationship between level of activity and CHD risk is strong. The relative risk of inactivity varies in different studies but the median value (based on a review of 43 mainly cohort studies) is about 1.9 for CHD event or CHD death, with methodologically superior studies tending to report higher values (Powell *et al.*, 1987). The relative risk associated with low (compared with high) fitness is somewhat higher (Blair *et al.*, 1996), possibly because measuring fitness reduces misclassification. Thus the magnitude of the increase in CHD risk associated with physical inactivity and low fitness is of the same order of magnitude as that conferred by smoking, hypertension and hypercholesterolaemia (Powell *et al.*, 1987).

The relationship between activity or fitness and CHD risk is dose-related (Morris *et al.*, 1990; Blair *et al.,* 1996), has been observed in populations worldwide (for review see Morris *et al.*, 1990), is independent of other major risk factors, including BMI (Figure 30) (Morris *et al.*, 1990; Haapanen *et al.*, 1997b) and is evident among women (Lemaitre *et al.*, 1995; Manson *et al.*, 1999; Haapanen-Niemi *et al.*, 2000) as well as men. Most information, however, relates to white Europeans and North Americans.

Everyday activities such as regular walking and cycling are associated with CHD risk. Among British civil servants, those who rated their regular walking as fast (over 6.4 km/h) or who did

Table 52. Prospective studies of total mortality in relation to physical activity or fitness in men

Reference	Population	Country	Measure of activity/ fitness	Analysis	Main findings	Notes
Sandvik et al. (1993)	1960 men aged 40–59 y, average follow-up 16 y	Norway	Fitness, measured as total work on a cycle ergometer during symptom-limited exercise tolerance test	Adjusted relative risk, highest vs lowest quartile	RR = 0.54 (0.32–0.89); $p = 0.015$ Mortality similar in fitness quartiles 1, 2 and 3	Data adjusted for many potential confounders. Fitness measured on cycle ergometer may not relate well to day-to-day activities where body weight is supported
Lee et al. (1995)	17 321 men, mean age 46 y, follow-up 22–26 y	USA (Harvard Alumni Study)	Physical activity by questionnaire	Relative risk for energy expended highest (≥ 6300 kJ/week) vs lowest (< 630 kJ/week) quintile	Total activity RR = 0.91 (0.82–1.0), p for trend < 0.05 Vigorous activity RR = 0.87 (0.78–0.97), p for trend = 0.007 Non-vigorous activity RR = 0.92 (0.82–1.0), p for trend = 0.36	Activity information very detailed. Analysis for different intensities mutually adjusted
Blair et al. (1996)	25 341 men, 7080 women, aged 20–88 y, average follow-up 8 y	USA	Fitness, time on maximal treadmill test, i.e., surrogate for maximal oxygen uptake	Adjusted relative risk, medium and highest vs lowest quintile	Men: RR = 0.66 (0.55–0.78) Women: RR = 0.48 (0.31–0.74)	Effects of fitness held independent of smoking, high cholesterol or high systolic blood pressure. Moderate and high fitness seemed to protect against influence of these other predictors
Kampert et al. (1996)	25 341 men, 7080 women aged 20–88 y, average follow-up ~ 8 y	USA	Fitness, time on maximal treadmill test, and physical activity by questionnaire	Trends across quintiles	Inverse association between level of physical fitness and mortality in men and women (p for for trend < 0.001) Inverse association between level of physical activity and mortality in men (p for trend 0.01), but not in women	Lack of relationship with physical activity in women may result from greater misclassification

Table 52 (contd)

Reference	Country	Population	Measure of activity/fitness	Analysis	Main findings	Notes
Hakim et al. (1998)	USA (Hawaii)	707 men aged 61–81 y, follow-up 12 y	Self-reported regular walking distance	Age-adjusted mortality rate	< 1.6 km/day = 40.5% > 3.2 km/day = 23.8% p for trend = 0.002	One of few studies specifically in elderly
Kujala et al. (1998)	Finland	7925 men 7977 women aged 25–64 y, follow-up 17 y	Physical activity by questionnaire	Adjusted relative risk, compared with sedentary (no leisure activity)	Occasional exercisers RR = 0.71 (0.62–0.81) Conditioning exercisers (at least vigorous walking > 6 times/month) RR = 0.57 (0.45–0.74) (p for trend < 0.001)	Twin study, examining potential modification of the effects of physical activity by genetic factors
Bijnen et al. (1999)	Netherlands	472 men, mean age 75 y, follow-up 5 y.	Physical activity by questionnaire	Adjusted relative risk, highest vs lowest tertile	RR = 0.44 (0.25–0.80); p for trend = 0.004 No association with intensity or type of exercise	Time in physical activity at baseline; low tertile 20 min/day; middle tertile 60 min/day; high tertile 150 min/day Activity at baseline not related to risk

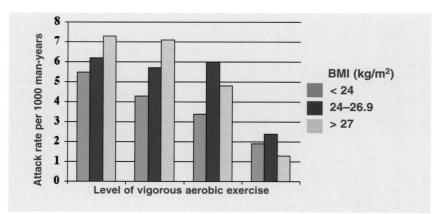

Figure 30   Rate of coronary heart disease attacks (1976–1986) in male executive-grade civil servants (rates per 1000 man-years) and levels of vigorous aerobic exercise, at different BMI (adapted from Morris *et al.*, 1990).

considerable amounts (≥ 40 km/week) of cycling experienced less than half the fatal and non-fatal CHD of the other men (Morris *et al.*, 1990). Among women who did not engage in vigorous exercise, those who walked the equivalent of three or more hours per week at a brisk pace had a multivariate relative risk of 0.65 (95 % CI 0.47–0.91) compared with those who walked infrequently (Manson *et al.*, 1999).

Evidence from cohort studies, with follow-up periods of between five and 26 years, shows a lower risk of stroke in physically active men and women, but data are less extensive and less consistent than for CHD. In the US Nurses' Health Study ($n \cong 72\,500$ women), there was an inverse gradient of risk with volume of activity assessed as MET × h per week (a measure of 'volume' of physical activity) (*p* for trend = 0.003) (Hu *et al.*, 2000): this was primarily due to the relation with ischaemic (thromboembolytic) stroke, women in the highest activity category exhibiting only half the risk of the least active. Among male Harvard alumni, total stroke incidence was inversely associated with energy expenditure in physical activity after adjustment for confounding factors but, as in some other studies, there was an

indication that this relationship might be U-shaped (Lee & Paffenbarger, 1998). All studies have related a single baseline measure of activity to incidence of stroke some or many years later. No studies of physical fitness are available.

Regular physical activity decreases the risk of developing hypertension. In a representative sample of the Finnish population, age-adjusted rates were 60–70% higher for sedentary men than for the most active men (estimated total energy expenditure) (Haapanen *et al.*, 1997b). Participation in vigorous sports was associated with a 35% lower risk among Harvard alumni, but chiefly among men who were overweight (Paffenbarger *et al.*, 1983). Information on women and on dose–response issues is lacking.

Intervention studies show that physical training decreases resting arterial blood pressure. A meta-analysis of more than 40 randomized, controlled trials found that decreases are greater in hypertensive subjects (defined as ≥ 140 mm Hg systolic or ≥ 90 mm Hg diastolic) (mean negative values 7.4/5.8 mm Hg) than in normotensives (mean value 2.6/1.8 mm Hg) (Fagard, 1999). These findings may in part reflect the acute effects of exercise, i.e., 'post-exercise

hypotension'. Blood pressure is reduced following a single session of exercise for up to 16 hours. In hypertensive men, mean arterial pressure was lowered by an average of 8 mm Hg for more than 12 hours after cycling for 30 minutes than on control days when only normal daily activities were performed (Pescatello *et al.*, 1991). This is a low-threshold phenomenon and has been noted after exercise at only 40% of maximal oxygen uptake. Like other acute effects, it may be enhanced in people who are regularly active at a high level because they generally expend more energy in a session (Haskell, 1994).

Type II diabetes

A relationship between risk of type II diabetes and physical activity level has been demonstrated in a number of prospective studies. Helmrich *et al.* (1991) assessed the physical activity levels of some 6000 male alumni of the University of Pennsylvania by questionnaire in 1962 and again in 1976. Age-adjusted incidence rates declined as energy expenditure in exercise increased. This relationship remained significant after adjustment for current BMI, history of hypertension and parental history of diabetes. Low physical fitness has also been associated with increased risk. Among American men who had attended a preventive medicine clinic, the least fit 20% had a 3.7-fold higher risk of becoming diabetic during a six-year follow-up than the most fit 40% (Wei *et al.*, 1999). In both these studies, the protective effect was strongest in men at high risk because of overweight, hypertension and a parental history of diabetes. It was evident for non-vigorous as well as vigorous exercise, when the total energy expended was high. Among women participating in the US Nurses' Health Study who did not report engaging in vigorous exercise (Hu *et al.*, 1999b), the risk of developing type II diabetes was inversely related to the volume of walking

(MET × h per week), even after adjustment for potential confounders (including BMI) (*p* for trend = 0.01). Faster usual walking pace was also independently associated with lower risk.

Hip fracture

Physical activity decreases the risk of hip fracture. Among 9516 healthy white women of average age 72 years, risk of hip fracture during a four-year follow-up was 30% lower in those who reported regularly walking for exercise than in those who did not walk regularly (Cummings *et al.*, 1995). Risk tended to decrease as the distance walked increased and the effect remained significant even after adjustment for physical frailty and the presence of other chronic diseases. In a case–control study, increased daily activity (including standing, walking, climbing stairs, carrying, housework and gardening) protected against fracture in elderly men and women (Cooper *et al.*, 1988). This effect was not greatly affected by controlling for BMI, smoking, alcohol consumption, history of stroke and use of corticosteroids.

Most hip fractures are precipitated by a fall and regular physical activity may decrease the risk of falling by improving balance and/or lower limb strength. In premenopausal women, a 1.5-year programme of high-impact exercise (three times per week) increased bone mineral density at the femoral neck, compared with the control group (Heinonen *et al.*, 1996); muscle power and dynamic balance were also improved. In another randomized controlled trial over one year (Nelson *et al.*, 1994), postmenopausal women (50–70 years) performed high-intensity strength exercises on two days per week. Not only was bone mineral density at the femoral neck and lumbar spine increased but muscle mass, muscle strength and dynamic balance were increased in exercisers and decreased in controls. A meta-analysis of data from seven randomized, controlled trials con-

cluded that exercise programmes alone appear to reduce the risk of falls by 10%; combining these programmes with balance training reduced the risk by a further 7% (Province *et al.*, 1995).

Other health outcomes

Several studies have found a lower incidence of gallbladder disease in physically active individuals. Among women in the US Nurses' Health Study, for example, physical activity was inversely associated with the risk of cholecystectomy (Leitzmann *et al.*, 1999). Compared with women in the lowest quintile of activity, women in the highest quintile had a multivariate relative risk of 0.69 (95% CI 0.61–0.78). Adjusting for BMI and weight change in the previous two years attenuated the association only slightly (multivariate relative risk 0.79). Not all studies have observed an association between physical activity level and gallbladder disease, however. After adjustment for potential confounders, no association was found among 16 785 men participating in the Harvard Alumni Study (Sahi *et al.*, 1998).

High levels of physical activity maintain functional capacities such as muscular strength, endurance and mobility (Figure 31). Among older persons, this improves measures of quality of life (King *et al.*, 2000), is associated with

a reduced likelihood of hospitalization for cardiovascular disease (LaCroix *et al.*, 1996) and helps maintain a capacity for independent living. Even the frail elderly can achieve important (>100%) gains in muscle strength through regular chair-based exercises (Fiatarone *et al.*, 1994). These gains were associated with significant increases in gait velocity and stair-climbing power.

Physical activity is related to psychological health. It is an effective treatment for mild-to-moderate depression and may reduce symptoms of anxiety (Martinsen & Stephens, 1994). Cross-sectional, population-based studies have shown significant positive associations between physical activity and general well-being and mood and negative associations with depression and anxiety (Stephens, 1988). Limited evidence from prospective studies supports these findings. For example, in a Canadian study with a seven-year follow-up of some 2500 people, baseline physical activity level was predictive of mental health at follow-up (Martinsen & Stephens, 1994). These analyses took into account age, sex, educational level, physical health and baseline psychological status and so constitute strong evidence that physical activity is predictive of future mental health. In one of a number of

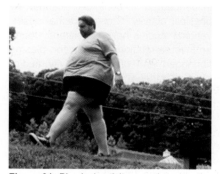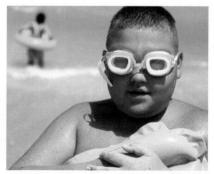

Figure 31 Physical activity may decrease the appetite, especially in obese individuals. Physical activity at a moderate rate does not increase the appetite. In some situations, the appetite will actually decrease. Research indicates that the decrease in appetite after physical activity is greater in individuals who are obese than in individuals who are at their desirable body weight.

randomized, controlled intervention trials, moderate-intensity training improved anxiety levels and perceived ability to cope with stress (Moses et al., 1989).

Effects on surrogate markers
Lipids

Regular physical activity leads to changes in blood lipids, particularly increases in HDL cholesterol and decreases in triglyceride levels. Cross-sectional comparisons of endurance athletes with sedentary men and women have typically found HDL cholesterol more than 20% higher in athletes (Durstine & Haskell, 1994). Differences have been related to distance run in both men and women, suggesting a dose-dependence. Among men, every 16-km increment in weekly distance run (up to 64 to 79 km/week) was associated with significant increases in HDL cholesterol (Williams, 1997). These findings may be confounded by genetic and/or other lifestyle characteristics, especially a lower total body and abdominal fat mass. Randomized intervention studies, mainly of moderate-intensity exercise (3–5 days per week, ≥ 30 minutes per session), have yielded less consistent results, from a decrease of 5.8% to an increase of about 25%, with a mean increase of 4.6%. Changes tend to be greater when weight loss accompanies training (Tran & Weltman, 1985). Other reasons for this variability probably include genetic predisposition, inadequate control of dietary habits (energy value and diet composition), blood volume changes, proximity of last exercise session and, in women, phase of the menstrual cycle.

Acute effects of exercise may contribute to the more favourable blood lipid characteristics of physically active people. One session of exercise markedly reduces both fasting and post-prandial triglyceride levels (Gill & Hardman, 2000), possibly by enhancing clearance of triglyceride-rich lipoproteins. This effect appears to depend on the energy expended in exercise, rather than on its intensity or pattern. Thirty minutes of brisk walking decreased day-long plasma triglyceride levels in sedentary men and women (compared with an inactive day), whether this was performed in one session before breakfast or in three 10-minute sessions (Murphy et al., 2000b). Faster clearance of triglycerides probably leads to higher HDL cholesterol.

Insulin sensitivity

The mechanisms underlying the enhanced insulin sensitivity in active people were discussed in Chapter 4. Insulin sensitivity appears to increase in relation to the volume of training undertaken (Mayer-Davis et al., 1998), but the benefit of exercise is lost within a few days when training is interrupted. For example, middle-aged men and women who were regularly active in moderate exercise showed a marked deterioration in their response to an oral glucose tolerance test after just three days without exercise (King et al., 1995). This suggests that the acute effects of exercise may account for some of the difference in insulin sensitivity in trained individuals.

Coagulation

Several aspects of haemostasis may be influenced in a beneficial manner by physical activity. Cross-sectional observational studies have consistently found an inverse relationship between plasma fibrinogen and physical activity and/or physical fitness. For example, in men from ten general practices in the United Kingdom, plasma fibrinogen decreased with the frequency of reported participation in vigorous exercise (Connelly et al., 1992). This epidemiological finding could partly explain the lower risk of CHD in active persons, but has not been reproduced consistently in randomized intervention trials. One reason may be that study designs have seldom taken proper account of the acute effects of the last exercise session.

People who are physically active do not experience the platelet activation and platelet hyperreactivity seen in sedentary individuals (Kestin et al., 1993). A possible reason is the less marked catecholamine response to exercise in habitually active people.

Flow-mediated dilatation

Physical activity may also influence the acute phase of cardiovascular disease by reducing endothelial dysfunction. Among asymptomatic men known to exhibit features of the metabolic syndrome, 12 weeks of training significantly increased flow-mediated dilatation measured at rest in the brachial artery (Lavrencic et al., 2000). In men with coronary artery disease, a brief (four-week) period of exercise training improved endothelium-dependent vasodilatation in both epicardial coronary vessels and in resistance vessels (Hambrecht et al., 2000). Both studies were randomized, controlled trials.

Bone mineral density

Physical activity may influence the risk of osteoporotic fracture through effects on bone mineral density, the microarchitecture of bone and/or the risk of falls. Bone mineral density at age 70 years is determined both by peak bone mass accumulated in youth and the subsequent rate of bone loss. Athletes, particularly those whose sports are associated with high impact, are consistently reported to have higher bone mineral density than sedentary counterparts (for review, see Suominen, 1993). This effect is a local response to local loading and may be most potent during growth. Bone mineral density in arm sites showed significantly greater side-to-side differences (higher in playing arms) in female tennis and squash players than in sedentary controls (Kannus et al., 1995). The difference was four to five times greater in those who started their playing careers before or at menarche than in those who started more than 15 years after menarche.

Prospective studies show that physical activity is a determinant of peak bone mass. In US college-aged women participating in recreational sports followed up for up to five years, physical activity was monitored at six-month intervals (Recker *et al.*, 1992). Level of activity was positively related to the rate of increase in spinal bone mineral density. Bone may be particularly sensitive to mechanical loading during the adolescent growth spurt (Haapasalo *et al.*, 1998).

Randomized intervention trials show that physical activity can be effective in maintaining bone mass in pre- menopausal women and substantially decreasing bone loss in postmenopausal women. The effect is small (typically about 1% per year) and seen in both the lumbar spine and femoral neck.

Chapter 7
Carcinogenicity

Human studies

As reviewed in Chapter 5, the associations between cancer risk and both overweight and physical activity suggest that weight control and physical activity generally offer benefits in terms of cancer risk rather than hazards.

The observational epidemiology of the relationship between BMI and cancer risk is sufficient to describe the possible adverse effects of lifetime weight control. Studying the consequences of intentional weight loss on cancer risk among persons who are overweight or obese has been more difficult because few people in the population have lost substantial amounts of weight and maintained that weight loss over time. The limited evidence available does not suggest an adverse effect of intentional weight loss on cancer risk, however. In addition, short-term studies of weight loss show that intermediate markers of cancer risk, such as estrogen levels, are affected in directions that would be likely to reduce long-term cancer risk.

Epidemiological studies that have examined long-term associations between changes in body weight in adulthood and overall mortality risk have not shown increased cancer risk from intentional weight loss (Williamson & Pamuk, 1993). Weight fluctuation resulting from repeated attempts to lose weight, a common finding among those who are overweight, is associated with increased risk for heart disease, stroke, diabetes and hip fracture, but has not been found to be consistently associated with increased risk of cancer (Lindblad et al., 1994; French et al., 1997).

For some cancer sites for which there is an inverse association between adiposity and cancer risk, factors such as alcohol, tobacco and/or pre-existing illness are likely to confound the associations. For example, overweight is associated with reduced risk for lung cancer and for cancers of the head and neck largely because those who abuse tobacco or alcohol are both less obese and at increased cancer risk due to their tobacco and alcohol habits. Reduced body weight can also be a sign of pre-existing cancer or of illnesses that increase cancer risk. Weight loss due to occult malignancies can be substantial for months or years before cancer diagnosis, and chronic conditions such as cirrhosis and chronic lung disease can lead to both chronic weight loss and increased risk for cancers at sites such as the lung, oral cavity and liver.

Among premenopausal women, there is an inverse association between BMI and breast cancer risk (see Chapter 5). The mechanisms responsible for this association are uncertain, but may well be related to the anovulation that accompanies excess weight. Reducing the prevalence of overweight among premenopausal women in the population by avoiding excess weight gain and/or by maintaining weight loss might improve the anovulation associated with overweight and thereby result in increased rates of premenopausal breast cancer.

The existing evidence on the relationship between physical activity and cancer risk shows either benefits or no association in nearly all studies. Evidence for an adverse effect of physical activity is seen rarely in epidemiological studies (for example, Mink et al., 1996).

Experimental models

While no evidence was available to the Working Group that either energy restriction or conditions of physical activity are capable of inducing cancer per se, conditions of restriction and exercise have been reported to increase the carcinogenic response in some defined model systems of chemical induction of cancer.

Weight control

Energy restriction, but not restriction of total diet, in the range of 10–40% of ad-libitum intake, when imposed chronically, is associated with inhibition of tumour development in most but not all experimental model systems in which it has been evaluated. On the other hand, there are several reports that when energy restriction was interrupted with periods of refeeding, loss of the protective effect against cancer and/or enhancement of tumour development occurred in model systems for breast, colon and liver cancer (Pollard et al., 1984; Lagopoulos et al., 1991; Mehta et al., 1993; Harris et al., 1995; Tagliaferro et al., 1996). Studies showing enhancement of tumours or of tumour markers are summarized in Table 53. Such experimental protocols have been referred to as energy cycling, patterned calorie restriction or cyclic food restriction, and such patterns of eating have parallels in human populations. In these studies, all of which involved the promotion phase of tumorigenesis, a variety of cyclic feeding patterns were investigated, but invariably

Table 53. Studies of increased mammary cancer and liver foci in cyclic-fed rodents

Organ site/ species/ strain (sex)	Age at beginning of study (wk)	No. of animals per group	Carcinogen exposure	Dietary restriction	Timing of restriction	Carcinogenic effect	Summarized effect	Reference
Mammary cancer								
Rat								
Sprague-Dawley (F)	3	50–56	25 mg/kg bw MNU at 50 days of age, i.p.	33% energy restricted	11 days following MNU, for 18 weeks AL control Meal-fed Meal-fed, cyclic restricted	Mammary cancer incidence: 54% 57% 63% ($p <$ 0.0001 vs AL)	Increased cancer incidence with meal-fed cyclic restricted	Tagliaferro et al. (1996)
Liver foci								
Mouse								
Swiss OF1 (M/F)	Weanling	16–18	0.5 µmol/g bw NDEA at wk 0, i.p.	Cereal-based diet, 30% diet restricted	Up to 36 weeks AL throughout DR throughout AL-24 wk/DR-12 wk DR-24 wk/AL-12 wk	No. of foci/group 338 115 175 173	DR throughout inhibited DR-24 wk/AL-12 wk increased compared with DR throughout	Lagopoulos et al. (1991)

MNU, *N*-methyl-*N*-nitrosourea; NDEA, *N*-nitrosodiethylamine; i.p., intraperitoneal; DR, dietary restriction; AL, *ad libitum*

led to loss of protective activity against cancer relative to that which was observed in chronically restricted controls. In other fields of inquiry, a similar pattern of energy cycling is referred to as weight cycling. Rodent models have been used to study the effects of weight cycling on propensity for obesity, development of insulin resistance, effects on diabetes and cardiovascular disease (Lu *et al.*, 1995; Lauer *et al.*, 1999; Sea *et al.*, 2000).

Physical activity

While physical activity protocols have resulted in inhibition of experimentally induced carcinogenesis, certain protocols have led to enhancement of the carcinogenic response (Table 54).

Thompson *et al.* (1988) investigated the effects of low-intensity, short-duration treadmill running on induction of mammary carcinogenesis. Female Sprague-Dawley rats were maintained on a 5% (w/w) corn oil diet (AIN-76A) from 21 to 64 days of age. At 50 days of age, they received either 5 mg 7,12-dimethyl-benz[*a*]anthracene (DMBA) or the vehicle. Fourteen days after DMBA intubation, they were randomized into three groups: 5% fat (w/w), sedentary; 24.6% fat (w/w), sedentary; or 24.6% fat (w/w), exercised on a motor-driven treadmill at a belt speed of 20 m/min and a 1° incline for 15 min per day on five days per week for 18 weeks (moderate exercise). Animals fed the high-fat diet had higher incidence and multiplicity of breast cancers than the low-fat group. Moderate treadmill exercise increased the inci-

dence and number of cancers and shortened latency in comparison with the sedentary high-fat and low-fat diet groups. Body composition was not altered by the exercise regime imposed, although the exercised animals weighed more than either sedentary group.

To control better for the non-training effects of treadmill running, Thompson *et al.* (1989b) fed female Sprague-Dawley rats a purified 5% fat diet (AIN-76A) from 21 to 64 days of age. At 50 days of age, they were administered 5 mg DMBA intragastrically. Fourteen days later, they were divided into three diet groups: 5% fat as corn oil, 24.6% fat as corn oil, or 24.6% fat as a mixture of palm (21.8%) and corn oil (2.8%). The combination of palm and corn oil provided the same amount of linoleic acid per gram as the 5% corn oil diet. Half of the animals receiving each diet were exercised on a treadmill at a speed of 20 m/min with a 1° incline for 15 min per day on five days per week, and were designated as the moderate-intensity treadmill exercise group. The remaining half were exercised at a speed of 2 m/min with a 1° incline for 15 min per day on five days per week, and were designated as a low-intensity sham control. The experiment was terminated 154 days after DMBA treatment. The median tumour-free time was significantly shortened by moderate-intensity exercise in rats receiving the 24.6% fat, corn oil-formulated diet in comparison with the sham-treated rats receiving the same diet (43 days versus 62 days, $p = 0.028$). Similarly, tumour appearance was more rapid in rats that

exercised at moderate intensity and consumed the low-fat corn oil diet than in the low-fat diet-fed sham-exercised group (57 days versus 67 days, $p = 0.046$). Exercise exerted no effect on the rate of tumour appearance in rats that received the 24.6% palm and corn oil mixture. Mean body weight gains were similar in all groups, although moderate-intensity exercised rats consistently weighed more than sham-exercised rats consuming the same diet. Gross carcass composition was unaffected by either the level of exercise or the amount of dietary fat consumed.

In another study, female Sprague-Dawley rats were subjected to an exercise protocol (treadmill 18 m/min at 15% incline for 60 min per day five times per week) from 21 to 50 days of age and given one injection of 37.5 mg/kg bw *N*-methyl-*N*-nitrosourea (MNU) at 50 days of age. At 22 weeks after MNU treatment, the tumour incidence, multiplicity and latency period were not different, but the growth rate of tumours in the exercise group was significantly greater than in the sedentary group (0.107 ± 0.025 versus 0.043 ± 0.009 g/day) and the final tumour weights were greater after exercise (3.2 ± 0.74 versus 1.2 ± 0.34 g) (Whittal-Strange *et al.*, 1998).

Using a different model system, Craven-Giles *et al.* (1994) investigated the modulation of pancreatic foci, an intermediate biomarker for pancreatic cancer, by treadmill running. As reported in Chapter 5, the burden of pancreatic foci was increased by treadmill running.

Table 54. Studies of increased carcinogen-induced tumours due to physical activity and exercise in experimental animals

Organ site/ species/strain (sex)	Age at beginning of study (wk)	Study type	No. per group	Carcinogen exposure/ diet	Type of exercise	Results	Reference
Mammary gland							
Rat							
Sprague-Dawley (F)	3	Post-initiation	28–35	5 mg DMBA at 50 days, p.o. 24.6% fat	Treadmill at 64 days for 18 weeks	Increase of tumour incidence	Thompson *et al.* (1988)
Sprague-Dawley (F)	3	Post-initiation	34–55	5 mg DMBA at 50 days, p.o. Corn oil 5% fat Corn oil 24.6% fat Corn/palm oil 24.6% fat	Treadmill at 64 days for 140 days High versus low High versus low High versus low	Decrease of latency Decrease of latency No effect	Thompson *et al.* (1989b)
Sprague-Dawley (F)	3	Pre-initiation	40	37.5 mg/kg bw MNU at 50 days, i.p., killed at 24 weeks	Treadmill from 21 to 50 days	Increase of tumour growth	Whittal-Strange *et al.* (1998)
Pancreas							
Rat							
Lewis (M)	2	Post-initiation	10–19	30 mg/kg azaserine at 14 days, i.p.	Treadmill from 13 to 31 weeks	Increase of acidophilic acinar cell foci	Craven-Giles *et al.* (1994)

Experiments in which decreased tumour incidence was observed are presented in Chapter 5.
DMBA, 7,12-dimethylbenz[a]anthracene; MNU, *N*-methyl-*N*-nitrosourea; i.p., intraperitoneal; p.o., orally

Chapter 8

Other adverse effects of weight control and physical activity

Health effects

Human studies

Weight control and weight loss

Data on effects of weight control in humans have been considered mainly in Chapter 6, in which risk modification due to BMI status and weight change was reviewed for all-cause mortality, other chronic diseases and surrogate markers. Keeping BMI within the normal range and weight stability over lifetime seem to constitute the optimal approach.

Adverse effects need to be considered in relation to various aspects of weight control, such as weight stability, small constant losses over time and heavy losses due to energy restriction. Not all of these aspects are relevant to each of the following sections. The induction of weight cycling deserves particular attention in connection with unsuccessful weight reduction. Long-term weight cycling has often been found to be associated with increased risk (Chapter 6). However, neither the reasons for increased risk in connection with weight cycling in the observational setting nor the underlying biological mechanisms are well understood.

Osteoporosis and fractures

Many studies have examined relationships of BMI or other measures of fatness in adult life to bone mineral density (Holbrook & Barrett-Connor, 1993; Mussolino et al., 1998; Kroke et al., 2000) and subsequent risk of fractures (Meyer et al., 1995; Ensrud et al., 1997a; Joakimsen et al., 1998; Owusu et al., 1998; Kato et al., 2000; Margolis et al.,

2000). Increased BMI has usually been found to be associated with improved bone mineral density and decreased risk of fracture. Of particular interest are studies that looked at the effect of weight change in adult life on risk of osteoporosis and fractures. Most of these found that weight gain is associated with a decreased risk of hip fracture (Grisso et al., 1994; Cummings et al., 1995; Meyer et al., 1995; Langlois et al., 1996; Ensrud et al., 1997b; French et al., 1997; Joakimsen et al., 1998; Langlois et al., 1998; Meyer et al., 1998) and that weight loss increases risk for hip fracture. However, further evaluation is needed of whether the increased fracture risk affects all bone sites similarly, whether mild weight losses and intentional weight reduction are associated with a substantial risk for fracture and whether exercise-induced weight reduction has effects different from those achieved by dietary weight reduction. For example, Ensrud et al. (1997b) found in a cohort study of 6754 non-black women that weight loss of more than 10% in the preceding six years induced higher risk of frailty fractures such as those of the proximal femur, pelvis and proximal humerus among thin women and those with unintentional weight loss. Intentional loss and mild losses were not linked with higher fracture risk in this study. However, intervention studies for weight reduction with middle-aged and older women have also showed a decrease in bone mineral density (Compston et al., 1992; Jensen et al., 1994; Chao et al., 2000). In connection with weight reduc-

tion, the beneficial effect of exercise as a means to reduce weight also needs to be taken into account.

Weight cycling is also linked to increased risk for hip fracture (Meyer et al., 1998: RR = 2.1 (95% CI 1.2–3.5) in Norwegian women and 2.7 (95% CI 1.2–5.9) in men; French et al., 1997: 1.6 (95% CI 0.96–2.8) in Iowa women). This observation from prospective cohort studies is supported by results of a cross-sectional survey of 169 pre-menopausal women in Finland (Fogelholm et al., 1997), which indicated that lower bone mineral density after weight cycling significantly affects the lumbar spine and distal radius (data adjusted for weight and age at menarche). Other bones such as the femoral neck and trochanter were not significantly affected in this study. These observations are consistent with those from another cross-sectional study on 1043 older white men and women, with particular emphasis on site-specific effects (Holbrook & Barrett-Connor, 1993). There is currently no plausible biological explanation for the lowering effect of weight cycling on weight-adjusted bone mineral density. This association contrasts with the fact that weight cycling is often linked with subsequent increase in weight, a well established protective factor.

Eating disorders

Epidemiological studies of anorexia nervosa, bulimia nervosa, binge-eating disorder and other eating disorders in different populations are hampered by inadequate reporting and case definition. Anorexia nervosa seems to affect 0.5% of young women and bulimia nervosa 2% in western societies (Hsu, 1996). The male-to-female ratio of anorexia nervosa is one to ten. Although anorexia and bulimia nervosa are still uncommon disorders, they are among the most common psychiatric disorders affecting young women in developed countries. In these societies, a preoccupation with thinness and sociocultural pressures to diet have often been regarded as playing an etiological role in the pathogenesis of anorexia nervosa (Hsu, 1997). However, even in developing countries where obesity is socially acceptable, the prevalence of anorexia nervosa has been reported to be within the range seen in western countries (Hoek et al., 1998). Severe dieting in adolescents is a predictor of anorexia nervosa and should be discouraged (Patton et al., 1999). There are no indications that recommendations to maintain BMI within the range of 18.5 and 25 kg/m^2 and moderate and gradual weight gain in adults who are already overweight induce the onset of eating disorders.

Sarcopenia

In the context of weight control and particular weight-reduction programmes addressed to the general population, the effect of age on body composition needs to be considered. The ratio of body fat mass to lean body mass gradually changes with age and fat is redistributed towards the abdominal cavity (Seidell & Visscher, 2000). At older ages, weight loss often particularly involves lean body mass, so that the percentage of fat increases (Poehlmann et al., 1995). While the reason for such changes is poorly understood, nutritional inadequacy and sarcopenia (loss of muscle) are clearly a problem in the oldest age groups (Baumgartner, 2000). Older adults with inadequate energy intake are more likely to develop acute illness and chronic disease (Mowe et al., 1994;

Naber et al., 1997). There is also evidence that unintentional weight loss in elderly subjects is often caused by acute or chronic diseases (Fischer & Johnson, 1990). It is not known whether such changes of body composition with age may be responsible for the finding in some prospective observational studies, often comprising older age groups, that weight loss was associated with increased all-cause mortality and disease risk.

Gallstones

Obesity is a risk factor for gallstones in women (less so in men) and this risk increases with weight loss and weight cycling. It is unclear what mechanisms in gallstone formation are responsible for the increased risk associated with weight changes; the fat and total energy contents of a weight-loss diet seem to have an important role. In the Nurses' Health Study I (Syngal et al., 1999) including 47 153 women, the relative risk for cholecystectomy was 1.2 (95% CI 0.96–1.5) among light weight cyclers (5–9 lb [2.3–4.1 kg] weight loss and gain within a 16-year period), 1.3 (95% CI 1.0–1.6) among moderate cyclers (10–19 lb [4.5–8.6 kg] weight gain and loss) and 1.7 (95% CI 1.3–2.1) among severe cyclers (≥20 lb [9.1 kg] weight loss and gain). Weight gainers had an increased risk for cholecystectomy (RR = 1.1; 95% CI 0.92–1.4), as did weight losers (RR = 1.6; 95% CI 1.2–2.1), compared with weight maintainers (who comprised only 11% of the population). Several clinical studies of obese individuals who achieved rapid weight loss with very low-energy diets have shown that up to one fourth of weight losers develop new gallstones after beginning a supervised very low-energy diet (Everhart, 1993). A third of these were symptomatic. In about half of the asymptomatic individuals, gallstones spontaneously disappeared within 1–2 years. The main risk factors for gallstone development were high BMI and high rate of weight

loss (caused by a very low-energy diet). One study compared two different very low-energy diets (with 3.0 g and 12.2 g of fat/day) and reported that new (asymptomatic) gallstones developed in 55% of subjects following the lower-fat diet, but in none with the higher-fat diet (Festi et al., 1998). Relatively high fat content of very low-energy diets may prevent gallstone formation by maintaining adequate gallbladder emptying, which counterbalances possible lithogenic mechanisms during weight loss.

Nutritional deficiencies

Dietary changes to lose weight can be associated with nutrient deficiencies. Elderly persons are particularly vulnerable to this (Mowe et al., 1994; Naber et al., 1997). Older versions of very low-energy diets have resulted in extreme malnutrition with some deaths reported. Modern very low-energy diets include sufficient amounts of nutrients during weight reduction under supervised conditions.

Drug treatment of obesity

Some drugs can help to promote weight loss and prevent weight regain in obese patients The most frequent adverse effects of orlistat are gastrointestinal (for example, oily stools, faecal urgency and faecal spotting) (Sjöström et al., 1998). These side-effects usually appear early during treatment and are mild and transient. Consumption of a diet rich in fat markedly increases the risk of these side-effects. Mean plasma levels of vitamins A, D, E and K and β-carotene are reduced, but remain within the reference range during prolonged orlistat treatment. Sibutramine may increase heart rate and blood pressure. Other common adverse effects are dry mouth, nausea and insomnia (Lean, 1997; James et al., 2000). Fenfluramine and dexfenfluramine have been reported to be associated with heart valve abnormalities, and these drugs were withdrawn from the market in 1997. One post hoc study suggests that prior use of dexfenfluramine or phentermine/fenfluramine may be associated with higher prevalence of aortic regurgitation compared with untreated matched controls (Gardin *et al.*, 2000).

Weight loss and cigarette smoking

The weight loss that is often associated with cigarette smoking is accompanied by increased risk for all of the many tobacco-related diseases including cardiovascular disease and cancer, although this cannot be regarded as an adverse effect of weight loss per se.

Conclusion

Weight loss can have adverse effects on bone that may be counteracted by increased physical activity. Other adverse effects of weight loss include eating disorders, loss of muscle mass (if physical activity is not sufficient), nutritional deficiencies and gallstones. For the few individuals for whom drug therapy is indicated, there are adverse effects that range from mild to severe or even life-threatening.

Physical activity

Ordinary physical activities, for example walking for personal transportation or climbing stairs, are seldom associated with adverse effects (at least in persons of 'healthy', 'normal' or 'acceptable' weight) (Figure 32). Adverse effects are mainly incurred during participation in structured exercise to improve fitness or through sports participation.

Cardiovascular risks

Although the absolute level of risk is small (for example, one sudden death per 1.5 million episodes of vigorous exercise in the US Physicians' Health Study (Albert *et al.*, 2000)), the risk of heart attack or sudden cardiac death is increased during exercise. Specifically, the risk during vigorous exercise (≥ 6 METs) (or up to one hour after it) is between two times greater (Willich *et al.*,

1993) and six times greater (Mittleman *et al.*, 1993) than during less strenuous activities or no activity. In these studies, both with around 1200 subjects, of whom some 70% were men, the excess risk was, however, mostly limited to persons who did not exercise regularly. Among those who exercised at least four or five times per week, there was little or no excess risk during exercise, compared with all other times. As reviewed in Chapter 6, however, the protective effect of regular exercise is very strong and appears to outweigh the transient increase during vigorous exercise.

Exercise, even strenuous exercise, is not harmful to the healthy cardiovascular system. Studies of young persons (< 30 years) dying during exercise have invariably found structural, usually congenital, cardiovascular disease (Maron *et al.*, 1996). Among older persons, severe atherosclerotic coronary artery disease is found in the majority of cases of exercise-related sudden death (Waller & Roberts, 1980). The increases in heart rate and blood pressure during exercise may give rise to haemodynamic shear stresses that disrupt a vulnerable plaque, setting in motion a chain of events (including platelet activation) culminating in acute infarction. An important factor may be the intensity of exercise, because moderate levels do not increase platelet adhesion and coagulability (Wang *et al.*, 1994; Weiss *et al.*, 1998). To minimize the risks of acute exercise, sedentary people should progress gradually from light to moderate exercise and avoid sudden, unaccustomed heavy exertion (US Department of Health and Human Services, 1996).

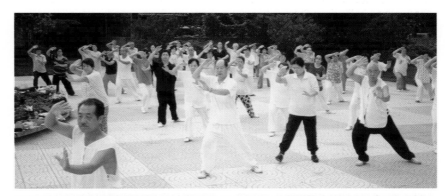

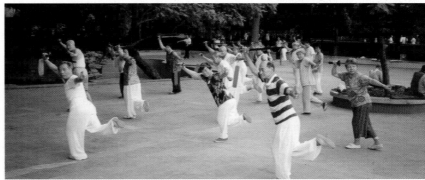

Figure 32 Older adults can benefit from regular physical activity, which needs not to be strenuous to achieve health benefits

Injuries

Injuries associated with exercise fall into two categories, overuse and acute traumatic. Incidence rates for acute sport and exercise-related injuries are probably rather low in the general population. For example, about 5% of adults who participated in a telephone survey reported an injury in the previous month (Uitenbroek, 1996). Rates are higher, of course, among sportsmen and women. For example, about half of 1391 surveyed participants in sports (Australian football, field hockey, basketball, netball) reported sustaining one or more injuries over a five-month winter season (Stevenson et al., 2000). At Groningen University Hospital in the Netherlands, sports injuries comprised about one fifth of all injuries treated over a seven-year period, making these the second highest cause of accidental injuries after home and leisure accidents (Dekker et al., 2000).

The majority of sports injuries are of low severity (Stevenson et al., 2000), but a minority (9% in the Groningen study (Dekker et al., 2000)) require hospitalization. Injuries are mainly musculoskeletal, the majority to the lower limb (e.g., ligament sprains, meniscus tear) (Baquie & Brukner, 1997), but cervical spinal injuries are occasionally incurred in sports such as rugby, trampolining, gymnastics and horse-riding (Silver, 1993). Two out of three sports injuries occur during team sports (Ytterstad, 1996), with soccer/football giving rise to a high number of injuries, even when corrected for exposure (Ytterstad, 1996; Stevenson et al., 2000).

Injuries to a lower limb are common in runners. Based on a review of 10 surveys, between 24% and 65% of runners sustained one or more injuries during a year (Hoeberigs, 1992). Fifty to 75% of injuries appear to be due to overuse, i.e., constant repetition of the same movement (van Mechelen, 1992). Weekly distance run is the most important determinant of these injuries, for women as well as for men (Hoeberigs, 1992). Other predisposing factors are probably high intensity, a rapid increase in training distance or intensity (impact forces increase with running speed), running on hard surfaces and in poor shoes. In beginners, the frequency of injuries increases when the duration of running sessions exceeds 30 minutes (Colbert et al., 2000b). Impact forces are much lower during walking, so the risk of injury is lower for walking than running (Colbert et al., 2000b). Even among older persons, walking for exercise carries a low risk for injury; among 21 men and women aged 70–79 years walking briskly for three sessions per week, increasing to 45 min per session, only one injury was sustained over 13 weeks (4.8%) (Pollock et al., 1991).

Bicycling (including on-road and off-road cycling) is associated with significant morbidity and mortality. Head injuries account for three quarters of deaths related to bicycling (Rivara et al., 1997a). Injuries during swimming – another common aerobic activity – are few, but deaths do occur from drowning in swimming pools, mainly among young children (Rivara et al., 1997b).

There is considerable inter-individual variation in predisposition to exercise-related illnesses such as hypothermia or hyperthermia and these may be exacerbated by environmental conditions, according to the fitness level of the individual. For example, slow runners and swimmers may experience net heat loss in conditions where those who can achieve a faster pace maintain thermal balance. Increased ventilation of the lungs during exercise increases the risk of exposure to environmental pollutants and can trigger environmentally-induced asthma (Utell & Looney, 1995). Exercise in a cold environment, particularly running, can also provoke asthma in susceptible individuals (Giesbrecht, 1995).

Osteoarthritis

The risk of articular surface damage or degeneration associated with repetitive stresses during exercise depends largely on the rate of loading and the number of loading cycles. The prevalence of osteoarthritis is increased among athletes in a number of sports disciplines, mainly those involving high loading (most ball games and competitive running) (Buckwalter & Lane, 1997). Performing more than three to four hours per day of heavy physical activity significantly increases the risk of developing osteoarthritis of the knee and running at least 20 miles per week increases the risk of osteoarthritis of the hip or knee (Vuori, 2001). Moderate levels of physical activity have not been found to be associated with risk.

Prior sports-related injuries may predispose to osteoarthritis. One study of 1321 former medical students with 36-year follow-up found that the risks of developing osteoarthritis of the knee or hip were > 5-fold and 3.5-fold higher in those reporting injury on the corresponding joint at entry or during follow-up, compared with those not reporting injury (Gelber et al., 2000).

Athletic amenorrhoea and low bone mineral density

Menstrual dysfunction can be induced by strenuous aerobic exercise, particularly in individuals with low levels of body fatness who undergo a rather sudden increase in training load. There is no evidence to suggest adverse effects on fertility in the long term.

However, young women with athletic amenorrhoea have been reported to have lower vertebral bone mineral density than their normally-menstruating peers (Cann et al., 1984). It was subsequently reported that this effect is not limited to the vertebra, but is evident at many skeletal sites (Rencken et al., 1996). Cross-sectional studies suggest an inverse relationship between lumbar spine mineral density and the degree of menstrual disorder (Drinkwater et al., 1990). As 64% of 97 young female athletes studied experienced one or more episodes of amenorrhoea lasting for more than six months (Drinkwater et al., 1990), many individuals may be at increased risk for running-related stress fractures and subsequent osteoporosis.

It is not known whether vertebral bone loss is reversible. Vertebral bone mineral density has been observed to remain low in formerly oligo/amenorrhoeic athletes despite several years of normal menses or use of oral contraceptives (Keen & Drinkwater, 1997). Amenorrhoeic athletes exhibit higher bone mineral density than anorexics, however (Marcus et al., 1985), presumably because the osteogenic effect of the exercise offsets the adverse effects of low estrogen levels.

Upper respiratory tract infection

Unusually high incidence rates for upper respiratory tract infections have been reported among individuals participating in large volumes of vigorous exercise (Nieman, 1994), as reviewed in Chapter 4.

Experimental studies
Weight control

In general, overnutrition resulting in obesity and undernutrition resulting in malnutrition are associated with increased morbidity and mortality. However, some investigators have coined the phrase 'undernutrition without malnutrition' to describe a degree of energy restriction associated with health benefits, including a reduction in the risk for cancer.

While such an eating pattern has many potential health benefits, there are some possible drawbacks, such as the potential toxicity of glucocorticoids that are elevated with underfeeding and with administered micronutrient intake in dietary restriction protocols that reduce intake of all constituents.

Several studies have suggested that elevated glucocorticoid hormone levels in underfed rodents may contribute to the effect of underfeeding on cancer prevention (see Chapter 5). Elevated levels of primary glucocorticoid hormones in mice (Yaktine et al., 1998), rats (Morimoto et al., 1977) and humans (Chiappelli et al., 1991; Kennedy et al., 1991) have been reported and many studies have suggested that glucocorticoid hormones may have cancer-preventive potential. However, they also have well known toxic effects, including reduced bone mineral content (Weiler et al., 1995) and blockage of cell cycle (Rhee et al., 1995). The blockage of cell cycle may be beneficial in relation to the prevention of cancer, but cell cycle blockage of normal cells could be detrimental.

Other effects of dietary restriction with uncertain health impacts include smaller heart, (Oscai & Holloszy, 1970), bradycardia, decreased rate of cardiac contraction and relaxation (Hilderman et al., 1996) and impaired cold thermoregulation (Banu et al., 1999). Dietary restriction can also lead to reduced cortical bone mass and mineralization (Banu et al., 1999).

Reducing food intake has the potential to reduce consumption of health-promoting dietary constituents. Evidence that diet restriction by reducing all dietary components may not optimize cancer prevention, reported by Birt et al. (1991), is presented in Chapter 5.

Physical activity

Studies in humans have indicated various potential adverse effects of excessive exercise training programmes, as reviewed above, but none of these effects have been studied in animal models under conditions of exercise that have been shown to prevent the development of cancer in an experimental tumour model system. [The Working Group noted that the available data from experimental studies do not permit generalizable conclusions about conditions of exercise (duration, intensity, and frequency) that are clearly protective against cancer in most model systems used to study the genesis of cancer and its prevention.]

Reproductive and developmental effects
Human studies

Excessive leanness (as indicated by a very low BMI, i.e., below 18.5 kg/m^2) and large weight loss have been associated with increased likelihood of anovulatory menstrual cycles or a shortened luteal phase. Women with very low or high BMI have been found to have reduced conception rates under controlled circumstances (Zaadstra et al., 1993). These disruptions are due to hypothalamic dysfunction. Frisch (1987) proposed that a minimum ratio of fat to lean mass is normally necessary for menarche, fitness and fertility. Weight gain usually restores fertility in underweight women.

Weight

Severe weight loss can result in functional hypogonadotropic hypogonadism, which plays a major part in the amenorrhoea that is characteristic of anorexia nervosa. The plasma levels of follicle-stimulating hormone, luteinizing hormone (LH), estradiol and urinary gonadotropins are low, as is the plasma level of leptin. Adult women can develop pubertal and even pre-pubertal patterns of LH secretion (Marshall & Kelch, 1979). In addition, the gonadal response to gonadotropin-releasing hormone (GnRH) is a function of body-weight loss (Beumont et al., 1976). In men with anorexia nervosa, LH and testosterone levels are low and can be in the pre-pubertal range. Fasting reduces LH pulse amplitude (Veldhuis et al., 1993) and increases response to exogenous GnRH. This may indicate a decrease in this pituitary hormone (Rojdmark, 1987).

Physical activity

Amenorrhoea in marathon runners and delayed menarche in ballet dancers, figure skaters and gymnasts have been reported (Constantini & Warren, 1994). When the activity is interrupted (e.g., by an injury), menarche may occur even before body composition changes significantly (Warren, 1990).

Heavy training before puberty can lead to blunted growth velocity and stunted leg length growth, suggesting that it can decrease ultimate height (Lindholm *et al.*, 1994). Although in the general population scoliosis is associated with earlier menarche, in a study of ballet dancers, there were both delayed puberty and scoliosis (Goldberg *et al.*, 1993).

Experimental studies
Weight

The effect of dietary restriction in blocking the ability of female mice to breed has long been known (Nelson *et al.*, 1982). The major effect is on GnRH, with attendant decreases in circulating levels of LH and estrogen. When body weight in mice was lowered by 10–30% compared with controls, there was a decrease in numbers of pups per male and of implants per female in a dose-related manner (Chapin *et al.*, 1993). Female Sprague-Dawley rats had a 20% decrease in the number of corpora lutea at 30% dietary restriction and had lower ovarian weight. The percentage of motile sperm in males was decreased by dietary restriction of approximately 10%.

Physical activity (exercise)

Given the level of interest in the effects of exercise on reproductive end-points in humans, surprisingly little work has been done in animal models.

Moderate exercise reduced ovarian steroid levels and disrupted vaginal cycles in rats (Axelson, 1987). Also in rats, plasma testosterone levels were reduced by exhausting acute exercise,

with little change in LH. In chronic treadmill training, there were inconsistent effects on testosterone levels, but the capacity of interstitial cell suspensions *in vitro* to produce testosterone after stimulation by gonadotropin increased by 20% (Harkonen *et al.*, 1990).

Genetic effects

There have been no studies on induction of heritable damage by dietary restriction or weight loss. A few studies have examined the reduction of DNA damage resulting from dietary restriction. However, if there is an increase in formation of oxidative radicals, it may be presumed that this will lead to increased potential to attack the genome (Marnett, 2000).

Human studies

Treadmill exercise to exhaustion increased measurable DNA damage in human lymphocytes (Hartmann *et al.*, 1994).

Experimental studies
Weight

A few studies have indicated that either dietary or energy restriction decreases the amount of oxidative damage products in organs such as the liver or heart of rodents (see the discussion of mechanisms in Chapter 5). This effect appears to be reversible with feeding *ad libitum* (Forster *et al.*, 2000). Additionally, long-term dietary restriction appears to lead to lower levels of oxidative products in muscle in old monkeys (Zainal *et al.*, 2000).

However, little is known on the total amount of damage in diet-restricted animals. Taylor *et al.* (1995) found significantly increased levels of oxidative damage (8-hydroxydeoxyguanosine and 8-hydroxyguanine) in the urine of diet-restricted mice compared with mice fed *ad libitum*. There is evidence that enzymes which protect against free radical damage, such as superoxide dismutase, glutathione peroxidase, catalase

and haem oxygenase are induced and the activities of these enzymes appear to increase (Feuers *et al.*, 1995; Taylor *et al.*, 1995; and Chapter 5). Inducible DNA repair is also elevated in rodents (see Chapter 5). Some endogenous factors, such as increased oxidative damage, are possibly inducing these enzymes.

Studies of spontaneous mutation rates in transgenic mice (presumably driven by oxidative processes) showed little change due to dietary restriction (Stuart *et al.*, 2000). However mutation rate is a result of both genetic damage and the fixation of that damage through replication and 40% dietary restriction (with supplementation) significantly inhibits cellular replication (Lu *et al.*, 1993). Diet-restricted animals increase their level of activity by more than 50% around feeding time (Duffy *et al.*, 1989, 1990a, b). This increased activity (see below) may be important in the generation of increased oxidative damage.

Physical activity

Exercise results in increased oxygen utilization and it is not unexpected that it also leads to increased oxygen-related damage, especially in the mitochondria (Radak *et al.*, 2000).

With forced training, elevated mitochondrial reactive species (i.e., oxidative damage) and increased lipid peroxidation were found in rat muscle (Bejma & Ji, 1999), consistent with the elevated glutathione levels found earlier (Kim *et al.*, 1996). Increased carbonyl derivatives were found in rat mitochondria, compared with cytosol, after swimming (Radak *et al.*, 2000).

Since muscle is considered non-replicative, a focus on muscle provides little information on heritable effects. However, with increased metabolism and oxidation throughout the body, the effects of oxygen-related damage on tissues that replicate remain an open question.

Chapter 9
Summary of data

Characteristics, occurrence, trends and analysis of weight and physical activity

The prevalence of overweight (body mass index (BMI) between 25 and 30 kg/m^2) and obesity (BMI of 30 kg/m^2 or higher) is increasing rapidly worldwide. In many countries overweight and obesity co-exist with undernutrition. The increase in prevalence is especially rapid in developing countries undergoing an economic transition to a market economy. Obesity is largely preventable through changes in lifestyle. The fundamental causes of the obesity epidemic are societal, resulting from an environment that promotes sedentary lifestyles and over-consumption of energy.

These changes in lifestyle and the resulting positive energy balance leading to weight gain and increased rates of obesity are all implicated in the changing patterns of morbidity, that usually start with a rapid increase in diseases such as type II diabetes mellitus and cardiovascular diseases, followed later by an increase in rates of various types of cancer such as cancer of the breast and colon.

The BMI provides the most widely accepted measure of the degree of overweight and obesity. It can be used to estimate the prevalence of obesity within a population and to estimate the health risks associated with it. However, the BMI may represent different levels of fatness and body fat distribution depending on age, sex and ethnicity.

Accumulation of body fat in the abdominal area (abdominal fat distribution) represents a particular risk for many of the metabolic consequences of obesity. Therefore, measurement of the waist circumference provides a simple and practical method, in addition to BMI, to identify individuals and populations at risk for obesity-associated illness.

The classification of overweight and obesity by BMI categories is complicated in children and adolescents by rapid changes of height and weight during growth. There is an emerging consensus on how to use BMI in children and adolescents, but there is still little comparable information on prevalence. Despite the methodological problems, the available cross-sectional and longitudinal data suggest that the prevalence of overweight and obesity are also rapidly increasing in these age-groups all over the world.

There are many ways to assess physical activity, ranging from precise techniques such as calorimetry and direct observation, to electronic monitoring devices. However, usually only job classification has been used to describe physical activity behaviours in large, representative populations. Job classifications of employed adults, however, are of limited value when misclassification is known to exist, or in populations where work-related energy expenditure is not very prevalent, as in developed countries. Recall surveys for occupational, leisure-time and household activity have been devised with a variety of time-frames from one week to a lifetime. Such surveys range in complexity from global attributions of activity and other single-item reports of general activity participation, to detailed quantitative histories.

Elucidation of the associations of physical activity with disease risk and with weight control depends crucially on having reliable valid measures of the major types of physical activity in its various contexts. It is known that strenuous physical activity is recalled with greater accuracy than light or moderate activity, while recall of recent activities is more accurate than that of activities at an earlier point in time.

Data on the prevalence and time-trends in physical activity patterns and sedentary behaviour are available mainly from affluent industrialized societies. These data focus mainly on participation in leisure-time physical activity. For the vast majority of countries worldwide, notably most developing nations, population data on physical activity participation are unavailable. In these countries, economic transition involves large numbers of people moving away from traditionally active rural lifestyles to cities and other urban environments. In such settings, they are likely to be much less physically active. Such changes in physical activity are affecting an increasing proportion of the world's population.

Intervention trials aimed at promoting weight reduction or physical activity have so far yielded disappointing results in terms of long-term changes, probably because of the complex range of social and behavioural factors that interact in determining the relevant habits. However, it is generally agreed that prevention of overweight and obesity and promotion of physical activity should receive high priority in the public health area. Prevention of overweight and obesity and promotion of physical activity should begin early in life and require individual action and responsibility, but also structural changes in the physical, economic, political and socioeconomic environments.

At present, our limited understanding of variation in susceptibility to obesity is a powerful justification for the development of strategies which are population-based rather than selectively targeted at high-risk individuals.

Metabolic consequences of overweight and physical activity

Human studies

Weight reduction and physical activity have strong and independent effects on various metabolic factors related to cancer risk. These effects vary somewhat by age, gender and menopausal status. Furthermore, physical activity has effects that are unrelated to those of body weight. Most studies have been conducted in Caucasian persons residing in western countries.

BMI

BMI is positively associated with insulin and inversely with IGFBP-1 and IGFBP-2 levels, in men and in both pre- and postmenopausal women. However, a BMI above 30 kg/m^2 ("obesity") is associated with a mild decrease in absolute IGF-I concentrations, compared with normally nourished but non-obese subjects. BMI is positively related to plasma-free IGF-I, unbound to any IGF-binding protein.

In both men and women, BMI is inversely related to plasma levels of sex-hormone-binding globulin (SHBG). However, the relationships of BMI to total and bioavailable androgens and estrogens depend on gender and menopausal status. In men and postmenopausal women, BMI correlates directly with estrone and with total and bioavailable estradiol levels. In premenopausal women, it is also related to higher estrone concentrations, but not to total or bioavailable estradiol levels. In men, increasing BMI is associated with decreased levels of total plasma testosterone, and a BMI above 30 kg/m^2 is also

associated with a decrease in bioavailable testosterone, unbound to SHBG. In women, BMI shows no clear association with plasma total testosterone, except in women with polycystic ovary syndrome (PCOS), in whom obesity increases total plasma androgen levels. However, BMI is positively associated with free testosterone concentrations in both pre- and postmenopausal women.

Weight reduction

Weight reduction in overweight and obese men and women has consistently been shown to lead to reduced insulin and glucose levels and to improve insulin sensitivity; it is accompanied by a rise in SHBG levels. Such findings were observed in both men and women and whatever method was used to reduce weight (low-energy or very low-energy diets, other changes in dietary composition, exercise, drugs or by-pass surgery). In obese women with PCOS, weight loss is usually associated with reduced plasma concentrations of total and bioavailable androgens (androstenedione, testosterone) as well as estrone. However, inconsistent effects on androgens and estrogens have been observed

with weight reduction in normo-androgenic premenopausal women.

Physical activity

Most studies on the effects of physical activity on hormone concentrations have addressed the short-term consequences (0–2 hours after exercise). Strenuous aerobic exercise acutely decreases plasma insulin and increases serum SHBG and total and free testosterone concentrations. In the longer term, an increase in physical activity lowers fasting plasma insulin concentration and improves insulin sensitivity, but long-term effects on SHBG and total or bioavailable sex steroids are less clear. Exercise acutely increases absolute concentrations of IGF-I and IGFBP-1, while the longer-term effects of increased regular exercise are unclear.

Experimental models

Physiological, metabolic and hormonal changes occur in experimental systems when energy balance is modulated either by altering energy intake using dietary approaches or by increasing energy expenditure through modulation of physical activity.

Metabolic syndrome – important to act on !

'Metabolic syndrome' occurs commonly in middle-aged men. It is variously defined as a combination of elevated blood glucose, elevated triglycerides, low levels of HDL cholesterol, systolic or diastolic hypertension, and obesity. Other characteristics included in the definition are central obesity (waist circumference or waist hip circumference ratio) and elevated levels of insulin (hyperinsulinaemia).

This 'metabolic syndrome' is important, as this clustering of risk factors is associated with increased risk of the development of coronary heart disease, type II diabetes and certain types of cancer. The favourable trends in the reduction in the rate of heart attack and stroke over the past 30 years in western countries may ultimately be reversed as the consequences of the increase in diabetes and obesity become manifest in middle-aged and older adults.

Weight control

Physiological changes associated with lowering dietary intake include a lower body weight with lower adiposity or fat mass, extended mean and maximal life-span, increased water consumption, decreased urinary output, decreased average body temperature, improved tolerance of high temperatures, decreased ability to withstand cold, decreased blood pressure with brady-cardia and delayed puberty. Metabolic effects include lower activity of the enzymes involved in glycolysis, an increase in enzymes involved in gluconeogenesis and changes in fatty acid metabolism. Endocrine effects include reduced levels of growth hormone, prolactin and sex-steroids, inhibition of sex-specific cytochrome P450s and elevated levels of gluco-corticoids.

Physical activity

Physiological changes accompanying increased physical activity include loss of body weight and adiposity, reduced blood pressure, a relative increase in heart size as body weight decreases and delayed puberty.

Metabolic effects include inhibition of glycolysis in trained animals, and increased plasma levels of fatty acids and protein. Endocrine effects include alterations in growth hormone dependent on type of activity, acute increases in catecholamines and glucocorticoids, reductions in sex steroids (dependent on the intensity and duration of the activity), increased gluco-corticoids and catecholamines and reduced sex steroids (with exhausting exercise).

A lack of long-term studies evaluating combinations of controlled dietary intake and controlled physical activity is noted. This is especially important since combinations of physical activity and dietary restriction may influence mortality rates.

Cancer-preventive effects
Human studies
Body weight

Colon cancer. Both case–control and cohort studies have shown positive associations between various measures of adiposity and risk of colorectal neoplasia. Studies have been consistent in many, mostly developed, countries. The association is much less evident for rectal cancer than for colon cancers. There is an approximately linear trend of colon cancer risk from BMI 23 to 30 kg/m^2, with a risk increase across this range of about 25% among women and about 50% among men. A similar relationship is seen also for colon adenomas, the precursor lesions for colon cancer, but the association is stronger for larger adenomas than for smaller adenomas. The association is similar for time periods early and late in adulthood and is largely independent of other known risk factors for colon cancer. These patterns suggest an effect of factors related to adiposity on the promotion of colon cancer.

Premenopausal breast cancer. In populations with a high incidence of breast cancer, the overall association between BMI and breast cancer risk among premenopausal women is inverse. This has been documented in numerous cohort and case–control studies that have carefully controlled for many reproductive and lifestyle factors. This reduction in risk with overweight is modest and does not appear to be observed until a BMI of 28 kg/m^2. Despite this reduced breast cancer incidence risk, however, the breast cancer mortality rate is not lower among heavier premenopausal women.

Postmenopausal breast cancer. More than 100 studies over nearly 30 years in populations in many countries have established that increased body weight increases breast cancer risk among postmenopausal women. Nearly all of these studies have shown that this association is largely independent of a wide variety of reproductive and lifestyle risk factors, and recent studies have indicated that it is independent of the effect of physical activity. The associationbetween overweight and breast cancer appears to increase in a stepwise fashion with advancing age after the menopause.

The large majority of cohort and case–control studies have shown positive associations, although the increase in risk with BMI has been somewhat modest. Above a BMI of 24 kg/m^2, breast cancer incidence rates increase among postmenopausal women, with the greatest slope of increase in risk across higher BMI levels being seen in low- and moderate-risk countries. This suggests that increases in BMI now being observed in countries previously at low risk for breast cancer may be a major factor contributing to future increases in breast cancer rates in those countries. Further, while risk ratios have levelled off at BMI levels near 28 kg/m^2 in high-risk countries, this is not the case in low- to moderate-risk countries, where risk has continued to increase across a wider range of body weight. The association between BMI and breast cancer is stronger among women who have never used postmenopausal hormone replacement therapy, suggesting that the increased breast cancer risk from overweight may be mediated by the elevations in endogenous estrogen production among heavier women.

Adult weight gain has been shown to be a strong and consistent predictor of postmenopausal breast cancer risk. As with the studies on BMI and breast cancer, adjustment for many breast cancer risk factors, including physical activity, does not weaken this association, which is particularly strong among women who have never used hormone replacement therapy.

Endometrial cancer. A positive association of endometrial cancer with body weight has been observed in nearly all of 25 epidemiological studies, including in studies conducted in Asia, Europe and North America, and among pre- and postmenopausal women. Overweight or obese women appear to be at a 2–3-fold increased risk of endometrial cancer. Adult weight gain appears to be a better predictor of risk than current weight and to be associated with risk in a linear dose-dependent fashion.

Prostate cancer. Among more than 25 studies that have examined the association between body weight and prostate cancer, no consistent pattern of association has emerged. These studies have included a variety of populations in North America, Europe and Asia, and considered weight at different life periods and body fat distribution. Some studies also focused on the more aggressive forms of the disease which may be less subject to screening detection bias. In sum, the absence of a clear pattern of association across many studies suggests the absence of an important association between body weight and the risk of prostate cancer.

Kidney cancer. Nearly all studies of renal-cell cancer (17 out of 19) have observed a more than twofold higher risk among obese men and women compared with persons of normal weight. This association is not seen in studies of cancer of the renal pelvis. The studies have been conducted in Australia, China, Europe and the United States. Obesity has been consistently observed to be associated with increased renal cancer risk in a dose-related manner among both men and women, with an approximately 2–3-fold increase in risk among those with BMI of 30 kg/m² or greater.

Lung cancer. Body weight has been observed to be inversely associated with lung cancer. However, in most studies, this association is substantially confounded by cigarette smoking history, and in some studies this inverse association was less consistently shown among never-smokers. Thus, the inverse association between body weight and lung cancer risk is difficult to interpret as causal because of the interrelationships between weight and the use of tobacco and tobacco-related chronic lung disease.

Oesophageal cancer. Obesity has been shown to be associated with increased risk for adenocarcinomas of the lower oesophagus and of the gastric cardia. There have been few such studies, but their findings have been consistent, suggesting a two-fold or greater increased risk for those with BMI over 25 kg/m².

Thyroid cancer. Obesity has been suggested to be associated with a modest increase in risk for cancer of the thyroid in a majority of 13 studies, mostly conducted among women.

Other cancers. There is a paucity of epidemiological data on body weight and cancers of the ovary, testis, liver, pancreas, gallbladder, head and neck cancers, and cancers at many other sites. The evidence from studies conducted in various countries for these sites is inconsistent and does not allow any conclusion to be drawn on possible associations with overweight or obesity.

Intervention trials with intermediate-effect biomarkers. Weight reduction in postmenopausal women has been shown to be associated with reduction of dense areas in mammograms in one clinical trial of a low-fat diet with minimal weight loss.

Physical activity

Colorectal cancer. Approximately 50 studies have examined the association between physical activity and colon cancer and some of these examined both colon and rectal cancer. These studies have almost uniformly shown that increasing levels of activity are associated with an approximately 40% reduction in risk of colon cancer, independent of BMI. Studies including rectal cancer indicate much weaker associations. Considerable consistency in associations has been detected using different methods for estimation of activity in many different populations, in America, Asia and Europe. Increasing levels of activity, whether in intensity, frequency or duration, seem to be associated with greater reduction in risk. It appears that activities performed at a more intense levels and sustained over many years are associated with the greatest risk reduction. The precise amount of activity needed to reduce colon cancer risk is not clear, however, due to the variety of methods used to estimate activity. It has been estimated that at least 30 minutes per day of more than moderate-level physical activity might be needed to see the greatest effect in risk reduction.

Breast cancer. Most of the more than 30 epidemiological studies, conducted in Asia, Europe and North America, demonstrated lower breast cancer risk among the most physically active women. In 8 of 14 cohort studies and in 14 of 19 case–control studies, lower breast cancer risk was seen among women who were most active. The decrease in risk of breast cancer was, on average, about 20–40%. Evidence for a linear trend in effect of increasing activity with decreasing risk of breast cancer was found in most of the studies that examined the dose–response relationship. These associations were observed for both occupational and recreational activity, among pre- and postmenopausal women, for activity measured at different periods in life and for different levels of intensity of activity. Activity that is sustained throughout lifetime, or at a minimum performed after menopause, may be particularly beneficial in reducing breast cancer risk. Although there are only limited data on the effect of physical activity in different ethnic and racial groups, it appears that physical activity does have similar effects within different populations. An effect of physical activity on breast cancer risk is biologically plausible since physical activity has a direct effect on the prevention of weight gain and postmenopausal obesity, both established breast cancer risk factors, but physical activity seems to have an effect on breast cancer risk independent of that of body weight. It has been estimated that breast cancer risk reduction begins at levels of 30–60 minutes per day of moderate-intensity to vigorous activity in addition to the usual levels of occupational and household activity of most women. Although lifetime physical activity is desirable, beginning recreational physical activity after menopause can probably be beneficial for both weight control and breast cancer risk reduction.

Endometrial cancer. Ten studies of populations in Asia, Europe and North America have been quite consistent in suggesting a moderately strong protective effect of physical activity on endometrial cancer. In most studies, this effect appeared to be independent of the association with body weight. An effect of physical activity on endometrial cancer is biologically plausible since it has a direct effect on the prevention of weight gain, an established risk factor for this disease.

Prostate cancer. About twenty epidemiological studies conducted in North America, Europe and Asia were considered in assessing the relationship of physical activity to prostate cancer. Although the data are inconsistent, a majority of studies found an inverse association with physical activity. The observed effect has been moderately strong and sometimes observed only in subgroups. Although additional data are needed, the available evidence suggests that physical activity may protect against prostate cancer.

Kidney cancer. The results of studies regarding the association between physical activity and renal-cell cancer are inconsistent for both occupational and leisure physical activity.

Lung cancer. Five of seven studies of physical activity and lung cancer demonstrated a decreased risk of lung cancer among the most physically active subjects. This effect could well be confounded by smoking and/or by chronic lung disease, as these factors both tend to reduce physical activity and are associated with increased lung cancer risk. Given these factors, and the limited amount of data available, the evidence for an association between physical activity and lung cancer is inconclusive.

Other cancers. The few epidemiological data on physical activity and cancers of the ovary, testis, liver, oesophagus, pancreas, gall-bladder and other cancer sites are inconsistent and do not allow any conclusion to be drawn on possible associations with physical activity.

Intervention trials with intermediate effect biomarkers. The data on effects of physical activity on intermediate effect markers for cancer from intervention studies are limited. Results of several intervention studies on training effects on menstrual and reproductive factors in girls and young women have been published. Most were very small and uncontrolled studies. In general, it appears that a greater effect of training is observed when body weight is decreased and when exercise is strenuous and prolonged. Data on exercise effects on other biomarkers of cancers from intervention studies are not available.

Population attributable risk

The proportions of some common cancers that are attributable to elevated body weight and to inadequate physical activity are substantial. The population attributable risk estimates for elevated BMI and for inadequate physical activity are derived from relative risk estimates that have been adjusted using multivariate methods, with many of the relative risks for elevated BMI having been adjusted for physical activity, and most of the physical activity estimates having been adjusted for BMI. To the extent that the measures of BMI and physical activity are accurate, those attributable risks should be largely independent, so that the attributable risk estimates for BMI and physical activity can be approximately summed to express an estimate of their joint impact on cancer risk. If physical activity is imprecisely measured, the amount of cancer risk attributable to physical activity will be underestimated, and residual confounding is possible. Nevertheless, the sum of the effects of elevated body weight and inadequate physical activity for many cancer sites is clearly substantial. For colon cancer, for which approximately 11% is attributable to BMI and 13–14% to physical inactivity, the combined effect of these two factors accounts for about a quarter of the cases. For postmenopausal breast cancer, for which 9–11% is attributable to BMI and 11% to physical inactivity, the combined effects account for about one fifth of the cases. Although the risks attributable to physical activity have not been quantitatively estimated for endometrial cancer, it is likely that with a 39% attributable risk for BMI alone, the combined effects might well account for approximately half of the cases. The attributable risks for BMI alone are 25% for kidney cancer and 37% for oesophageal cancer. Therefore, for many of the common cancers, between one quarter and one third of the cases may be attributable to the combined effects of elevated body weight and inadequate physical activity.

Experimental studies
Weight control
Cancer and premalignant lesions
Restriction of energy intake in the range of 10–40% of the amount consumed by control animals fed *ad libitum* inhibited the development of cancer in the majority of experimental model systems for carcinogenesis, including spontaneous and chemically induced cancers of the mammary gland, liver and pituitary gland, chemically induced cancers of the colon and skin, as well as spontaneous and genetically induced lymphomas. However, some types of tumour were not inhibited by energy restriction, including chemically induced ductular carcinomas of the pancreas. Limited evidence of cancer prevention was available for chemically induced tumours of the prostate and spontaneous and chemically induced tumours of the acinar pancreas. The inhibitory activity in these models has been reported to be proportional to the duration and magnitude of the restriction imposed. It is important to note that cancer-preventive activity generally coincided with a slower rate of growth or the absence of weight gain rather than with weight loss. While some evidence implies a role of body fat in accounting for these effects, other results suggest that the effects are not due to body fat *per se*. Thus, in terms of the cancer-preventive effects of weight control, the role of energy restriction is prominent. Both the initiation and the post-initiation stages of chemically induced mammary carcinogenesis have been reported to be inhibited by energy restriction. However, the protective effects of energy restriction maintained during the post-initiation stage of carcinogenesis are greater in magnitude and have been most consistently observed in a wide spectrum of model systems. The effects of dietary restriction on carcinogenesis closely parallel the

effects of energy restriction observed for the mammary gland, acinar pancreas and liver. Further, energy restriction, irrespective of whether fat or carbohydrate is reduced, is more effective than a simple reduction in fat intake at constant energy intake in preventing mammary and skin carcinogenesis. However, feeding a high-fat restricted diet generally dampens prevention by underfeeding of cancer at these sites. Overall, the available evidence indicates that a reduced rate of growth and a smaller size for age as achieved by restricting energy intake prevent the development of cancer in laboratory animal models.

Intermediate biomarkers
The effects of energy restriction on intermediate biomarkers have been investigated for colon, liver, pancreas and mammary gland. Markers studied included cell proliferation, aberrant crypt foci, glutathione *S*-transferase-positive foci, pancreatic acinar foci and epidermal growth factor. In general, changes in these markers paralleled the reported effects of energy restriction on cancer end-points.

Physical activity
Cancer and premalignant lesions.
Investigations of the effect of physical activity on cancer prevention in chemically induced or spontaneous tumour models have relied primarily on providing animals with access to an activity wheel (voluntary activity) or on exercising animals using a treadmill (involuntary activity). The effects of such activity on tumour development have varied, with reports of inhibition, no effect and enhancement of the carcinogenic response. Chemically induced rat mammary tumour induction was inhibited by voluntary but not involuntary activity. Colon tumour yield was reduced by voluntary activity in rats in two studies. Spontaneous intestinal tumours in Min mice were not affected by in-

voluntary activity. In one study, rat liver tumour induction was clearly inhibited by involuntary exercise. Pancreatic ductular tumour induction was not inhibited by voluntary exercise. In general, when physical activity has been shown to protect against cancer, the magnitude of the effect has been modest. Studies of voluntary activity have more commonly reported protection than studies in which treadmill running was investigated. However, clear-cut exercise dose effects have not been shown. Thus, from experimental studies, the type of physical activity and the conditions of exercise intensity, duration and frequency that consistently and reproducibly inhibit tumour development have yet to be defined.

Intermediate biomarkers
The effects of two types of physical activity, free access to an activity wheel and treadmill running, on intermediate biomarkers for liver, pancreatic or mammary gland cancer have been investigated. The markers studied include glutathione *S*-transferase-positive hepatic foci, pancreatic acidophilic and basophilic foci and cell proliferation and development in the mammary gland. Whereas changes in marker activity generally reflected a protective effect of access to a running wheel against liver cancer, marker responses in pancreas and mammary gland failed to provide clear evidence for protection by physical activity in these organs.

Mechanisms of cancer prevention
Weight control
Humans
One major class of mechanisms that may form a physiological and causal link between excess body weight, physical inactivity and cancer risk is alterations in endogenous hormone metabolism.

Obesity and lack of physical activity are causes of insulin resistance and chronic hyperinsulinaemia. Chronic hyperinsulinaemia, in turn, is related to a host of metabolic alterations including elevated blood glucose levels, decreased levels of IGF-binding proteins (IGFBP-1 and -2) and of SHBG, and increases in free plasma IGF-I unbound to IGF-binding proteins and bioavailable androgens and estrogens unbound to SHBG. In addition, adiposity leads to increased peripheral formation of estrogens from androgen precursors, and hence to higher absolute estrogen concentrations in men and postmenopausal women. In some premenopausal women, hyperinsulinaemia may lead to ovarian overproduction of androgens and, in extreme cases, to chronic anovulation and a drop in ovarian progesterone production.

This global pattern of obesity-associated endocrine alterations, or specific aspects of it, may be causally related to increased risk of cancers of the endometrium and breast. The most firmly established epidemiological evidence is for a relationship between bioavailable estrogens in postmenopausal women and breast cancer risk. In addition, there is substantial evidence that elevated estrogen concentrations also increase endometrial cancer risk in postmenopausal women. Before menopause, endometrial cancer risk appears to be increased especially in women with severe ovarian hyperandrogenism, who have frequent anovulatory cycles and hence low ovarian progesterone production. The roles of endogenous sex hormones in the etiology of premenopausal breast cancer, and of endogenous hormones in general in relation to ovarian cancer, are less clear. Current evidence shows no clear relationship between total and bioavailable plasma androgens and risk of prostate cancer, nor with anthropometric indices of adiposity.

Exogenous hormones for postmenopausal replacement therapy have been generally found to increase breast cancer risk, but may either increase or decrease risk of endometrial cancer, depending on the type of hormone preparation used. This, combined with favourable hormonal changes observed after weight loss, strongly suggests that weight loss in obese postmenopausal women may decrease the risk of these cancers.

There is some evidence that chronic hyperinsulinaemia may increase the risk of colon cancer, and chronically elevated insulin levels may also contribute to the development of endometrial cancer. Furthermore, there is indirect evidence to suggest that chronic hyperinsulinaemia and related metabolic alterations may also increase risk of cancers of the pancreas and kidney.

Relatively independently of obesity, elevations in circulating IGF-I, either as absolute concentrations or relative to levels of IGFBP-3, its major plasmatic binding protein, appear to be related to increased risk of prostate cancer and premenopausal breast cancer, and possibly cancers of the colorectum and lung. Although prolonged fasting and energy malnutrition cause a dramatic drop in total IGF-I levels, obesity is not related to an increase, but rather also to a mild decrease in IGF-I, compared with the normally nourished non-obese state.

Frequent gastro-oesophageal reflux, which is often related to obesity, may increase the risk of Barrett's oesophagus and its progression towards oesophageal adenoma.

Experimental studies

Energy restriction has been reported to inhibit the initiation and post-initiation (promotion/progression) stages of carcinogenesis, although in some model systems it is without protective activity. Energy restriction modulates the activity of proteins in both phase I and phase II drug-metabolizing systems as well as the processes involved in DNA repair. Collectively, these effects are likely to work in concert to account, at least in part, for the inhibitory effects of energy reduction during carcinogenic initiation. In the majority of model systems evaluated, energy restriction modulates the post-initiation stages (promotion/progression) of carcinogenesis. Mechanisms likely to account for protective activity include inhibition of cell proliferation and/or the induction of apoptosis. Candidate molecules that may mediate these effects include sex steroids, glucocorticoids and insulin-like growth factors and their binding proteins. The signal transduction pathways and the specific components of cell cycle and cell death machinery involved in these processes are beginning to be elucidated. Limited information is available on the role of angiogenesis or modulation of the immune function in relation to the protective activity of energy restriction.

Physical activity
Humans
Mechanisms by which weight loss due to physical activity could have cancer-preventive effects have been described above. Other proposed mechanisms through which especially physical activity might decrease cancer risk, but for which there is no direct epidemiological evidence, include enhanced immune function, decreased intestinal transit time and effects on bile acid metabolism.

Experimental studies
While physical activity has been shown to inhibit the development of cancer in several model systems, the number of mechanistic investigations is limited. Areas investigated include modulation of immune function and endocrine status, but results are inconclusive. While other mechanisms have been hypothesized, relevant data from studies under experimental conditions of physical activity shown to inhibit tumour development were not available.

Other beneficial effects
Weight control
All-cause mortality

Studies on all-cause mortality in relation to BMI are associated with methodological problems. In the general population, the association between BMI and all-cause mortality follows a U-, J- or reverse J-shaped relationship. In studies with good control for confounding, BMI in the normal range showed the lowest risk. The current observational data do not indicate that weight loss lowers risk of all-cause mortality.

Cardiovascular disease

High BMI and weight gain increase risk for cardiovascular diseases. Limited evidence exists from observational studies that weight loss decreases risk of cardiovascular disease. This is supported by the proven benefits of weight reduction in intervention trials among high-risk individuals.

Effects on morbidity

Both BMI status and weight gain increase risks of hypertension, type II diabetes, insulin resistance, dyslipidaemia and numerous other overweight-related conditions. Intentional weight loss of 5–10% resulting from lifestyle changes improves surrogate markers of cardiovascular diseases and reduces the risk of hypertension and type II diabetes in overweight high-risk individuals. Maintained weight loss also reduces risks of many other obesity-related diseases and quality of life.

Physical activity

Physical activity has important health benefits above and beyond improved weight control. The level of physical activity is inversely associated with all-cause mortality rates in middle-aged and older men and women. This relationship is linear, at least up to an energy expenditure in activity of about 14.7 MJ (3500 kcal) per week, with little further benefit at higher levels. This is equivalent to brisk walking at 6.4 km/h for about 8.5 h. Physical inactivity and low levels of fitness are also associated with higher rates of coronary heart disease, stroke, type II diabetes, hypertension and (in a smaller number of studies) gallbladder disease.

The compelling evidence related to coronary heart disease from studies published over more than 50 years in different populations is buttressed by evidence of plausible mechanisms. The relationship between level of physical activity or fitness is strong, graded and independent of other risk factors. Moderate-intensity activities such as cycling and brisk or fast walking decrease coronary heart disease risk, but more vigorous exercise probably confers more benefit. The dose–response relationships for the other health outcomes mentioned above are less clear. In women, physical activity may decrease the risk of hip fracture through effects on bone mineral density and/or through decreasing the risk of falls.

Carcinogenicity
Weight control
Human studies

The associations between cancer risk and both overweight and physical activity suggest generally that weight control and physical activity offer benefits in terms of cancer risk rather than hazards (see above). Although the observational epidemiology of the relationship between BMI and cancer risk is sufficient to conclude no adverse effects of lifetime weight control on cancer risk, there have been insufficient studies of the consequences on cancer risk of major intentional weight loss to estimate either the benefits or the risks. For some cancer sites for which an inverse association has been observed between adiposity and cancer risk, factors such as alcohol, tobacco and/or pre-existing illness probably confound the associations. Among premenopausal women, there is an inverse association between BMI and breast cancer risk, perhaps induced by mechanisms related to anovulation. Reducing the prevalence of overweight among premenopausal women improves the anovulation associated with overweight and might thereby result in increased rates of premenopausal breast cancer.

Experimental studies

Loss of cancer-preventive activity and/or frank enhancement of the carcinogenic response has been observed in model systems for the breast, colon and liver with some cyclic feeding protocols, in which periods of restricted energy intake were alternated with periods of *ad libitum* feeding.

Physical activity
Humans

No clear evidence is available of any increase in cancer risks directly associated with physical activity.

Experimental studies

While physical activity has generally been reported to either inhibit or have no effect on carcinogenesis in experimental models, conditions of treadmill running have been reported to increase the carcinogenic response in the mammary gland and the level of intermediate biomarkers in the pancreas.

Other adverse effects
Health effects
Weight control
Human studies

Adverse effects of weight loss include risk of gall-stones, eating disorders, malnutrition and sarcopenia, in addition to adverse effects specific to use of weight-loss drugs. Obesity and weight gain seem to protect against loss of bone mineral density, and weight loss decreases bone mineral density and may increase fracture risk.

Experimental studies

Few potential adverse conditions have been identified to be associated with underfeeding experimental animals to control weight gain. However, animals in these protocols have elevated glucocorticoid hormone levels that may negatively affect bone mineral density and cell cycle of normal cells. Furthermore, in some dietary restriction studies, animals exhibited bradycardia, leukopenia and an inability to tolerate cold. However, it is unclear if these observations are due to reduced energy intake or the reduction of other dietary constituents with these protocols. Dietary restriction may reduce intake of cancer-protective constituents to an extent that diminishes the cancer-preventive effect of the energy restriction.

Physical activity
Human studies

Most of the risks from physical activity are evident only when people engage in high volumes and/or intensities of exercise. Strenuous exercise can trigger myocardial infarction, but the short-term increase in risk during and soon after a session is largely restricted to individuals who are unaccustomed to this. The risk of orthopaedic injury seems to be related to volume and intensity of exercise. Prior sports-related injuries may predispose to the development of osteoarthritis of the knee and hip. Exercise, particularly running in a cold environment, may trigger exercise-induced asthma in susceptible individuals. Among young women, intensive training may lead to menstrual dysfunction characterized by oligomenorrhoea. Women reporting extended periods of oligomenorrhoea or amenorrhoea have lower vertebral bone mineral density which may increase their subsequent risk of osteoporotic fracture. The extent to which these changes are reversible is not known.

Experimental studies

None of the adverse effects of exercise training noted in humans has been studied in animal models under conditions of exercise that have been shown to prevent the development of cancer in an experimental tumour model system.

Reproductive and developmental effects
Weight control
Human studies

A minimum ratio of fat to lean mass is normally necessary for menarche and the maintenance of female reproduction. Excessive leanness (as indicated by a BMI below 18.5 kg/m^2) has been associated with a decreased likelihood of fecundity due to anovulatory menstrual cycles or a shortened luteal phase.

Experimental studies

In mice, dietary restriction can make female mice enter anestrus, by decreasing gonadotropin-releasing hormone with consequent decreases in the hormones it stimulates. Lower levels of dietary restriction can inhibit fertility in male and female mice. Higher levels are needed to depress fertility in rats.

Physical activity
Human studies

Physical activity can result in women becoming amenorrhoeal and puberty can be delayed. In men, heavy exercise can lead to drops in the reproductive axis hormones in the short-term, and in chronic exercisers there is also some evidence of a decrease.

Experimental studies

In rats, moderate exercise can disrupt estrous cycling. In male rats, the results for chronic effects are inconsistent.

Genetic and related effects

There are no data on effects of either weight control and/or exercise in inducing mutations or other genetic end-points. There is some evidence that, although specific organs can have lower levels of oxidative damage, plasma and urine measures of oxidative damage can be increased by dietary restriction in rats. Also, increased mitochondrial DNA damage and lipid peroxidation have been found after training to exhaustion in humans and in chronic training in rats.

Chapter 10
Recommendations

Recommendations for research

Critically evaluate existing and new methods for assessment of body composition, physical activity and diet.

- *Physical activity*: Develop standardized, validated methods to assess physical activity that will capture different dimensions of activity, such as duration, frequency and intensity, to allow comparisons between epidemiological and population studies.

- *Body composition*: Develop standardized, validated methods to measure body composition and evaluate the need for ethnic-specific and age-specific BMI and waist cut-points.
- *Diet*: develop methods to assess aspects of dietary habits that influence weight gain. This includes development of biomarkers and questionnaires that capture aspects such as macronutrient composition, energy density, glycaemic index, dietary patterns, palatability and portion sizes.

Maintain and enhance systems for monitoring trends in body composition and physical activity in various populations

- Develop national surveillance programmes that allow global monitoring of indicators of body composition and physical activity in men and women.
- Develop methods to study environmental factors (physical, economic and socio-cultural) that determine behaviour in populations undergoing various stages of economic development.

- Develop strategies for using data from population monitoring to evaluate potential changes in physical activity and dietary patterns resulting from interventions and policy initiatives.

Conduct observational epidemiological studies using improved and standardized measures of physical activity and indicators of body composition and fat distribution in diverse populations (by age, sex and ethnicity) of sufficient sample size to assess cancer risk

- Study the relationship between different indicators of body composition and fat distribution and cancer risk.
- Study the relationship between physical activity patterns and cancer risk.
- Study the interactions between physical activity and dietary habits and body composition in relation to cancer risk.
- Study the interactions between genetic variation and physical activity patterns in relation to weight gain and body composition.
- Study the effect of voluntary weight reduction on cancer risk in overweight and obese individuals in different subgroups of sex and age.
- Establish the association between putative cancer biomarkers with cancer risk. The link between a biomarker and cancer should be firmly established before testing intervention effects on the biomarkers.

Conduct long-term clinical intervention studies in subgroups of age, sex and ethnicity to alter behavioural patterns (dietary and physical activity) which may influence weight gain. Specific circumstances of high risk for weight gain (such as smoking cessation and pregnancy) should be addressed in interventions.

- Conduct long-term (more than one year) intervention studies on dietary modification (e.g., changing macro-nutrient composition, energy density, glycaemic index, dietary patterns, palatability and portion sizes) in relation to weight gain.
- Conduct long-term (more than one year) intervention studies on changing physical activity patterns (modu-lations of intensity, frequency and duration of various sorts of physical activity) in relation to weight gain.
- Conduct long-term (more than one year) intervention studies on the interaction between dietary modifica-tion and physical activity in relation to weight gain.
- Conduct long-term (at least 1–2 years) intervention studies of dietary modification and physical activity to prevent excessive weight gain and to treat obesity, in relation to cancer risk.
- Conduct intervention studies to deter-mine whether hormonal, biochemical and molecular mechanisms identified in animals are similarly affected by energy intake, physical activity and their interaction in humans.

Conduct community intervention studies to prevent weight gain and promote physical activity

- Establish the effectiveness and effi-ciency of various community strate-gies to prevent weight gain and pro-mote physical activity.
- Develop effective strategies for the prevention of overweight and obesity at three levels: community (directed at everyone in the population); selec-tive (directed at subgroups of the populations with above-average risk of developing obesity); targeted (directed at high-risk individuals with existing weight problems but who are not yet obese).
- Determine the characteristics of sub-stantial and sustainable interventions to promote physical activity. For example, a comprehensive interven-tion to promote bicycle use for trans-portation might be tested with multiple components such as bicycle paths, relief of taxes on bicycle purchases, secure bicycle storage and other measures.
- Determine whether physical activity and weight control strategies can be replicated under different situations and in different populations.

Carry out studies in humans to establish the mechanisms by which weight gain and physical activity are related to cancer development (at least for all sites reviewed in this volume)

- Conduct studies of the effects of physical activity on menarche, men-strual cycle characteristics and endo-genous sex hormones in girls and young women.
- Evaluate the acute versus chronic effects of physical activity on mechanistic pathways related to cancer, especially for moderate-intensity activity, the level most likely to be adopted by individuals.
- Carry out mechanistic studies to identify physiological processes that can be used as biomarkers of energy status in relation to cancer prevention.
- Identify surrogate end-point markers for cancer risk that are modulated by either the level of energy intake and/or the level of physical activity, such as polyps or breast density.
- Study the long-term effects of physi-cal activity and weight control on sex hormones and insulin-like growth factor 1 (IGF-1).
- Study the role of prostaglandins in the mediation of the association between physical activity and weight gain and as intermediate indicators of cancer development.

Conduct experimental and mechanistic studies relevant to the circumstances of human activity to clarify the mechanisms by which weight gain and lack of physical activity lead to cancer development in animal models.

- Develop animal models, including genetically modified animals, that replicate patho-physiological pro-cesses related to cancer in humans such as pre- and postmenopausal breast cancer.
- Use existing and new animal models to explore the hormonal, biochemical, and molecular mechanisms of can-cer prevention by maintaining body weight through energy intake, physi-cal activity and their interactions.

- Conduct research with animal models to establish the components of exercise such as duration, frequency and intensity that influence cancer end-points.
- Develop biomarkers for evaluating the interactions between reducing energy intake (via dietary restriction) and increasing energy expenditure (by physical activity) in various combinations.
- Examine whether antagonistic interactions exist between reducing energy intake via dietary restriction and increasing energy expenditure by physical activity that could nullify the beneficial effects of either type of intervention for cancer prevention.

Recommendations for public health[1]

Obesity cannot be prevented or managed, nor physical activity promoted, solely at the level of the individual. Governments, the food industry, international agencies, the media, communities and individuals all need to work together to modify the environment so that it is less conducive to weight gain.

A number of recommendations assume a certain level of infrastructure which may not exist in developing countries. However, the underlying targets to improve dietary quality and ensure appropriate levels of physical activity for healthy weight are relevant for developing countries and should be incorporated into strategies to prevent the situation from worsening.

The health consequences and economic costs of weight gain and physical inactivity are enormous. Thus, substantial public investment is both appropriate and necessary in order to have a major impact on these problems.

Most current weight guidelines indicate a desirable BMI range of 18.5 to 25 kg/m^2, based primarily on the relationships of body weight to risks of cardiovascular diseases, diabetes and total mortality. The benefits of maintaining weight in this range clearly extend to reduced risks of important cancers. This relatively wide range of BMI is used because the ratio of fat to lean mass can vary among individuals of the same weight. However, within this range of BMI, the degree of adiposity varies substantially and is influenced by metabolic abnormalities. Most individuals will experience lower risks of cardiovascular disease and diabetes if they maintain their weight within the lower part of this range.

For persons who are already overweight or obese, most current recommendations first emphasize that additional weight gain should be avoided, and then that weight reductions of 5 to 10% are desirable. Direct evidence does not exist at present that weight reduction will lead to reduced risks of cancer. However, hormonal changes produced by weight loss seem likely to reduce risks of some cancers, and epidemiological evidence suggests that loss of weight even late in life would favourably affect the risks of breast and endometrial cancer.

Governmental and non-governmental organizations

- Public education should provide timely and accurate information on the epidemic of obesity and inactivity, and on ways this can be addressed.
- Governments at local and national levels should ensure that schoolchildren at all stages have proper access at school to healthy meals and to recreation and sports facilities.
- Governments at local and national levels, as well as non-governmental organizations, should provide adequate funding for effective physical education programmes in schools.
- Communities and buildings should be designed to encourage use of stairs and walking. A proportion of transportation budgets should be allocated for development of bicycle and pedestrian facilities, notably in urban areas.
- In developing countries there are dietary traditions, behavioural patterns and infrastructures that potentially could aid programmes for prevention of weight gain. Efforts should be made to prevent the loss of cultural traditions that promote healthy diets and physical activity.

---

[1] In general, the following recommendations are relevant to adults up to the age of 75 years, though this age limit may rise as populations improve in their lifetime adherence to healthy lifestyles. Where relevant, they have been drawn from a number of source documents (e.g. World Cancer Research Fund, 1997; WHO Consultations on Obesity, 1998).

Worksites and schools

- Employers should encourage physical activity and weight control by all employees. Methods can include provisions for exercise areas at work, showers, financial incentives to walk, bicycle or use public transportation rather than cars.

- School curricula should include adequate teaching on food, nutrition and health, and on the importance of active living.

- Schools should include one hour of physical education on most days.

Health professionals and educators

- Health professionals should counsel individuals about a healthy range of body weight. For persons currently within the healthy range, it is recommended that weight gain during adult life should not exceed 5 kg.

- Medical schools and other health science professional programmes should make the study of food, nutrition and physical activity and their relation to health and disease an integral part of the training of health professionals.

- Physicians and health-care providers should counsel their patients on the need for an active lifestyle for the prevention of cancer and other non-communicable diseases.

- Health-care providers and educators should set a personal example by engaging in regular physical activity and controlling their weight to the best of their ability.

- Health-care providers and and teachers should take an active role in their communities to support regular physical activity and weight control.

- Maternal and child-health programmes can provide a suitable context for promoting awareness of the need for physical activity and preventing weight gain, particularly in developing countries.

Families and individuals

- Prevention of overweight and obesity should begin early in life. It should be based on the development of life-long healthy eating and physical activity patterns. However, it is never too late to benefit from starting to be more active.

- Individuals should be encouraged to maintain physical activity in order to promote energy balance and weight control. The primary goal should be to perform continuous physical activity on most days of the week. At total of one hour per day of moderate-intensity activity such as walking may be needed to maintain a healthy body weight, particularly for people with sedentary occupations. More vigorous activity, such as fast walking, several times per week may give some additional benefits regarding cancer prevention. Therefore, planned vigorous activities such as sports should be undertaken according to individual interests and capabilities.

- Individuals should where possible give priority to the more active alternatives in their daily lives.

- Parents and individuals should limit the purchase and availability at home of high-energy foods and beverages with low nutritional value, such as soda beverages and baked snacks and instead provide healthy foods, in particular an abundant supply of fruits and vegetables and whole grain products.

Chapter 11
Evaluation

Cancer-preventive activity

Humans

There is *sufficient evidence* in humans for a cancer-preventive effect of avoidance of weight gain. This evidence has been obtained for cancers of the colon, breast (post-menopausal), endometrium, kidney (renal-cell) and oesophagus (adenocarcinoma).

For premenopausal breast cancer, the available evidence on the avoidance of weight gain *suggests lack of a cancer-preventive effect.*

For all other sites, the evidence is *inadequate.*

There is *inadequate evidence* in humans for a cancer-preventive effect of intentional weight loss for any cancer site.

There is *sufficient evidence* in humans for a cancer-preventive effect of physical activity. This has been obtained for cancers of the colon and breast.

For cancers of the endometrium and prostate, there is *limited evidence* for a cancer-preventive effect of physical activity.

For all other sites, the evidence is *inadequate.*

Experimental animals

There is *sufficient evidence* in experimental animals for a cancer-preventive effect of avoidance of weight gain by restriction of dietary energy intake. This evidence has been obtained for spontaneous and chemically induced cancers of the mammary gland, liver and pituitary gland (adenoma), for chemically induced cancers of the colon and the skin (non-melanoma) and for spontaneous and genetically induced lymphoma.

For chemically induced cancers of the prostate, and for spontaneous and chemically induced cancers of the acinar pancreas, there is *limited evidence* in experimental animals for a cancer-preventive effect of avoidance of weight gain by restriction of dietary energy intake.

There is *limited evidence* in experimental animals for a cancer-preventive effect of avoidance of weight gain by physical activity for spontaneous mammary tumours and for chemically induced mammary and colon cancers. For all other cancer sites, the evidence is *inadequate.*

There are data in experimental animals indicating that diet restriction (reduction of all dietary components but with vitamin supplements) gives rise to a decrease in the spontaneous incidence of tumours in lung, testis, thyroid follicular cells, preputial and clitoral gland, and of adrenal phaeochromocytomas.

Overall evaluation

The prevalence of overweight and obesity in adults and children has increased rapidly over the last two decades in most countries. In many developed countries half or more of the adult population is now overweight or obese, and similar prevalence rates have been reached in urban areas of some developing countries.

- Decreased levels of overall physical activity are a major contributor to the rise in rates of overweight and obesity.

- Epidemiological studies, animal experiments and mechanistic investigations all support a beneficial effect of weight control and physical activity in the prevention of cancer.

- Limiting weight gain during adult life, thereby avoiding overweight and obesity, reduces the risk of post-menopausal breast cancer, and cancers of the colon, uterus (endometrium), kidney (renal cell) and oesophagus (adenocarcinoma).

- Weight loss among overweight or obese persons possibly reduces risks of these cancers, but no firm conclusion can be drawn because of the sparsity of the epidemiological evidence.

- Regular physical activity reduces the risk of breast and colon cancer, and possibly reduces risk of uterine (endometrial) and prostate cancers. These effects seem to be in part independent of that of weight control.

- Taken together, excess body weight and physical inactivity account for approximately one fourth to one third of breast cancer, and cancers of the colon, endometrium, kidney (renal cell) and oesophagus (adenocarcinoma). Thus adiposity and inactivity appear to be the most important avoidable causes of postmenopausal breast cancer, endometrial cancer, renal-cell cancer, and adenocarcinoma of the oesophagus, and among the most important avoidable causes of colon cancer.

- In addition to the important reductions in cancer incidence, weight control and regular physical activity will lead to substantial decreases in cardiovascular disease, type II diabetes, and other chronic diseases.

- Control of the obesity epidemic will require the participation of all segments of society and substantial investments, particularly in public education, community environments that promote walking and other physical activities, work-site and school programmes that include at least one hour of physical activity on most days, and transportation systems that encourage walking and use of bicycles.

References

Adami, H.O., McLaughlin, J., Ekbom, A., Berne, C., Silverman, D., Hacker, D. & Persson, I. (1991) Cancer risk in patients with diabetes mellitus. *Cancer Causes Control*, **2**, 307–314

Ainsworth, B.E. (2000) Issues in the assessment of physical activity in women. *Res. Q. Exerc. Sport*, **71**, S37–S42

Ainsworth, B.E., Haskell, W.L., Leon, A.S., Jacobs, D.R., Jr, Montoye, H.J., Sallis, J.F. & Paffenbarger, R.S., Jr (1993) Compendium of physical activities: classification of energy costs of human physical activities. *Med. Sci. Sports Exerc.*, **25**, 71–80

Ainsworth, B.E., Montoye, H.J. & Leon, A.S. (1994) Methods of assessing physical activity during leisure and work. In: Bouchard, C., Shephard, R.J. & Stephens, T., eds, *Physical Activity, Fitness, and Health: A Consensus of Current Knowledge,* Champaign, Human Kinetics Publishers, pp. 146–159

Ainsworth, B.E., Haskell, W.L., Whitt, M.C., Irwin, M.L., Swartz, A.M., Strath, S.J., O'Brien, W.L., Bassett, D.R., Jr, Schmitz, K.H., Emplaincourt, P.O., Jacobs, D.R., Jr & Leon, A.S. (2000) Compendium of physical activities: an update of activity codes and MET intensities. *Med. Sci. Sports Exerc.*, **32**, S498–S504

Akre, O., Ekbom, A., Sparen, P. & Tretli, S. (2000) Body size and testicular cancer. *J. Natl Cancer Inst.*, **92**, 1093–1096

Al-Isa, A.N. (1995) Prevalence of obesity among adult Kuwaitis: a cross-sectional study. *Int. J. Obes. Relat. Metab. Disord.*, **19**, 431–433

Al-Mannai, A., Dickerson, J.W., Morgan, J.B. & Khalfan, H. (1996) Obesity in Bahraini adults. *J. R. Soc. Health*, **116**, 30–40

Al Nuaim, A. *et al.* (1996) Prevalence of diabetes mellitus, obesity and hypercholesterolemia in Saudi Arabia. In: Musaiger, A.O. & Miladi, S.S., eds, *Diet-related Non-communicable Diseases in the Arab Countries in the Gulf,* Cairo, FAO, UN, pp. 73–81

Albanes, D., Blair, A. & Taylor, P.R. (1989) Physical activity and risk of cancer in the NHANES I population. *Am. J. Public Health*, **79**, 744–750

Albanes, D., Conway, J.M., Taylor, P.R., Moe, P.W. & Judd, J. (1990) Validation and comparison of eight physical activity questionnaires. *Epidemiology*, **1**, 65–71

Albert, C.M., Mittleman, M.A., Chae, C.U., Lee, I.M., Hennekens, C.H. & Manson, J.E. (2000) Triggering of sudden death from cardiac causes by vigorous exertion. *New Engl. J. Med.*, **343**, 1355–1361

Albright, A., Franz, M., Hornsby, G., Kriska, A., Marrero, D., Ullrich, I. & Verity, L.S. (2000) American College of Sports Medicine position stand. Exercise and type 2 diabetes. *Med. Sci. Sports Exerc.*, **32**, 1345–1360

Allaben, W.T., Chou, M., Pegram, R.A., Leakey, J., Feuers, R.J., Duffy, P.H., Turturro, A. & Hart, R.W. (1990) Modulation of toxicity and carcinogenesis by caloric restriction. *Korean J. Toxicol.*, **6**, 167–182

Allison, D.B., Faith, M.S., Heo, M. & Kotler, D.P. (1997) Hypothesis concerning the U-shaped relation between body mass index and mortality. *Am. J. Epidemiol.*, **146**, 339–349

Allison, D.B., Faith, M.S., Heo, M., Townsend-Butterworth, D. & Williamson, D.F. (1999a) Meta-analysis of the effect of excluding early deaths on the estimated relationship between body mass index and mortality. *Obes. Res.*, **7**, 342–354

Allison, D.B., Zannolli, R., Faith, M.S., Heo, M., Pietrobelli, A., VanItallie, T.B., Pi-Sunyer, F.X. & Heymsfield, S.B. (1999b) Weight loss increases and fat loss decreases all-cause mortality rate: results from two independent cohort studies. *Int. J. Obes. Relat. Metab. Disord.*, **23**, 603–611

Amemiya, T., Kawahara, R., Yoshino, M., Komori, K. & Hirata, Y. (1990) Population study on the adipose tissue distribution in Japanese women born in 1948. *Diabetes Res. Clin. Pract.*, **10 Suppl. 1**, S71–S76

American College of Sports Medicine (ACSM) (1990) American College of Sports Medicine position stand. The recommended quantity and quality of exercise for developing and maintaining cardiorespiratory and muscular fitness in healthy adults. *Med. Sci. Sports Exerc.*, **22**, 265–274

Amiel, S.A., Sherwin, R.S., Simonson, D.C., Lauritano, A.A. & Tamborlane, W.V. (1986) Impaired insulin action in puberty. A contributing factor to poor glycemic control in adolescents with diabetes. *New Engl. J. Med.*, **315**, 215–219

An, P., Rice, T., Gagnon, J., Hong, Y., Leon, A.S., Skinner, J.S., Wilmore, J.H., Bouchard, C. & Rao, D.C. (2000) A genetic study of sex hormone-binding globulin measured before and after a 20-week endurance exercise training program: the HERITAGE Family Study. *Metabolism*, **49**, 1014–1020

Andersen, R.E., Wadden, T.A., Bartlett, S.J., Zemel, B., Verde, T.J. & Franckowiak, S.C. (1999) Effects of lifestyle activity vs structured aerobic exercise in obese women: a randomized trial. *JAMA*, **281**, 335–340

Andersen, L.B., Schnohr, P., Schroll, M. & Hein, H.O. (2000) All-cause mortality associated with physical activity during leisure time, work, sports, and cycling to work. *Arch. Intern. Med.*, **160**, 1621–1628

Anderssen, N., Jacobs, D.R., Sidney, S., Bild, D.E., Sternfeld, B., Slattery, M.L. & Hannan, P. (1996) Change and secular trends in physical activity patterns in young adults: a seven-year longitudinal follow-up in the Coronary Artery Risk Development in Young Adults Study (CARDIA). *Am. J. Epidemiol.*, **143**, 351–362

Anderssen, S.A., Holme, I., Urdal, P. & Hjermann, I. (1998) Associations between central obesity and indexes of hemostatic, carbohydrate and lipid metabolism. Results of a 1-year intervention from the Oslo Diet and Exercise Study. *Scand. J. Med. Sci. Sports*, **8**, 109–115

Andersson, B., Mårin, P., Lissner, L., Vermeulen, A. & Björntorp, P. (1994) Testosterone concentrations in women and men with NIDDM. *Diabetes Care*, **17**, 405–411

Andersson, S.O., Baron, J., Wolk, A., Lindgren, C., Bergström, R. & Adami, H.O. (1995) Early life risk factors for prostate cancer: a population-based case-control study in Sweden. *Cancer Epidemiol. Biomarkers Prev.*, **4**, 187–192

Andersson, S.O., Baron, J., Bergström, R., Lindgren, C., Wolk, A. & Adami, H.O. (1996) Lifestyle factors and prostate cancer risk: a case-control study in Sweden. *Cancer Epidemiol. Biomarkers Prev.*, **5**, 509–513

Andersson, S.O., Wolk, A., Bergström, R., Adami, H.O., Engholm, G., Englund, A. & Nyrén, O. (1997) Body size and prostate cancer: a 20-year follow-up study among 135006 Swedish construction workers. *J. Natl Cancer Inst.*, **89**, 385–389

Andres, R. (1985) Mortality and obesity: the rationale for age-group specific weight-height tables. In: Andres, R., Bierman, E.L. & Hazzard, W.R., eds, *Principles of Geriatric Medicine,* New York, McGraw Hill, pp. 311–318

Andres, R., Muller, D.C. & Sorkin, J.D. (1993) Long-term effects of change in body weight on all-cause mortality. A review. *Ann. Intern. Med.*, **119**, 737–743

Andrianopoulos, G., Nelson, R.L., Bombeck, C.T. & Souza, G. (1987) The influence of physical activity in 1,2-dimethylhydrazine induced colon carcinogenesis in the rat. *Anticancer Res.*, **7**, 849–852

Apter, D. (1996) Hormonal events during female puberty in relation to breast cancer risk. *Eur. J. Cancer Prev.*, **5**, 476–482

Arce, J.C., De Souza, M.J., Pescatello, L.S. & Luciano, A.A. (1993) Subclinical alterations in hormone and semen profile in athletes. *Fertil. Steril.*, **59**, 398–404

Argente, J., Caballo, N., Barrios, V., Muñoz, M.T., Pozo, J., Chowen, J.A., Morandé, G. & Hernández, M. (1997a) Multiple endocrine abnormalities of the growth hormone and insulin-like growth factor axis in patients with anorexia nervosa: effect of short- and long-term weight recuperation. *J. Clin. Endocrinol. Metab.*, **82**, 2084–2092

Argente, J., Caballo, N., Barrios, V., Pozo, J., Muñoz, M.T., Chowen, J.A. & Hernández, M. (1997b) Multiple endocrine abnormalities of the growth hormone and insulin-like growth factor axis in prepubertal children with exogenous obesity: effect of short- and long-term weight reduction. *J. Clin. Endocrinol. Metab.*, **82**, 2076–2083

Armario, A., Montero, J.L. & Jolin, T. (1987) Chronic food restriction and the circadian rhythms of pituitary-adrenal hormones, growth hormone and thyroid-stimulating hormone. *Ann. Nutr. Metab.*, **31**, 81–87

Armstrong, T., Bauman, A. & Davies, J. (2000) *Physical Activity Patterns of Australian Adults. Results of the 1999 National Physical Activity Survey,* Canberra, Australian Institute of Health and Welfare, pp. 1–68

Arvola, P., Wu, X., Kahonen, M., Makynen, H., Riutta, A., Mucha, I., Solakivi, T., Kainulainen, H. & Porsti, I. (1999) Exercise enhances vasorelaxation in experimental obesity associated hypertension. *Cardiovasc. Res.*, **43**, 992–1002

Asal, N.R., Risser, D.R., Kadamani, S., Geyer, J.R., Lee, E.T. & Cherng, N. (1988) Risk factors in renal cell carcinoma: I. Methodology, demographics, tobacco, beverage use, and obesity. *Cancer Detect. Prev.*, **11**, 359–377

Attia, N., Tamborlane, W.V., Heptulla, R., Maggs, D., Grozman, A., Sherwin, R.S. & Caprio, S. (1998) The metabolic syndrome and insulin-like growth factor I regulation in adolescent obesity. *J. Clin. Endocrinol. Metab.*, **83**, 1467–1471

Aubert, M.L., Pierroz, D.D., Gruaz, N.M., d'Alleves, V., Vuagnat, B.A., Pralong, F.P., Blum, W.F. & Sizonenko, P.C. (1998) Metabolic control of sexual function and growth: role of neuropeptide Y and leptin. *Mol. Cell Endocrinol.*, **140**, 107–113

Austin, H., Austin, J.M., Jr, Partridge, E.E., Hatch, K.D. & Shingleton, H.M. (1991) Endometrial cancer, obesity, and body fat distribution. *Cancer Res.*, **51**, 568–572

Asia-Pacific Perspective (2000) *The Asia-Pacific Perspective: Redefining Obesity and its Treatment,* Health Communications Australia

Axelson, J.F. (1987) Forced swimming alters vaginal estrous cycles, body composition, and steroid levels without disrupting lordosis behavior or fertility in rats. *Physiol. Behav.*, **41**, 471–479

Ayabe, T., Tsutsumi, O., Sakai, H., Yoshikawa, H., Yano, T., Kurimoto, F. & Taketani, Y. (1997) Increased circulating levels of insulin-like growth factor-I and decreased circulating levels of insulin-like growth factor binding protein-1 in postmenopausal women with endometrial cancer. *Endocr. J.*, **44**, 419–424

Ayatollahi, S.M. & Carpenter, R.G. (1993) Height, weight, BMI and weight-for-height of adults in southern Iran: how should obesity be defined? *Ann. Hum. Biol.*, **20**, 13–19

Azziz, R. (1989) Reproductive endocrinologic alterations in female asymptomatic obesity. *Fertil. Steril.*, **52**, 703–725

Azziz, R., Potter, H.D., Bradley, E.L., Jr & Boots, L.R. (1994) D^5-Androstene-3b,17b-diol in healthy eumenorrheic women: relationship to body mass and hormonal profile. *Fertil. Steril.*, **62**, 321–326

Baecke, J.A., Burema, J. & Frijters, J.E. (1982) A short questionnaire for the measurement of habitual physical activity in epidemiological studies. *Am. J. Clin. Nutr.*, **36**, 936–942

Bagatell, C.J. & Bremner, W.J. (1990) Sperm counts and reproductive hormones in male marathoners and lean controls. *Fertil. Steril.*, **53**, 688–692

Bagga, D., Ashley, J.M., Geffrey, S.P., Wang, H.J., Barnard, R.J., Korenman, S. & Heber, D. (1995) Effects of a very low fat, high fiber diet on serum hormones and menstrual function. Implications for breast cancer prevention. *Cancer*, **76**, 2491–2496

Baik, M., Choi, C.B., Keller, W.L. & Park, C.S. (1992) Developmental stages and energy restriction affect cellular oncogene expression in tissues of female rats. *J. Nutr.*, **122**, 1614–1619

Baik, I., Ascherio, A., Rimm, E.B., Giovannucci, E., Spiegelman, D., Stampfer, M.J. & Willett, W.C. (2000) Adiposity and mortality in men. *Am. J. Epidemiol.*, **152**, 264-271

Baker, E.A., Brennan, L.K., Brownson, R. & Houseman, R.A. (2000) Measuring the determinants of physical activity in the community: current and future directions. *Res. Q. Exerc. Sport*, **71**, S146–S158

Ball, M.J., Wilson, B.D., Robertson, I.K., Wilson, N. & Russell, D.G. (1993) Obesity and body fat distribution in New Zealanders: a pattern of coronary heart disease risk. *N.Z. Med. J.*, **106**, 69–72

Ballard-Barbash, R., Schatzkin, A., Taylor, P.R. & Kahle, L.L. (1990a) Association of change in body mass with breast cancer. *Cancer Res.*, **50**, 2152–2155

Ballard-Barbash, R., Schatzkin, A., Carter, C.L., Kannel, W.B., Kreger, B.E., D'Agostino, R.B., Splansky, G.L., Anderson, K.M. & Helsel, W.E. (1990b) Body fat distribution and breast cancer in the Framingham Study. *J. Natl Cancer Inst.*, **82**, 286–290

Ballard-Barbash, R., Schatzkin, A., Albanes, D., Schiffman, M.H., Kreger, B.E., Kannel, W.B., Anderson, K.M. & Helsel, W.E. (1990c) Physical activity and risk of large bowel cancer in the Framingham Study. *Cancer Res*, **50**, 3610–3613

Ballor, D.L. (1991) Effect of dietary restriction and/or exercise on 23-h metabolic rate and body composition in female rats. *J. Appl. Physiol.*, **71**, 801–806

Banerjee, S., Saenger, P., Hu, M., Chen, W. & Barzilai, N. (1997) Fat accretion and the regulation of insulin-mediated glycogen synthesis after puberty in rats. *Am. J. Physiol.*, **273**, R1534–R1539

Bang, P., Brandt, J., Degerblad, M., Enberg, G., Kaijser, L., Thorén, M. & Hall, K. (1990) Exercise-induced changes in insulin-like growth factors and their low molecular weight binding protein in healthy subjects and patients with growth hormone deficiency. *Eur. J. Clin. Invest.*, **20**, 285–292

Banu, M.J., Orhii, P.B., Mejia, W., McCarter, R.J., Mosekilde, L., Thomsen, J.S. & Kalu, D.N. (1999) Analysis of the effects of growth hormone, voluntary exercise, and food restriction on diaphyseal bone in female F344 rats. *Bone*, **25**, 469–480

Baquie, P. & Brukner, P. (1997) Injuries presenting to an Australian sports medicine centre: a 12-month study. *Clin. J. Sport Med.*, **7**, 28–31

Barbe, P., Bennet, A., Stebenet, M., Perret, B. & Louvet, J.P. (1993) Sex-hormone-binding globulin and protein-energy malnutrition indexes as indicators of nutritional status in women with anorexia nervosa. *Am. J. Clin. Nutr.*, **57**, 319–322

Barefoot, J.C., Heitmann, B.L., Helms, M.J., Williams, R.B., Surwit, R.S. & Siegler, I.C. (1998) Symptoms of depression and changes in body weight from adolescence to mid-life. *Int. J. Obes. Relat. Metab. Disord.*, **22**, 688–694

Bastarrachea, J., Hortobagyi, G.N., Smith, T.L., Kau, S.W. & Buzdar, A.U. (1994) Obesity as an adverse prognostic factor for patients receiving adjuvant chemotherapy for breast cancer. *Ann. Intern. Med.*, **120**, 18–25

Bates, G.W. & Whitworth, N.S. (1982) Effect of body weight reduction on plasma androgens in obese, infertile women. *Fertil. Steril.*, **38**, 406–409

Bauman, A., Smith, B., Stoker, L., Bellew, B. & Booth, M. (1999) Geogra-phical influences upon physical activity participation: evidence of a 'coastal effect'. *Aust. N.Z. J. Public Health*, **23**, 322–324

Baumgartner, R.N. (2000) Body composition in healthy aging. *Ann. NY Acad. Sci.*, **904**, 437–448

Baxter, R.C. (2000) Insulin-like growth factor (IGF)-binding proteins: interactions with IGFs and intrinsic bioactivities. *Am. J. Physiol. Endocrinol. Metab.*, **278**, E967–E976

Baxter, R.C. & Turtle, J.R. (1978) Regulation of hepatic growth hormone receptors by insulin. *Biochem. Biophys. Res. Commun.*, **84**, 350–357

Beer-Borst, S., Morabia, A., Hercberg, S., Vitek, O., Bernstein, M.S., Galan, P., Galasso, R., Giampaoli, S., Houterman, S., McCrum, E., Panico, S., Pannozzo, F., Preziosi, P., Ribas, L., Serra-Majem, L., Verschuren, W.M., Yarnell, J. & Northridge, M.E. (2000) Obesity and other health determinants across Europe: the EURALIM project. *J. Epidemiol. Community Health*, **54**, 424–430

Beitins, I.Z., McArthur, J.W., Turnbull, B.A., Skrinar, G.S. & Bullen, B.A. (1991) Exercise induces two types of human luteal dysfunction: confirmation by urinary free progesterone. *J. Clin. Endocrinol. Metab.*, **72**, 1350–1358

Bejma, J. & Ji, L.L. (1999) Aging and acute exercise enhance free radical generation in rat skeletal muscle. *J. Appl. Physiol.*, **87**, 465–470

Bell, A.W., Bassett, J.M., Chandler, K.D. & Boston, R.C. (1983) Fetal and maternal endocrine responses to exercise in the pregnant ewe. *J. Dev. Physiol.*, **5**, 129–141

Benhamou, S., Lenfant, M.H., Ory-Paoletti, C. & Flamant, R. (1993) Risk factors for renal-cell carcinoma in a French case-control study. *Int. J. Cancer*, **55**, 32–36

Benito, E., Obrador, A., Stiggelbout, A., Bosch, F.X., Mulet, M., Muñoz, N. & Kaldor, J. (1990) A population-based case-control study of colorectal cancer in Majorca. I. Dietary factors. *Int. J. Cancer*, **45**, 69–76

Benito, M., Valverde, A.M. & Lorenzo, M. (1996) IGF-I: a mitogen also involved in differentiation processes in mammalian cells. *Int. J. Biochem. Cell Biol.*, **28**, 499–510

Bennett, S.A. & Magnus, P. (1994) Trends in cardiovascular risk factors in Australia. Results from the National Heart Foundation's Risk Factor Prevalence Study, 1980–1989. *Med. J. Aust.*, **161**, 519–527

Bennett, A., Tacca, M.D., Stamford, I.F. & Zebro, T. (1977) Prostaglandins from tumours of human large bowel. *Br. J. Cancer*, **35**, 881–884

Bereket, A., Lang, C.H., Blethen, S.L., Gelato, M.C., Fan, J., Frost, R.A. & Wilson, T.A. (1995) Effect of insulin on the insulin-like growth factor system in children with new-onset insulin-dependent diabetes mellitus. *J. Clin. Endocrinol. Metab.*, **80**, 1312–1317

Bereket, A., Lang, C.H. & Wilson, T.A. (1999) Alterations in the growth hormone-insulin-like growth factor axis in insulin dependent diabetes mellitus. *Horm. Metab. Res.*, **31**, 172–181

Bergström, A. (2001) Thesis. Renal cell cancer: the role of physical activity and body size. Karolinska Institutet, Stockholm, pp. 1–62

Bergström, A., Moradi, T., Lindblad, P., Nyrén, O., Adami, H.O. & Wolk, A. (1999) Occupational physical activity and renal cell cancer: a nationwide cohort study in Sweden. *Int. J. Cancer*, **83**, 186–191

Bergström, A., Pisani, P., Tenet, V., Wolk, A. & Adami, H.O. (2001) Overweight as an avoidable cause of cancer in Europe. *Int. J. Cancer*, **91**, 421–430

Berlin, J.A. & Colditz, G.A. (1990) A meta-analysis of physical activity in the prevention of coronary heart disease. *Am. J. Epidemiol.*, **132**, 612–628

Bermon, S., Ferrari, P., Bernard, P., Altare, S. & Dolisi, C. (1999) Responses of total and free insulin-like growth factor-I and insulin-like growth factor binding protein-3 after resistance exercise and training in elderly subjects. *Acta Physiol. Scand.*, **165**, 51–56

Bernasconi, D., Del Monte, P., Meozzi, M., Randazzo, M., Marugo, A., Badaracco, B. & Marugo, M. (1996) The impact of obesity on hormonal parameters in hirsute and nonhirsute women. *Metabolism*, **45**, 72–75

Bernstein, L. & Ross, R.K. (1993) Endogenous hormones and breast cancer risk. Epidemiol. Rev., 15, 48–65

Bernstein, L., Ross, R.K., Lobo, R.A., Hanisch, R., Krailo, M.D. & Henderson, B.E. (1987) The effects of moderate physical activity on menstrual cycle patterns in adolescence: implications for breast cancer prevention. Br. J. Cancer, 55, 681–685

Bernstein, L., Henderson, B.E., Hanisch, R., Sullivan-Halley, J. & Ross, R.K. (1994) Physical exercise and reduced risk of breast cancer in young women. J. Natl Cancer Inst., 86, 1403–1408

Bernstein, C., Bernstein, H., Garewal, H., Dinning, P., Jabi, R., Sampliner, R.E., McCuskey, M.K., Panda, M., Roe, D.J., L'Heureux, L. & Payne, C. (1999) A bile acid-induced apoptosis assay for colon cancer risk and associated quality control studies. Cancer Res., 59, 2353–2357

Berrino, F., Bellati, C., Secreto, G., Camerini, E., Pala, V., Panico, S., Allegro, G. & Kaaks, R. (2001) Reducing bioavailable sex hormones through a comprehensive change in diet: the DIANA (Diet and Androgens) randomized trial. Cancer Epidemiol. Biomarkers Prev., 10, 25–33

Berrios, X., Koponen, T., Huiguang, T., Khaltaev, N., Puska, P. & Nissinen, A. (1997) Distribution and prevalence of major risk factors of noncommunicable diseases in selected countries: the WHO Inter-Health Programme. Bull. World Health Organ., 75, 99–108

Berstein, L.M. (1988) Newborn macrosomy and cancer. Adv. Cancer Res., 50, 231–278

Beumont, P.J.V., George, G.C.W., Pimstone, B.L. & Vinik, A.I. (1976) Body weight and the pituitary response to hypothalamic-releasing hormones in patients with anorexia nervosa. J. Clin. Endocrinol. Metab., 43, 487–496

Bhagavathi, R. & Devi, S.A. (1993) Interaction of exercise and age on substrates of carbohydrate metabolism. Indian J. Exp. Biol., 31, 72–75

Bijnen, F.C., Feskens, E.J., Caspersen, C.J., Nagelkerke, N., Mosterd, W.L. & Kromhout, D. (1999) Baseline and previous physical activity in relation to mortality in elderly men: the Zutphen Elderly Study. Am. J. Epidemiol., 150, 1289–1296

Bild, D.E., Sholinsky, P., Smith, D.E., Lewis, C.E., Hardin, J.M. & Burke, G.L. (1996) Correlates and predictors of weight loss in young adults: the CARDIA study. Int. J. Obes. Relat. Metab. Disord., 20, 47–55

Bird, C.L., Frankl, H.D., Lee, E.R. & Haile, R.W. (1998) Obesity, weight gain, large weight changes, and adenomatous polyps of the left colon and rectum. Am. J. Epidemiol., 147, 670–680

Birt, D.F. (1987) Fat and calorie effects on carcinogenesis at sites other than the mammary gland. Am. J. Clin. Nutr., 45, 203–209

Birt, D.F., Julius, A.D., White, L.T. & Pour, P.M. (1989) Enhancement of pancreatic carcinogenesis in hamsters fed a high-fat diet ad libitum and at a controlled calorie intake. Cancer Res., 49, 5848–5851

Birt, D.F., Pelling, J.C., White, L.T., Dimitroff, K. & Barnett, T. (1991) Influence of diet and calorie restriction on the initiation and promotion of skin carcinogenesis in the SENCAR mouse model. Cancer Res., 51, 1851–1854

Birt, D.F., Pinch, H.J., Barnett, T., Phan, A. & Dimitroff, K. (1993) Inhibition of skin tumor promotion by restriction of fat and carbohydrate calories in SENCAR mice. Cancer Res., 53, 27–31

Birt, D.F., Pelling, J.C., Anderson, J. & Barnett, T. (1994a) Consumption of reduced-energy/low-fat diet or constant-energy/high-fat diet during mezerein treatment inhibited mouse skin tumor promotion. Carcinogenesis, 15, 2341–2345

Birt, D.F., Copenhaver, J., Pelling, J.C. & Anderson, J. (1994b) Dietary energy restriction and fat modulation of protein kinase C isoenzymes and phorbol ester binding in Sencar mouse epidermis. Carcinogenesis, 15, 2727–2732

Birt, D.F., Kris, E.S. & Luthra, R. (1995) Modification of murine skin tumor promotion by dietary energy and fat. In: Mukhtar, H., ed., Skin Cancer: Mechanisms and Human Relevance, Boca Raton, CRC Press, pp. 371–381

Birt, D.F., Barnett, T., Pour, P.M. & Copenhaver, J. (1996) High-fat diet blocks the inhibition of skin carcinogenesis and reductions in protein kinase C by moderate energy restriction. Mol. Carcinog., 16, 115–120

Birt, D.F., Pour, P.M., Nagel, D.L., Barnett, T., Blackwood, D. & Duysen, E. (1997) Dietary energy restriction does not inhibit pancreatic carcinogenesis by N-nitrosobis-2-(oxopropyl)amine in the Syrian hamster. Carcinogenesis, 18, 2107–2111

Birt, D.F., Yaktine, A. & Duysen, E. (1999) Glucocorticoid mediation of dietary energy restriction inhibition of mouse skin carcinogenesis. J. Nutr., 129, 571S–574S

Birt, D.F., Duysen, E., Wang, W. & Yaktine, A. (2001) Corticosterone supplementation reduced selective protein kinase c isoform expression in the epidermis of adrenalectomized mice. Cancer Epidemiol. Biomarkers Prev., 10, 679–685

Björntorp, P. (1990) "Portal" adipose tissue as a generator of risk factors for cardiovascular disease and diabetes. Arteriosclerosis, 10, 493–496

Björntorp, P. (1997) Body fat distribution, insulin resistance, and metabolic diseases. Nutrition, 13, 795–803

Blaakaer, J. (1997) The pituitary-gonadal function in postmenopausal women with epithelial ovarian tumors. APMIS Suppl., 74, 1–27

Blair, S.N., Shaten, J., Brownell, K., Collins, G. & Lissner, L. (1993) Body weight change, all-cause mortality, and cause-specific mortality in the Multiple Risk Factor Intervention Trial. Ann. Intern. Med., 119, 749–757

Blair, S.N., Kohl, H.W., III, Barlow, C.E., Paffenbarger, R.S., Jr, Gibbons, L.W. & Macera, C.A. (1995) Changes in physical fitness and all-cause mortality. A prospective study of healthy and unhealthy men. JAMA, 273, 1093-1098

Blair, S.N., Kampert, J.B., Kohl, H.W., III, Barlow, C.E., Macera, C.A., Paffenbarger, R.S., Jr. & Gibbons, L.W. (1996) Influences of cardiorespiratory fitness and other precursors on cardiovascular disease and all-cause mortality in men and women. JAMA, 276, 205–210

Blitzer, P.H., Blitzer, E.C. & Rimm, A.A. (1976) Association between teen-age obesity and cancer in 56,111 women: all cancers and endometrial carcinoma. Prev. Med., 5, 20–31

Bloch, C.A., Clemons, P. & Sperling, M.A. (1987) Puberty decreases insulin sensitivity. J. Pediatr., 110, 481–487

Boeing, H., Schlehofer, B. & Wahrendorf, J. (1997) Diet, obesity and risk for renal cell carcinoma: results from a case control-study in Germany. Z. Ernahrungswiss., 36, 3–11

Boeing, H., Weisgerber, U.M., Jeckel, A., Rose, H.J. & Kroke, A. (2000) Association between glycated hemoglobin and diet and other lifestyle factors in a nondiabetic population: cross-sectional evaluation of data from the Potsdam cohort of the European Prospective Investigation into Cancer and Nutrition Study. *Am. J. Clin. Nutr.*, **71**, 1115–1122

Boissonneault, G.A., Elson, C.E. & Pariza, M.W. (1986) Net energy effects of dietary fat on chemically induced mammary carcinogenesis in F344 rats. *J. Natl Cancer Inst.*, **76**, 335–338

Bona, G., Petri, A., Rapa, A., Conti, A. & Sartorio, A. (1999) The impact of gender, puberty and body mass on reference values for urinary growth hormone (GH) excretion in normally growing non-obese and obese children. *Clin. Endocrinol. (Oxf.)*, **50**, 775–781

Bonen, A. (1992) Recreational exercise does not impair menstrual cycles: a prospective study. *Int. J. Sports Med.*, **13**, 110–120

Bonen, A. (1995) Benefits of exercise for type II diabetics: convergence of epidemiologic, physiologic, and molecular evidence. *Can. J. Appl. Physiol.*, **20**, 261–279

Bonnefoy, M., Kostka, T., Patricot, M.C., Berthouze, S.E., Mathian, B. & Lacour, J.R. (1999) Influence of acute and chronic exercise on insulin-like growth factor-I in healthy active elderly men and women. *Aging (Milano)*, **11**, 373–379

Booth, M.L., Hunter, C., Gore, C.J., Bauman, A. & Owen, N. (2000) The relationship between body mass index and waist circumference: implications for estimates of the population prevalence of overweight. *Int. J. Obes. Relat. Metab. Disord.*, **24**, 1058–1061

Borghouts, L.B. & Keizer, H.A. (2000) Exercise and insulin sensitivity: a review. *Int. J. Sports Med.*, **21**, 1–12

Bosland, M.C. (2000) The role of steroid hormones in prostate carcinogenesis. *J. Natl Cancer Inst. Monogr.*, **27**, 39–66

Bostick, R.M., Potter, J.D., Kushi, L.H., Sellers, T.A., Steinmetz, K.A., McKenzie, D.R., Gapstur, S.M. & Folsom, A.R. (1994) Sugar, meat, and fat intake, and non-dietary risk factors for colon cancer incidence in Iowa women (United States). *Cancer Causes Control*, **5**, 38–52

Bouchard, C. (1994) Genetics of obesity: overview and research directions. In: Bouchard, C., ed., *The Genetics of Obesity*, Boca Raton, CRC Press, pp. 223–233

Bouchardy, C., Lê, M.G. & Hill, C. (1990) Risk factors for breast cancer according to age at diagnosis in a French case-control study. *J. Clin. Epidemiol.*, **43**, 267–275

Boutwell, R.K., Brush, M.K. & Rusch, H.P. (1948) Some physiological effects associated with chronic caloric restriction. *Am. J. Physiol.*, **154**, 517

Boutwell, R.K., Brush, M.K. & Rusch, H.P. (1949) The stimulating effect of dietary fat on carcinogenesis. *Cancer Res.*, **9**, 741–746

Boyar, A.P., Rose, D.P., Loughridge, J.R., Engle, A., Palgi, A., Laakso, K., Kinne, D. & Wynder, E.L. (1988) Response to a diet low in total fat in women with postmenopausal breast cancer: a pilot study. *Nutr. Cancer*, **11**, 93–99

Boyd, N.F., Greenberg, C., Lockwood, G., Little, L., Martin, L., Byng, J., Yaffe, M. & Tritchler, D. (1997) Effects at two years of a low-fat, high-carbohydrate diet on radiologic features of the breast: results from a randomized trial. Canadian Diet and Breast Cancer Prevention Study Group. *J. Natl Cancer Inst.*, **89**, 488–496

Boyle, C.A., Dobson, A.J., Egger, G. & Magnus, P. (1994) Can the increasing weight of Australians be explained by the decreasing prevalence of cigarette smoking? *Int. J. Obes. Relat. Metab. Disord.*, **18**, 55–60

Bradlow, H.L., Hershcopf, R.E. & Fishman, J.F. (1986) Oestradiol 16 α-hydroxylase: a risk marker for breast cancer. *Cancer Surv.*, **5**, 573–583

Bratusch-Marrain, P.R., Smith, D. & DeFronzo, R.A. (1982) The effect of growth hormone on glucose metabolism and insulin secretion in man. *J. Clin. Endocrinol. Metab.*, **55**, 973–982

Brind, J., Strain, G., Miller, L., Zumoff, B., Vogelman, J. & Orentreich, N. (1990) Obese men have elevated plasma levels of estrone sulfate. *Int. J. Obes.*, **14**, 483–486

Brinton, L.A. & Swanson, C.A. (1992) Height and weight at various ages and risk of breast cancer. *Ann. Epidemiol.*, **2**, 597–609

Brinton, L.A., Berman, M.L., Mortel, R., Twiggs, L.B., Barrett, R.J., Wilbanks, G.D., Lannom, L. & Hoover, R.N. (1992) Reproductive, menstrual, and medical risk factors for endometrial cancer: results from a case-control study. *Am. J. Obstet. Gynecol.*, **167**, 1317–1325

Brown, L.M., Swanson, C.A., Gridley, G., Swanson, G.M., Schoenberg, J.B., Greenberg, R.S., Silverman, D.T., Pottern, L.M., Hayes, R.B., Schwartz, A.G., Liff, J.M., Fraumeni, J.F., Jr & Hoover, R.N. (1995) Adenocarcinoma of the esophagus: role of obesity and diet. *J. Natl Cancer Inst.*, **87**, 104–109

Brown, S.A., Upchurch, S., Anding, R., Winter, M. & Ramirez, G. (1996) Promoting weight loss in type II diabetes. *Diabetes Care*, **19**, 613–624

Brown, C.D., Higgins, M., Donato, K.A., Rohde, F.C., Garrison, R., Obarzanek, E., Ernst, N.D. & Horan, M. (2000) Body mass index and the prevalence of hypertension and dyslipidemia. *Obes. Res.*, **8**, 605–619

Brownson, R.C., Zahm, S.H., Chang, J.C. & Blair, A. (1989) Occupational risk of colon cancer. An analysis by anatomic subsite. *Am. J. Epidemiol.*, **130**, 675–687

Brownson, R.C., Chang, J.C., Davis, J.R. & Smith, C.A. (1991) Physical activity on the job and cancer in Missouri. *Am. J. Public Health*, **81**, 639–642

Brownson, R.C., Smith, C.A., Pratt, M., Mack, N.E., Jackson-Thompson, J., Dean, C.G., Dabney, S. & Wilkerson, J.C. (1996) Preventing cardiovascular disease through community-based risk reduction: the Bootheel Heart Health Project. *Am. J. Public Health*, **86**, 206–213

Bruning, P.F., Bonfrer, J.M., Hart, A.A., Van Noord, P.A., van der Hoeven, H., Collette, H.J., Battermann, J.J., Jong-Bakker, M., Nooijen, W.J. & de Waard, F. (1992a) Body measurements, estrogen availability and the risk of human breast cancer: a case-control study. *Int. J. Cancer*, **51**, 14–19

Bruning, P.F., Bonfrer, J.M., Van Noord, P.A., Hart, A.A., Jong-Bakker, M. & Nooijen, W.J. (1992b) Insulin resistance and breast-cancer risk. *Int. J. Cancer*, **52**, 511–516

Bruning, P.F., Van Doorn, J., Bonfrer, J.M., Van Noord, P.A., Korse, C.M., Linders, T.C. & Hart, A.A. (1995) Insulin-like growth-factor-binding protein 3 is decreased in early-stage operable pre-menopausal breast cancer. *Int. J. Cancer*, **62**, 266–270

Bruunsgaard, H., Hartkopp, A., Mohr, T., Konradsen, H., Heron, I., Mordhorst, C.H. & Pedersen, B.K. (1997) *In vivo* cell-mediated immunity and vaccination response following prolonged, intense exercise. *Med. Sci. Sports Exerc.*, **29**, 1176–1181

Buckwalter, J.A. & Lane, N.E. (1997) Athletics and osteoarthritis. *Am. J. Sports Med.*, **25**, 873–881

Buemann, B. & Tremblay, A. (1996) Effects of exercise training on abdominal obesity and related metabolic complications. *Sports Med.*, **21**, 191–212

Bueno de Mesquita, H.B., Moerman, C.J., Runia, S. & Maisonneuve, P. (1990) Are energy and energy-providing nutrients related to exocrine carcinoma of the pancreas? *Int. J. Cancer*, **46**, 435–444

Build and Blood Pressure Study (1959) Chicago, Society of Actuaries

Build and Blood Pressure Study 1979 (1980) Chicago, Society of Actuaries and Association of Life Insurance Medical Directors of America

Bullen, B.A., Skrinar, G.S., Beitins, I.Z., Carr, D.B., Reppert, S.M., Dotson, C.O., Fencl, M.D., Gervino, E.V. & McArthur, J.W. (1984) Endurance training effects on plasma hormonal responsiveness and sex hormone excretion. *J. Appl. Physiol.*, **56**, 1453–1463

Bullen, B.A., Skrinar, G.S., Beitins, I.Z., von Mering, G., Turnbull, B.A. & McArthur, J.W. (1985) Induction of menstrual disorders by strenuous exercise in untrained women. *New Engl. J. Med.*, **312**, 1349–1353

Burghen, G.A., Givens, J.R. & Kitabchi, A.E. (1980) Correlation of hyperandrogenism with hyperinsulinism in polycystic ovarian disease. *J. Clin. Endocrinol. Metab.,* **50**, 113–116

Burks, D.J., de Mora, J.F., Schubert, M., Withers, D.J., Myers, M.G., Towery, H.H., Altamuro, S.L., Flint, C.L. & White, M.F. (2000) IRS-2 pathways integrate female reproduction and energy homeostasis. *Nature*, **407**, 377–382

Burnet, F.M. (1970) The concept of immunological surveillance. *Prog. Exp. Tumor Res.,* **13**, 1–27

Burroughs, K.D., Dunn, S.E., Barrett, J.C. & Taylor, J.A. (1999) Insulin-like growth factor-I: a key regulator of human cancer risk? *J. Natl Cancer Inst.*, **91**, 579–581

Butkus, J.A., Brogan, R.S., Giustina, A., Kastello, G., Sothmann, M. & Wehrenberg, W.B. (1995) Changes in the growth hormone axis due to exercise training in male and female rats: secretory and molecular responses. *Endocrinology*, **136**, 2664–2670

Byers, T., Marshall, J., Graham, S., Mettlin, C. & Swanson, M. (1983) A case-control study of dietary and nondietary factors in ovarian cancer. *J. Natl Cancer Inst.*, **71**, 681–686

Caan, B.J., Coates, A.O., Slattery, M.L., Potter, J.D., Quesenberry, C.P., Jr & Edwards, S.M. (1998) Body size and the risk of colon cancer in a large case-control study. *Int. J. Obes. Relat. Metab. Disord.*, **22**, 178–184

Calle, E.E., Miracle-McMahill, H.L., Thun, M.J. & Heath, C.W., Jr (1995) Estrogen replacement therapy and risk of fatal colon cancer in a prospective cohort of postmenopausal women. *J. Natl Cancer Inst.*, **87**, 517–523

Calle, E.E., Murphy, T.K., Rodriguez, C., Thun, M.J. & Heath, C.W. Jr (1998a) Occupation and breast cancer mortality in a prospective cohort of US women. *Am. J. Epidemiol.*, **148**, 191–197

Calle, E.E., Murphy, T.K., Rodriguez, C., Thun, M.J. & Heath, C.W. Jr (1998b) Diabetes mellitus and pancreatic cancer mortality in a prospective cohort of United States adults. *Cancer Causes Control*, **9**, 403–410

Calle, E.E., Thun, M.J., Petrelli, J.M., Rodriguez, C. & Heath, C.W., Jr (1999) Body-mass index and mortality in a prospective cohort of U.S. adults. *New Engl. J. Med.*, **341**, 1097–1105

Camargo, C.A., Jr, Weiss, S.T., Zhang, S., Willett, W.C. & Speizer, F.E. (1999) Prospective study of body mass index, weight change, and risk of adult-onset asthma in women. *Arch. Intern. Med.*, **159**, 2582–2588

Camoriano, J.K., Loprinzi, C.L., Ingle, J.N., Therneau, T.M., Krook, J.E. & Veeder, M.H. (1990) Weight change in women treated with adjuvant therapy or observed following mastectomy for node-positive breast cancer. *J. Clin. Oncol.*, **8**, 1327–1334

Cann, C.E., Martin, M.C., Genant, H.K. & Jaffe, R.B. (1984) Decreased spinal mineral content in amenorrheic women. *JAMA*, **251**, 626–629

Cappon, J., Brasel, J.A., Mohan, S. & Cooper, D.M. (1994) Effect of brief exercise on circulating insulin-like growth factor I. *J. Appl. Physiol.*, **76**, 2490–2496

Cappuccio, F.P. (1997) Ethnicity and cardio-vascular risk: variations in people of African ancestry and South Asian origin. *J. Hum. Hypertens.*, **11**, 571–576

Caprio, S., Plewe, G., Diamond, M.P., Simonson, D.C., Boulware, S.D., Sherwin, R.S. & Tamborlane, W.V. (1989) Increased insulin secretion in puberty: a compensatory response to reductions in insulin sensitivity. *J. Pediatr.*, **114**, 963–967

Carpenter, C.L., Ross, R.K., Paganini-Hill, A. & Bernstein, L. (1999) Lifetime exercise activity and breast cancer risk among post-menopausal women. *Br. J. Cancer*, **80**, 1852–1858

Cartee, G.D. (1994) Aging skeletal muscle: response to exercise. *Exerc. Sport Sci. Rev.*, **22**, 91–120

Casagrande, J.T., Louie, E.W., Pike, M.C., Roy, S., Ross, R.K. & Henderson, B.E. (1979) "Incessant ovulation" and ovarian cancer. *Lancet*, **2**, 170–173

CASH (1987) The reduction in risk of ovarian cancer associated with oral-contraceptive use. The Cancer and Steroid Hormone Study of the Centers for Disease Control and the National Institute of Child Health and Human Development. *New Engl. J. Med.*, **316**, 650–655

Caspersen, C.J. (1989) Physical activity epidemiology: concepts, methods, and applications to exercise science. *Exerc. Sport Sci. Rev.*, **17**, 423–473

Caspersen, C.J. (1994) What are the lessons from the US approach to setting targets? In: Killoran, A.J., Fentem, P. & Caspersen, C.J., eds, *Moving on: International Perspectives on Promoting Physical Activity,* London, Health Education Authority, pp. 35–55

Caspersen, C.J., Powell, K.E. & Christenson, G.M. (1985) Physical activity, exercise, and physical fitness: definitions and distinctions for health-related research. *Public Health Rep.*, **100**, 126–131

Caspersen, C.J., Merritt, R.K. & Stephens, T. (1994) International physical activity patterns: A methodological perspective. In: Dishman, R.K., ed., *Advances in Exercise Adherence*, Champaign, Human Kinetics Publishers, pp. 71–110

Caspersen, C.J., Pereira, M.A. & Curran, K.M. (2000) Changes in physical activity patterns in the United States, by sex and cross-sectional age. *Med. Sci. Sports Exerc.*, **32**, 1601–1609

Caufriez, A., Golstein, J., Lebrun, P., Herchuelz, A., Furlanetto, R. & Copinschi, G. (1984) Relations between immunoreactive somato-medin C, insulin and T3 patterns during fasting in obese subjects. *Clin. Endocrinol. (Oxf.)*, **20**, 65–70

Cauley, J.A., Gutai, J.P., Kuller, L.H., LeDonne, D. & Powell, J.G. (1989) The epidemiology of serum sex hormones in postmenopausal women. *Am. J. Epidemiol.*, **129**, 1120–1131

Centers for Disease Control (1997) Monthly estimates of leisure-time physical inactivity—United States, 1994. *MMWR Morb. Mortal. Wkly Rep.*, **46**, 393–397

Cerhan, J.R., Torner, J.C., Lynch, C.F., Rubenstein, L.M., Lemke, J.H., Cohen, M.B., Lubaroff, D.M. & Wallace, R.B. (1997) Association of smoking, body mass, and physical activity with risk of prostate cancer in the Iowa 65+ Rural Health Study (United States). *Cancer Causes Control*, **8**, 229–238

Chadan, S.G., Dill, R.P., Vanderhoek, K. & Parkhouse, W.S. (1999) Influence of physical activity on plasma insulin-like growth factor-1 and insulin-like growth factor binding proteins in healthy older women. *Mech. Ageing Dev.*, **109**, 21–34

Chagnon, Y.C., Pérusse, L., Weisnagel, S.J., Rankinen, T. & Bouchard, C. (2000) The human obesity gene map: the 1999 update. *Obes. Res.*, **8**, 89–117

Chan, J.M., Stampfer, M.J., Giovannucci, E., Gann, P.H., Ma, J., Wilkinson, P., Hennekens, C.H. & Pollak, M. (1998) Plasma insulin-like growth factor-I and prostate cancer risk: a prospective study. *Science*, **279**, 563–566

Chandra, R.K. & Kutty, K.M. (1980) Immunocompetence in obesity. *Acta Paediatr. Scand.*, **69**, 25–30

Chang, W.Y. & Prins, G.S. (1999) Estrogen receptor-β: implications for the prostate gland. *Prostate*, **40**, 115–124

Chang, R.J., Laufer, L.R., Meldrum, D.R., DeFazio, J., Lu, J.K., Vale, W.W., Rivier, J.E. & Judd, H.L. (1983) Steroid secretion in polycystic ovarian disease after ovarian suppression by a long-acting gonadotropin-releasing hormone agonist. *J. Clin. Endocrinol. Metab.*, **56**, 897–903

Chao, D., Espeland, M.A., Farmer, D., Register, T.C., Lenchik, L., Applegate, W.B. & Ettinger, W.H. (2000) Effect of voluntary weight loss on bone mineral density in older overweight

women. *J. Am. Geriatr. Soc.*, **48**, 753–759

Chapin, R.E., Gulati, D.K., Barnes, L.H. & Teague, J.L. (1993) The effects of feed restriction on reproductive function in Sprague-Dawley rats. *Fundam. Appl. Toxicol.*, **20**, 23–29

Chapman, I.M., Hartman, M.L., Pieper, K.S., Skiles, E.H., Pezzoli, S.S., Hintz, R.L. & Thorner, M.O. (1998) Recovery of growth hormone release from suppression by exogenous insulin-like growth factor I (IGF-I): evidence for a suppressive action of free rather than bound IGF-I. *J. Clin. Endocrinol. Metab.*, **83**, 2836–2842

Chasan-Taber, S., Rimm, E.B., Stampfer, M.J., Spiegelman, D., Colditz, G.A., Giovannucci, E., Ascherio, A. & Willett, W.C. (1996) Reproducibility and validity of a self-administered physical activity questionnaire for male health professionals. *Epidemiology*, **7**, 81–86

Chaturvedi, N. & Fuller, J.H. (1995) Mortality risk by body weight and weight change in people with NIDDM. The WHO Multinational Study of Vascular Disease in Diabetes. *Diabetes Care*, **18**, 766–774

Chen, J., Campbell, T.C., Junyao, L. & Peto, R. (1990) *Diet, Life-Style, and Mortality in China: A Study of the Characteristics of 65 Chinese Counties*, Oxford, Oxford University Press

Chen, W., Nichols, J., Zhou, Y., Chung, K.T., Hart, R.W. & Chou, M.W. (1995) Effect of dietary restriction on glutathione S-transferase activity specific toward aflatoxin B1-8,9-epoxide. *Toxicol. Lett*, **78**, 235–243

Chen, W., Zhou, Y., Nichols, J., Chung, K.T., Hart, R.W. & Chou, M.W. (1996) Effect of dietary restriction on benzo[a]pyrene (BaP) metabolic activation and pulmonary BaP-DNA adduct formation in mouse. *Drug Chem. Toxicol.*, **19**, 21–39

Chen, C.L., White, E., Malone, K.E. & Daling, J.R. (1997) Leisure-time physical activity in relation to breast cancer among young women (Washington, United States). *Cancer Causes Control*, **8**, 77–84

Cheney, K.E., Liu, R.K., Smith, G.S., Meredith, P.J., Mickey, M.R. & Walford, R.L. (1983) The effect of dietary restriction of varying duration on survival, tumor patterns, immune function, and body temperature in B10C3F1 female mice. *J. Gerontol.*, **38**, 420–430

Cheng, K.K., Sharp, L., McKinney, P.A., Logan, R.F., Chilvers, C.E., Cook-Mozaffari, P., Ahmed, A. & Day, N.E. (2000) A case-control study of oesophageal adenocarcinoma in women: a preventable disease. *Br J Cancer*, **83**, 127–132

Chiappelli, F., Gwirtsman, H.E., Lowy, M., Gormley, G., Nguyen, L.D., Nguyen, L., Popow, J., Esmail, I., Fahey, J.L. & Strober, M. (1991) Pituitary-adrenal-immune system in normal subjects and in patients with anorexia nervosa: the number of circulating helper T lymphocytes (CD4) expressing the homing receptor Leu8 is regulated in part by pituitary-adrenal products. *Psychoneuroendocrinology*, **16**, 423–432

Chie, W.C., Chen, C.F., Lee, W.C. & Chen, C.J. (1996) Body size and risk of pre- and post-menopausal breast cancer in Taiwan. *Anticancer Res.*, **16**, 3129–3132

Chie, W.C., Li, C.Y., Huang, C.S., Chang, K.J. & Lin, R.S. (1998) Body size as a factor in different ages and breast cancer risk in Taiwan. *Anticancer Res.*, **18**, 565–570

Ching, P.L., Willett, W.C., Rimm, E.B., Colditz, G.A., Gortmaker, S.L. & Stampfer, M.J. (1996) Activity level and risk of overweight in male health professionals. *Am. J. Public Health*, **86**, 25–30

Choban, P.S., Onyejekwe, J., Burge, J.C. & Flancbaum, L. (1999) A health status assessment of the impact of weight loss following Roux-en-Y gastric bypass for clinically severe obesity. *J. Am. Coll. Surg.*, **188**, 491–497

Chou, M.W., Kong, J., Chung, K.T. & Hart, R.W. (1993a) Effect of caloric restriction on the metabolic activation of xenobiotics. *Mutat. Res.*, **295**, 223–235

Chou, M.W., Pegram, R.A., Turturro, A., Holson, R. & Hart, R.W. (1993b) Effect of caloric restriction on the induction of hepatic cytochrome P-450 and Ah receptor binding in C57BL/6N and DBA/2J mice. *Drug Chem. Toxicol.*, **16**, 1–19

Chou, M.W., Chen, W., Mikhailova, M.V., Nichols, J., Weis, C., Jackson, C.D., Hart, R.W. & Chung, K.T. (1997) Dietary restriction modulated carcinogen-DNA adduct formation and the carcinogen-induced DNA strand breaks. *Toxicol. Lett.*, **92**, 21–30

Chow, W.H., Dosemeci, M., Zheng, W., Vetter, R., McLaughlin, J.K., Gao, Y.T. & Blot, W.J. (1993) Physical activity and occupational risk of colon cancer in Shanghai, China. *Int. J. Epidemiol.*, **22**, 23–29

Chow, W.H., Malker, H.S., Hsing, A.W., McLaughlin, J.K., Weiner, J.A., Stone, B.J., Ericsson, J.L. & Blot, W.J. (1994) Occupational risks for colon cancer in Sweden. *J. Occup. Med*, **36**, 647–651

Chow, W.H., Finkle, W.D., McLaughlin, J.K., Frankl, H., Ziel, H.K. & Fraumeni, J.F. (1995) The relation of gastroesophageal reflux disease and its treatment to adenocarcinomas of the esophagus and gastric cardia. *JAMA*, **274**, 474–477

Chow, W.H., McLaughlin, J.K., Mandel, J.S., Wacholder, S., Niwa, S. & Fraumeni, J.F., Jr (1996) Obesity and risk of renal cell cancer. *Cancer Epidemiol. Biomarkers Prev.*, **5**, 17–21

Chow, W.H., Blot, W.J., Vaughan, T.L., Risch, H.A., Gammon, M.D., Stanford, J.L., Dubrow, R., Schoenberg, J.B., Mayne, S.T., Farrow, D.C., Ahsan, H., West, A.B., Rotterdam, H., Niwa, S. & Fraumeni, J.F., Jr (1998) Body mass index and risk of adenocarcinomas of the esophagus and gastric cardia. *J. Natl Cancer Inst.*, **90**, 150–155

Chow, W.H., Gridley, G., Fraumeni, J.F., Jr & Järvholm, B. (2000) Obesity, hypertension, and the risk of kidney cancer in men. *New Engl. J. Med.*, **343**, 1305–1311

Chu, S.Y., Lee, N.C., Wingo, P.A., Senie, R.T., Greenberg, R.S. & Peterson, H.B. (1991) The relationship between body mass and breast cancer among women enrolled in the Cancer and Steroid Hormone Study. *J. Clin. Epidemiol.*, **44**, 1197–1206

Chung, M.H., Kasai, H., Nishimura, S. & Yu, B.P. (1992) Protection of DNA damage by dietary restriction. *Free Radic. Biol. Med.*, **12**, 523–525

Chyou, P.H., Nomura, A.M. & Stemmermann, G.N. (1994) A prospective study of weight, body mass index and other anthropometric measurements in relation to site-specific cancers. *Int. J. Cancer*, **57**, 313–317

Cigolini, M., Seidell, J.C., Targher, G., Deslypere, J.P., Ellsinger, B.M., Charzewska, J., Cruz, A. & Björntorp, P. (1995) Fasting serum insulin in relation to components of the metabolic syndrome in European healthy men: the European Fat Distribution Study. *Metabolism*, **44**, 35–40

Clarke, G. & Whittemore, A.S. (2000) Prostate cancer risk in relation to anthropometry and physical activity: the National Health and Nutrition Examination Survey I

Epidemiological Follow-Up Study. *Cancer Epidemiol. Biomarkers Prev.*, **9**, 875–881

Clemmons, D.R. & Underwood, L.E. (1991) Nutritional regulation of IGF-I and IGF binding proteins. *Annu. Rev. Nutr.*, **11**, 393–412

Clemmons, D.R., Klibanski, A., Underwood, L.E., McArthur, J.W., Ridgway, E.C., Beitins, I.Z. & Van Wyk, J.J. (1981) Reduction of plasma immunoreactive somatomedin C during fasting in humans. *J. Clin. Endocrinol. Metab.*, **53**, 1247–1250

Clemmons, D.R., Snyder, D.K. & Busby, W.H. (1991) Variables controlling the secretion of insulin-like growth factor binding protein-2 in normal human subjects. *J. Clin. Endocrinol. Metab.*, **73**, 727–733

Coakley, E.H., Rimm, E.B., Colditz, G., Kawachi, I. & Willett, W. (1998) Predictors of weight change in men: results from the Health Professionals Follow-up Study. *Int. J. Obes. Relat. Metab. Disord.*, **22**, 89–96

Coates, R.J., Clark, W.S., Eley, J.W., Greenberg, R.S., Huguley, C.M., Jr & Brown, R.L. (1990) Race, nutritional status, and survival from breast cancer. *J. Natl Cancer Inst.*, **82**, 1684–1692

Coates, R.J., Uhler, R.J., Hall, H.I., Potischman, N., Brinton, L.A., Ballard-Barbash, R., Gammon, M.D., Brogan, D.R., Daling, J.R., Malone, K.E., Schoenberg, J.B. & Swanson, C.A. (1999) Risk of breast cancer in young women in relation to body size and weight gain in adolescence and early adulthood. *Br. J. Cancer*, **81**, 167–174

Coenen, C., Wegener, M., Wedmann, B., Schmidt, G. & Hoffmann, S. (1992) Does physical exercise influence bowel transit time in healthy young men? *Am. J. Gastroenterol.*, **87**, 292–295

Cohen, N.D. & Hilf, R. (1974) Influence of insulin on growth and metabolism of 7,12-dimethylbenz(alpha)anthracene-induced mammary tumors. *Cancer Res.*, **34**, 3245–3252

Cohen, L.A., Choi, K.W. & Wang, C.X. (1988) Influence of dietary fat, caloric restriction, and voluntary exercise on N-nitrosomethylurea-induced mammary tumorigenesis in rats. *Cancer Res.*, **48**, 4276–4283

Cohen, L.A., Choi, K., Backlund, J.Y., Harris, R. & Wang, C.X. (1991) Modulation of N-nitrosomethylurea induced mammary tumorigenesis by dietary fat and voluntary exercise. *In Vivo*, **5**, 333–344

Cohen, L.A., Boylan, E., Epstein, M. & Zang, E. (1992) Voluntary exercise and experimental mammary cancer. *Adv Exp Med Biol*, **322**, 41–59

Cohen, L.A., Kendall, M.E., Meschter, C., Epstein, M.A., Reinhardt, J. & Zang, E. (1993) Inhibition of rat mammary tumorigenesis by voluntary exercise. *In Vivo*, **7**, 151–158

Coiro, V., Passeri, M., Capretti, L., Speroni, G., Davoli, C., Marchesi, C., Rossi, G., Camellini, L., Volpi, R., Roti, E. & Chiodera, P. (1990) Serotonergic control of TSH and PRL secretion in obese men. *Psychoneuroendocrinology*, **15**, 261–268

Colbert, L.H., Davis, J.M., Essig, D.A., Ghaffar, A. & Mayer, E.P. (2000a) Exercise and tumor development in a mouse predisposed to multiple intestinal adenomas. *Med. Sci. Sports Exerc.*, **32**, 1704–1708

Colbert, L.H., Hootman, J.M. & Macera, C.A. (2000b) Physical activity-related injuries in walkers and runners in the aerobics center longitudinal study. *Clin. J. Sport Med.*, **10**, 259–263

Colditz, G.A., Willett, W.C., Stampfer, M.J., Manson, J.E., Hennekens, C.H., Arky, R.A. & Speizer, F.E. (1990) Weight as a risk factor for clinical diabetes in women. *Am. J. Epidemiol.*, **132**, 501–513

Cole, T.J., Bellizzi, M.C., Flegal, K.M. & Dietz, W.H. (2000) Establishing a standard definition for child overweight and obesity worldwide: international survey. *BMJ*, **320**, 1240–1243

Collaborative Group on Hormonal Factors in Breast Cancer (1997) Breast cancer and hormone replacement therapy: collaborative reanalysis of data from 51 epidemiological studies of 52,705 women with breast cancer and 108,411 women without breast cancer. *Lancet*, **350**, 1047–1059

Colman, E., Katzel, L.I., Rogus, E., Coon, P., Muller, D. & Goldberg, A.P. (1995) Weight loss reduces abdominal fat and improves insulin action in middle-aged and older men with impaired glucose tolerance. *Metabolism*, **44**, 1502–1508

Compston, J.E., Laskey, M.A., Croucher, P.I., Coxon, A. & Kreitzman, S. (1992) Effect of diet-induced weight loss on total body bone mass. *Clin. Sci. (Colch.)*, **82**, 429–432

Connelly, J.B., Cooper, J.A. & Meade, T.W. (1992) Strenuous exercise, plasma fibrinogen, and factor VII activity. *Br. Heart J.*, **67**, 351–354

Conover, C.A. & Lee, P.D. (1990) Insulin regulation of insulin-like growth factor-binding protein production in cultured HepG2 cells. *J. Clin. Endocrinol. Metab.*, **70**, 1062–1067

Conover, C.A., Lee, P.D., Kanaley, J.A., Clarkson, J.T. & Jensen, M.D. (1992) Insulin regulation of insulin-like growth factor binding protein-1 in obese and nonobese humans. *J. Clin. Endocrinol. Metab.*, **74**, 1355–1360

Constantini, N.W. & Warren, M.P. (1994) Special problems of the female athlete. *Baillieres Clin. Rheumatol.*, **8**, 199–219

Coogan, P.F. & Aschengrau, A. (1999) Occupational physical activity and breast cancer risk in the upper Cape Cod cancer incidence study. *Am. J. Ind. Med.*, **36**, 279–285

Coogan, P.F., Clapp, R.W., Newcomb, P.A., Mittendorf, R., Bogdan, G., Baron, J.A. & Longnecker, M.P. (1996) Variation in female breast cancer risk by occupation. *Am. J. Ind. Med.*, **30**, 430–437

Coogan, P.F., Newcomb, P.A., Clapp, R.W., Trentham-Dietz, A., Baron, J.A. & Longnecker, M.P. (1997) Physical activity in usual occupation and risk of breast cancer (United States). *Cancer Causes Control*, **8**, 626–631

Cooper, C., Barker, D.J. & Wickham, C. (1988) Physical activity, muscle strength, and calcium intake in fracture of the proximal femur in Britain. *BMJ*, **297**, 1443–1446

Cook, J.C., Klinefelter, G.R., Hardisty, J.F., Sharpe, R.M. & Foster, P.M. (1999) Rodent Leydig cell tumorigenesis: a review of the physiology, pathology, mechanisms, and relevance to humans. *Crit. Rev. Toxicol.*, **29**, 169–261

Copeland, K.C., Colletti, R.B., Devlin, J.T. & McAuliffe, T.L. (1990) The relationship between insulin-like growth factor-I, adiposity, and aging. *Metabolism*, **39**, 584–587

Cordain, L., Latin, R.W. & Behnke, J.J. (1986) The effects of an aerobic running program on bowel transit time. *J. Sports Med. Phys. Fitness*, **26**, 101–104

Cottreau, C.M., Ness, R.B., Kriska, A.M. (2000) Physical activity and reduced risk of ovarian cancer. *Obstet. Gynecol.*, **96**, 609–614

Coughlin, S.S., Neaton, J.D., Randall, B. & Sengupta, A. (1997) Predictors of mortality from kidney cancer in 332,547 men screened for the Multiple Risk Factor Intervention Trial. *Cancer*, **79**, 2171–2177

Coulam, C.B., Annegers, J.F. & Kranz, J.S. (1983) Chronic anovulation syndrome and associated neoplasia. *Obstet. Gynecol.*, **61**, 403–407

Counts, D.R., Gwirtsman, H., Carlsson, L.M., Lesem, M. & Cutler, G.B. (1992) The effect of anorexia nervosa and refeeding on growth hormone-binding protein, the insulin-like growth factors (IGFs), and the IGF-binding proteins. *J. Clin. Endocrinol. Metab.*, **75**, 762–767

Cramer, D.W. & Welch, W.R. (1983) Determinants of ovarian cancer risk. II. Inferences regarding pathogenesis. *J. Natl Cancer Inst.*, **71**, 717–721

Cramer, D.W., Hutchison, G.B., Welch, W.R., Scully, R.E. & Ryan, K.J. (1983) Determinants of ovarian cancer risk. I. Reproductive experiences and family history. *J. Natl Cancer Inst.*, **71**, 711–716

Crandall, C.J. (1999) Estrogen replacement therapy and colon cancer: a clinical review. *J. Womens Health Gend. Based Med.*, **8**, 1155–1166

Crave, J.C., Lejeune, H., Brébant, C., Baret, C. & Pugeat, M. (1995a) Differential effects of insulin and insulin-like growth factor I on the production of plasma steroid-binding globulins by human hepatoblastoma-derived (Hep G2) cells. *J. Clin. Endocrinol. Metab.*, **80**, 1283–1289

Crave, J.C., Fimbel, S., Lejeune, H., Cugnardey, N., Déchaud, H. & Pugeat, M. (1995b) Effects of diet and metformin administration on sex hormone-binding globulin, androgens, and insulin in hirsute and obese women. *J. Clin. Endocrinol. Metab.*, **80**, 2057–2062

Craven-Giles, T., Tagliaferro, A.R., Ronan, A.M., Baumgartner, K.J. & Roebuck, B.D. (1994) Dietary modulation of pancreatic carcinogenesis: calories and energy expenditure. *Cancer Res.*, **54**, 1964s–1968s

Crawford, D.A., Jeffery, R.W. & French, S.A. (1999) Television viewing, physical inactivity and obesity. *Int. J. Obes. Relat. Metab. Disord.*, **23**, 437–440

Cummings, S.R., Nevitt, M.C., Browner, W.S., Stone, K., Fox, K.M., Ensrud, K.E., Cauley, J., Black, D. & Vogt, T.M. (1995) Risk factors for hip fracture in white women. Study of Osteoporotic Fractures Research Group. *New Engl. J. Med.*, **332**, 767-773

Curtis, A.B., Strogatz, D.S., James, S.A. & Raghunathan, T.E. (1998) The contribution of baseline weight and weight gain to blood pressure change in African Americans: the Pitt County Study. *Ann. Epidemiol.*, **8**, 497-503

Dahlgren, E., Friberg, L.G., Johansson, S., Lindström, B., Odén, A., Samsioe, G. & Janson, P.O. (1991) Endometrial carcinoma; ovarian dysfunction — a risk factor in young women. *Eur. J. Obstet. Gynecol. Reprod. Biol.*, **41**, 143–150

Dal Maso, L., La Vecchia, C., Franceschi, S., Preston-Martin, S., Ron, E., Levi, F., Mack, W., Mark, S.D., McTiernan, A., Kolonel, L., Mabuchi, K., Jin, F., Wingren, G., Galanti, M.R., Hallquist, A., Glattre, E., Lund, E., Linos, D. & Negri, E. (2000) A pooled analysis of thyroid cancer studies. V. Anthropometric factors. *Cancer Causes Control*, **11**, 137–144

Daneryd, P.L., Hafstrom, L.R. & Karlberg, I.H. (1990) Effects of spontaneous physical exercise on experimental cancer anorexia and cachexia. *Eur. J. Cancer*, **26**, 1083–1088

Dattilo, A.M. & Kris-Etherton, P.M. (1992) Effects of weight reduction on blood lipids and lipoproteins: a meta-analysis. *Am. J. Clin. Nutr.*, **56**, 320–328

D'Avanzo, B., La Vecchia, C., Talamini, R. & Franceschi, S. (1996a) Anthropometric measures and risk of cancers of the upper digestive and respiratory tract. *Nutr. Cancer*, **26**, 219–227

D'Avanzo, B., Nanni, O., La Vecchia, C., Franceschi, S., Negri, E., Giacosa, A., Conti, E., Montella, M., Talamini, R. & Decarli, A. (1996b) Physical activity and breast cancer risk. *Cancer Epidemiol. Biomarkers Prev.*, **5**, 155–160

Davidow, A.L., Neugut, A.I., Jacobson, J.S., Ahsan, H., Garbowski, G.C., Forde, K.A., Treat, M.R. & Waye, J.D. (1996) Recurrent adenomatous polyps and body mass index. *Cancer Epidemiol. Biomarkers Prev.*, **5**, 313–315

Davidson, M.H., Hauptman, J., DiGirolamo, M., Foreyt, J.P., Halsted, C.H., Heber, D., Heimburger, D.C., Lucas, C.P., Robbins, D.C., Chung, J. & Heymsfield, S.B. (1999) Weight control and risk factor reduction in obese subjects treated for 2 years with orlistat: a randomized controlled trial. *JAMA*, **281**, 235–242

Davis, R.B., Boyd, D.G., McKinney, M.E. & Jones, C.C. (1990) Effects of exercise and exercise conditioning on blood platelet function. *Med. Sci. Sports Exerc.*, **22**, 49–53

Day, G.L., Blot, W.J., Austin, D.F., Bernstein, L., Greenberg, R.S., Preston-Martin, S., Schoenberg, J.B., Winn, D.M., McLaughlin, J.K. & Fraumeni, J.F., Jr (1993) Racial differences in risk of oral and pharyngeal cancer: alcohol, tobacco, and other determinants. *J. Natl Cancer Inst.*, **85**, 465–473

de Castro, J.J., Aleixo Dias, J., Baptista, F., Garcia e Costa, Galvao-Teles, A. & Camilo-Alves, A. (1998) Secular trends of weight, height and obesity in cohorts of young Portuguese males in the District of Lisbon: 1960–1990. *Eur J. Epidemiol.*, **14**, 299–303

De Crée, C., Van Kranenburg, G., Geurten, P., Fujimori, Y. & Keizer, H.A. (1997a) 4-Hydroxycatecholestrogen metabolism responses to exercise and training: possible implications for menstrual cycle irregularities and breast cancer. *Fertil. Steril.*, **67**, 505–516

De Crée, C., Van Kranenburg, G., Geurten, P., Fujimura, Y. & Keizer, H.A. (1997b) Exercise-induced changes in enzymatic O-methylation of catecholestrogens by erythrocytes of eumenorrheic women. *Med. Sci. Sports Exerc.*, **29**, 1580–1587

De Crée, C., Ball, P., Seidlitz, B., Van Kranenburg, G., Geurten, P. & Keizer, H.A. (1997c) Responses of catecholestrogen metabolism to acute graded exercise in normal menstruating women before and after training. *J. Clin. Endocrinol. Metab.*, **82**, 3342–3348

De Pergola, G., Triggiani, V., Giorgino, F., Cospite, M.R., Garruti, G., Cignarelli, M., Guastamacchia, E. & Giorgino, R. (1994) The free testosterone to dehydroepiandrosterone sulphate molar ratio as a marker of visceral fat accumulation in premenopausal obese women. *Int. J. Obes. Relat. Metab. Disord.*, **18**, 659–664

De Pergola, G., Zamboni, M., Pannacciulli, N., Turcato, E., Giorgino, F., Armellini, F.,

Logoluso, F., Sciaraffia, M., Bosello, O. & Giorgino, R. (1998) Divergent effects of short-term, very-low-calorie diet on insulin-like growth factor-I and insulin-like growth factor binding protein-3 serum concentrations in premenopausal women with obesity. *Obes. Res.*, **6**, 408–415

de Ridder, C.M., Bruning, P.F., Zonderland, M.L., Thijssen, J.H., Bonfrer, J.M., Blankenstein, M.A., Huisveld, I.A. & Erich, W.B. (1990) Body fat mass, body fat distribution, and plasma hormones in early puberty in females. *J. Clin. Endocrinol. Metab.*, **70**, 888–893

De Souza, M.J., Arce, J.C., Pescatello, L.S., Scherzer, H.S. & Luciano, A.A. (1994) Gonadal hormones and semen quality in male runners. A volume threshold effect of endurance training. *Int. J. Sports Med.*, **15**, 383–391

De Stavola, B.L., Hardy, R., Kuh, D., dos Santos Silva, I., Wadsworth, M. & Swerdlow, A.J. (2000) Birthweight, childhood growth and risk of breast cancer in a British cohort. *Br. J. Cancer*, **83**, 964–968

de Waard, F. & Baanders-van Halewijn, E.A. (1974) A prospective study in general practice on breast-cancer risk in postmenopausal women. *Int. J. Cancer*, **14**, 153–160

de Waard, F., Ramlau, R., Mulders, Y., de Vries, T. & van Waveren, S. (1993) A feasibility study on weight reduction in obese postmenopausal breast cancer patients. *Eur. J. Cancer Prev.*, **2**, 233–238

Dean, D.J. & Cartee, G.D. (2000) Calorie restriction increases insulin-stimulated tyrosine phosphorylation of insulin receptor and insulin receptor substrate-1 in rat skeletal muscle. *Acta Physiol. Scand.*, **169**, 133–139

Dean, D.J., Gazdag, A.C., Wetter, T.J. & Cartee, G.D. (1998) Comparison of the effects of 20 days and 15 months of calorie restriction on male Fischer 344 rats. *Aging (Milano)*, **10**, 303–307

Decarli, A., Favero, A., La Vecchia, C., Russo, A., Ferraroni, M., Negri, E. & Franceschi, S. (1997) Macronutrients, energy intake, and breast cancer risk: implications from different models. *Epidemiology*, **8**, 425–428

Deeg, D.J.H., Miles, T.P., Van Zonneveld, R.J. & Curb, J.D. (1990) Weight change, survival time and cause of death in Dutch elderly. *Arch. Gerontol. Geriatr.*, **10**, 97–111

DeFronzo, R.A. (1988) Lilly lecture 1987. The triumvirate: β-cell, muscle, liver. A collusion responsible for NIDDM. *Diabetes*, **37**, 667–687

Dekker, R., Kingma, J., Groothoff, J.W., Eisma, W.H. & Ten Duis, H.J. (2000) Measurement of severity of sports injuries: an epidemiological study. *Clin. Rehabil.*, **14**, 651–656

Del Giudice, M.E., Fantus, I.G., Ezzat, S., McKeown-Eyssen, G., Page, D. & Goodwin, P.J. (1998) Insulin and related factors in premenopausal breast cancer risk. *Breast Cancer Res. Treat.*, **47**, 111–120

Demark-Wahnefried, W., Winer, E.P. & Rimer, B.K. (1993) Why women gain weight with adjuvant chemotherapy for breast cancer. *J. Clin. Oncol.*, **11**, 1418–1429

Demark-Wahnefried, W., Rimer, B.K. & Winer, E.P. (1997) Weight gain in women diagnosed with breast cancer. *J. Am. Diet. Assoc.*, **97**, 519–529

Demers, L.M., Harrison, T.S., Halbert, D.R. & Santen, R.J. (1981) Effect of prolonged exercise on plasma prostaglandin levels. *Prostaglandins Med.*, **6**, 413–418

den Tonkelaar, I., Seidell, J.C. & Collette, H.J. (1995a) Body fat distribution in relation to breast cancer in women participating in the DOM-project. *Breast Cancer Res. Treat.*, **34**, 55–61

den Tonkelaar, I., de Waard, F., Seidell, J.C. & Fracheboud, J. (1995b) Obesity and subcutaneous fat patterning in relation to survival of postmenopausal breast cancer patients participating in the DOM-project. *Breast Cancer Res. Treat.*, **34**, 129–137

Dengel, D.R., Pratley, R.E., Hagberg, J.M., Rogus, E.M. & Goldberg, A.P. (1996) Distinct effects of aerobic exercise training and weight loss on glucose homeostasis in obese sedentary men. *J. Appl. Physiol.*, **81**, 318–325

Denti, L., Pasolini, G., Sanfelici, L., Ablondi, F., Freddi, M., Benedetti, R. & Valenti, G. (1997) Effects of aging on dehydroepiandrosterone sulfate in relation to fasting insulin levels and body composition assessed by bioimpedance analysis. *Metabolism*, **46**, 826–832

Després, J.P., Moorjani, S., Lupien, P.J., Tremblay, A., Nadeau, A. & Bouchard, C. (1990) Regional distribution of body fat, plasma lipoproteins, and cardiovascular disease. *Arteriosclerosis*, **10**, 497–511

Després, J.P., Pouliot, M.C., Moorjani, S., Nadeau, A., Tremblay, A., Lupien, P.J., Thériault, G. & Bouchard, C. (1991) Loss of abdominal fat and metabolic response to exercise training in obese women. *Am. J. Physiol.*, **261**, E159–E167

Deurenberg, P., Weststrate, J.A. & Seidell, J.C. (1991) Body mass index as a measure of body fatness: age- and sex-specific prediction formulas. *Br. J. Nutr.*, **65**, 105–114

Deurenberg-Yap, M., Schmidt, G., van Staveren, W.A. & Deurenberg, P. (2000) The paradox of low body mass index and high body fat percentage among Chinese, Malays and Indians in Singapore. *Int. J. Obes. Relat. Metab. Disord.*, **24**, 1011–1017

Dhahbi, J.M., Mote, P.L., Wingo, J., Tillman, J.B., Walford, R.L. & Spindler, S.R. (1999) Calories and aging alter gene expression for gluconeogenic, glycolytic, and nitrogen-metabolizing enzymes. *Am. J. Physiol.*, **277**, E352–E360

Dhurandhar, N.V. & Kulkarni, P.R. (1992) Prevalence of obesity in Bombay. *Int. J. Obes. Relat. Metab. Disord.*, **16**, 367–375

Di Luigi, L., Conti, F.G., Casini, A., Guidetti, L., Zezze, G., Pigozzi, F., Spera, G., Fortunio, G. & Romanelli, F. (1997) Growth hormone and insulin-like growth factor I responses to moderate submaximal acute physical exercise in man: effects of octreotide, a somatostatin analogue, administration. *Int. J. Sports Med.*, **18**, 257–263

Dickson, R.B., Thompson, E.W. & Lippman, M.E. (1990) Regulation of proliferation, invasion and growth factor synthesis in breast cancer by steroids. *J. Steroid Biochem. Mol. Biol.*, **37**, 305–316

Dietz, W.H. (1994) Critical periods in childhood for the development of obesity. *Am. J. Clin. Nutr.*, **59**, 955–959

Dietz, A.T., Newcomb, P.A., Marcus, P.M. & Storer, B.E. (1995) The association of body size and large bowel cancer risk in Wisconsin (United States) women. *Cancer Causes Control*, **6**, 30–36

Dishman, R.K. & Buckworth, J. (1996) Increasing physical activity: a quantitative synthesis. *Med. Sci. Sports Exerc.*, **28**, 706–719

Dishman, R.K., Oldenburg, B., O'Neal, H. & Shephard, R.J. (1998) Worksite physical activity interventions. *Am. J. Prev. Med.*, **15**, 344–361

Djuric, Z., Lu, M.H., Lewis, S.M., Luongo, D.A., Chen, X.W., Heilbrun, L.K., Reading, B.A., Duffy, P.H. & Hart, R.W. (1992) Oxidative DNA damage levels in rats fed low-fat, high-fat, or calorie-restricted diets. *Toxicol. Appl. Pharmacol.*, **115**, 156–160

Doak, C.M., Adair, L.S., Monteiro, C. & Popkin, B.M. (2000) Overweight and underweight coexist within households in Brazil, China and Russia. *J. Nutr.*, **130**, 2965–2971

Dolan, K., Sutton, R., Walker, S.J., Morris, A.I., Campbell, F. & Williams, E.M. (1999) New classification of oesophageal and gastric carcinomas derived from changing patterns in epidemiology. *Br. J. Cancer*, **80**, 834–842

Doll, H.A., Petersen, S.E. & Stewart-Brown, S.L. (2000) Obesity and physical and emotional well-being: associations between body mass index, chronic illness, and the physical and mental components of the SF-36 questionnaire. *Obes. Res.*, **8**, 160–170

Dorgan, J.F., Brown, C., Barrett, M., Splansky, G.L., Kreger, B.E., D'Agostino, R.B., Albanes, D. & Schatzkin, A. (1994) Physical activity and risk of breast cancer in the Framingham Heart Study. *Am. J. Epidemiol.*, **139**, 662–669

Dosemeci, M., Hayes, R.B., Vetter, R., Hoover, R.N., Tucker, M., Engin, K., Unsal, M. & Blair, A. (1993) Occupational physical activity, socioeconomic status, and risks of 15 cancer sites in Turkey. *Cancer Causes Control*, **4**, 313–321

Dowell, R.T., Tipton, C.M. & Tomanek, R.J. (1976) Cardiac enlargement mechanisms with exercise training and pressure overload. *J Mol. Cell Cardiol.*, **8**, 407–418

Drinkard, C.R., Sellers, T.A., Potter, J.D., Zheng, W., Bostick, R.M., Nelson, C.L. & Folsom, A.R. (1995) Association of body mass index and body fat distribution with risk of lung cancer in older women. *Am. J. Epidemiol.*, **142**, 600–607

Drinkwater, B.L., Bruemner, B. & Chesnut, C.H., III (1990) Menstrual history as a determinant of current bone density in young athletes. *JAMA*, **263**, 545–548

Dubin, N., Moseson, M. & Pasternack, B.S. (1986) Epidemiology of malignant melanoma: pigmentary traits, ultraviolet radiation, and the identification of high-risk populations. *Recent Results Cancer Res.*, **102**, 56–75

Dublin, L.I. (1953) Relation of obesity to longevity. *New Engl. J. Med.*, **248**, 971–974

Duffy, P.H., Feuers, R.J., Leakey, J.A., Nakamura, K., Turturro, A. & Hart, R.W. (1989) Effect of chronic caloric restriction on physiological variables related to energy metabolism in the male Fischer 344 rat. *Mech. Ageing Dev.*, **48**, 117–133

Duffy, P.H., Feuers, R., Nakamura, K.D., Leakey, J. & Hart, R.W. (1990a) Effect of chronic caloric restriction on the synchronization of various physiological measures in old female Fischer 344 rats. *Chronobiol. Int.*, **7**, 113–124

Duffy, P.H., Feuers, R.J. & Hart, R.W. (1990b) Effect of chronic caloric restriction on the circadian regulation of physiological and behavioral variables in old male B6C3F1 mice. *Chronobiol. Int.*, **7**, 291–303

Duffy, P.H., Feuers, R.J., Pipkin, J., Berg, T.F., Divine, B., Leakey, J., Turturro, A. & Hart, R.W. (1995) The effect of caloric modulation and aging on the physiological response of rodents to drug toxicity. In: Hart, R., Neuman, D. & Robertson, R., eds, *Dietary Restriction: Implications for the Design and Interpretation of Toxicity and Carcinogenicity Studies,* Washington, DC, ILSI Press, pp. 127–140

Duncan, K., Harris, S. & Ardies, C.M. (1997) Running exercise may reduce risk for lung and liver cancer by inducing activity of antioxidant and phase II enzymes. *Cancer Lett.*, **116**, 151–158

Dunn, S.E., Kari, F.W., French, J., Leininger, J.R., Travlos, G., Wilson, R. & Barrett, J.C. (1997) Dietary restriction reduces insulin-like growth factor I levels, which modulates apoptosis, cell proliferation, and tumor progression in p53-deficient mice. *Cancer Res.*, **57**, 4667–4672

Dunn, A.L., Andersen, R.E. & Jakicic, J.M. (1998) Lifestyle physical activity interventions. History, short- and long-term effects, and recommendations. *Am. J. Prev. Med.*, **15**, 398–412

Dunn, A.L., Marcus, B.H., Kampert, J.B., Garcia, M.E., Kohl, H.W. & Blair, S.N. (1999) Comparison of lifestyle and structured interventions to increase physical activity and cardiorespiratory fitness: a randomized trial. *JAMA*, **281**, 327–334

Durstine, J.L. & Haskell, W.L. (1994) Effects of exercise training on plasma lipids and lipoproteins. *Exerc. Sport Sci. Rev.*, **22**, 477–521

Dyer, A.R., Stamler, J. & Greenland, P. (2000) Associations of weight change and weight variability with cardiovascular and all-cause mortality in the Chicago Western Electric Company Study. *Am. J. Epidemiol.*, **152**, 324–333

Eaton, N.E., Reeves, G.K., Appleby, P.N. & Key, T.J. (1999) Endogenous sex hormones and prostate cancer: a quantitative review of prospective studies. *Br. J. Cancer*, **80**, 930–934

Ebeling, P. & Koivisto, V.A. (1994) Non-esterified fatty acids regulate lipid and glucose oxidation and glycogen synthesis in healthy man. *Diabetologia*, **37**, 202–209

Egger, G. & Swinburn, B. (1997) An "ecological" approach to the obesity pandemic. *BMJ*, **315**, 477–480

Ehrmann, D.A. (1999) Insulin-lowering therapeutic modalities for polycystic ovary syndrome. *Endocrinol. Metab. Clin. North Am.*, **28**, 423–438

Ehrmann, D.A., Barnes, R.B. & Rosenfield, R.L. (1995) Polycystic ovary syndrome as a form of functional ovarian hyperandrogenism due to dysregulation of androgen secretion. *Endocr. Rev.*, **16**, 322–353

Ekbom, A., Trichopoulos, D., Adami, H.O., Hsieh, C.C. & Lan, S.J. (1992) Evidence of prenatal influences on breast cancer risk. *Lancet*, **340**, 1015–1018

Ekbom, A., Hsieh, C.C., Lipworth, L., Adami, H.O. & Trichopoulos, D. (1997) Intrauterine environment and breast cancer risk in women: a population-based study. *J. Natl Cancer Inst.*, **89**, 71–76

Eliakim, A., Wolach, B., Kodesh, E., Gavrieli, R., Radnay, J., Ben-Tovim, T., Yarom, Y. & Falk, B. (1997) Cellular and humoral immune response to exercise among gymnasts and untrained girls. *Int. J. Sports Med.*, **18**, 208–212

Elias, A.N., Pandian, M.R., Wang, L., Suarez, E., James, N. & Wilson, A.F. (2000) Leptin and IGF-I levels in unconditioned male volunteers after short-term exercise. *Psychoneuroendocrinology*, **25**, 453–461

Elliott, E.A., Matanoski, G.M., Rosenshein, N.B., Grumbine, F.C. & Diamond, E.L. (1990) Body fat patterning in women with endometrial cancer. *Gynecol. Oncol.*, **39**, 253–258

Elwood, J.M., Cole, P., Rothman, K.J. & Kaplan, S.D. (1977) Epidemiology of endometrial cancer. *J. Natl Cancer Inst.*, **59**, 1055–1060

Engelman, R.W., Day, N.K. & Good, R.A. (1993) Calories, parity, and prolactin influence mammary epithelial kinetics and differentiation and alter mouse mammary tumor risk. *Cancer Res.*, **53**, 1188–1194

Engelman, R.W., Day, N.K. & Good, R.A. (1994) Calorie intake during mammary development influences cancer risk: lasting inhibition of C3H/HeOu mammary tumorigenesis by peripubertal calorie restriction. *Cancer Res.*, **54**, 5724–5730

Engelman, R.W., Owens, U.E., Bradley, W.G., Day, N.K. & Good, R.A. (1995) Mammary and submandibular gland epidermal growth factor expression is reduced by calorie restriction. *Cancer Res.*, **55**, 1289–1295

Enger, S.M., Ross, R.K., Paganini-Hill, A., Carpenter, C.L. & Bernstein, L. (2000) Body size, physical activity, and breast cancer hormone receptor status: results from two case-control studies. *Cancer Epidemiol. Biomarkers Prev.*, **9**, 681–687

Enriori, C.L., Orsini, W., del Carmen Cremona, M., Etkin, A.E., Cardillo, L.R. & Reforzo-Membrives, J. (1986) Decrease of circulating level of SHBG in postmenopausal obese women as a risk factor in breast cancer: reversible effect of weight loss. *Gynecol. Oncol.*, **23**, 77–86

Ensrud, K.E., Lipschutz, R.C., Cauley, J.A., Seeley, D., Nevitt, M.C., Scott, J., Orwoll, E.S., Genant, H.K. & Cummings, S.R. (1997a) Body size and hip fracture risk in older women: a prospective study. Study of Osteoporotic Fractures Research Group. *Am. J. Med.*, **103**, 274–280

Ensrud, K.E., Cauley, J., Lipschutz, R. & Cummings, S.R. (1997b) Weight change and fractures in older women. Study of Osteoporotic Fractures Research Group. *Arch. Intern. Med.*, **157**, 857–863

Erfurth, E.M., Hagmar, L.E., Saaf, M. & Hall, K. (1996) Serum levels of insulin-like growth factor I and insulin-like growth factor-binding protein 1 correlate with serum free testosterone and sex hormone binding globulin levels in healthy young and middle-aged men. *Clin. Endocrinol. (Oxf.)*, **44**, 659–664

Eriksson, J., Taimela, S., Eriksson, K., Parviainen, S., Peltonen, J. & Kujala, U. (1997) Resistance training in the treatment of non-insulin-dependent diabetes mellitus. *Int. J. Sports Med.*, **18**, 242–246

Ershler, W.B., Berman, E. & Moore, A.L. (1986) Slower B16 melanoma growth but greater pulmonary colonization in calorie-restricted mice. *J. Natl Cancer Inst.*, **76**, 81–85

Estivariz, C.F. & Ziegler, T.R. (1997) Nutrition and the insulin-like growth factor system. *Endocrine*, **7**, 65–71

European Commission (1999) *A Pan-EU Survey on Consumer Attitudes to Physical Activity, Body Weight and Health*. Luxembourg, Office for Official Publications of the European Communities

Evans, D.J., Hoffmann, R.G., Kalkhoff, R.K. & Kissebah, A.H. (1983) Relationship of androgenic activity to body fat topography, fat cell morphology, and metabolic aberrations in premenopausal women. *J. Clin. Endocrinol. Metab.*, **57**, 304–310

Evans, D.J., Barth, J.H. & Burke, C.W. (1988) Body fat topography in women with androgen excess. *Int. J. Obes.*, **12**, 157–162

Everhart, J.E. (1993) Contributions of obesity and weight loss to gallstone disease. *Ann. Intern. Med.*, **119**, 1029–1035

Everhart, J. & Wright, D. (1995) Diabetes mellitus as a risk factor for pancreatic cancer. A meta-analysis. *JAMA*, **273**, 1605–1609

Everitt, A.V., Seedsman, N.J. & Jones, F. (1980) The effects of hypophysectomy and continuous food restriction, begun at ages 70 and 400 days, on collagen aging, proteinuria, incidence of pathology and longevity in the male rat. *Mech. Ageing Dev.*, **12**, 161–172

Ewbank, P.P., Darga, L.L. & Lucas, C.P. (1995) Physical activity as a predictor of weight maintenance in previously obese subjects. *Obes. Res.*, **3**, 257–263

Ewertz, M., Machado, S.G., Boice, J.D., Jr & Jensen, O.M. (1984) Endometrial cancer following treatment for breast cancer: a case-control study in Denmark. *Br. J. Cancer*, **50**, 687–692

Fagard, R.H. (1999) Physical activity in the prevention and treatment of hypertension in the obese. *Med. Sci. Sports Exerc.*, **31**, S624–S630

Fahrner, C.L. & Hackney, A.C. (1998) Effects of endurance exercise on free testosterone concentration and the binding affinity of sex hormone binding globulin (SHBG). *Int. J. Sports Med.,* **19**, 12–15

Falkner, K.L., Trevisan, M. & McCann, S.E. (1999) Reliability of recall of physical activity in the distant past. *Am. J. Epidemiol.,* **150**, 195–205

Falorni, A., Bini, V., Cabiati, G., Papi, F., Arzano, S., Celi, F. & Sanasi, M. (1997) Serum levels of type I procollagen C-terminal propeptide, insulin-like growth factor-I (IGF-I), and IGF binding protein-3 in obese children and adolescents: relationship to gender, pubertal development, growth, insulin, and nutritional status. *Metabolism,* **46**, 862–871

Farnsworth, W.E. (1996) Roles of estrogen and SHBG in prostate physiology. *Prostate,* **28**, 17–23

Farrow, D.C., Weiss, N.S., Lyon, J.L. & Daling, J.R. (1989) Association of obesity and ovarian cancer in a case-control study. *Am. J. Epidemiol.,* **129**, 1300–1304

Farrow, D.C., Vaughan, T.L., Sweeney, C., Gammon, M.D., Chow, W.H., Risch, H.A., Stanford, J.L., Hansten, P.D., Mayne, S.T., Schoenberg, J.B., Rotterdam, H., Ahsan, H., West, A.B., Dubrow, R., Fraumeni, J.F. & Blot, W.J. (2000) Gastroesophageal reflux disease, use of H2 receptor antagonists, and risk of esophageal and gastric cancer. *Cancer Causes Control,* **11**, 231–238

Fathalla, M.F. (1971) Incessant ovulation—a factor in ovarian neoplasia? *Lancet,* **2**, 163

Felig, P., Pozefsky, T., Marliss, E. & Cahill, G.F. (1970) Alanine: key role in gluconeogenesis. *Science,* **167**, 1003–1004

Felson, D.T., Zhang, Y., Anthony, J.M., Naimark, A. & Anderson, J.J. (1992) Weight loss reduces the risk for symptomatic knee osteoarthritis in women. The Framingham Study. *Ann. Intern. Med.,* **116**, 535–539

Fernandes, G., Chandrasekar, B., Troyer, D.A., Venkatraman, J.T. & Good, R.A. (1995) Dietary lipids and calorie restriction affect mammary tumor incidence and gene expression in mouse mammary tumor virus/v-Ha-ras transgenic mice. *Proc. Natl Acad. Sci. USA,* **92**, 6494–6498

Fernandes, G., Venkatraman, J.T., Turturro, A., Attwood, V.G. & Hart, R.W. (1997) Effect of food restriction on life span and immune functions in long-lived Fischer-344 x Brown

Norway F1 rats. *J. Clin. Immunol.,* **17**, 85–95

Ferry, R.J., Jr, Katz, L.E., Grimberg, A., Cohen, P. & Weinzimer, S.A. (1999) Cellular actions of insulin-like growth factor binding proteins. *Horm. Metab. Res.,* **31**, 192–202

Feskens, E.J., Loeber, J.G. & Kromhout, D. (1994) Diet and physical activity as determinants of hyperinsulinemia: the Zutphen Elderly Study. *Am. J. Epidemiol.,* **140**, 350–360

Festi, D., Colecchia, A., Orsini, M., Sangermano, A., Sottili, S., Simoni, P., Mazzella, G., Villanova, N., Bazzoli, F., Lapenna, D., Petroni, M.L., Pavesi, S., Neri, M. & Roda, E. (1998) Gallbladder motility and gallstone formation in obese patients following very low calorie diets. Use it (fat) to lose it (well). *Int. J. Obes. Relat. Metab. Disord.,* **22**, 592–600

Feuers, R.J., Duffy, P.H., Leakey, J.A., Turturro, A., Mittelstaedt, R.A. & Hart, R.W. (1989) Effect of chronic caloric restriction on hepatic enzymes of intermediary metabolism in the male Fischer 344 rat. *Mech. Ageing Dev.,* **48**, 179–189

Feuers, R.J., Duffy, P.H., Chen, F., Desai, V., Oriake, E., Shaddock, J.G., Pipkin, J.W., Weindruch, R. & Hart, R.W. (1995) Intermediary metabolism and antioxidant systems. In: Hart, R., Neuman, D. & Robertson, R., eds, *Dietary Restriction: Implications for the Design and Interpretation of Toxicity and Carcinogenicity Studies,* Washington, DC, ILSI Press, pp. 181–195

Fiatarone, M.A., O'Neill, E.F., Ryan, N.D., Clements, K.M., Solares, G.R., Nelson, M.E., Roberts, S.B., Kehayias, J.J., Lipsitz, L.A. & Evans, W.J. (1994) Exercise training and nutritional supplementation for physical frailty in very elderly people. *New Engl. J. Med.,* **330**, 1769–1775

Field, C.J., Gougeon, R. & Marliss, E.B. (1991) Changes in circulating leukocytes and mitogen responses during very-low-energy all-protein reducing diets. *Am. J. Clin. Nutr.,* **54**, 123–129

Field, A.E., Colditz, G.A., Willett, W.C., Longcope, C. & McKinlay, J.B. (1994) The relation of smoking, age, relative weight, and dietary intake to serum adrenal steroids, sex hormones, and sex hormone-binding globulin in middle-aged men. *J. Clin. Endocrinol. Metab.,* **79**, 1310–1316

Field, A.E., Byers, T., Hunter, D.J., Laird, N.M., Manson, J.E., Williamson, D.F., Willett,

W.C. & Colditz, G.A. (1999) Weight cycling, weight gain, and risk of hypertension in women. *Am. J. Epidemiol.,* **150**, 573–579

Finkle, W.D., McLaughlin, J.K., Rasgon, S.A., Yeoh, H.H. & Low, J.E. (1993) Increased risk of renal cell cancer among women using diuretics in the United States. *Cancer Causes Control,* **4**, 555–558

Fischer, J. & Johnson, M.A. (1990) Low body weight and weight loss in the aged. *J. Am. Diet. Assoc.,* **90**, 1697–1706

Fischer, W.H. & Lutz, W.K. (1994) Mouse skin papilloma formation by chronic dermal application of 7,12-dimethylbenz[a]anthracene is not reduced by diet restriction. *Carcinogenesis,* **15**, 129–131

Fisher, R.P., Falkner, K.L., Trevisan, M. & McCauley, M.R. (2000) Adapting the cognitive interview to enhance long-term (35 years) recall of physical activities. *J. Appl. Psychol.,* **85**, 180–189

Fishman, J., Boyar, R.M. & Hellman, L. (1975) Influence of body weight on estradiol metabolism in young women. *J. Clin. Endocrinol. Metab.,* **41**, 989–991

Flegal, K.M., Troiano, R.P., Pamuk, E.R., Kuczmarski, R.J. & Campbell, S.M. (1995) The influence of smoking cessation on the prevalence of overweight in the United States. *New Engl. J. Med.,* **333**, 1165–1170

Flegal, K.M., Carroll, M.D., Kuczmarski, R.J. & Johnson, C.L. (1998) Overweight and obesity in the United States: prevalence and trends, 1960–1994. *Int. J. Obes. Relat. Metab. Disord.,* **22**, 39–47

Flier, J.S. (1983) Insulin receptors and insulin resistance. *Annu. Rev. Med.,* **34**, 145–160

Flood, V., Webb, K., Lazarus, R. & Pang, G. (2000) Use of self-report to monitor overweight and obesity in populations: some issues for consideration. *Aust. N.Z. J. Public Health,* **24**, 96–99

Foekens, J.A., Portengen, H., Janssen, M. & Klijn, J.G. (1989) Insulin-like growth factor-1 receptors and insulin-like growth factor-1-like activity in human primary breast cancer. *Cancer,* **63**, 2139–2147

Fogelholm, M. & Hiilloskorpi, H. (1999) Weight and diet concerns in Finnish female and male athletes. *Med. Sci. Sports Exerc.,* **31**, 229–235

Fogelholm, M. & Kukkonen-Harjula, K. (2000) Does physical activity prevent weight gain – a systematic review. *Obes. Rev.*, **1**, 95–111

Fogelholm, M., Männistö, S., Vartiainen, E. & Pietinen, P. (1996a) Determinants of energy balance and overweight in Finland 1982 and 1992. *Int. J. Obes. Relat. Metab. Disord.*, **20**, 1097–1104

Fogelholm, M., Van Marken-Lichtenbelt, W., Ottenheijm, R. & Westerterp, K. (1996b) Amenorrhea in ballet dancers in the Netherlands. *Med. Sci. Sports Exerc.*, **28**, 545–550

Fogelholm, M., Sievänen, H., Heinonen, A., Virtanen, M., Uusi-Rasi, K., Pasanen, M. & Vuori, I. (1997) Association between weight cycling history and bone mineral density in premenopausal women. *Osteopor. Int.*, **7**, 354–358

Fogelholm, M., Kujala, U., Kaprio, J. & Sarna, S. (2000a) Predictors of weight change in middle-aged and old men. *Obes. Res.*, **8**, 367–373

Fogelholm, M., Kukkonen-Harjula, K., Nenonen, A. & Pasanen, M. (2000b) Effects of walking training on weight maintenance after a very-low-energy diet in pre-menopausal obese women: a randomized controlled trial. *Arch. Intern. Med.*, **160**, 2177–2184

Folsom, A.R., Kaye, S.A., Potter, J.D. & Prineas, R.J. (1989) Association of incident carcinoma of the endometrium with body weight and fat distribution in older women: early findings of the Iowa Women's Health Study. *Cancer Res.*, **49**, 6828–6831

Folsom, A.R., Kaye, S.A., Prineas, R.J., Potter, J.D., Gapstur, S.M. & Wallace, R.B. (1990) Increased incidence of carcinoma of the breast associated with abdominal adiposity in postmenopausal women. *Am. J. Epidemiol.*, **131**, 794–803

Folsom, A.R., French, S.A., Zheng, W., Baxter, J.E. & Jeffery, R.W. (1996) Weight variability and mortality: the Iowa Women's Health Study. *Int. J. Obes. Relat. Metab. Disord.*, **20**, 704–709

Folsom, A.R., Kushi, L.H., Anderson, K.E., Mink, P.J., Olson, J.E., Hong, C.P., Sellers, T.A., Lazovich, D. & Prineas, R.J. (2000) Associations of general and abdominal obesity with multiple health outcomes in older women: the Iowa Women's Health Study. *Arch. Intern. Med.*, **160**, 2117–2128

Fontaine, K.R., Bartlett, S.J. & Barofsky, I. (2000) Health-related quality of life among obese persons seeking and not currently seeking treatment. *Int. J. Eating Disord.*, **27**, 101–105

Ford, E.S. (1999) Body mass index and colon cancer in a national sample of adult US men and women. *Am. J. Epidemiol.*, **150**, 390–398

Forrester, T., Wilks, R., Bennett, F., McFarlane-Anderson, N., McGee, D., Cooper, R. & Fraser, H. (1996) Obesity in the Caribbean. *Ciba Found. Symp.*, **201**, 17–31

Forster, M.J., Sohal, B.H. & Sohal, R.S. (2000) Reversible effects of long-term caloric restriction on protein oxidative damage. *J. Gerontol. A Biol. Sci. Med. Sci.*, **55**, B522–B529

Fortmann, S.P., Winkleby, M.A., Flora, J.A., Haskell, W.L. & Taylor, C.B. (1990) Effect of long-term community health education on blood pressure and hypertension control. The Stanford Five-City Project. *Am. J. Epidemiol.*, **132**, 629–646

Frame, L.T., Hart, R.W. & Leakey, J.E. (1998) Caloric restriction as a mechanism mediating resistance to environmental disease. *Environ. Health Perspect.*, **106, Suppl. 1**, 313–324

Franceschi, S., Favero, A., La Vecchia, C., Baron, A.E., Negri, E., Dal Maso, L., Giacosa, A., Montella, M., Conti, E. & Amadori, D. (1996) Body size indices and breast cancer risk before and after menopause. *Int. J. Cancer*, **67**, 181–186

Franceschi, S., Dal Maso, L., Levi, F., Conti, E., Talamini, R. & La Vecchia, C. (2001) Leanness as early marker of cancer of the oral cavity and pharynx. *Ann. Oncol.*, **12**, 331–336

Franz, M.J., Monk, A., Barry, B., McClain, K., Weaver, T., Cooper, N., Upham, P., Bergenstal, R. & Mazze, R.S. (1995) Effectiveness of medical nutrition therapy provided by dietitians in the management of non-insulin-dependent diabetes mellitus: a randomized, controlled clinical trial. *J. Am. Diet. Assoc.*, **95**, 1009-1017

Fraser, G. & Pearce, N. (1993) Occupational physical activity and risk of cancer of the colon and rectum in New Zealand males. *Cancer Causes Control*, **4**, 45–50

Fraser, G.E. & Shavlik, D. (1997) Risk factors, lifetime risk, and age at onset of breast cancer. *Ann. Epidemiol.*, **7**, 375–382

Fredriks, A.M., van Buuren, S., Wit, J.M. & Verloove-Vanhorick, S.P. (2000) Body index measurements in 1996–7 compared with 1980. *Arch. Dis. Child.*, **82**, 107–112

Fredriksson, M., Bengtsson, N.O., Hardell, L. & Axelson, O. (1989) Colon cancer, physical activity, and occupational exposures. A case-control study. *Cancer*, **63**, 1838–1842

Freedman, L.S., Clifford, C. & Messina, M. (1990) Analysis of dietary fat, calories, body weight, and the development of mammary tumors in rats and mice: a review. *Cancer Res.*, **50**, 5710–5719

French, S.A., Jeffery, R.W., Folsom, A.R., Williamson, D.F. & Byers, T. (1995) History of intentional and unintentional weight loss in a population-based sample of women aged 55 to 69 years. *Obes. Res.*, **3**, 163-170

French, S.A., Folsom, A.R., Jeffery, R.W., Zheng, W., Mink, P.J. & Baxter, J.E. (1997) Weight variability and incident disease in older women: the Iowa Women's Health Study. *Int. J. Obes. Relat. Metab. Disord.*, **21**, 217-223

French, S.A., Jeffery, R.W. & Murray, D. (1999a) Is dieting good for you? Prevalence, duration and associated weight and behaviour changes for specific weight loss strategies over four years in US adults. *Int. J. Obes. Relat. Metab. Disord.*, **23**, 320–327

French, S.A., Folsom, A.R., Jeffery, R.W. & Williamson, D.F. (1999b) Prospective study of intentionality of weight loss and mortality in older women: the Iowa Women's Health Study. *Am. J. Epidemiol.*, **149**, 504-514

Friedenreich, C.M. & Rohan, T.E. (1995) Physical activity and risk of breast cancer. *Eur. J. Cancer Prev.*, **4**, 145–151

Friedenreich, C.M., Courneya, K.S. & Bryant, H.E. (1998) The lifetime total physical activity questionnaire: development and reliability. *Med. Sci. Sports Exerc.*, **30**, 266–274

Friedenreich, C.M., Bryant, H.E. & Courneya, K.S. (2001a) Case-control study of lifetime physical activity and breast cancer risk. *Am. J. Epidemiol.*, **154**, 336–347

Friedenreich, C.M., Courneya, K.S. & Bryant, H.E. (2001b) Influence of physical activity in different age and life periods on the risk of breast cancer. *Epidemiology*, **12**, 604–612

Friedenreich, C.M., Courneya, K.S. & Bryant, H.E. (2001c) Relation between intensity of physical activity and breast cancer risk reduction. *Med. Sci. Sports Exerc.* **33**, 1538–1545

Friedman, G.D. & van den Eeden, S.K. (1993) Risk factors for pancreatic cancer: an exploratory study. *Int. J. Epidemiol., 22,* 30–37

Friedman, J.M. & Halaas, J.L. (1998) Leptin and the regulation of body weight in mammals. *Nature*, **395**, 763–770

Frisch, R.E. (1987) Body fat, menarche, fitness and fertility. *Hum. Reprod.*, **2**, 521–533

Frisch, R.E., Wyshak, G. & Vincent, L. (1980) Delayed menarche and amenorrhea in ballet dancers. *New Engl. J. Med.*, **303**, 17–19

Frisch, R.E., Gotz-Welbergen, A.V., McArthur, J.W., Albright, T., Witschi, J., Bullen, B., Birnholz, J., Reed, R.B. & Hermann, H. (1981) Delayed menarche and amenorrhea of college athletes in relation to age of onset of training. *JAMA*, **246**, 1559–1563

Frisch, R.E., Wyshak, G., Albright, N.L., Albright, T.E., Schiff, I., Jones, K.P., Witschi, J., Shiang, E., Koff, E. & Marguglio, M. (1985) Lower prevalence of breast cancer and cancers of the reproductive system among former college athletes compared to non-athletes. *Br. J. Cancer*, **52**, 885–891

Frystyk, J., Vestbo, E., Skjaerbaek, C., Mogensen, C.E. & Orskov, H. (1995) Free insulin-like growth factors in human obesity. *Metabolism*, **440**, 37–44

Fujimoto, W.Y. (1996) Overview of non-insulin-dependent diabetes mellitus (NIDDM) in different population groups. *Diabet. Med.,* **13**, S7–S10

Fujioka, S., Matsuzawa, Y., Tokunaga, K., Kawamoto, T., Kobatake, T., Keno, Y., Kotani, K., Yoshida, S. & Tarui, S. (1991) Improvement of glucose and lipid metabolism associated with selective reduction of intra-abdominal visceral fat in premenopausal women with visceral fat obesity. *Int. J. Obes.*, **15**, 853–859

Fulton, J.E. & Shekelle, R.B. (1997) Cigarette smoking, weight gain, and coronary mortality: results from the Chicago Western Electric Study. *Circulation*, **96**, 1438–1444

Gabriel, H. & Kindermann, W. (1997) The acute immune response to exercise: what does it mean? *Int. J. Sports Med.,* **18 Suppl. 1**, S28–S45

Galanis, D.J., Kolonel, L.N., Lee, J. & Le Marchand, L. (1998a) Anthropometric predictors of breast cancer incidence and survival in a multi-ethnic cohort of female residents of Hawaii, United States. *Cancer Causes Control*, **9**, 217–224

Galanis, D.J., Harris, T., Sharp, D.S. & Petrovitch, H. (1998b) Relative weight, weight change, and risk of coronary heart disease in the Honolulu Heart Program. *Am. J. Epidemiol.*, **147**, 379–386

Gallagher, R.P., Elwood, J.M., Hill, G.B., Coldman, A.J., Threlfall, W.J. & Spinelli, J.J. (1985) Reproductive factors, oral contraceptives and risk of malignant melanoma: Western Canada Melanoma Study. *Br. J. Cancer*, **52**, 901–907

Gallagher, R.P., Huchcroft, S., Phillips, N., Hill, G.B., Coldman, A.J., Coppin, C. & Lee, T. (1995) Physical activity, medical history, and risk of testicular cancer (Alberta and British Columbia, Canada). *Cancer Causes Control*, **6**, 398–406

Gallagher, D., Visser, M., Sepulveda, D., Pierson, R.N., Harris, T. & Heymsfield, S.B. (1996) How useful is body mass index for comparison of body fatness across age, sex, and ethnic groups? *Am. J. Epidemiol.*, **143**, 228–239

Gama, R., Teale, J.D. & Marks, V. (1990) The effect of synthetic very low calorie diets on the GH-IGF-1 axis in obese subjects. *Clin. Chim. Acta*, **188**, 31–38

Gammon, M.D., Schoenberg, J.B., Britton, J.A., Kelsey, J.L., Coates, R.J., Brogan, D., Potischman, N., Swanson, C.A., Daling, J.R., Stanford, J.L. & Brinton, L.A. (1998) Recreational physical activity and breast cancer risk among women under age 45 years. *Am. J. Epidemiol.*, **147**, 273–280

Gann, P.H., Hennekens, C.H., Ma, J., Longcope, C. & Stampfer, M.J. (1996) Prospective study of sex hormone levels and risk of prostate cancer. *J. Natl Cancer Inst.*, **88**, 1118–1126

Gapstur, S.M., Gann, P.H., Lowe, W., Liu, K., Colangelo, L. & Dyer, A. (2000) Abnormal glucose metabolism and pancreatic cancer mortality. *JAMA*, **283**, 2552–2558

Garabrant, D.H., Peters, J.M., Mack, T.M. & Bernstein, L. (1984) Job activity and colon cancer risk. *Am. J. Epidemiol.*, **119**, 1005–1014

Garcia-Palmieri, M.R., Costas, R., Jr., Cruz-Vidal, M., Sorlie, P.D. & Havlik, R.J. (1982) Increased physical activity: a protective factor against heart attacks in Puerto Rico. *Am. J. Cardiol.*, **50**, 749–755

Gardin, J.M., Schumacher, D., Constantine, G., Davis, K.D., Leung, C. & Reid, C.L. (2000) Valvular abnormalities and cardiovascular status following exposure to dexfenfluramine or phentermine/fenfluramine. *JAMA*, **283**, 1703–1709

Garfinkel, L. (1985) Overweight and cancer. *Ann. Intern. Med.*, **103**, 1034–1036

Garfinkel, L. & Stellman, S.D. (1988) Mortality by relative weight and exercise. *Cancer*, **62**, 1844–1850

Garrow, J.S. & Summerbell, C.D. (1995) Meta-analysis: effect of exercise, with or without dieting, on the body composition of overweight subjects. *Eur. J. Clin. Nutr.*, **49**, 1–10

Garthwaite, S.M., Cheng, H., Bryan, J.E., Craig, B.W. & Holloszy, J.O. (1986) Ageing, exercise and food restriction: effects on body composition. *Mech. Ageing Dev.*, **36**, 187–196

Gelber, A.C., Hochberg, M.C., Mead, L.A., Wang, N.Y., Wigley, F.M. & Klag, M.J. (2000) Joint injury in young adults and risk for subsequent knee and hip osteoarthritis. *Ann. Intern. Med.*, **133**, 321–328

Gerhardsson, M., Norell, S.E., Kiviranta, H., Pedersen, N.L. & Ahlbom, A. (1986) Sedentary jobs and colon cancer. *Am. J. Epidemiol., 123*, 775–780

Gerhardsson, M., Floderus, B. & Norell, S.E. (1988) Physical activity and colon cancer risk. *Int. J. Epidemiol.*, **17**, 743–746

Gerhardsson de Verdier, M., Steineck, G., Hagman, U., Rieger, A. & Norell, S.E. (1990a) Physical activity and colon cancer: a case-referent study in Stockholm. *Int. J. Cancer*, **46**, 985–989

Gerhardsson de Verdier, M., Hagman, U., Steineck, G., Rieger, A. & Norell, S.E. (1990b) Diet, body mass and colorectal cancer: a case-referent study in Stockholm. *Int. J. Cancer*, **46**, 832–838

Ghadirian, P., Simard, A., Baillargeon, J., Maisonneuve, P. & Boyle, P. (1991) Nutritional factors and pancreatic cancer in the francophone community in Montreal, Canada. *Int. J. Cancer*, **47**, 1–6

Ghannem, H., Maarouf, R., Tabka, A., Haj, F.A. & Marzouki, M. (1993) La triade obésité, hypertension et troubles de la glycorégulation dans une population semi-urbaine du Sahel Tunisien. *Diabete Metab.*, **19**, 310–314

Giagulli, V.A., Kaufman, J.M. & Vermeulen, A. (1994) Pathogenesis of the decreased androgen levels in obese men. *J. Clin. Endocrinol. Metab.*, **79**, 997–1000

Gibson, S.L. & Hilf, R. (1980) Regulation of estrogen-binding capacity by insulin in 7,12-dimethylbenz(a)anthracene-induced mammary tumors in rats. *Cancer Res.*, **40**, 2343–2348

Giesbrecht, G.G. (1995) The respiratory system in a cold environment. *Aviat. Space Environ. Med.*, **66**, 890–902

Gill, J.M. & Hardman, A.E. (2000) Postprandial lipemia: effects of exercise and restriction of energy intake compared. *Am. J. Clin. Nutr.*, **71**, 465-471

Gillette, C.A., Zhu, Z., Westerlind, K.C., Melby, C.L., Wolfe, P. & Thompson, H.J. (1997) Energy availability and mammary carcinogenesis: effects of calorie restriction and exercise. *Carcinogenesis*, **18**, 1183–1188

Giovannucci, E. (1995) Insulin and colon cancer. *Cancer Causes Control*, **6**, 164–179

Giovannucci, E. (1999) Insulin-like growth factor-I and binding protein-3 and risk of cancer. *Horm. Res.*, **51 Suppl. 3**, 34–41

Giovannucci, E., Ascherio, A., Rimm, E.B., Colditz, G.A., Stampfer, M.J. & Willett, W.C. (1995) Physical activity, obesity, and risk for colon cancer and adenoma in men. *Ann. Intern. Med.*, **122**, 327–334

Giovannucci, E., Colditz, G.A., Stampfer, M.J. & Willett, W.C. (1996) Physical activity, obesity, and risk of colorectal adenoma in women (United States). *Cancer Causes Control*, **7**, 253–263

Giovannucci, E., Rimm, E.B., Stampfer, M.J., Colditz, G.A. & Willett, W.C. (1997) Height, body weight, and risk of prostate cancer. *Cancer Epidemiol. Biomarkers Prev.*, **6**, 557–563

Giovannucci, E., Leitzmann, M., Spiegelman, D., Rimm, E.B., Colditz, G.A., Stampfer, M.J. & Willett, W.C. (1998) A prospective study of physical activity and prostate cancer in male health professionals. *Cancer Res.*, **58**, 5117–5122

Giovannucci, E., Pollak, M.N., Platz, E.A.,

Willett, W.C., Stampfer, M.J., Majeed, N., Colditz, G.A., Speizer, F.E. & Hankinson, S.E. (2000) A prospective study of plasma insulin-like growth factor-1 and binding protein-3 and risk of colorectal neoplasia in women. *Cancer Epidemiol. Biomarkers Prev.*, **9**, 345–349

Giuffrida, D., Lupo, L., La Porta, G.A., La Rosa, G.L., Padova, G., Foti, E., Marchese, V. & Belfiore, A. (1992) Relation between steroid receptor status and body weight in breast cancer patients. *Eur. J. Cancer*, **28**, 112–115

Gleeson, M. (2000) Mucosal immunity and respiratory illness in elite athletes. *Int. J. Sports Med.*, **21 Suppl. 1**, S33–S43

Glenny, A.M., O'Meara, S., Melville, A., Sheldon, T.A. & Wilson, C. (1997) The treatment and prevention of obesity: a systematic review of the literature. *Int. J. Obes. Relat. Metab. Disord.*, **21**, 715–737

Godin, G. & Shephard, R.J. (1985) A simple method to assess exercise behavior in the community. *Can. J. Appl. Sport Sci.*, **10**, 141–146

Godsland, I.F., Leyva, F., Walton, C., Worthington, M. & Stevenson, J.C. (1998) Associations of smoking, alcohol and physical activity with risk factors for coronary heart disease and diabetes in the first follow-up cohort of the Heart Disease and Diabetes Risk Indicators in a Screened Cohort study (HDDRISC-1). *J. Intern. Med.*, **244**, 33–41

Gofin, J., Abramson, J.H., Kark, J.D. & Epstein, L. (1996) The prevalence of obesity and its changes over time in middle-aged and elderly men and women in Jerusalem. *Int. J. Obes. Relat. Metab. Disord.*, **20**, 260–266

Goldberg, C.J., Dowling, F.E. & Fogarty, E.E. (1993) Adolescent idiopathic scoliosis — early menarche, normal growth. *Spine*, **18**, 529–535

Golden, N.H., Kreitzer, P., Jacobson, M.S., Chasalow, F.I., Schebendach, J., Freedman, S.M. & Shenker, I.R. (1994) Disturbances in growth hormone secretion and action in adolescents with anorexia nervosa. *J. Pediatr.*, **125**, 655–660

Goldstein, D.J. (1992) Beneficial health effects of modest weight loss. *Int. J. Obes. Relat. Metab. Disord.*, **16**, 397–415

Golland, L.C., Evans, D.L., Stone, G.M., Tyler-McGowan, C.M., Hodgson, D.R. & Rose, R.J. (1999) Maximal exercise transiently disrupts hormonal secretory patterns

in standardbred geldings. *Equine Vet. J. Suppl.*, **30**, 581–585

Good, R.A. & Fernandes, G. (1981) Enhancement of immunologic function and resistance to tumor growth in Balb/c mice by exercise. *Fed. Proc.*, **40**, 1040

Good, R., Hanson, L. & Edelman, R. (1982) Infections and undernutrition. *Nutr. Rev.*, **40**, 119–128

Goodman, M.T. & Wilkens, L.R. (1993) Relation of body size and the risk of lung cancer. *Nutr. Cancer*, **20**, 179–186

Goodman, M.T., Morgenstern, H. & Wynder, E.L. (1986) A case-control study of factors affecting the development of renal cell cancer. *Am. J. Epidemiol.*, **124**, 926–941

Goodman, M.T., Kolonel, L.N. & Wilkens, L.R. (1992) The association of body size, reproductive factors and thyroid cancer. *Br. J. Cancer*, **66**, 1180–1184

Goodman, M.T., Hankin, J.H., Wilkens, L.R., Lyu, L.C., McDuffie, K., Liu, L.Q. & Kolonel, L.N. (1997) Diet, body size, physical activity, and the risk of endometrial cancer. *Cancer Res.*, **57**, 5077–5085

Goodman-Gruen, D. & Barrett-Connor, E. (1997) Epidemiology of insulin-like growth factor-I in elderly men and women. The Rancho Bernardo Study. *Am. J. Epidemiol.*, **145**, 970–976

Goodpaster, B.H., Kelley, D.E., Wing, R.R., Meier, A. & Thaete, F.L. (1999) Effects of weight loss on regional fat distribution and insulin sensitivity in obesity. *Diabetes*, **48**, 839–847

Goodrick, C.L. (1974) The effects of exercise on longevity and behavior of hybrid mice which differ in coat color. *J. Gerontol.*, **29**, 129–133

Goodwin, P.J., Panzarella, T. & Boyd, N.F. (1988) Weight gain in women with localized breast cancer—a descriptive study. *Breast Cancer Res. Treat.*, **11**, 59–66

Goodwin, P., Esplen, M.J., Butler, K., Winocur, J., Pritchard, K., Brazel, S., Gao, J. & Miller, A. (1998) Multidisciplinary weight management in locoregional breast cancer: results of a phase II study. *Breast Cancer Res. Treat.*, **48**, 53–64

Goodyear, L.J. & Kahn, B.B. (1998) Exercise, glucose transport, and insulin sensitivity. *Annu. Rev. Med.*, **49**, 235–261

Grady, D. & Ernster, V.L. (1996) Endometrial cancer. In: Schottenfeld, D. & Fraumeni, J.F., Jr, eds, *Cancer Epidemiology and Prevention*, New York, Oxford University Press, pp. 1058–1089

Graham, T.E. & MacLean, D.A. (1998) Ammonia and amino acid metabolism in skeletal muscle: human, rodent and canine models. *Med. Sci. Sports Exerc.*, **30**, 34–46

Graham, S., Haughey, B., Marshall, J. Priore, R., Byers, T, Rzepka, T. Mettlin. C. & Pontes, J.E. (1983) Diet in the epidemiology of carcinoma of the prostate gland. *J. Natl. Cancer Inst.*, **70**, 687-692

Graham, S., Marshall, J., Haughey, B., Mittelman, A., Swanson, M., Zielezny, M., Byers, T., Wilkinson, G. & West, D. (1988) Dietary epidemiology of cancer of the colon in western New York. *Am. J. Epidemiol.*, **128**, 490–503

Gram, I.T., Funkhouser, E. & Tabar, L. (1999) Moderate physical activity in relation to mammographic patterns. *Cancer Epidemiol. Biomarkers Prev.*, **8**, 117–122

Grant, M.B., Mames, R.N., Fitzgerald, C., Ellis, E.A., Caballero, S., Chegini, N. & Guy, J. (1993) Insulin-like growth factor I as an angiogenic agent. *In vivo* and *in vitro* studies. *Ann. N.Y. Acad. Sci.*, **692**, 230–242

Grasl-Kraupp, B., Bursch, W., Ruttkay-Nedecky, B., Wagner, A., Lauer, B. & Schulte-Hermann, R. (1994) Food restriction eliminates preneoplastic cells through apoptosis and antagonizes carcinogenesis in rat liver. *Proc. Natl Acad. Sci. USA*, **91**, 9995–9999

Gray, A.B., Telford, R.D. & Weidemann, M.J. (1993) Endocrine response to intense interval exercise. *Eur. J. Appl. Physiol*, **66**, 366–371

Greenberg, E.R., Vessey, M.P., McPherson, K., Doll, R. & Yeates, D. (1985) Body size and survival in premenopausal breast cancer. *Br. J. Cancer*, **51**, 691–697

Greene, J.W. (1993) Exercise-induced menstrual irregularities. *Compr. Ther.*, **19**, 116–120

Greenwald, P., Damon, A., Kirmss, V. & Polan, A.K. (1974) Physical and demographic features of men before developing cancer of the prostate. *J. Natl Cancer Inst.*, **53**, 341–346

Grenman, S., Rönnemaa, T., Irjala, K., Kaihola, H.L. & Grönroos, M. (1986) Sex steroid, gonadotropin, cortisol, and prolactin levels in healthy, massively obese women: correlation with abdominal fat cell size and effect of weight reduction. *J. Clin. Endocrinol. Metab.*, **63**, 1257–1261

Grimm, J.J. (1999) Interaction of physical activity and diet: implications for insulin-glucose dynamics. *Public Health Nutr.*, **2**, 363–368

Grisso, J.A., Kelsey, J.L., Strom, B.L., O'Brien, L.A., Maislin, G., LaPann, K., Samelson, L. & Hoffman, S. (1994) Risk factors for hip fracture in black women. The Northeast Hip Fracture Study Group. *New Engl. J. Med.*, **330**, 1555–1559

Grol, M.E., Eimers, J.M., Alberts, J.F., Bouter, L.M., Gerstenbluth, I., Halabi, Y., van Sonderen, E. & van den Heuvel, W.J. (1997) Alarmingly high prevalence of obesity in Curacao: data from an interview survey stratified for socioeconomic status. *Int. J. Obes. Relat. Metab. Disord.*, **21**, 1002–1009

Grönberg, H., Damber, L. & Damber, J.E. (1996) Total food consumption and body mass index in relation to prostate cancer risk: a case-control study in Sweden with prospectively collected exposure data. *J. Urol.*, **155**, 969–974

Gross, L.D., Sallis, J.F., Buono, M.J., Roby, J.J. & Nelson, J.A. (1990) Reliability of interviewers using the Seven-Day Physical Activity Recall. *Res. Q. Exerc. Sport*, **61**, 321–325

Guagnano, M.T., Ballone, E., Pace-Palitti, V., Vecchia, R.D., D'Orazio, N., Manigrasso, M.R., Merlitti, D. & Sensi, S. (2000) Risk factors for hypertension in obese women. The role of weight cycling. *Eur. J. Clin. Nutr.*, **54**, 356-360

Guare, J.C., Wing, R.R. & Grant, A. (1995) Comparison of obese NIDDM and nondiabetic women: short- and long-term weight loss. *Obes. Res.*, **3**, 329-335

Guest, C.S., O'Dea, K., Hopper, J.L. & Larkins, R.G. (1993) Hyperinsulinaemia and obesity in aborigines of south-eastern Australia, with comparisons from rural and urban Europid populations. *Diabetes Res. Clin. Pract.*, **20**, 155–164

Guo, W.D., Hsing, A.W., Li, J.Y., Chen, J.S., Chow, W.H. & Blot, W.J. (1994) Correlation of cervical cancer mortality with reproductive and dietary factors, and serum markers in China. *Int. J. Epidemiol.*, **23**, 1127–1132

Guo, S.S., Zeller, C., Chumlea, W.C. & Siervogel, R.M. (1999) Aging, body composition, and lifestyle: the Fels Longitudinal Study. *Am. J. Clin. Nutr.*, **70**, 405–411

Guzick, D.S., Wing, R., Smith, D., Berga, S.L. & Winters, S.J. (1994) Endocrine consequences of weight loss in obese, hyperandrogenic, anovulatory women. *Fertil. Steril.*, **61**, 598–604

Haapanen, N., Miilunpalo, S., Pasanen, M., Oja, P. & Vuori, I. (1997a) Association between leisure time physical activity and 10-year body mass change among working-aged men and women. *Int. J. Obes. Relat. Metab. Disord.*, **21**, 288–296

Haapanen, N., Miilunpalo, S., Vuori, I., Oja, P. & Pasanen, M. (1997b) Association of leisure time physical activity with the risk of coronary heart disease, hypertension and diabetes in middle-aged men and women. *Int. J. Epidemiol.*, **26**, 739–747

Haapanen-Niemi, N., Miilunpalo, S., Pasanen, M., Vuori, I., Oja, P. & Malmberg, J. (2000) Body mass index, physical inactivity and low level of physical fitness as determinants of all-cause and cardiovascular disease mortality—16 y follow-up of middle-aged and elderly men and women. *Int. J. Obes. Relat. Metab. Disord.*, **24**, 1465–1474

Haapasalo, H., Kannus, P., Sievanen, H., Pasanen, M., Uusi-Rasi, K., Heinonen, A., Oja, P. & Vuori, I. (1998) Effect of long-term unilateral activity on bone mineral density of female junior tennis players. *J. Bone Miner. Res.*, **13**, 310-319

Haddad, F., Bodell, P.W., McCue, S.A., Herrick, R.E. & Baldwin, K.M. (1993) Food restriction-induced transformations in cardiac functional and biochemical properties in rats. *J. Appl. Physiol.*, **74**, 606–612

Hadden, D.R., Blair, A.L., Wilson, E.A., Boyle, D.M., Atkinson, A.B., Kennedy, A.L., Buchanan, K.D., Merrett, J.D., Montgomery, D.A. & Weaver, J.A. (1986) Natural history of diabetes presenting age 40-69 years: a prospective study of the influence of intensive dietary therapy. *Q. J. Med.*, **59**, 579–598

Haffner, S.M. (2000) Sex hormones, obesity, fat distribution, type 2 diabetes and insulin resistance: epidemiological and clinical correlation. *Int. J. Obes. Relat. Metab. Disord.*, **24 Suppl. 2**, S56–S58

Haffner, S.M., Mykkanen, L., Valdez, R.A. & Katz, M.S. (1993a) Relationship of sex hormones to lipids and lipoproteins in nondiabetic men. *J. Clin. Endocrinol. Metab.*, **77**, 1610–1615

Haffner, S.M., Valdez, R.A., Stern, M.P. & Katz, M.S. (1993b) Obesity, body fat distribution and sex hormones in men. *Int. J. Obes. Relat. Metab. Disord.*, **17**, 643–649

Haffner, S.M., Karhapää, P., Mykkänen, L. & Laakso, M. (1994a) Insulin resistance, body fat distribution, and sex hormones in men. *Diabetes*, **43**, 212–219

Haffner, S.M., Valdez, R.A., Mykkänen, L., Stern, M.P. & Katz, M.S. (1994b) Decreased testosterone and dehydroepiandrosterone sulfate concentrations are associated with increased insulin and glucose concentrations in nondiabetic men. *Metabolism*, **43**, 599–603

Haffner, S.M., Miettinen, H., Karhapaa, P., Mykkanen, L. & Laakso, M. (1997) Leptin concentrations, sex hormones, and cortisol in nondiabetic men. *J. Clin. Endocrinol. Metab.*, **82**, 1807–1809

Hagen, J., Deitel, M., Khanna, R.K. & Ilves, R. (1987) Gastroesophageal reflux in the massively obese. *Int. Surg.*, **72**, 1–3

Hainer, V., Stich, V., Kunesova, M., Parizkova, J., Zak, A., Wernischova, V. & Hrabak, P. (1992) Effect of 4-wk treatment of obesity by very-low-calorie diet on anthropometric, metabolic, and hormonal indexes. *Am. J. Clin. Nutr.*, **56**, 281S–282S

Hakim, A.A., Petrovitch, H., Burchfiel, C.M., Ross, G.W., Rodriguez, B.L., White, L.R., Yano, K., Curb, J.D. & Abbott, R.D. (1998) Effects of walking on mortality among nonsmoking retired men. *New Engl. J. Med.*, **338**, 94-99

Häkkinen, K., Pakarinen, A., Kraemer, W.J., Newton, R.U. & Alen, M. (2000) Basal concentrations and acute responses of serum hormones and strength development during heavy resistance training in middle-aged and elderly men and women. *J. Gerontol. A Biol. Sci. Med. Sci.*, **55**, B95–B105

Hall, D.M., Oberley, T.D., Moseley, P.M., Buettner, G.R., Oberley, L.W., Weindruch, R. & Kregel, K.C. (2000a) Caloric restriction improves thermotolerance and reduces hyperthermia-induced cellular damage in old rats. *FASEB J.*, **14**, 78–86

Hall, I.J., Newman, B., Millikan, R.C. & Moorman, P.G. (2000b) Body size and breast cancer risk in black women and white women. The Carolina Breast Cancer Study. *Am. J. Epidemiol.*, **151**, 754–764

Hambrecht, R., Wolf, A., Gielen, S., Linke, A., Hofer, J., Erbs, S., Schoene, N. & Schuler, G. (2000) Effect of exercise on coronary endothelial function in patients with coronary artery disease. *New Engl. J. Med.*, **342**, 454–460

Hamilton-Fairley, D., Kiddy, D., Anyaoku, V., Koistinen, R., Seppälä, M. & Franks, S. (1993) Response of sex hormone binding globulin and insulin-like growth factor binding protein-1 to an oral glucose tolerance test in obese women with polycystic ovary syndrome before and after calorie restriction. *Clin. Endocrinol. (Oxf.)*, **39**, 363–367

Hamm, P., Shekelle, R.B. & Stamler, J. (1989) Large fluctuations in body weight during young adulthood and twenty-five-year risk of coronary death in men. *Am. J. Epidemiol.*, **129**, 312-318

Hammerman, M.R. (1999) The growth hormone-insulin-like growth factor axis in kidney re-revisited. *Nephrol. Dial. Transplant.*, **14**, 1853–1860

Hammond, E.C. & Garfinkel, L. (1969) Coronary heart disease, stroke, and aortic aneurysm. Factors in the etiology. *Arch. Environ. Health*, **19**, 167–182

Han, T.S., van Leer, E.M., Seidell, J.C. & Lean, M.E. (1995) Waist circumference action levels in the identification of cardiovascular risk factors: prevalence study in a random sample. *BMJ*, **311**, 1401–1405

Handa, K., Ishii, H., Kono, S., Shinchi, K., Imanishi, K., Mihara, H. & Tanaka, K. (1997) Behavioral correlates of plasma sex hormones and their relationships with plasma lipids and lipoproteins in Japanese men. *Atherosclerosis*, **130**, 37–44

Hankinson, S.E., Willett, W.C., Manson, J.E., Colditz, G.A., Hunter, D.J., Spiegelman, D., Barbieri, R.L. & Speizer, F.E. (1998a) Plasma sex steroid hormone levels and risk of breast cancer in postmenopausal women. *J. Natl Cancer Inst.*, **90**, 1292–1299

Hankinson, S.E., Willett, W.C., Colditz, G.A., Hunter, D.J., Michaud, D.S., Deroo, B., Rosner, B., Speizer, F.E. & Pollak, M. (1998b) Circulating concentrations of insulin-like growth factor-I and risk of breast cancer. *Lancet*, **351**, 1393–1396

Hanson, R.L., McCance, D.R., Jacobsson, L.T., Narayan, K.M., Nelson, R.G., Pettitt, D.J., Bennett, P.H. & Knowler, W.C. (1995) The U-shaped association between body mass index and mortality: relationship with weight gain in a Native American population. *J. Clin. Epidemiol.*, **48**, 903–916

Hargreaves, M. (1998) 1997 Sir William Refshauge Lecture. Skeletal muscle glucose metabolism during exercise: implications for health and performance. *J. Sci. Med. Sport*, **1**, 195–202

Harkonen, M., Naveri, H., Kuoppasalmi, K. & Huhtaniemi, I. (1990) Pituitary and gonadal function during physical exercise in the male rat. *J. Steroid Biochem.*, **35**, 127–132

Harlass, F.E., Plymate, S.R., Fariss, B.L. & Belts, R.P. (1984) Weight loss is associated with correction of gonadotropin and sex steroid abnormalities in the obese anovulatory female. *Fertil. Steril.*, **42**, 649–652

Harman, S.M., Metter, E.J., Blackman, M.R., Landis, P.K. & Carter, H.B. (2000) Serum levels of insulin-like growth factor I (IGF-I), IGF-II, IGF-binding protein-3, and prostate-specific antigen as predictors of clinical prostate cancer. *J. Clin. Endocrinol. Metab.*, **85**, 4258–4265

Harris, T., Cook, E.F., Garrison, R., Higgins, M., Kannel, W. & Goldman, L. (1988) Body mass index and mortality among nonsmoking older persons. The Framingham Heart Study. *JAMA*, **259**, 1520-1524

Harris, R.E., Namboodiri, K.K. & Wynder, E.L. (1992) Breast cancer risk: effects of estrogen replacement therapy and body mass. *J. Natl Cancer Inst.*, **84**, 1575–1582

Harris, S.R., Brix, A.E., Broderson, J.R. & Bunce, O.R. (1995) Chronic energy restriction versus energy cycling and mammary tumor promotion. *Proc. Soc. Exp. Biol. Med.*, **209**, 231-236

Hartge, P., Schiffman, M.H., Hoover, R., McGowan, L., Lesher, L. & Norris, H.J. (1989) A case-control study of epithelial ovarian cancer. *Am. J. Obstet. Gynecol.*, **161**, 10–16

Hartman, W.M., Stroud, M., Sweet, D.M. & Saxton, J. (1993) Long-term maintenance of weight loss following supplemented fasting. *Int. J. Eat. Disord.*, **14**, 87–93

Hartman, T.J., Albanes, D., Rautalahti, M., Tangrea, J.A., Virtamo, J., Stolzenberg, R. & Taylor, P.R. (1998) Physical activity and prostate cancer in the Alpha-Tocopherol, Beta-Carotene (ATBC) Cancer Prevention Study (Finland). *Cancer Causes Control*, **9**, 11–18

Hartmann, A., Plappert, U., Raddatz, K., Grunert-Fuchs, M. & Speit, G. (1994) Does physical activity induce DNA damage? *Mutagenesis*, **9**, 269–272

Harvell, D.M., Strecker, T.E., Xie, B., Buckles, L.K., Tochacek, M., McComb, R.D. & Shull, J.D. (2001a) Diet/gene interactions in estrogen-induced mammary carcinogenesis in the ACI rat. *J. Nutr.,* **131**, 3087–3091

Harvell, D.M., Spady, T.J., Strecker, T.E., Lemus-Wilson, A.M., Pennington, K.L., Shen, F., Birt, D.F., McComb, R.D. & Shull, J.D. (2001b) Dietary energy restriction inhibits estrogen induced pituitary tumorigenesis in a rat strain specific manner. In: Li, J.J., Li, S.A. & Daling, J.R., eds, *Hormonal Carcinogenesis III,* New York, Springer Verlag, pp. 496–501

Haskell, W.L. (1994) J.B. Wolffe Memorial Lecture. Health consequences of physical activity: understanding and challenges regarding dose-response. *Med. Sci. Sports Exerc.,* **26**, 649–660

Hatta, H., Atomi, Y., Shinohara, S., Yamamoto, Y. & Yamada, S. (1988) The effects of ovarian hormones on glucose and fatty acid oxidation during exercise in female ovariectomized rats. *Horm. Metab. Res.,* **20**, 609–611

Hautanen, A. (2000) Synthesis and regulation of sex hormone-binding globulin in obesity. *Int. J. Obes. Relat. Metab. Disord.,* **24 Suppl. 2**, S64–S70

Health Canada (1999) *Physical Activity of Canadians.* 2.1 Description of the survey and reports. National Population Health Survey Highlights, Ottawa, Health Canada

Heasman, K.Z., Sutherland, H.J., Campbell, J.A., Elhakim, T. & Boyd, N.F. (1985) Weight gain during adjuvant chemotherapy for breast cancer. *Breast Cancer Res. Treat.,* **5**, 195–200

Heath, C.W., Jr, Lally, C.A., Calle, E.E., McLaughlin, J.K. & Thun, M.J. (1997) Hypertension, diuretics, and antihypertensive medications as possible risk factors for renal cell cancer. *Am. J. Epidemiol.,* **145**, 607–613

Heber, D., Ashley, J.M., Leaf, D.A. & Barnard, R.J. (1991) Reduction of serum estradiol in postmenopausal women given free access to low-fat high-carbohydrate diet. *Nutrition,* **7**, 137–139

Hebert, J.R., Augustine, A., Barone, J., Kabat, G.C., Kinne, D.W. & Wynder, E.L. (1988) Weight, height and body mass index in the prognosis of breast cancer: early results of a prospective study. *Int. J. Cancer,* **42**, 315–318

Hebert, P.R., Ajani, U., Cook, N.R., Lee, I.M., Chan, K.S. & Hennekens, C.H. (1997) Adult height and incidence of cancer in male physicians (United States). *Cancer Causes Control,* **8**, 591–597

Heilbronn, L.K., Noakes, M. & Clifton, P.M. (1999) Effect of energy restriction, weight loss, and diet composition on plasma lipids and glucose in patients with type 2 diabetes. *Diabetes Care,* **22**, 889–895

Heinonen, A., Kannus, P., Sievanen, H., Oja, P., Pasanen, M., Rinne, M., Uusi-Rasi, K. & Vuori, I. (1996) Randomised controlled trial of effect of high-impact exercise on selected risk factors for osteoporotic fractures. *Lancet,* **348**, 1343-1347

Heitmann, B.L. (2000) Ten-year trends in overweight and obesity among Danish men and women aged 30–60 years. *Int. J. Obes. Relat. Metab. Disord.,* **24**, 1347–1352

Heitmann, B.L., Kaprio, J., Harris, J.R., Rissanen, A., Korkeila, M. & Koskenvuo, M. (1997) Are genetic determinants of weight gain modified by leisure-time physical activity? A prospective study of Finnish twins. *Am. J. Clin. Nutr.,* **66**, 672–678

Helakorpi, S., Uutela, A., Prättälä, R. & Puska, P. (1999) *Health Behaviour and Health Among Finnish Adult Population, Spring 1999,* Helsinki, National Public Health Institute

Hellénius, M.L., Brismar, K.E., Berglund, B.H. & de Faire, U.H. (1995) Effects on glucose tolerance, insulin secretion, insulin-like growth factor 1 and its binding protein, IGFBP-1, in a randomized controlled diet and exercise study in healthy, middle-aged men. *J. Intern. Med.,* **238**, 121–130

Heller, S.R., Clarke, P., Daly, H., Davis, I., McCulloch, D.K., Allison, S.P. & Tattersall, R.B. (1988) Group education for obese patients with type 2 diabetes: greater success at less cost. *Diabet. Med.,* **5**, 552–556

Helmrich, S.P., Ragland, D.R., Leung, R.W. & Paffenbarger, R.S., Jr (1991) Physical activity and reduced occurrence of non-insulin-dependent diabetes mellitus. *New Engl. J. Med.,* **325**, 147–152

Helzlsouer, K.J., Alberg, A.J., Gordon, G.B., Longcope, C., Bush, T.L., Hoffman, S.C. & Comstock, G.W. (1995) Serum gonadotropins and steroid hormones and the development of ovarian cancer. *JAMA,* **274**, 1926–1930

Henderson, B.E., Casagrande, J.T., Pike, M.C., Mack, T., Rosario, I. & Duke, A. (1983) The epidemiology of endometrial cancer in young women. *Br. J. Cancer,* **47**, 749–756

Henderson, B.E., Ross, R. & Bernstein, L. (1988) Estrogens as a cause of human cancer: the Richard and Hinda Rosenthal Foundation award lecture. *Cancer Res.,* **48**, 246–253

Heuson, J.C. & Legros, N. (1972) Influence of insulin deprivation on growth of the 7,12-dimethylbenz(a)anthracene-induced mammary carcinoma in rats subjected to alloxan diabetes and food restriction. *Cancer Res.,* **32**, 226–232

Heymsfield, S.B., Segal, K.R., Hauptman, J., Lucas, C.P., Boldrin, M.N., Rissanen, A., Wilding, J.P. & Sjöström, L. (2000) Effects of weight loss with orlistat on glucose tolerance and progression to type 2 diabetes in obese adults. *Arch. Intern. Med.,* **160**, 1321–1326

Hiatt, R.A., Tolan, K. & Quesenberry, C.P., Jr (1994) Renal cell carcinoma and thiazide use: a historical, case-control study (California, USA). *Cancer Causes Control,* **5**, 319–325

Higgins, M., D'Agostino, R., Kannel, W., Cobb, J. & Pinsky, J. (1993) Benefits and adverse effects of weight loss. Observations from the Framingham Study. *Ann. Intern. Med.,* **119**, 758-763

Hikita, H., Vaughan, J. & Pitot, H.C. (1997) The effect of two periods of short-term fasting during the promotion stage of hepatocarcinogenesis in rats: the role of apoptosis and cell proliferation. *Carcinogenesis,* **18**, 159–166

Hikita, H., Vaughan, J., Babcock, K. & Pitot, H.C. (1999) Short-term fasting and the reversal of the stage of promotion in rat hepatocarcinogenesis: role of cell replication, apoptosis, and gene expression. *Toxicol. Sci.,* **52**, 17–23

Hilderman, T., McKnight, K., Dhalla, K.S., Rupp, H. & Dhalla, N.S. (1996) Effects of long-term dietary restriction on cardiovascular function and plasma catecholamines in the rat. *Cardiovasc. Drugs Ther.,* **10 Suppl. 1**, 247–250

Hilf, R., Hissin, P.J. & Shafie, S.M. (1978) Regulatory interrelationships for insulin and estrogen action in mammary tumors. *Cancer Res.,* **38**, 4076–4085

Hill, M.J. (1998) Energy intake, physical exercise, overweight and cancer. *Eur. J. Cancer Prev.*, **7**, 251–252

Hill, R.N., Crisp, T.M., Hurley, P.M., Rosenthal, S.L. & Singh, D.V. (1998) Risk assessment eating of thyroid follicular cell tumors. *Environ. Health Perspect.*, **106**, 447–457

Himeno, Y., Engelman, R.W. & Good, R.A. (1992) Influence of calorie restriction on oncogene expression and DNA synthesis during liver regeneration. *Proc. Natl Acad. Sci. USA*, **89**, 5497–5501

Hindmarsh, P., Di Silvio, L., Pringle, P.J., Kurtz, A.B. & Brook, C.G. (1988) Changes in serum insulin concentration during puberty and their relationship to growth hormone. *Clin. Endocrinol. (Oxf.)*, **28**, 381–388

Hirose, K., Tajima, K., Hamajima, N., Inoue, M., Takezaki, T., Kuroishi, T., Yoshida, M. & Tokudome, S. (1995) A large-scale, hospital-based case-control study of risk factors of breast cancer according to menopausal status. *Jpn J. Cancer Res.*, **86**, 146–154

Hirose, K., Tajima, K., Hamajima, N., Takezaki, T., Inoue, M., Kuroishi, T., Kuzuya, K., Nakamura, S. & Tokudome, S. (1996) Subsite (cervix/endometrium)-specific risk and protective factors in uterus cancer. *Jpn J. Cancer Res.*, **87**, 1001–1009

Hislop, T.G., Coldman, A.J., Elwood, J.M., Brauer, G. & Kan, L. (1986) Childhood and recent eating patterns and risk of breast cancer. *Cancer Detect. Prev.*, **9**, 47–58

Ho, S.C., Woo, J. & Sham, A. (1994) Risk factor change in older persons, a perspective from Hong Kong: weight change and mortality. *J. Gerontol.*, **49**, M269–M272

Hochberg, Z., Hertz, P., Colin, V., Ish-Shalom, S., Yeshurun, D., Youdim, M.B. & Amit, T. (1992) The distal axis of growth hormone (GH) in nutritional disorders: GH-binding protein, insulin-like growth factor-I (IGF-I), and IGF-I receptors in obesity and anorexia nervosa. *Metabolism*, **41**, 106–112

Hodge, A.M. & Zimmet, P.Z. (1994) The epidemiology of obesity. *Baillieres Clin. Endocrinol. Metab.*, **8**, 577–599

Hodge, A.M., Dowse, G.K., Zimmet, P.Z. & Collins, V.R. (1995) Prevalence and secular trends in obesity in Pacific and Indian Ocean island populations. *Obes. Res.*, **3 Suppl. 2**, 77s–87s

Hodge, A.M., Dowse, G.K., Gareeboo, H., Tuomilehto, J., Alberti, K.G. & Zimmet, P.Z. (1996) Incidence, increasing prevalence, and predictors of change in obesity and fat distribution over 5 years in the rapidly developing population of Mauritius. *Int. J. Obes. Relat. Metab. Disord.*, **20**, 137–146

Hodgson, D.M., Chiappelli, F., Kung, M., Tio, D.L., Morrow, N.S. & Taylor, A.N. (1996) Effect of acute dietary restriction on the colonization of MADB106 tumor cells in the rat. *Neuroimmunomodulation*, **3**, 371–380

Hodgson, D.M., Chiappelli, F., Morrow, N.S. & Taylor, A.N. (1997) Chronic dietary restriction influences tumor metastasis in the rat: parametric considerations. *Nutr. Cancer*, **28**, 189–198

Hoeberigs, J.H. (1992) Factors related to the incidence of running injuries. A review. *Sports Med.*, **13**, 408–422

Hoek, H.W., van Harten, P.N., van Hoeken, D. & Susser, E. (1998) Lack of relation between culture and anorexia nervosa—results of an incidence study on Curacao. *New Engl. J. Med.*, **338**, 1231–1232

Hoffman, S.A., Paschkis, K.E., DeBias, D.A., Cantarow, A. & Williams, T.L. (1962) The influence of exercise on the growth of transplanted rat tumors. *Cancer Res.*, **22**, 597–599

Hoffman-Goetz, L. (1998) Influence of physical activity and exercise on innate immunity. *Nutr. Rev.*, **56**, S126–S130

Hoffman-Goetz, L., MacNeil, B., Arumugam, Y. & Randall Simpson, J. (1992) Differential effects of exercise and housing condition on murine natural killer cell activity and tumor growth. *Int. J. Sports Med.*, **13**, 167–171

Hoffman-Goetz, L., May, K.M. & Arumugam, Y. (1994) Exercise training and mouse mammary tumour metastasis. *Anticancer Res.*, **14**, 2627–2631

Hoffman-Goetz, L., Apter, D., Demark-Wahnefried, W., Goran, M.I., McTiernan, A. & Reichman, M.E. (1998) Possible mechanisms mediating an association between physical activity and breast cancer. *Cancer*, **83**, 621–628

Holbrook, T.L. & Barrett-Connor, E. (1993) The association of lifetime weight and weight control patterns with bone mineral density in an adult community. *Bone Miner.*, **20**, 141–149

Holdstock, D.J., Misiewicz, J.J., Smith, T. & Rowlands, E.N. (1970) Propulsion (mass movements) in the human colon and its relationship to meals and somatic activity. *Gut*, **11**, 91–99

Hollander, P.A., Elbein, S.C., Hirsch, I.B., Kelley, D., McGill, J., Taylor, T., Weiss, S.R., Crockett, S.E., Kaplan, R.A., Comstock, J., Lucas, C.P., Lodewick, P.A., Canovatchel, W., Chung, J. & Hauptman, J. (1998) Role of orlistat in the treatment of obese patients with type 2 diabetes. A 1-year randomized double-blind study. *Diabetes Care*, **21**, 1288–1294

Holloszy, J.O. (1997) Mortality rate and longevity of food-restricted exercising male rats: a reevaluation. *J. Appl. Physiol.*, **82**, 399–403

Holloszy, J.O. & Schechtman, K.B. (1991) Interaction between exercise and food restriction: effects on longevity of male rats. *J. Appl. Physiol.*, **70**, 1529–1535

Holloszy, J.O., Smith, E.K., Vining, M. & Adams, S. (1985) Effect of voluntary exercise on longevity of rats. *J. Appl. Physiol.*, **59**, 826–831

Holme, I., Helgeland, A., Hjermann, I., Leren, P. & Lund-Larsen, P.G. (1981) Physical activity at work and at leisure in relation to coronary risk factors and social class. A 4-year mortality follow-up. The Oslo study. *Acta Med. Scand.*, **209**, 277–283

Holte, J., Bergh, T., Gennarelli, G. & Wide, L. (1994) The independent effects of polycystic ovary syndrome and obesity on serum concentrations of gonadotrophins and sex steroids in premenopausal women. *Clin. Endocrinol. (Oxf.)*, **41**, 473–481

Holte, J., Bergh, T., Berne, C., Wide, L. & Lithell, H. (1995) Restored insulin sensitivity but persistently increased early insulin secretion after weight loss in obese women with polycystic ovary syndrome. *J. Clin. Endocrinol. Metab.*, **80**, 2586–2593

Hopkins, W.G., Wilson, N.C., Russell, D.G. & Herbison, G.P. (1991) *Life in New Zealand Commission Report*. Volume III: *Physical Activity*, Dunedin, University of Otago, pp. 1–54

Hopkins, N.J., Jakeman, P.M., Hughes, S.C. & Holly, J.M. (1994) Changes in circulating insulin-like growth factor-binding protein-1 (IGFBP-1) during prolonged exercise: effect of carbohydrate feeding. *J. Clin. Endocrinol. Metab.*, **79**, 1887–1890

Hornum, M., Cooper, D.M., Brasel, J.A., Bueno, A. & Sietsema, K.E. (1997) Exercise-induced changes in circulating growth factors with cyclic variation in plasma estradiol in women. *J. Appl. Physiol.*, **82**, 1946–1951

Host, C.R., Norton, K.I., Olds, T.S., Lowe, E.L. & Mulligan, S.P. (1995) The effects of altered exercise distribution on lymphocyte subpopulations. *Eur. J. Appl. Physiol.*, **72**, 157–164

Houmard, J.A., McCulley, C., Shinebarger, M.H. & Bruno, N.J. (1994) Effects of exercise training on plasma androgens in men. *Horm. Metab. Res.*, **26**, 297–300

Houmard, J.A., Shaw, C.D., Hickey, M.S. & Tanner, C.J. (1999) Effect of short-term exercise training on insulin-stimulated PI 3-kinase activity in human skeletal muscle. *Am. J. Physiol.*, **277**, E1055–E1060

Hsieh, C.C., Trichopoulos, D., Katsouyanni, K. & Yuasa, S. (1990) Age at menarche, age at menopause, height and obesity as risk factors for breast cancer: associations and interactions in an international case-control study. *Int. J. Cancer*, **46**, 796–800

Hsieh, C.C., Signorello, L.B., Lipworth, L., Lagiou, P., Mantzoros, C.S. & Trichopoulos, D. (1998) Predictors of sex hormone levels among the elderly: a study in Greece. *J. Clin. Epidemiol.*, **51**, 837–841

Hsieh, C.C., Thanos, A., Mitropoulos, D., Deliveliotis, C., Mantzoros, C.S. & Trichopoulos, D. (1999) Risk factors for prostate cancer: a case-control study in Greece. *Int. J. Cancer*, **80**, 699–703

Hsing, A.W., McLaughlin, J.K., Zheng, W., Gao, Y.T. & Blot, W.J. (1994) Occupation, physical activity, and risk of prostate cancer in Shanghai, People's Republic of China. *Cancer Causes Control*, **5**, 136–140

Hsing, A.W., McLaughlin, J.K., Cocco, P., Co-Chien, H.T. & Fraumeni, J.F., Jr (1998a) Risk factors for male breast cancer (United States). *Cancer Causes Control*, **9**, 269–275

Hsing, A.W., McLaughlin, J.K., Chow, W.H., Schuman, L.M., Co-Chien, H.T., Gridley, G., Bjelke, E., Wacholder, S. & Blot, W.J. (1998b) Risk factors for colorectal cancer in a prospective study among U.S. white men. *Int. J. Cancer*, **77**, 549–553

Hsing, A.W., Deng, J., Sesterhenn, I.A., Mostofi, F.K., Stanczyk, F.Z., Benichou, J., Xie, T. & Gao, Y.T. (2000) Body size and prostate cancer: a population-based case-control study in China. *Cancer Epidemiol. Biomarkers Prev.*, **9**, 1335–1341

Hsu, L.K. (1996) Epidemiology of the eating disorders. *Psychiatr. Clin. North Am.*, **19**, 681–700

Hsu, L.K. (1997) Can dieting cause an eating disorder? *Psychol. Med.*, **27**, 509–513

Hsu-Hage, B.H. & Wahlqvist, M.L. (1993) Cardiovascular risk in adult Melbourne Chinese. *Aust. J. Public Health*, **17**, 306–313

Hu, Y.H., Nagata, C., Shimizu, H., Kaneda, N. & Kashiki, Y. (1997) Association of body mass index, physical activity, and reproductive histories with breast cancer: a case-control study in Gifu, Japan. *Breast Cancer Res. Treat.*, **43**, 65–72

Hu, F.B., Manson, J.E., Liu, S., Hunter, D., Colditz, G.A., Michels, K.B., Speizer, F.E. & Giovannucci, E. (1999a) Prospective study of adult onset diabetes mellitus (type 2) and risk of colorectal cancer in women. *J. Natl Cancer Inst.*, **91**, 542–547

Hu, F.B., Sigal, R.J., Rich-Edwards, J.W., Colditz, G.A., Solomon, C.G., Willett, W.C., Speizer, F.E. & Manson, J.E. (1999b) Walking compared with vigorous physical activity and risk of type 2 diabetes in women: a prospective study. *JAMA*, **282**, 1433–1439

Hu, F.B., Stampfer, M.J., Colditz, G.A., Ascherio, A., Rexrode, K.M., Willett, W.C. & Manson, J.E. (2000) Physical activity and risk of stroke in women. *JAMA*, **283**, 2961-2967

Huang, Z., Hankinson, S.E., Colditz, G.A., Stampfer, M.J., Hunter, D.J., Manson, J.E., Hennekens, C.H., Rosner, B., Speizer, F.E. & Willett, W.C. (1997) Dual effects of weight and weight gain on breast cancer risk. *JAMA*, **278**, 1407–1411

Huang, Z., Willett, W.C., Manson, J.E., Rosner, B., Stampfer, M.J., Speizer, F.E. & Colditz, G.A. (1998) Body weight, weight change, and risk for hypertension in women. *Ann. Intern. Med.*, **128**, 81-88

Huang, Z., Willett, W.C., Colditz, G.A., Hunter, D.J., Manson, J.E., Rosner, B., Speizer, F.E. & Hankinson, S.E. (1999) Waist circumference, waist:hip ratio, and risk of breast cancer in the Nurses' Health Study. *Am. J. Epidemiol.*, **150**, 1316–1324

Hurel, S.J., Koppiker, N., Newkirk, J., Close, P.R., Miller, M., Mardell, R., Wood, P.J. &

Kendall-Taylor, P. (1999) Relationship of physical exercise and ageing to growth hormone production. *Clin. Endocrinol. (Oxf.)*, **51**, 687–691

Hurley, B.F., Nemeth, P.M., Martin, W.H., Hagberg, J.M., Dalsky, G.P. & Holloszy, J.O. (1986) Muscle triglyceride utilization during exercise: effect of training. *J. Appl. Physiol.*, **60**, 562–567

Hursting, S.D., Switzer, B.R., French, J.E. & Kari, F.W. (1993) The growth hormone: insulin-like growth factor 1 axis is a mediator of diet restriction-induced inhibition of mononuclear cell leukemia in Fischer rats. *Cancer Res.*, **53**, 2750–2757

Hursting, S.D., Perkins, S.N. & Phang, J.M. (1994) Calorie restriction delays spontaneous tumorigenesis in p53-knockout transgenic mice. *Proc. Natl Acad Sci U S A*, **91**, 7036–7040

Hursting, S.D., Perkins, S.N., Brown, C.C., Haines, D.C. & Phang, J.M. (1997) Calorie restriction induces a p53-independent delay of spontaneous carcinogenesis in p53-deficient and wild-type mice. *Cancer Res.*, **57**, 2843–2846

IARC (1986) *IARC Monographs on the Evaluation of Carcinogenic Risks to Humans.* Vol. 38, *Tobacco Smoking,* Lyon, International Agency for Research on Cancer

IARC (1988) *IARC Monographs on the Evaluation of Carcinogenic Risks to Humans.* Vol. 44, *Alcohol Drinking,* Lyon, International Agency for Research on Cancer

IARC (1999) *IARC Monographs on the Evaluation of Carcinogenic Risks to Humans.* Vol. 72, *Hormonal Contraception and Post-Menopausal Hormonal Therapy,* Lyon, IARC

Iatropoulos, M.J., Williams, G.M., Abdo, K.M., Kari, F.W. & Hart, R.W. (1997) Mechanistic studies on genotoxicity and carcinogenicity of salicylazosulfapyridine, an anti-inflammatory medicine. *Exp. Toxicol. Pathol.*, **49**, 15–28

Ikuyama, T., Watanabe, T., Minegishi, Y. & Osanai, H. (1993) Effect of voluntary exercise on 3'-methyl-4-dimethylaminoazobenzene-induced hepatomas in male Jc1:Wistar rats. *Proc. Soc. Exp. Biol. Med.*, **204**, 211–215

Ilic, M., Vlajinac, H. & Marinkovic, J. (1996) Case-control study of risk factors for prostate cancer. *Br. J. Cancer*, **74**, 1682–1686

Imai, K., Matsuyama, S., Miyake, S., Suga, K. & Nakachi, K. (2000) Natural cytotoxic activity of peripheral-blood lymphocytes and cancer incidence: an 11-year follow-up study of a general population. *Lancet*, **356**, 1795–1799

Innes, K., Byers, T. & Schymura, M. (2000) Birth characteristics and subsequent risk for breast cancer in very young women. *Am. J. Epidemiol.*, **152**, 1121–1128

Inoue, M., Okayama, A., Fujita, M., Enomoto, T., Tanizawa, O. & Ueshima, H. (1994) A case–control study on risk factors for uterine endometrial cancer in Japan. *Jpn J. Cancer Res.*, **85**, 346–350

Ip, C. (1990) Quantitative assessment of fat and calorie as risk factors in mammary carcinogenesis in an experimental model. *Prog. Clin. Biol. Res.*, **346**, 107–117

Iranmanesh, A., Lizarralde, G. & Veldhuis, J.D. (1991) Age and relative adiposity are specific negative determinants of the frequency and amplitude of growth hormone (GH) secretory bursts and the half-life of endogenous GH in healthy men. *J. Clin. Endocrinol. Metab.*, **73**, 1081–1088

Iribarren, C., Sharp, D.S., Burchfiel, C.M. & Petrovitch, H. (1995) Association of weight loss and weight fluctuation with mortality among Japanese American men. *New Engl. J. Med.*, **333**, 686-692

Irish Heart Foundation (1994) *Happy Heart National Survey: A Report on Health Behaviour in Ireland*, Dublin, Irish Heart Foundation

Ismail, M.N., Zawiah, H., Chee, S.S. & Ng, K.K. (1995) Prevalence of obesity and chronic energy deficiency (CED) in adult Malaysians. *Malaysian J. Nutr.*, **1**, 1–10

Ivandic, A., Prpic-Krizevac, I., Sucic, M. & Juric, M. (1998) Hyperinsulinemia and sex hormones in healthy premenopausal women: relative contribution of obesity, obesity type, and duration of obesity. *Metabolism*, **47**, 13–19

Ivy, J.L. (1997) Role of exercise training in the prevention and treatment of insulin resistance and non-insulin-dependent diabetes mellitus. *Sports Med.*, **24**, 321–336

Iwasaki, K., Gleiser, C.A., Masoro, E.J., McMahan, C.A., Seo, E.J. & Yu, B.P. (1988) The influence of dietary protein source on longevity and age-related disease processes of Fischer rats. *J. Gerontol.*, **43**, B5–12

Jacobs, D.R., Jr, Hahn, L.P., Haskell, W.L., Pirie, P. & Sidney, S. (1989) Validity and reliability of short physical activity history: CARDIA and the Minnesota Heart Health Program. *J. Cardiopulm. Rehabil.*, **9**, 448–459

Jacobs, D.R., Jr, Ainsworth, B.E., Hartman, T.J. & Leon, A.S. (1993) A simultaneous evaluation of 10 commonly used physical activity questionnaires. *Med. Sci. Sports Exerc.*, **25**, 81–91

Jakicic, J.M., Wing, R.R., Butler, B.A. & Robertson, R.J. (1995) Prescribing exercise in multiple short bouts versus one continuous bout: effects on adherence, cardiorespiratory fitness, and weight loss in overweight women. *Int. J. Obes. Relat. Metab. Disord.*, **19**, 893–901

Jakicic, J.M., Winters, C., Lang, W. & Wing, R.R. (1999) Effects of intermittent exercise and use of home exercise equipment on adherence, weight loss, and fitness in overweight women: a randomized trial. *JAMA*, **282**, 1554–1560

Jakubowicz, D.J. & Nestler, J.E. (1997) 17α-Hydroxyprogesterone responses to leuprolide and serum androgens in obese women with and without polycystic ovary syndrome offer dietary weight loss. *J. Clin. Endocrinol. Metab.*, **82**, 556–560

James, S.J. & Muskhelishvili, L. (1994) Rates of apoptosis and proliferation vary with caloric intake and may influence incidence of spontaneous hepatoma in C57BL/6 x C3H F_1 mice. *Cancer Res.*, **54**, 5508–5510

James, W.P., Astrup, A., Finer, N., Hilsted, J., Kopelman, P., Rossner, S., Saris, W.H. & Van Gaal, L.F. (2000) Effect of sibutramine on weight maintenance after weight loss: a randomised trial. STORM Study Group. Sibutramine Trial of Obesity Reduction and Maintenance. *Lancet*, **356**, 2119–2125

Jäpel, M., Lötzerich, H. & Appell, H.J. (1992) Physical exercise may improve macrophage phagocytic activity of tumor bearing mice. *In Vivo*, **6**, 215–218

Jasper, H., Pennisi, P., Vitale, M., Mella, A., Ropelato, G. & Chervin, A. (1999) Evaluation of disease activity by IGF-I and IGF binding protein-3 (IGFBP3) in acromegaly patients distributed according to a clinical score. *J. Endocrinol. Invest.*, **22**, 29–34

Jebb, S.A. & Moore, M.S. (1999) Contribution of a sedentary lifestyle and inactivity to the etiology of overweight and obesity: current evidence and research issues. *Med. Sci. Sports Exerc.*, **31**, S534–S541

Jeffery, R.W., Bjornson-Benson, W.M., Rosenthal, B.S., Lindquist, R.A., Kurth, C.L. & Johnson, S.L. (1984) Correlates of weight loss and its maintenance over two years of follow-up among middle-aged men. *Prev. Med.*, **13**, 155–168

Jeffery, R.W., Gray, C.W., French, S.A., Hellerstedt, W.L., Murray, D., Luepker, R.V. & Blackburn, H. (1995) Evaluation of weight reduction in a community intervention for cardiovascular disease risk: changes in body mass index in the Minnesota Heart Health Program. *Int. J. Obes. Relat. Metab. Disord.*, **19**, 30–39

Jeffery, R.W., Drewnowski, A., Epstein, L.H., Stunkard, A.J., Wilson, G.T., Wing, R.R. & Hill, D.R. (2000) Long-term maintenance of weight loss: current status. *Health Psychol.*, **19**, 5–16

Jensen, L.B., Quaade, F. & Sørensen, O.H. (1994) Bone loss accompanying voluntary weight loss in obese humans. *J. Bone Miner. Res.*, **9**, 459–463

Ji, B.T., Hatch, M.C., Chow, W.H., McLaughlin, J.K., Dai, Q., Howe, G.R., Gao, Y.T. & Fraumeni, J.F., Jr (1996) Anthropometric and reproductive factors and the risk of pancreatic cancer: a case–control study in Shanghai, China. *Int. J. Cancer*, **66**, 432–437

Ji, B.T., Chow, W.H., Yang, G., McLaughlin, J.K., Gao, R.N., Zheng, W., Shu, X.O., Jin, F., Fraumeni, J.F., Jr & Gao, Y.T. (1997) Body mass index and the risk of cancers of the gastric cardia and distal stomach in Shanghai, China. *Cancer Epidemiol. Biomarkers Prev.*, **6**, 481–485

Joakimsen, R.M., Fonnebo, V., Magnus, J.H., Tollan, A. & Sogaard, A.J. (1998) The Tromso Study: body height, body mass index and fractures. *Osteopor. Int.*, **8**, 436–442

John, E.M., Schwartz, G.G., Dreon, D.M. & Koo, J. (1999) Vitamin D and breast cancer risk: the NHANES I epidemiologic follow-up study, 1971-1975 to 1992. National Health and Nutrition Examination Survey. *Cancer Epidemiol. Biomarkers Prev.*, **8**, 399–406

Jones, N.L. & Campbell, E.J. (1982) *Clinical Exercise Testing*, 2nd ed., Philadelphia, W.B. Saunders, pp. 1–249

Jones, C.O. & White, N.G. (1994) Adiposity in aboriginal people from Arnhem Land, Australia: variation in degree and distribution associated with age, sex and lifestyle. *Ann. Hum. Biol.*, **21**, 207–227

Jones, J.I. & Clemmons, D.R. (1995) Insulin-like growth factors and their binding proteins: biological actions. *Endocr. Rev.*, **16**, 3–34

Jonsdottir, I.H. (2000) Exercise immunology: neuroendocrine regulation of NK-cells. *Int. J. Sports Med.*, **21 Suppl. 1**, S20–S23

Jürimäe, T., Karelson, K., Smirnova, T. & Viru, A. (1990) The effect of a single-circuit weight-training session on the blood biochemistry of untrained university students. *Eur. J. Appl. Physiol*, **61**, 344–348

Juul, A., Main, K., Blum, W.F., Lindholm, J., Ranke, M.B. & Skakkebæk, N.E. (1994) The ratio between serum levels of insulin-like growth factor (IGF)-I and the IGF binding proteins (IGFBP-1, 2 and 3) decreases with age in healthy adults and is increased in acromegalic patients. *Clin. Endocrinol. (Oxf.)*, **41**, 85–93

Kaaks, R. (1996) Nutrition, hormones, and breast cancer: is insulin the missing link? *Cancer Causes Control*, **7**, 605–625

Kaaks, R. & Lukanova, A. (2001) Energy balance and cancer: the role of insulin and insulin-like growth factor-I. *Proc. Nutr. Soc.*, **60**, 1–16

Kaaks, R., Van Noord, P.A., den Tonkelaar, I., Peeters, P.J.H., Riboli, E. & Grobbee, D.E. (1998) Breast-cancer incidence in relation to height, weight and body-fat distribution in the Dutch "DOM" cohort. *Int. J. Cancer*, **76**, 647–651

Kaaks, R., Lukanova, A. & Sommersberg, B. (2000a) Plasma androgens, IGF-I, body size, and prostate cancer risk: a synthetic review. *Prostate Cancer Prostat. Dis.*, **3**, 157–172

Kaaks, R., Toniolo, P., Akhmedkhanov, A., Lukanova, A., Biessy, C., Déchaud, H., Rinaldi, S., Zeleniuch-Jacquotte, A., Shore, R.E. & Riboli, E. (2000b) Serum C-peptide, insulin-like growth factor (IGF)-I, IGF-binding proteins, and colorectal cancer risk in women. *J. Natl Cancer Inst.*, **92**, 1592–1600

Kabat, G.C. & Wynder, E.L. (1992) Body mass index and lung cancer risk. *Am. J. Epidemiol.*, **135**, 769–774

Kabat, G.C., Ng, S.K. & Wynder, E.L. (1993) Tobacco, alcohol intake, and diet in relation to adenocarcinoma of the esophagus and gastric cardia. *Cancer Causes Control*, **4**, 123–132

Kabat, G.C., Chang, C.J. & Wynder, E.L. (1994) The role of tobacco, alcohol use, and body mass index in oral and pharyngeal cancer. *Int. J. Epidemiol.*, **23**, 1137–1144

Kabat, G.C., Chang, C.J., Sparano, J.A., Sepkovie, D.W., Hu, X.P., Khalil, A., Rosenblatt, R. & Bradlow, H.L. (1997) Urinary estrogen metabolites and breast cancer: a case-control study. *Cancer Epidemiol. Biomarkers Prev.*, **6**, 505–509

Kabuto, M., Akiba, S., Stevens, R.G., Neriishi, K. & Land, C.E. (2000) A prospective study of estradiol and breast cancer in Japanese women. *Cancer Epidemiol. Biomarkers Prev.*, **9**, 575–579

Kadyrova, R.K. & Shakieva, R.A. (1986) Dynamics of changes in the lipid composition of bile in patients with alimentary obesity during treatment [in Russian]. *Ter. Arkh.*, **58**, 79–82

Kahn, H.S., Tatham, L.M., Rodriguez, C., Calle, E.E., Thun, M.J. & Heath, C.W. (1997) Stable behaviors associated with adults' 10-year change in body mass index and likelihood of gain at the waist. *Am. J. Public Health*, **87**, 747–754

Kaijser, M., Lichtenstein, P., Granath, F., Erlandsson, G., Cnattingius, S. & Ekbom, A. (2001) In utero exposures and breast cancer: a study of opposite-sexed twins. *J. Natl Cancer Inst.*, **93**, 60–62

Kakizawa, S., Kaneko, T., Hasegawa, S. & Hirano, T. (1995) Effects of feeding, fasting, background adaptation, acute stress, and exhaustive exercise on the plasma somatolactin concentrations in rainbow trout. *Gen. Comp. Endocrinol.*, **98**, 137–146

Kampert, J.B., Blair, S.N., Barlow, C.E. & Kohl, H.W.I. (1996) Physical activity, physical fitness, and all-cause and cancer mortality: a prospective study of men and women. *Ann. Epidemiol.*, **6**, 452–457

Kampman, E., Potter, J.D., Slattery, M.L., Caan, B.J. & Edwards, S. (1997) Hormone replacement therapy, reproductive history, and colon cancer: a multicenter, case-control study in the United States. *Cancer Causes Control*, **8**, 146–158

Kannus, P., Haapasalo, H., Sankelo, M., Sievänen, H., Pasanen, M., Heinonen, A., Oja, P. & Vuori, I. (1995) Effect of starting age of physical activity on bone mass in the dominant arm of tennis and squash players. *Ann. Intern. Med.*, **123**, 27-31

Kari, F.W., Dunn, S.E., French, J.E. & Barrett, J.C. (1999) Roles for insulin-like growth factor-1 in mediating the anti-carcinogenic effects of caloric restriction. *J. Nutr. Health Aging*, **3**, 92–101

Kark, J.D., Yaari, S., Rasooly, I. & Goldbourt, U. (1995) Are lean smokers at increased risk of lung cancer? The Israel Civil Servant Cancer Study. *Arch. Intern. Med.*, **155**, 2409–2416

Karlsson, J., Sjöström, L. & Sullivan, M. (1998) Swedish obese subjects (SOS) — an intervention study of obesity. Two-year follow-up of health-related quality of life (HRQL) and eating behavior after gastric surgery for severe obesity. *Int. J. Obes. Relat. Metab. Disord.*, **22**, 113-126

Kasim-Karakas, S.E., Almario, R.U., Mueller, W.M. & Peerson, J. (2000) Changes in plasma lipoproteins during low-fat, high-carbohydrate diets: effects of energy intake. *Am. J. Clin. Nutr.*, **71**, 1439–1447

Kato, I., Tominaga, S. & Ikari, A. (1990) A case-control study of male colorectal cancer in Aichi Prefecture, Japan: with special reference to occupational activity level, drinking habits and family history. *Jpn J. Cancer Res*, **81**, 115–121

Kato, I., Toniolo, P., Zeleniuch-Jacquotte, A., Shore, R.E., Koenig, K.L., Akhmedkhanov, A. & Riboli, E. (2000) Diet, smoking and anthropometric indices and postmenopausal bone fractures: a prospective study. *Int. J. Epidemiol.*, **29**, 85–92

Katsouyanni, K., Boyle, P. & Trichopoulos, D. (1991) Diet and urine estrogens among postmenopausal women. *Oncology*, **48**, 490–494

Katz, L.E., Satin-Smith, M.S., Collett-Solberg, P., Baker, L., Stanley, C.A. & Cohen, P. (1998) Dual regulation of insulin-like growth factor binding protein-1 levels by insulin and cortisol during fasting. *J. Clin. Endocrinol. Metab.*, **83**, 4426–4430

Kaye, S.A., Folsom, A.R., Soler, J.T., Prineas, R.J. & Potter, J.D. (1991) Associations of body mass and fat distribution with sex hormone concentrations in postmenopausal women. *Int. J. Epidemiol.*, **20**, 151–156

Kazakoff, K., Cardesa, T., Liu, J., Adrian, T.E., Bagchi, D., Bagchi, M., Birt, D.F. & Pour, P.M. (1996) Effects of voluntary physical exercise on high-fat diet-promoted pancreatic carcinogenesis in the hamster model. *Nutr. Cancer*, **26**, 265–279

Kearney, J.M., Kearney, M.J., McElhone, S. & Gibney, M.J. (1999) Methods used to conduct the pan-European Union survey on consumer attitudes to physical activity, body weight and health. *Public Health Nutr.*, **2**, 79–86

Keen, A.D. & Drinkwater, B.L. (1997) Irreversible bone loss in former amenorrheic athletes. *Osteopor. Int.*, **7**, 311–315

Keenan, K.P., Laroque, P., Soper, K.A., Morrissey, R.E. & Dixit, R. (1996) The effects of overfeeding and moderate dietary restriction on Sprague-Dawley rat survival, pathology, carcinogenicity, and the toxicity of pharmaceutical agents. *Exp. Toxicol. Pathol.*, **48**, 139–144

Keizer, H.A. & Rogol, A.D. (1990) Physical exercise and menstrual cycle alterations. What are the mechanisms? *Sports Med.*, **10**, 218–235

Kelder, S.H., Perry, C.L. & Klepp, K.I. (1993) Community-wide youth exercise promotion: long-term outcomes of the Minnesota Heart Health Program and the Class of 1989 Study. *J. School Health*, **63**, 218–223

Kelley, D.E. & Goodpaster, B.H. (1999) Effects of physical activity on insulin action and glucose tolerance in obesity. *Med. Sci. Sports Exerc.*, **31**, S619–S623

Kelley, D.S., Daudu, P.A., Branch, L.B., Johnson, H.L., Taylor, P.C. & Mackey, B. (1994) Energy restriction decreases number of circulating natural killer cells and serum levels of immunoglobulins in overweight women. *Eur. J. Clin. Nutr.*, **48**, 9–18

Kelsey, J.L., LiVolsi, V.A., Holford, T.R., Fischer, D.B., Mostow, E.D., Schwartz, P.E., O'Connor, T. & White, C. (1982) A case–control study of cancer of the endometrium. *Am. J. Epidemiol.*, **116**, 333–342

Kennedy, S.H., Brown, G.M., McVey, G. & Garfinkel, P.E. (1991) Pineal and adrenal function before and after refeeding in anorexia nervosa. *Biol. Psychiatry*, **30**, 216–224

Kestin, A.S., Ellis, P.A., Barnard, M.R., Errichetti, A., Rosner, B.A. & Michelson, A.D. (1993) Effect of strenuous exercise on platelet activation state and reactivity. *Circulation*, **88**, 1502–1511

Key, T.J. & Pike, M.C. (1988) The dose-effect relationship between 'unopposed' oestrogens and endometrial mitotic rate: its central role in explaining and predicting endometrial cancer risk. *Br. J. Cancer*, **57**, 205–212

Key, T.J., Silcocks, P.B., Davey, G.K., Appleby, P.N. & Bishop, D.T. (1997) A case-control study of diet and prostate cancer. *Br. J. Cancer*, **76**, 678–687

Khandwala, H.M., McCutcheon, I.E., Flyvbjerg, A. & Friend, K.E. (2000) The effects of insulin-like growth factors on tumorigenesis and neoplastic growth. *Endocr. Rev.*, **21**, 215–244

Kiddy, D.S., Hamilton-Fairley, D., Seppala, M., Koistinen, R., James, V.H., Reed, M.J. & Franks, S. (1989) Diet-induced changes in sex hormone binding globulin and free testosterone in women with normal or polycystic ovaries: correlation with serum insulin and insulin-like growth factor-I. *Clin. Endocrinol. (Oxf.)*, **31**, 757–763

Kiddy, D.S., Hamilton-Fairley, D., Bush, A., Short, F., Anyaoku, V., Reed, M.J. & Franks, S. (1992) Improvement in endocrine and ovarian function during dietary treatment of obese women with polycystic ovary syndrome. *Clin. Endocrinol. (Oxf.)*, **36**, 105–111

Kim, Y.I. (1998) Diet, lifestyle, and colorectal cancer: is hyperinsulinemia the missing link? *Nutr. Rev.*, **56**, 275–279

Kim, J.D., McCarter, R.J. & Yu, B.P. (1996) Influence of age, exercise, and dietary restriction on oxidative stress in rats. *Aging (Milano)*, **8**, 123–129

King, A.C., Frey-Hewitt, B., Dreon, D.M. & Wood, P.D. (1989) Diet vs exercise in weight maintenance. The effects of minimal intervention strategies on long-term outcomes in men. *Arch. Intern. Med.*, **149**, 2741–2746

King, A.C., Haskell, W.L., Taylor, C.B., Kraemer, H.C. & DeBusk, R.F. (1991) Group-vs home-based exercise training in healthy older men and women. A community-based clinical trial. *JAMA*, **266**, 1535–1542

King, D.S., Baldus, P.J., Sharp, R.L., Kesl, L.D., Feltmeyer, T.L. & Riddle, M.S. (1995) Time course for exercise-induced alterations in insulin action and glucose tolerance in middle-aged people. *J. Appl. Physiol.*, **78**, 17–22

King, A.C., Pruitt, L.A., Phillips, W., Oka, R., Rodenburg, A. & Haskell, W.L. (2000) Comparative effects of two physical activity programs on measured and perceived physical functioning and other health-related quality of life outcomes in older adults. *J. Gerontol. A Biol. Sci. Med. Sci.*, **55**, M74–M83

Kirkpatrick, C.S., White, E. & Lee, J.A. (1994) Case-control study of malignant melanoma in Washington State. II. Diet, alcohol, and obesity. *Am. J. Epidemiol.*, **139**, 869–880

Kirschner, M.A., Samojlik, E., Drejka, M., Szmal, E., Schneider, G. & Ertel, N. (1990) Androgen-estrogen metabolism in women with upper body *versus* lower body obesity. *J. Clin. Endocrinol. Metab.*, **70**, 473–479

Klesges, R.C., Klesges, L.M., Haddock, C.K. & Eck, L.H. (1992) A longitudinal analysis of the impact of dietary intake and physical activity on weight change in adults. *Am. J. Clin. Nutr.*, **55**, 818–822

Kluge, A., Zimmermann, R., Münkel, B., Mohri, M., Sack, S., Schaper, J. & Schaper, W. (1995) Insulin-like growth factor I is involved in inflammation linked angiogenic processes after microembolisation in porcine heart. *Cardiovasc. Res.*, **29**, 407–415

Klurfeld, D.M., Welch, C.B., Davis, M.J. & Kritchevsky, D. (1989a) Determination of degree of energy restriction necessary to reduce DMBA-induced mammary tumorigenesis in rats during the promotion phase. *J. Nutr.*, **119**, 286–291

Klurfeld, D.M., Welch, C.B., Lloyd, L.M. & Kritchevsky, D. (1989b) Inhibition of DMBA-induced mammary tumorigenesis by caloric restriction in rats fed high-fat diets. *Int. J. Cancer*, **43**, 922–925

Klurfeld, D.M., Lloyd, L.M., Welch, C.B., Davis, M.J., Tulp, O.L. & Kritchevsky, D. (1991) Reduction of enhanced mammary carcinogenesis in LA/N-cp (corpulent) rats by energy restriction. *Proc. Soc. Exp. Biol. Med.*, **196**, 381–384

Knatterud, G.L., Klimt, C.R., Goldner, M.G., Hawkins, B.S., Weisenfeld, S., Kreines, H. & Haddock, L. (1982) Effects of hypoglycemic agents on vascular complications in patients with adult-onset diabetes. VIII. Evaluation of insulin therapy: final report. *Diabetes*, **31, Suppl. 5**, 1–81

Knekt, P., Heliövaara, M., Rissanen, A., Aromaa, A., Seppänen, R., Teppo, L. & Pukkala, E. (1991) Leanness and lung-cancer risk. *Int. J. Cancer*, **49**, 208–213

Knip, M. & Nuutinen, O. (1993) Long-term effects of weight reduction on serum lipids and plasma insulin in obese children. *Am. J. Clin. Nutr.*, **57**, 490–493

Koffler, K.H., Menkes, A., Redmond, R.A., Whitehead, W.E., Pratley, R.E. & Hurley, B.F. (1992) Strength training accelerates gastrointestinal transit in middle-aged and older men. *Med. Sci. Sports Exerc.*, **24**, 415–419

Kohl, H.W., Fulton, J.E. & Caspersen, C.J. (2000) Physical activity assessment among children and adolescents. *Prev. Med.*, **31**, S54–S76

Koistinen, H., Koistinen, R., Selenius, L., Ylikorkala, Q. & Seppälä, M. (1996) Effect of marathon run on serum IGF-I and IGF-binding protein 1 and 3 levels. *J. Appl. Physiol.*, **80**, 760–764

Kolonel, L.N., Nomura, A.M., Lee, J. & Hirohata, T. (1986) Anthropometric indicators of breast cancer risk in post-menopausal women in Hawaii. *Nutr. Cancer*, **8**, 247–256

Kolonel, L.N., Yoshizawa, C.N. & Hankin, J.H. (1988) Diet and prostatic cancer: a case-control study in Hawaii. *Am. J. Epidemiol.*, **127**, 999–1012

Kono, S., Handa, K., Hayabuchi, H., Kiyohara, C., Inoue, H., Marugame, T., Shinomiya, S., Hamada, H., Onuma, K. & Koga, H. (1999) Obesity, weight gain and risk of colon adenomas in Japanese men. *Jpn J. Cancer Res.*, **90**, 805–811

Koohestani, N., Chia, M.C., Pham, N.A., Tran, T.T., Minkin, S., Wolever, T.M. & Bruce, W.R. (1998) Aberrant crypt focus promotion and glucose intolerance: correlation in the rat across diets differing in fat, n-3 fatty acids and energy. *Carcinogenesis*, **19**, 1679–1684

Kopelman, P.G., White, N., Pilkington, T.R. & Jeffcoate, S.L. (1981) The effect of weight loss on sex steroid secretion and binding in massively obese women. *Clin. Endocrinol. (Oxf.)*, **15**, 113–116

Koprowski, C., Ross, R.K., Mack, W.J., Henderson, B.E. & Bernstein, L. (1999) Diet, body size and menarche in a multiethnic cohort. *Br. J. Cancer*, **79**, 1907–1911

Kotake, K., Koyama, Y., Nasu, J., Fukutomi, T. & Yamaguchi, N. (1995) Relation of family history of cancer and environmental factors to the risk of colorectal cancer: a case-control study. *Jpn. J. Clin. Oncol.*, **25**, 195–202

Koumantaki, Y., Tzonou, A., Koumantakis, E., Kaklamani, E., Aravantinos, D. & Trichopoulos, D. (1989) A case-control study of cancer of endometrium in Athens. *Int. J. Cancer*, **43**, 795–799

Koziris, L.P., Hickson, R.C., Chatterton, R.T., Jr, Groseth, R.T., Christie, J.M., Goldflies, D.G. & Unterman, T.G. (1999) Serum levels of total and free IGF-I and IGFBP-3 are increased and maintained in long-term training. *J. Appl. Physiol.*, **86**, 1436–1442

Kraemer, R.R., Kilgore, J.L., Kraemer, G.R. & Castracane, V.D. (1992) Growth hormone, IGF-I, and testosterone responses to resistive exercise. *Med. Sci. Sports Exerc.*, **24**, 1346–1352

Kraemer, W.J., Fleck, S.J., Dziados, J.E., Harman, E.A., Marchitelli, L.J., Gordon, S.E., Mello, R., Frykman, P.N., Koziris, L.P. & Triplett, N.T. (1993) Changes in hormonal concentrations after different heavy-resistance exercise protocols in women. *J. Appl. Physiol.*, **75**, 594–604

Kraemer, W.J., Aguilera, B.A., Terada, M., Newton, R.U., Lynch, J.M., Rosendaal, G., McBride, J.M., Gordon, S.E. & Hakkinen, K. (1995) Responses of IGF-I to endogenous increases in growth hormone after heavy-resistance exercise. *J. Appl. Physiol.*, **79**, 1310–1315

Kraemer, W.J., Volek, J.S., Bush, J.A., Putukian, M. & Sebastianelli, W.J. (1998) Hormonal responses to consecutive days of heavy-resistance exercise with or without nutritional supplementation. *J. Appl. Physiol.*, **85**, 1544–1555

Kraemer, W.J., Häkkinen, K., Newton, R.U., Nindl, B.C., Volek, J.S., McCormick, M., Gotshalk, L.A., Gordon, S.E., Fleck, S.J., Campbell, W.W., Putukian, M. & Evans, W.J. (1999) Effects of heavy-resistance training on hormonal response patterns in younger vs. older men. *J. Appl. Physiol.*, **87**, 982–992

Kramer, T.R., Moore, R.J., Shippee, R.L., Friedl, K.E., Martinez-Lopez, L., Chan, M.M. & Askew, E.W. (1997) Effects of food restriction in military training on T-lymphocyte responses. *Int. J. Sports Med.*, **18 Suppl. 1**, S84–S90

Kreiger, N., Marrett, L.D., Dodds, L., Hilditch, S. & Darlington, G.A. (1993) Risk factors for renal cell carcinoma: results of a population-based case-control study. *Cancer Causes Control*, **4**, 101–110

Kritchevsky, D. (1992) Caloric restriction and experimental carcinogenesis. *Adv. Exp. Med. Biol.*, **322**, 131–141

Kritchevsky, D. (1997) Caloric restriction and experimental mammary carcinogenesis. *Breast Cancer Res. Treat.*, **46**, 161–167

Kritchevsky, D. (1999) Caloric restriction and experimental carcinogenesis. *Toxicol. Sci.*, **52**, 13–16

Kritchevsky, D., Welch, C.B. & Klurfeld, D.M. (1989) Response of mammary tumors to caloric restriction for different time periods during the promotion phase. *Nutr. Cancer*, **12**, 259–269

Kroke, A., Klipstein-Grobusch, K., Bergmann, M.M., Weber, K. & Boeing, H. (2000) Influence of body composition on quantitative ultrasound parameters of the os calcis in a population-based sample of pre- and postmenopausal women. *Calcif. Tissue Int.*, **66**, 5–10

Kronborg, O. & Fenger, C. (1999) Clinical evidence for the adenoma-carcinoma sequence. *Eur. J. Cancer Prev.*, **8**, Suppl. 1, S73–S86

Krotkiewski, M., Björntorp, P., Sjöström, L. & Smith, U. (1983) Impact of obesity on metabolism in men and women. Importance of regional adipose tissue distribution. *J. Clin. Invest.*, **72**, 1150–1162

Kujala, U.M., Kaprio, J., Sarna, S. & Koskenvuo, M. (1998) Relationship of leisure-time physical activity and mortality: the Finnish twin cohort. *JAMA*, **279**, 440-444

Kumae, T., Yamasaki, K., Ishizaki, K. & Ito, T. (1999) Effects of summer camp endurance training on non-specific immunity in long-distance runners. *Int. J. Sports Med.*, **20**, 390–395

Kumagai, S., Shono, N., Kondo, Y. & Nishizumi, M. (1994) The effect of endurance training on the relationships between sex hormone binding globulin, high density lipoprotein cholesterol, apoprotein A1 and physical fitness in pre-menopausal women with mild obesity. *Int. J. Obes. Relat. Metab. Disord.*, **18**, 249–254

Kumar, S.P., Roy, S.J., Tokumo, K. & Reddy, B.S. (1990) Effect of different levels of calorie restriction on azoxymethane-induced colon carcinogenesis in male F344 rats. *Cancer Res.*, **50**, 5761–5766

Kumari, B.S. & Chandra, R.K. (1993) Overnutrition and immune responses. *Nutr. Res.*, **13**, S3–S18

Kune, G.A., Kune, S. & Watson, L.F. (1990) Body weight and physical activity as predictors of colorectal cancer risk. *Nutr. Cancer*, **13**, 9–17

Kyogoku, S., Hirohata, T., Takeshita, S., Nomura, Y., Shigematsu, T. & Horie, A. (1990) Survival of breast-cancer patients and body size indicators. *Int. J. Cancer*, **46**, 824–831

La Vecchia, C., Franceschi, S., Gallus, G., Decarli, A., Colombo, E., Mangioni, C. & Tognoni, G. (1982) Oestrogens and obesity as risk factors for endometrial cancer in Italy. *Int. J. Epidemiol.*, **11**, 120–126

La Vecchia, C., Franceschi, S., Decarli, A., Gallus, G. & Tognoni, G. (1984) Risk factors for endometrial cancer at different ages. *J. Natl Cancer Inst.*, **73**, 667–671

La Vecchia, C., Parazzini, F., Negri, E., Fasoli, M., Gentile, A. & Franceschi, S. (1991) Anthropometric indicators of endometrial cancer risk. *Eur. J. Cancer*, **27**, 487–490

La Vecchia, C., Negri, E., Franceschi, S., Talamini, R., Bruzzi, P., Palli, D. & Decarli, A. (1997a) Body mass index and postmenopausal breast cancer: an age-specific analysis. *Br. J. Cancer*, **75**, 441–444

La Vecchia, C., Negri, E., Decarli, A. & Franceschi, S. (1997b) Diabetes mellitus and colorectal cancer risk. *Cancer Epidemiol. Biomarkers Prev.*, **6**, 1007–1010

La Vecchia, C., Ron, E., Franceschi, S., Dal Maso, L., Mark, S.D., Chatenoud, L., Braga, C., Preston-Martin, S., McTiernan, A., Kolonel, L., Mabuchi, K., Jin, F., Wingren, G., Galanti, M.R., Hallquist, A., Lund, E., Levi, F., Linos, D. & Negri, E. (1999a) A pooled analysis of case-control studies of thyroid cancer. III. Oral contraceptives, menopausal replacement therapy and other female hormones. *Cancer Causes Control*, **10**, 157–166

La Vecchia, C., Braga, C., Franceschi, S., Dal Maso, L. & Negri, E. (1999b) Population-attributable risk for colon cancer in Italy. *Nutr. Cancer*, **33**, 196–200

Laakso, M. & Lehto, M. (1997) Epidemiology of macrovascular disease in diabetes. *Diabetes Rev.*, **5**, 294-315

LaCroix, A.Z., Leveille, S.G., Hecht, J.A., Grothaus, L.C. & Wagner, E.H. (1996) Does walking decrease the risk of cardiovascular disease hospitalizations and death in older adults? *J. Am. Geriatr. Soc.*, **44**, 113–120

Lagergren, J., Bergström, R. & Nyrén, O. (1999a) Association between body mass and adenocarcinoma of the esophagus and gastric cardia. *Ann. Intern. Med.*, **130**, 883–890

Lagergren, J., Bergström, R., Lindgren, A. & Nyrén, O. (1999b) Symptomatic gastroesophageal reflux as a risk factor for esophageal adenocarcinoma. *New Engl. J. Med.*, **340**, 825–831

Lagergren, J., Bergström, R., Adami, H.O. & Nyrén, O. (2000) Association between medications that relax the lower esophageal sphincter and risk for esophageal adenocarcinoma. *Ann. Intern. Med.*, **133**, 165–175

Lagiou, P., Signorello, L.B., Trichopoulos, D., Tzonou, A., Trichopoulou, A. & Mantzoros, C.S. (1998) Leptin in relation to prostate cancer and benign prostatic hyperplasia. *Int. J. Cancer*, **76**, 25–28

Lagopoulos, L., Sunahara, G.I., Würzner, H., Dombrowsky, I. & Stalder, R. (1991) The effects of alternating dietary restriction and ad libitum feeding of mice on the development of diethylnitrosamine-induced liver tumours and its correlation to insulinaemia. *Carcinogenesis*, **12**, 311–315

Lahmann, P.H., Lissner, L., Gullberg, B. & Berglund, G. (2000) Sociodemographic factors associated with long-term weight gain, current body fatness and central adiposity in Swedish women. *Int. J. Obes. Relat. Metab. Disord.*, **24**, 685–694

Lahti-Koski, M., Vartiainen, E., Mannisto, S. & Pietinen, P. (2000) Age, education and occupation as determinants of trends in body mass index in Finland from 1982 to 1997. *Int. J. Obes. Relat. Metab. Disord.*, **24**, 1669–1676

Lane, H.W., Teer, P., Keith, R.E., White, M.T. & Strahan, S. (1991) Reduced energy intake and moderate exercise reduce mammary tumor incidence in virgin female BALB/c mice treated with 7,12-dimethylbenz(a)anthracene. *J. Nutr.*, **121**, 1883–1888

Langendonk, J.G., Meinders, A.E., Burggraaf, J., Frölich, M., Roelen, C.A., Schoemaker, R.C., Cohen, A.F. & Pijl, H. (1999) Influence of obesity and body fat distribution on growth hormone kinetics in humans. *Am. J. Physiol.*, **277**, E824–E829

Langlois, J.A., Harris, T., Looker, A.C. & Madans, J. (1996) Weight change between age 50 years and old age is associated with risk of hip fracture in white women aged 67 years and older. *Arch. Intern. Med.*, **156**, 989–994

Langlois, J.A., Visser, M., Davidovic, L.S., Maggi, S., Li, G. & Harris, T.B. (1998) Hip fracture risk in older white men is associated with change in body weight from age 50 years to old age. *Arch. Intern. Med.*, **158**, 990–996

Lanzone, A., Fulghesu, A.M., Andreani, C.L., Apa, R., Fortini, A., Caruso, A. & Mancuso, S. (1990) Insulin secretion in polycystic ovarian disease: effect of ovarian suppression by GnRH agonist. *Hum. Reprod.*, **5**, 143–149

LaPerriere, A., Antoni, M.H., Ironson, G., Perry, A., McCabe, P., Klimas, N., Helder, L., Schneiderman, N. & Fletcher, M.A. (1994) Effects of aerobic exercise training on lymphocyte subpopulations. *Int. J. Sports Med.*, **15 Suppl. 3**, S127–S130

Lapidus, L., Helgesson, O., Merck, C. & Björntorp, P. (1988) Adipose tissue distribution and female carcinomas. A 12-year follow-up of participants in the population study of women in Gothenburg, Sweden. *Int. J. Obes.*, **12**, 361–368

LaPorte, R.E., Black-Sandler, R., Cauley, J.A., Link, M., Bayles, C. & Marks, B. (1983) The assessment of physical activity in older women: analysis of the interrelationship and reliability of activity monitoring, activity surveys, and caloric intake. *J Gerontol.*, **38**, 394–397

Larsen, M.L. (1989) The utility of glycated hemoglobin in identification of impaired glucose tolerance. *Diabetes Res.*, **12**, 67–70

Larsson, B., Bengtsson, C., Björntorp, P., Lapidus, L., Sjöström, L., Svärdsudd, K., Tibblin, G., Wedel, H., Welin, L. & Wilhelmsen, L. (1992) Is abdominal body fat distribution a major explanation for the sex difference in the incidence of myocardial infarction? The study of men born in 1913 and the study of women, Goteborg, Sweden. *Am. J. Epidemiol.*, **135**, 266–273

Lasko, C.M. & Bird, R.P. (1995) Modulation of aberrant crypt foci by dietary fat and caloric restriction: the effects of delayed intervention. *Cancer Epidemiol Biomarkers Prev.*, **4**, 49–55

Lasko, C.M., Good, C.K., Adam, J. & Bird, R.P. (1999) Energy restriction modulates the development of advanced preneoplastic lesions depending on the level of fat in the diet. *Nutr Cancer*, **33**, 69–75

Lauer, J.B., Reed, G.W. & Hill, J.O. (1999) Effects of weight cycling induced by diet cycling in rats differing in susceptibility to dietary obesity. *Obes. Res.*, **7**, 215-222

Lavrencic, A., Salobir, B.G. & Keber, I. (2000) Physical training improves flow-mediated dilation in patients with the polymetabolic syndrome. *Arterioscler. Thromb. Vasc. Biol.*, **20**, 551-555

Lawrence, C., Tessaro, I., Durgerian, S., Caputo, T., Richart, R., Jacobson, H. & Greenwald, P. (1987) Smoking, body weight, and early-stage endometrial cancer. *Cancer*, **59**, 1665–1669

Lazarus, R., Wake, M., Hesketh, K. & Waters, E. (2000) Change in body mass index in Australian primary school children, 1985–1997. *Int. J. Obes. Relat. Metab. Disord.*, **24**, 679–684

Le Marchand, L., Kolonel, L.N., Earle, M.E. & Mi, M.P. (1988a) Body size at different periods of life and breast cancer risk. *Am. J. Epidemiol.*, **128**, 137–152

Le Marchand, L., Kolonel, L.N., Myers, B.C. & Mi, M.P. (1988b) Birth characteristics of premenopausal women with breast cancer. *Br. J. Cancer*, **57**, 437–439

Le Marchand, L., Wilkens, L.R. & Mi, M.P. (1991a) Early-age body size, adult weight gain and endometrial cancer risk. *Int. J. Cancer*, **48**, 807–811

Le Marchand, L., Kolonel, L.N. & Yoshizawa, C.N. (1991b) Lifetime occupational physical activity and prostate cancer risk. *Am. J. Epidemiol.*, **133**, 103–111

Le Marchand, L., Wilkens, L.R. & Mi, M.P. (1992) Obesity in youth and middle age and risk of colorectal cancer in men. *Cancer Causes Control*, **3**, 349–354

Le Marchand, L., Kolonel, L.N., Wilkens, L.R., Myers, B.C. & Hirohata, T. (1994) Animal fat consumption and prostate cancer: a prospective study in Hawaii. *Epidemiology*, **5**, 276–282

Le Marchand, L., Wilkens, L.R., Kolonel, L.N., Hankin, J.H. & Lyu, L.C. (1997) Associations of sedentary lifestyle, obesity, smoking, alcohol use, and diabetes with the risk of colorectal cancer. *Cancer Res.*, **57**, 4787–4794

Le Pen, C., Levy, E., Loos, F., Banzet, M.N. & Basdevant, A. (1998) "Specific" scale compared with "generic" scale: a double measurement of the quality of life in a French community sample of obese subjects. *J. Epidemiol. Community Health*, **52**, 445-450

Leakey, J.A., Cunny, H.C., Bazare, J., Jr, Webb, P.J., Lipscomb, J.C., Slikker, W., Jr, Feuers, R.J., Duffy, P.H. & Hart, R.W. (1989) Effects of aging and caloric restriction on hepatic drug metabolizing enzymes in the Fischer 344 rat. II: Effects on conjugating enzymes. *Mech. Ageing Dev.*, **48**, 157–166

Leakey, J., Seng, J., Manjgaladze, M., Kozlovskaya, N., Xia, S., Lee, M.Y., Frame, L., Chen, S., Rhodes, C., Duffy, P. & Hart, R. (1995) Influence of caloric intake on drug metabolizing enzyme expression: relevance to tumorigenesis and toxicity testing. In: Hart, R., Neuman, D. & Robertson, R., eds, *Dietary Restriction: Implications for the Design and Interpretation of Toxicity and Carcinogenicity Studies*, Washington, DC, ILSI Press, pp. 167–180

Leakey, J., Seng, J.E., Barnas, C., Baker, V. & Hart, R. (1998) A mechanistic basis for the beneficial effects of dietary restriction on longevity and disease. Consequences for the interpretation of rodent toxicity studies. *Int. J. Toxicol.*, **17**, 5–56

Lean, M.E. (1997) Sibutramine — a review of clinical efficacy. *Int. J. Obes. Relat. Metab. Disord.*, **21, Suppl. 1**, S30–S36

Lean, M.E., Han, T.S. & Morrison, C.E. (1995) Waist circumference as a measure for indicating need for weight management. *BMJ*, **311**, 158–161

Lean, M.E., Han, T.S. & Deurenberg, P. (1996) Predicting body composition by densitometry from simple anthropometric measurements. *Am. J. Clin. Nutr.*, **63**, 4–14

Lean, M.E., Han, T.S. & Seidell, J.C. (1998) Impairment of health and quality of life in people with large waist circumference. *Lancet*, **351**, 853-856

Lee, I.M. & Paffenbarger, R.S., Jr (1992a) Quetelet's index and risk of colon cancer in college alumni. *J. Natl Cancer Inst.*, **84**, 1326–1331

Lee, I.M. & Paffenbarger, R.S., Jr (1992b) Re: "Body mass index and lung cancer risk". *Am. J. Epidemiol.*, **136**, 1417–1419

Lee, I.M. & Paffenbarger, R.S., Jr (1992c) Change in body weight and longevity. *JAMA*, **268**, 2045–2049

Lee, I.M. & Paffenbarger, R.S., Jr (1994) Physical activity and its relation to cancer risk: a prospective study of college alumni. *Med. Sci. Sports Exerc.*, **26**, 831–837

Lee, I.M. & Paffenbarger, R.S., Jr (1996) Is weight loss hazardous? *Nutr. Rev.*, **54**, S116-S124

Lee, I.M. & Paffenbarger, R.S., Jr (1998) Physical activity and stroke incidence: the Harvard Alumni Health Study. *Stroke*, **29**, 2049–2054

Lee, I.M. & Paffenbarger, R.S., Jr (2000) Associations of light, moderate, and vigorous intensity physical activity with longevity. The Harvard Alumni Health Study. *Am. J. Epidemiol.*, **151**, 293–299

Lee, I.M., Paffenbarger, R.S., Jr & Hsieh, C. (1991) Physical activity and risk of developing colorectal cancer among college alumni. *J. Natl Cancer Inst.*, **83**, 1324–1329

Lee, I.M., Paffenbarger, R.S., Jr & Hsieh, C.C. (1992) Physical activity and risk of prostatic cancer among college alumni. *Am. J. Epidemiol.*, **135**, 169–179

Lee, I.M., Manson, J.A., Hennekens, C.H., Paffenbarger, R.S., Jr (1993) Body weight and mortality. *JAMA*, **270**, 2823–2828

Lee, I.M., Hsieh, C.C. & Paffenbarger, R.S., Jr (1995) Exercise intensity and longevity in men. The Harvard Alumni Health Study. *JAMA*, **273**, 1179–1184

Lee, I.M., Manson, J.E., Ajani, U., Paffenbarger, R.S.J., Hennekens, C.H. & Buring, J.E. (1997a) Physical activity and risk of colon cancer: the Physicians' Health Study (United States). *Cancer Causes Control*, **8**, 568–574

Lee, P.D., Giudice, L.C., Conover, C.A. & Powell, D.R. (1997b) Insulin-like growth factor binding protein-1: recent findings and new directions. *Proc. Soc. Exp. Biol. Med.*, **216**, 319–357

Lee, I.M., Sesso, H.D. & Paffenbarger, R.S.J. (1999a) Physical activity and risk of lung cancer. *Int. J. Epidemiol.*, **28**, 620–625

Lee, D.Y., Kim, S.J. & Lee, Y.C. (1999b) Serum insulin-like growth factor (IGF)-I and IGF-binding proteins in lung cancer patients. *J. Korean Med. Sci.*, **14**, 401–404

Lee, C.K., Klopp, R.G., Weindruch, R. & Prolla, T.A. (1999c) Gene expression profile of aging and its retardation by caloric restriction. *Science*, **285**, 1390–1393

Lee, C.D., Blair, S.N. & Jackson, A.S. (1999d) Cardiorespiratory fitness, body composition, and all-cause and cardiovascular disease mortality in men. *Am. J. Clin. Nutr.*, **69**, 373–380

Leenen, R., van der Kooy, K., Seidell, J.C., Deurenberg, P. & Koppeschaar, H.P. (1994) Visceral fat accumulation in relation to sex hormones in obese men and women undergoing weight loss therapy. *J. Clin. Endocrinol. Metab.*, **78**, 1515–1520

Leermakers, E.A., Perri, M.G., Shigaki, C.L. & Fuller, P.R. (1999) Effects of exercise-focused versus weight-focused maintenance programs on the management of obesity. *Addict. Behav.*, **24**, 219–227

Lees, A.W., Jenkins, H.J., May, C.L., Cherian, G., Lam, E.W. & Hanson, J. (1989) Risk factors and 10-year breast cancer survival in northern Alberta. *Breast Cancer Res. Treat.*, **13**, 143–151

Leitzmann, M.F., Rimm, E.B., Willett, W.C., Spiegelman, D., Grodstein, F., Stampfer, M.J., Colditz, G.A. & Giovannucci, E. (1999) Recreational physical activity and the risk of cholecystectomy in women. *New Engl. J. Med.*, **341**, 777–784

Lemaitre, R.N., Heckbert, S.R., Psaty, B.M. & Siscovick, D.S. (1995) Leisure-time physical activity and the risk of nonfatal myocardial infarction in postmenopausal women. *Arch. Intern. Med.*, **155**, 2302-2308

Lemieux, S., Prud'homme, D., Bouchard, C., Tremblay, A. & Després, J.P. (1996) A single threshold value of waist girth identifies normal-weight and overweight subjects with excess visceral adipose tissue. *Am. J. Clin. Nutr.*, **64**, 685–693

Leung, K.C., Waters, M.J., Markus, I., Baumbach, W.R. & Ho, K.K. (1997) Insulin and insulin-like growth factor-I acutely inhibit surface translocation of growth hormone receptors in osteoblasts: a novel mechanism of growth hormone receptor regulation. *Proc. Natl Acad. Sci. USA*, **94**, 11381–11386

Leung, K.C., Doyle, N., Ballesteros, M., Waters, M.J. & Ho, K.K. (2000) Insulin regulation of human hepatic growth hormone receptors: divergent effects on biosynthesis and surface translocation. *J. Clin. Endocrinol. Metab.*, **85**, 4712–4720

Levi, F., La Vecchia, C., Negri, E. & Franceschi, S. (1993) Selected physical activities and the risk of endometrial cancer. *Br. J. Cancer*, **67**, 846–851

Levi, F., Pasche, C., Lucchini, F., Tavani, A. & La Vecchia, C. (1999a) Occupational and leisure-time physical activity and the risk of colorectal cancer. *Eur. J. Cancer Prev.*, **8**, 487–493

Levi, F., Pasche, C., Lucchini, F. & La Vecchia, C. (1999b) Occupational and leisure time physical activity and the risk of breast cancer. *Eur. J. Cancer*, **35**, 775–778

Lew, E.A. & Garfinkel, L. (1979) Variations in mortality by weight among 750,000 men and women. *J. Chronic. Dis.*, **32**, 563–576

Lin, S.J., Defossez, P.A. & Guarente, L. (2000) Requirement of NAD and SIR2 for life-span extension by calorie restriction in Saccharomyces cerevisiae. *Science*, **289**, 2126–2128

Lindblad, P., Wolk, A., Bergström, R., Persson, I. & Adami, H.O. (1994) The role of obesity and weight fluctuations in the etiology of renal cell cancer: a population-based case-control study. *Cancer Epidemiol. Biomarkers Prev.*, **3**, 631–639

Lindblad, P., Chow, W.H., Chan, J., Bergström, A., Wolk, A., Gridley, G., McLaughlin, J.K., Nyrén, O. & Adami, H.O. (1999) The role of diabetes mellitus in the aetiology of renal cell cancer. *Diabetologia*, **42**, 107–112

Lindgarde, F. & Saltin, B. (1981) Daily physical activity, work capacity and glucose tolerance in lean and obese normoglycaemic middle-aged men. *Diabetologia*, **20**, 134–138

Lindholm, C., Hagenfeldt, K. & Ringertz, B.M. (1994) Pubertal development in elite juvenile gymnasts. Effects of physical training. *Acta Obstet. Gynecol. Scand.*, **73**, 269–273

Lipman, J.M., Turturro, A. & Hart, R.W. (1989) The influence of dietary restriction on DNA repair in rodents: a preliminary study. *Mech. Ageing Dev.*, **48**, 135–143

Lissner, L., Andres, R., Muller, D.C. & Shimokata, H. (1990) Body weight variability in men: metabolic rate, health and longevity. *Int. J. Obes.*, **14**, 373–383

Lissner, L., Odell, P.M., D'Agostino, R.B., Stokes, J., Kreger, B.E., Belanger, A.J. & Brownell, K.D. (1991) Variability of body weight and health outcomes in the Framingham population. *New Engl. J. Med.*, **324**, 1839–1844

Little, J., Logan, R.F., Hawtin, P.G., Hardcastle, J.D. & Turner, I.D. (1993) Colorectal adenomas and energy intake, body size and physical activity: a case-control study of subjects participating in the Nottingham faecal occult blood screening programme. *Br. J. Cancer*, **67**, 172–176

Liu, G.C., Coulston, A.M., Lardinois, C.K., Hollenbeck, C.B., Moore, J.G. & Reaven, G.M. (1985) Moderate weight loss and sulfonylurea treatment of non-insulin-dependent diabetes mellitus. Combined effects. *Arch. Intern. Med.*, **145**, 665–669

Liu, S., Lee, I.M., Linson, P., Ajani, U., Buring, J.E. & Hennekens, C.H. (2000) A prospective study of physical activity and risk of prostate cancer in US physicians. *Int. J. Epidemiol.*, **29**, 29–35

Liu, Y., Duysen, E., Yaktine, A.L., Au, A., Wang, W. & Birt, D.F. (2001) Dietary energy restriction inhibits ERK but not JNK or p38 activity in the epidermis of SENCAR mice. *Carcinogenesis*, **22**, 607–612

Livingstone, B. (2000) Epidemiology of childhood obesity in Europe. *Eur. J. Pediatr.*, **159**, S14–S34

Lobo, R.A., Granger, L., Goebelsmann, U. & Mishell, D.R., Jr (1981) Elevations in unbound serum estradiol as a possible mechanism for inappropriate gonadotropin secretion in women with PCO. *J. Clin. Endocrinol. Metab.*, **52**, 156–158

Løchen, M.L. & Rasmussen, K. (1992) The Tromsø study: physical fitness, self reported physical activity, and their relationship to other coronary risk factors. *J. Epidemiol. Community Health*, **46**, 103–107

Lojander, J., Mustajoki, P., Rönkä, S., Mecklin, P. & Maasilta, P. (1998) A nurse-managed weight reduction programme for obstructive sleep apnoea syndrome. *J. Intern. Med.*, **244**, 251–255

Lok, E., Scott, F.W., Mongeau, R., Nera, E.A., Malcolm, S. & Clayson, D.B. (1990) Calorie restriction and cellular proliferation in various tissues of the female Swiss Webster mouse. *Cancer Lett.*, **51**, 67–73

London, S.J., Colditz, G.A., Stampfer, M.J., Willett, W.C., Rosner, B. & Speizer, F.E. (1989) Prospective study of relative weight, height, and risk of breast cancer. *JAMA*, **262**, 2853–2858

Long, S.D., O'Brien, K., MacDonald, K.G., Leggett-Frazier, N., Swanson, M.S., Pories, W.J. & Caro, J.F. (1994) Weight loss in severely obese subjects prevents the progression of impaired glucose tolerance to type II diabetes. A longitudinal interventional study. *Diabetes Care*, **17**, 372–375

Longnecker, M.P., Gerhardsson de Verdier, M., Frumkin, H. & Carpenter, C. (1995) A case-control study of physical activity in relation to risk of cancer of the right colon and rectum in men. *Int. J. Epidemiol.*, **24**, 42–50

Loprinzi, C.L., Athmann, L.M., Kardinal, C.G., O'Fallon, J.R., See, J.A., Bruce, B.K., Dose, A.M., Miser, A.W., Kern, P.S., Tschetter, L.K. & Rayson, S. (1996) Randomized trial of dietician counseling to try to prevent weight gain associated with breast cancer adjuvant chemotherapy. *Oncology*, **53**, 228–232

Losonczy, K.G., Harris, T.B., Cornoni-Huntley, J., Simonsick, E.M., Wallace, R.B., Cook, N.R., Ostfeld, A.M. & Blazer, D.G. (1995) Does weight loss from middle age to old age explain the inverse weight mortality relation in old age? *Am. J. Epidemiol.*, **141**, 312–321

Loucks, A.B. (1990) Effects of exercise training on the menstrual cycle: existence and mechanisms. *Med. Sci. Sports Exerc.*, **22**, 275–280

Loucks, A.B., Verdun, M. & Heath, E.M. (1998) Low energy availability, not stress of exercise, alters LH pulsatility in exercising women. *J. Appl. Physiol.*, **84**, 37–46

Lu, M.H., Hinson, W.G., Turturro, A., Anson, J. & Hart, R.W. (1991) Cell cycle analysis in bone marrow and kidney tissues of dietary restricted rats. *Mech. Ageing Dev.*, **59**, 111–121

Lu, M.H., Hinson, W.G., Turturro, A., Sheldon, W.G. & Hart, R.W. (1993) Cell proliferation by cell cycle analysis in young and old dietary restricted mice. *Mech. Ageing Dev.*, **68**, 151–162

Lu, H., Buison, A., Uhley, V. & Jen, K.L. (1995) Long-term weight cycling in female Wistar rats: effects on metabolism. *Obes. Res.*, **3**, 521–530

Lubin, F., Ruder, A.M., Wax, Y. & Modan, B. (1985) Overweight and changes in weight throughout adult life in breast cancer etiology. A case-control study. *Am. J. Epidemiol.*, **122**, 579–588

Lubin, F., Rozen, P., Arieli, B., Farbstein, M., Knaani, Y., Bat, L. & Farbstein, H. (1997) Nutritional and lifestyle habits and water-fiber interaction in colorectal adenoma etiology. *Cancer Epidemiol. Biomarkers Prev.*, **6**, 79–85

Luepker, R.V., Murray, D.M., Jacobs, D.R.J., Mittelmark, M.B., Bracht, N., Carlaw, R., Crow, R., Elmer, P., Finnegan, J., Folsom, A.R., Grimm, R., Hannan, P.J., Jeffrey, R., Lando, H., McGovern, P., Mullis, R., Perry, C.L., Pechacek, T., Pirie, P., Sprafka, J.M., Weisbrod, R. & Blackburn, H. (1994) Community education for cardiovascular disease prevention: risk factor changes in the Minnesota Heart Health Program. *Am. J. Public Health*, **84**, 1383–1393

Lukanova, A., Toniolo, P., Akhmedkhanov, A., Biessy, C., Haley, N.J., Shore, R.E., Riboli, E., Rinaldi, S. & Kaaks, R. (2001) A prospective study of insulin-like growth factor-I, IGF-binding proteins-1, -2 and -3 and lung cancer risk in women. *Int. J. Cancer*, **92**, 888–892

Lund Nilsen, T.I. & Vatten, L.J. (1999) Anthropometry and prostate cancer risk: a prospective study of 22,248 Norwegian men. *Cancer Causes Control*, **10**, 269–275

Lund Nilsen, T.I., Johnsen, R. & Vatten, L.J. (2000) Socio-economic and lifestyle factors associated with the risk of prostate cancer. *Br. J. Cancer*, **82**, 1358–1363

Ma, J., Pollak, M.N., Giovannucci, E., Chan, J.M., Tao, Y., Hennekens, C.H. & Stampfer, M.J. (1999) Prospective study of colorectal cancer risk in men and plasma levels of insulin-like growth factor (IGF)-I and IGF-binding protein-3. *J. Natl Cancer Inst.*, **91**, 620–625

Macera, C.A. & Pratt, M. (2000) Public health surveillance of physical activity. *Res. Q. Exerc. Sport*, **71**, 97–103

Mackinnon, L.T. (2000) Chronic exercise training effects on immune function. *Med. Sci. Sports Exerc.*, **32**, S369–S376

Maclure, M. & Willett, W. (1990) A case-control study of diet and risk of renal adenocarcinoma. *Epidemiology*, **1**, 430–440

Maclure, M., Travis, L.B., Willett, W. & MacMahon, B. (1991) A prospective cohort study of nutrient intake and age at menarche. *Am. J. Clin. Nutr.*, **54**, 649–656

Maehle, B.O. & Tretli, S. (1996) Pre-morbid body-mass-index in breast cancer: reversed effect on survival in hormone receptor negative patients. *Breast Cancer Res. Treat.*, **41**, 123–130

Maggio, C.A. & Pi-Sunyer, F.X. (1997) The prevention and treatment of obesity. Application to type 2 diabetes. *Diabetes Care*, **20**, 1744–1766

Magnusson, C., Baron, J., Persson, I., Wolk, A., Bergström, R., Trichopoulos, D. & Adami, H.O. (1998) Body size in different periods of life and breast cancer risk in postmenopausal women. *Int. J. Cancer*, **76**, 29–34

Magnusson, C., Baron, J.A., Correia, N., Bergström, R., Adami, H.O. & Persson, I. (1999) Breast-cancer risk following long-term oestrogen- and oestrogen-progestin-replacement therapy. *Int. J. Cancer*, **81**, 339–344

Malkinson, A.M. (1992) Primary lung tumors in mice: an experimentally manipulable model of human adenocarcinoma. *Cancer Res.*, **52**, 2670s–2676s

Mandarino, L.J. (1999) Skeletal muscle insulin resistance in humans. In: Reaven, G.M. & Laws, A., eds, *Insulin Resistance*, Totowa, NJ, Humana Press, pp. 179–195

Manjgaladze, M., Chen, S., Frame, L.T., Seng, J.E., Duffy, P.H., Feuers, R.J., Hart, R.W. & Leakey, J.E. (1993) Effects of caloric restriction on rodent drug and carcinogen metabolizing enzymes: implications for mutagenesis and cancer. *Mutat. Res.*, **295**, 201–222

Mann, J.I. (2000) Can dietary intervention produce long-term reduction in insulin resistance? *Br. J. Nutr.*, **83 Suppl. 1**, S169–S172

Manning, J.M. & Bronson, F.H. (1991) Suppression of puberty in rats by exercise: effects on hormone levels and reversal with GnRH infusion. *Am. J. Physiol.*, **260**, R717–R723

Manning, R.M., Jung, R.T., Leese, G.P. & Newton, R.W. (1995) The comparison of four weight reduction strategies aimed at overweight diabetic patients. *Diabet. Med.*, **12**, 409–415

Männistö, S., Pietinen, P., Pyy, M., Palmgren, J., Eskelinen, M. & Uusitupa, M. (1996) Body-size indicators and risk of breast cancer according to menopause and estrogen-receptor status. *Int. J. Cancer*, **68**, 8–13

Manousos, O., Souglakos, J., Bosetti, C., Tzonou, A., Chatzidakis, V., Trichopoulos, D., Adami, H.O. & Mantzoros, C. (1999) IGF-I and IGF-II in relation to colorectal cancer. *Int. J. Cancer*, **83**, 15–17

Manson, J.E., Willett, W.C., Stampfer, M.J., Colditz, G.A., Hunter, D.J., Hankinson, S.E., Hennekens, C.H. & Speizer, F.E. (1995) Body weight and mortality among women. *New Engl. J. Med.*, **333**, 677–685

Manson, J.E., Hu, F.B., Rich-Edwards, J.W., Colditz, G.A., Stampfer, M.J., Willett, W.C., Speizer, F.E. & Hennekens, C.H. (1999) A prospective study of walking as compared with vigorous exercise in the prevention of coronary heart disease in women. *New Engl. J. Med.*, **341**, 650–658

Mantzoros, C.S., Tzonou, A., Signorello, L.B., Stampfer, M., Trichopoulos, D. & Adami, H.O. (1997) Insulin-like growth factor 1 in relation to prostate cancer and benign prostatic hyperplasia. *Br. J. Cancer*, **76**, 1115–1118

Mantzoros, C.S., Bolhke, K., Moschos, S. & Cramer, D.W. (1999) Leptin in relation to carcinoma *in situ* of the breast: a study of pre-menopausal cases and controls. *Int. J. Cancer*, **80**, 523–526

Marcos, A., Varela, P., Toro, O., Lopez-Vidriero, I., Nova, E., Madruga, D., Casas, J. & Morande, G. (1997a) Interactions between nutrition and immunity in anorexia nervosa: a 1-y follow-up study. *Am. J. Clin. Nutr.*, **66**, 485S–490S

Marcos, A., Varela, P., Toro, O., Nova, E., Lopez-Vidriero, I. & Morande, G. (1997b) Evaluation of nutritional status by immunologic assessment in bulimia nervosa: influence of body mass index and vomiting episodes. *Am. J. Clin. Nutr.*, **66**, 491S–497S

Marcus, R., Cann, C., Madvig, P., Minkoff, J., Goddard, M., Bayer, M., Martin, M., Gaudiani, L., Haskell, W. & Genant, H. (1985) Menstrual function and bone mass in elite women distance runners. Endocrine and metabolic features. *Ann. Intern. Med.*, **102**, 158–163

Marcus, P.M., Newcomb, P.A. & Storer, B.E. (1994) Early adulthood physical activity and colon cancer risk among Wisconsin women. *Cancer Epidemiol. Biomarkers Prev.*, **3**, 641–644

Marcus, B.H., Owen, N., Forsyth, L.H., Cavill, N.A. & Fridinger, F. (1998) Physical activity interventions using mass media, print media, and information technology. *Am. J. Prev. Med.*, **15**, 362–378

Marcus, P.M., Newman, B., Moorman, P.G., Millikan, R.C., Baird, D.D., Qaqish, B. & Sternfeld, B. (1999) Physical activity at age 12 and adult breast cancer risk (United States). *Cancer Causes Control*, **10**, 293–302

Margetts, B.M., Rogers, E., Widhal, K., Remaut de Winter, A.M. & Zunft, H.J. (1999) Relationship between attitudes to health, body weight and physical activity and level of physical activity in a nationally representative sample in the European Union. *Public Health Nutr.*, **2**, 97–103

Margolis, K.L., Ensrud, K.E., Schreiner, P.J. & Tabor, H.K. (2000) Body size and risk for clinical fractures in older women. Study of Osteoporotic Fractures Research Group. *Ann. Intern. Med.*, **133**, 123–127

Mårin, P., Kvist, H., Lindstedt, G., Sjöström, L. & Björntorp, P. (1993) Low concentrations of insulin-like growth factor-I in abdominal obesity. *Int. J. Obes. Relat. Metab. Disord.*, **17**, 83–89

Markovic, T.P., Jenkins, A.B., Campbell, L.V., Furler, S.M., Kraegen, E.W. & Chisholm, D.J. (1998) The determinants of glycemic responses to diet restriction and weight loss in obesity and NIDDM. *Diabetes Care*, **21**, 687–694

Markowitz, S., Morabia, A., Garibaldi, K. & Wynder, E. (1992) Effect of occupational and recreational activity on the risk of colorectal cancer among males: a case-control study. *Int. J. Epidemiol.*, **21**, 1057–1062

Marks, S.J., Moore, N.R., Clark, M.L., Strauss, B.J. & Hockaday, T.D. (1996) Reduction of visceral adipose tissue and improvement of metabolic indices: effect of dexfenfluramine in NIDDM. *Obes. Res.*, **4**, 1–7

Marnett, L.J. (2000) Oxyradicals and DNA damage. *Carcinogenesis*, **21**, 361–370

Maron, B.J., Shirani, J., Poliac, L.C., Mathenge, R., Roberts, W.C. & Mueller, F.O. (1996) Sudden death in young competitive athletes. Clinical, demographic, and pathological profiles. *JAMA*, **276**, 199–204

Marshall, J.C. & Kelch, R.P. (1979) Low dose pulsatile gonadotropin-releasing hormone in anorexia nervosa: a model of human pubertal development. *J. Clin. Endocrinol. Metab.*, **49**, 712–718

Marshall, J.R., Graham, S., Haughey, B.P., Shedd, D., O'Shea, R., Brasure, J., Wilkinson, G.S. & West, D. (1992) Smoking, alcohol, dentition and diet in the epidemiology of oral cancer. *Eur. J. Cancer B, Oral Oncol*, **28B**, 9–15

Martha, P.M. & Reiter, E.O. (1991) Pubertal growth and growth hormone secretion. *Endocrinol. Metab. Clin. North Am.*, **20**, 165–182

Marti, B. & Minder, C.E. (1989) Physical occupational activity and colonic carcinoma mortality in Swiss men 1979-1982. *Soz. Präventivmed.*, **34**, 30–37

Martinez, M.E., Giovannucci, E., Spiegelman, D., Hunter, D.J., Willett, W.C. & Colditz, G.A. (1997) Leisure-time physical activity, body size, and colon cancer in women. Nurses' Health Study Research Group. *J. Natl Cancer Inst.*, **89**, 948–955

Martinez, J.A., Kearney, J.M., Kafatos, A., Paquet, S. & Martinez-Gonzalez, M.A. (1999a) Variables independently associated with self-reported obesity in the European Union. *Public Health Nutr.*, **2**, 125–133

Martinez, M.E., Heddens, D., Earnest, D.L., Bogert, C.L., Roe, D., Einspahr, J., Marshall, J.R. & Alberts, D.S. (1999b) Physical activity, body mass index, and prostaglandin E_2 levels in rectal mucosa. *J. Natl Cancer Inst.*, **91**, 950–953

Martinsen, E.V. & Stephens, T. (1994) Exercise and mental health in clinical and free-living populations. In: Dishman, R.K., ed., *Advances in Exercise Adherence*, Champaign, IL, Human Kinetics, pp. 55–72

Martorell, R., Kettel Khan, L., Hughes, M.L. & Grummer-Strawn, L.M. (2000a) Obesity in women from developing countries. *Eur. J. Clin. Nutr.*, **54**, 247–252

Martorell, R., Kettel Khan, L., Hughes, M.L. & Grummer-Strawn, L.M. (2000b) Overweight and obesity in preschool children from developing countries. *Int. J. Obes. Relat. Metab. Disord.*, **24**, 959–967

Mayer-Davis, E.J., D'Agostino, R., Karter, A.J., Haffner, S.M., Rewers, M.J., Saad, M. & Bergman, R.N. (1998) Intensity and amount of physical activity in relation to insulin sensitivity: the Insulin Resistance Atherosclerosis Study. *JAMA*, **279**, 669-674

McCredie, M. & Stewart, J.H. (1992) Risk factors for kidney cancer in New South Wales, Australia. II. Urologic disease, hypertension, obesity, and hormonal factors. *Cancer Causes Control*, **3**, 323–331

McGuire, M.T., Wing, R.R., Klem, M.L., Lang, W. & Hill, J.O. (1999) What predicts weight regain in a group of successful weight losers? *J. Consult. Clin. Psychol.*, **67**, 177–185

McKeown-Eyssen, G. (1994) Epidemiology of colorectal cancer revisited: are serum triglycerides and/or plasma glucose associated with risk? *Cancer Epidemiol. Biomarkers Prev., 3*, 687–695

McLaughlin, J.K., Mandel, J.S., Blot, W.J., Schuman, L.M., Mehl, E.S. & Fraumeni, J.F., Jr (1984) A population-based case-control study of renal cell carcinoma. *J. Natl Cancer Inst., 72*, 275–284

McLaughlin, J.K., Gridley, G., Block, G., Winn, D.M., Preston-Martin, S., Schoenberg, J.B., Greenberg, R.S., Stemhagen, A., Austin, D.F., Ershow, A.G., Blot, W.J. & Fraumeni, J.F., Jr (1988) Dietary factors in oral and pharyngeal cancer. *J. Natl Cancer Inst., 80*, 1237–1243

McLaughlin, J.K., Gao, Y.T., Gao, R.N., Zheng, W., Ji, B.T., Blot, W.J. & Fraumeni, J.F., Jr (1992) Risk factors for renal-cell cancer in Shanghai, China. *Int. J. Cancer, 52*, 562–565

McMurray, R.W., Bradsher, R.W., Steele, R.W. & Pilkington, N.S. (1990) Effect of prolonged modified fasting in obese persons on in vitro markers of immunity: lymphocyte function and serum effects on normal neutrophils. *Am. J. Med. Sci., 299*, 379–385

McNee, R.K., Mason, B.H., Neave, L.M. & Kay, R.G. (1987) Influence of height, weight, and obesity on breast cancer incidence and recurrence in Auckland, New Zealand. *Breast Cancer Res. Treat., 9*, 145–150

McTiernan, A., Stanford, J.L., Weiss, N.S., Daling, J.R. & Voigt, L.F. (1996) Occurrence of breast cancer in relation to recreational exercise in women age 50–64 years. *Epidemiology, 7*, 598–604

McTiernan, A., Ulrich, C., Kumai, C., Bean, D., Schwartz, R., Mahloch, J., Hastings, R., Gralow, J. & Potter, J.D. (1998) Anthropometric and hormone effects of an eight-week exercise-diet intervention in breast cancer patients: results of a pilot study. *Cancer Epidemiol. Biomarkers Prev., 7*, 477–481

Megia, A., Herranz, L., Luna, R., Gomez-Candela, C., Pallardo, F. & Gonzalez-Gancedo, P. (1993) Protein intake during aggressive calorie restriction in obesity determines growth hormone response to growth hormone-releasing hormone after weight loss. *Clin. Endocrinol. (Oxf.), 39*, 217–220

Mehta, R.S., Harris, S.R., Gunnett, C.A., Bunce, O.R. & Hartle, D.K. (1993) The effects of patterned calorie-restricted diets on mammary tumor incidence and plasma endothelin levels in DMBA-treated rats. *Carcinogenesis, 14*, 1693–1696

Meilahn, E.N., De Stavola, B., Allen, D.S., Fentiman, I., Bradlow, H.L., Sepkovic, D.W. & Kuller, L.H. (1998) Do urinary oestrogen metabolites predict breast cancer? Guernsey III cohort follow-up. *Br. J. Cancer, 78*, 1250–1255

Mellemgaard, A., Engholm, G., McLaughlin, J.K. & Olsen, J.H. (1994) Risk factors for renal-cell carcinoma in Denmark. III. Role of weight, physical activity and reproductive factors. *Int. J. Cancer, 56*, 66–71

Mellemgaard, A., Lindblad, P., Schlehofer, B., Bergström, R., Mandel, J.S., McCredie, M., McLaughlin, J.K., Niwa, S., Odaka, N., Pommer, W. & Olsen, J.H. (1995) International renal-cell cancer study. III. Role of weight, height, physical activity, and use of amphetamines. *Int. J. Cancer, 60*, 350–354

Mercer, C.D., Wren, S.F., DaCosta, L.R. & Beck, I.T. (1987) Lower esophageal sphincter pressure and gastroesophageal pressure gradients in excessively obese patients. *J. Med., 18*, 135–146

Merritt, R.J., Bistrian, B.R., Blackburn, G.L. & Suskind, R.M. (1980) Consequences of modified fasting in obese pediatric and adolescent patients. I. Protein-sparing modified fast. *J. Pediatr., 96*, 13–19

Merry, B.J. & Holehan, A.M. (1985) *In vivo* DNA synthesis in the dietary restricted long-lived rat. *Exp. Gerontol., 20*, 15–28

Merzenich, H., Boeing, H. & Wahrendorf, J. (1993) Dietary fat and sports activity as determinants for age at menarche. *Am. J. Epidemiol., 138*, 217–224

Messer, N.A. & l'Anson, H. (2000) The nature of the metabolic signal that triggers onset of puberty in female rats. *Physiol. Behav., 68*, 377–382

Meyer, F., Moisan, J., Marcoux, D. & Bouchard, C. (1990) Dietary and physical determinants of menarche. *Epidemiology, 1*, 377–381

Meyer, H.E., Tverdal, A. & Falch, J.A. (1995) Changes in body weight and incidence of hip fracture among middle aged Norwegians. *BMJ, 311*, 91–92

Meyer, H.E., Tverdal, A. & Selmer, R. (1998) Weight variability, weight change and the incidence of hip fracture: a prospective study of 39,000 middle-aged Norwegians. *Osteopor. Int., 8*, 373–378

Mezzetti, M., La Vecchia, C., Decarli, A., Boyle, P., Talamini, R. & Franceschi, S. (1998) Population attributable risk for breast cancer: diet, nutrition, and physical exercise. *J. Natl Cancer Inst., 90*, 389–394

Michels, K.B., Trichopoulos, D., Robins, J.M., Rosner, B.A., Manson, J.E., Hunter, D.J., Colditz, G.A., Hankinson, S.E., Speizer, F.E. & Willett, W.C. (1996) Birthweight as a risk factor for breast cancer. *Lancet, 348*, 1542–1546

Micic, D., Macut, D., Popovic, V., Kendereski, A., Sumarac-Dumanovic, M., Zoric, S., Dieguez, C. & Casanueva, F.F. (1999) Growth hormone (GH) response to GH-releasing peptide-6 and GH-releasing hormone in normal-weight and overweight patients with non-insulin-dependent diabetes mellitus. *Metabolism, 48*, 525–530

Mikkelsen, K.L., Heitmann, B.L., Keiding, N. & Sørensen, T.I. (1999) Independent effects of stable and changing body weight on total mortality. *Epidemiology, 10*, 671-678

Miles, M.P., Naukam, R.J., Hackney, A.C. & Clarkson, P.M. (1999) Blood leukocyte and glutamine fluctuations after eccentric exercise. *Int. J. Sports Med., 20*, 322–327

Miller, D.J., Freedson, P.S. & Kline, G.M. (1994) Comparison of activity levels using the Caltrac® accelerometer and five questionnaires. *Med. Sci. Sports Exerc., 26*, 376–382

Mills, P.K., Beeson, W.L., Phillips, R.L. & Fraser, G.E. (1989) Cohort study of diet, lifestyle, and prostate cancer in Adventist men. *Cancer, 64*, 598–604

Mink, P.J., Folsom, A.R., Sellers, T.A. & Kushi, L.H. (1996) Physical activity, waist-to-hip ratio, and other risk factors for ovarian cancer: a follow-up study of older women. *Epidemiology, 7*, 38–45

Mittal, A., Muthukumar, A., Jolly, C.A., Zaman, K. & Fernandes, G. (2000) Reduced food consumption increases water intake and modulates renal aquaporin-1 and -2 expression in autoimmune prone mice. *Life Sci., 66*, 1471–1479

Mittendorf, R., Longnecker, M.P., Newcomb, P.A., Dietz, A.T., Greenberg, E.R., Bogdan, G.F., Clapp, R.W. & Willett, W.C. (1995) Strenuous physical activity in young adulthood and risk of breast cancer (United States). *Cancer Causes Control*, 6, 347–353

Mittleman, M.A., Maclure, M., Tofler, G.H., Sherwood, J.B., Goldberg, R.J. & Muller, J.E. (1993) Triggering of acute myocardial infarction by heavy physical exertion. Protection against triggering by regular exertion. Determinants of Myocardial Infarction Onset Study Investigators. *New Engl. J. Med.*, 329, 1677–1683

Moens, G., van Gaal, L., Muls, E., Viaene, B. & Jacques, P. (1999) Body mass index and health among the working population. *Eur. J. Public Health*, 9, 119–123

Mohle-Boetani, J.C., Grosser, S., Whittemore, A.S., Malec, M., Kampert, J.B. & Paffenbarger, R.S., Jr (1988) Body size, reproductive factors, and breast cancer survival. *Prev. Med.*, 17, 634–642

Moisan, J., Meyer, F. & Gingras, S. (1991) Leisure physical activity and age at menarche. *Med. Sci. Sports Exerc.*, 23, 1170–1175

Molarius, A. & Seidell, J.C. (1998) Selection of anthropometric indicators for classification of abdominal fatness – a critical review. *Int. J. Obes. Relat. Metab. Disord.*, 22, 719–727

Molarius, A., Seidell, J.C., Kuulasmaa, K., Dobson, A.J. & Sans, S. (1997) Smoking and relative body weight: an international perspective from the WHO MONICA Project. *J. Epidemiol. Community Health*, 51, 252–260

Molarius, A., Seidell, J.C., Sans, S., Tuomilehto, J. & Kuulasmaa, K. (1999) Varying sensitivity of waist action levels to identify subjects with overweight or obesity in 19 populations of the WHO MONICA Project. *J. Clin. Epidemiol.*, 52, 1213–1224

Molarius, A., Seidell, J.C., Sans, S., Tuomilehto, J. & Kuulasmaa, K. (2000) Educational level, relative body weight, and changes in their association over 10 years: an international perspective from the WHO MONICA Project. *Am. J. Public Health*, 90, 1260–1268

Moldoveanu, A.I., Shephard, R.J. & Shek, P.N. (2000) Exercise elevates plasma levels but not gene expression of IL-1β, IL-6, and TNF-α in blood mononuclear cells. *J. Appl. Physiol.*, 89, 1499–1504

Møller, H., Mellemgaard, A., Lindvig, K. & Olsen, J.H. (1994) Obesity and cancer risk: a Danish record-linkage study. *Eur. J. Cancer*, 30A, 344–350

Möllerström, G., Carlström, K., Lagrelius, A. & Einhorn, N. (1993) Is there an altered steroid profile in patients with endometrial carcinoma? *Cancer*, 72, 173–181

Montagnani, C.F., Arena, B. & Maffulli, N. (1992) Estradiol and progesterone during exercise in healthy untrained women. *Med. Sci. Sports Exerc.*, 24, 764–768

Monteiro, C.A., D'A Benicio, M.H., Conde, W.L. & Popkin, B.M. (2000) Shifting obesity trends in Brazil. *Eur. J. Clin. Nutr.*, 54, 342–346

Moore, D.B., Folsom, A.R., Mink, P.J., Hong, C.P., Anderson, K.E. & Kushi, L.H. (2000a) Physical activity and incidence of postmenopausal breast cancer. *Epidemiology*, 11, 292–296

Moore, L.L., Visioni, A.J., Wilson, P.W., D'Agostino, R.B., Finkle, W.D. & Ellison, R.C. (2000b) Can sustained weight loss in overweight individuals reduce the risk of diabetes mellitus? *Epidemiology*, 11, 269–273

Moradi, T., Nyrén, O., Bergström, R., Gridley, G., Linet, M., Wolk, A., Dosemeci, M. & Adami, H.O. (1998) Risk for endometrial cancer in relation to occupational physical activity: a nationwide cohort study in Sweden. *Int. J. Cancer*, 76, 665–670

Moradi, T., Adami, H.O., Bergström, R., Gridley, G., Wolk, A., Gerhardsson, M., Dosemeci, M. & Nyrén, O. (1999) Occupational physical activity and risk for breast cancer in a nationwide cohort study in Sweden. *Cancer Causes Control*, 10, 423–430

Moradi, T., Nyrén, O., Zack, M., Magnusson, C., Persson, I. & Adami, H.O. (2000a) Breast cancer risk and lifetime leisure-time and occupational physical activity (Sweden). *Cancer Causes Control*, 11, 523–531

Moradi, T., Weiderpass, E., Signorello, L.B., Persson, I., Nyrén, O. & Adami, H.O. (2000b) Physical activity and postmenopausal endometrial cancer risk (Sweden). *Cancer Causes Control*, 11, 829–837

Morales, A.J., Laughlin, G.A., Butzow, T., Maheshwari, H., Baumann, G. & Yen, S.S. (1996) Insulin, somatotropic, and luteinizing hormone axes in lean and obese women with polycystic ovary syndrome: common and distinct features. *J. Clin. Endocrinol. Metab.*, 81, 2854–2864

Mori, M., Harabuchi, I., Miyake, H., Casagrande, J.T., Henderson, B.E. & Ross, R.K. (1988) Reproductive, genetic, and dietary risk factors for ovarian cancer. *Am. J. Epidemiol.*, 128, 771–777

Mori, M., Nishida, T., Sugiyama, T., Komai, K., Yakushiji, M., Fukuda, K., Tanaka, T., Yokoyama, M. & Sugimori, H. (1998) Anthropometric and other risk factors for ovarian cancer in a case-control study. *Jpn J. Cancer Res.*, 89, 246–253

Moriguchi, S., Oonishi, K., Kato, M. & Kishino, Y. (1995) Obesity is a risk factor for deteriorating cellular immune functions decreased with aging. *Nutr. Res.*, 15, 151–160

Morimoto, Y., Arisue, K. & Yamamura, Y. (1977) Relationship between circadian rhythm of food intake and that of plasma corticosterone and effect of food restriction on circadian adrenocortical rhythm in the rat. *Neuroendocrinology*, 23, 212–222

Morris, J.N., Clayton, D.G., Everitt, M.G., Semmence, A.M. & Burgess, E.H. (1990) Exercise in leisure time: coronary attack and death rates. *Br. Heart J.*, 63, 325–334

Moses, J., Steptoe, A., Mathews, A. & Edwards, S. (1989) The effects of exercise training on mental well-being in the normal population: a controlled trial. *J. Psychosom. Res.*, 33, 47–61

Moseson, M., Koenig, K.L., Shore, R.E. & Pasternack, B.S. (1993) The influence of medical conditions associated with hormones on the risk of breast cancer. *Int. J. Epidemiol.*, 22, 1000–1009

Mowat, M.R. (1998) p53 in tumor progression: life, death, and everything. *Adv. Cancer Res.*, 74, 25–48

Mowe, M., Bohmer, T. & Kindt, E. (1994) Reduced nutritional status in an elderly population (> 70 y) is probable before disease and possibly contributes to the development of disease. *Am. J. Clin. Nutr.*, 59, 317–324

Mukherjee, P., Sotnikov, A.V., Mangian, H.J., Zhou, J.R., Visek, W.J. & Clinton, S.K. (1999) Energy intake and prostate tumor growth, angiogenesis, and vascular endothelial growth factor expression. *J. Natl Cancer Inst.*, 91, 512–523

Mulrow, C.D., Chiquette, E., Angel, L., Cornell, J., Summerbell, C., Anagnostelis, B., Grimm, R. & Brand, M.B. (2000) Dieting to reduce body weight for controlling hypertension in adults. *Cochrane Database Syst. Rev.*, **21**, CD000484

Murphy, T.K., Calle, E.E., Rodriguez, C., Khan, H.S. & Thun, M.J. (2000a) Body mass index and colon cancer mortality in a large prospective study. *Am. J. Epidemiol.*, **152**, 847–854

Murphy, M.H., Nevill, A.M. & Hardman, A.E. (2000b) Different patterns of brisk walking are equally effective in decreasing postprandial lipaemia. *Int. J. Obes. Relat. Metab. Disord.*, **24**, 1303–1309

Murray, D.M., Kurth, C., Mullis, R. & Jeffery, R.W. (1990) Cholesterol reduction through low-intensity interventions: results from the Minnesota Heart Health Program. *Prev. Med.*, **19**, 181–189

Musaiger, A.O. & Gregory, W.B. (2000) Profile of body composition of school children (6–18 y) in Bahrain. *Int. J. Obes. Relat. Metab. Disord.*, **24**, 1093–1096

Muscat, J.E. & Wynder, E.L. (1992) Tobacco, alcohol, asbestos, and occupational risk factors for laryngeal cancer. *Cancer*, **69**, 2244–2251

Muscat, J.E., Hoffmann, D. & Wynder, E.L. (1995) The epidemiology of renal cell carcinoma. A second look. *Cancer*, **75**, 2552–2557

Musey, V.C., Goldstein, S., Farmer, P.K., Moore, P.B. & Phillips, L.S. (1993) Differential regulation of IGF-1 and IGF-binding protein-1 by dietary composition in humans. *Am. J. Med. Sci.*, **305**, 131–138

Muskhelishvili, L., Hart, R.W., Turturro, A. & James, S.J. (1995) Age-related changes in the intrinsic rate of apoptosis in livers of diet-restricted and ad libitum-fed B6C3F1 mice. *Am. J. Pathol.*, **147**, 20–24

Muskhelishvili, L., Turturro, A., Hart, R.W. & James, S.J. (1996) Pi-class glutathione-S-transferase-positive hepatocytes in aging B6C3F1 mice undergo apoptosis induced by dietary restriction. *Am. J. Pathol.*, **149**, 1585–1591

Mussolino, M.E., Looker, A.C., Madans, J.H., Langlois, J.A. & Orwoll, E.S. (1998) Risk factors for hip fracture in white men: the NHANES I Epidemiologic Follow-up Study. *J. Bone Miner. Res.*, **13**, 918–924

Must, A., Willett, W.C. & Dietz, W.H. (1993) Remote recall of childhood height, weight, and body build by elderly subjects. *Am. J. Epidemiol.*, **138**, 56–64

Muti, P., Bradlow, H.L., Micheli, A., Krogh, V., Freudenheim, J.L., Schunemann, H.J., Stanulla, M., Yang, J., Sepkovic, D.W., Trevisan, M. & Berrino, F. (2000) Estrogen metabolism and risk of breast cancer: a prospective study of the 2:16alpha-hydroxyestrone ratio in premenopausal and postmenopausal women. *Epidemiology*, **11**, 635–640

Naber, T.H., Schermer, T., de Bree, A., Nusteling, K., Eggink, L., Kruimel, J.W., Bakkeren, J., van Heereveld, H. & Katan, M.B. (1997) Prevalence of malnutrition in nonsurgical hospitalized patients and its association with disease complications. *Am. J. Clin. Nutr.*, **66**, 1232–1239

Nair, S.C., Toshkov, I.A., Yaktine, A.L., Barnett, T.D., Chaney, W.G. & Birt, D.F. (1995) Dietary energy restriction-induced modulation of protein kinase C zeta isozyme in the hamster pancreas. *Mol. Carcinog.*, **14**, 10–15

Nakamura, K.D., Duffy, P.H., Lu, M.H., Turturro, A. & Hart, R.W. (1989) The effect of dietary restriction on myc protooncogene expression in mice: a preliminary study. *Mech. Ageing Dev.*, **48**, 199–205

Nam, S.Y., Lee, E.J., Kim, K.R., Cha, B.S., Song, Y.D., Lim, S.K., Lee, H.C. & Huh, K.B. (1997) Effect of obesity on total and free insulin-like growth factor (IGF)-1, and their relationship to IGF-binding protein (BP)-1, IGFBP-2, IGFBP-3, insulin, and growth hormone. *Int. J. Obes. Relat. Metab. Disord.*, **21**, 355–359

National Institutes of Health and National Heart, Lung and Blood Institute (NHLBI) (1998) Clinical guidelines on the identification, evaluation, and treatment of overweight and obesity in adults—the evidence report. *Obes. Res.*, **6**, 51S–210S

National Task Force on the Prevention and Treatment of Obesity (2000) Overweight, obesity, and health risk. *Arch. Intern. Med.*, **160**, 898-904

National Toxicology Program (NTP) (1997) Toxicology and carcinogenesis studies of dietary restriction in F344/N rats and B6C3F$_1$ mice (Technical Report Series Number 460), Washington, DC, Department of Health and Human Services, NIH, NIEHS

Ndiaye, B., Cournot, G., Pelissier, M.A., Debray, O.W. & Lemonnier, D. (1995) Rat serum osteocalcin concentration is decreased by restriction of energy intake. *J. Nutr.*, **125**, 1283–1290

Negri, E., Ron, E., Franceschi, S., Dal Maso, L., Mark, S.D., Preston-Martin, S., McTiernan, A., Kolonel, L., Kleinerman, R., Land, C., Jin, F., Wingren, G., Galanti, M.R., Hallquist, A., Glattre, E., Lund, E., Levi, F., Linos, D., Braga, C. & La Vecchia, C. (1999) A pooled analysis of case-control studies of thyroid cancer. I. Methods. *Cancer Causes Control*, **10**, 131–142

Nehlsen-Cannarella, S.L., Nieman, D.C., Balk-Lamberton, A.J., Markoff, P.A., Chritton, D.B., Gusewitch, G. & Lee, J.W. (1991) The effects of moderate exercise training on immune response. *Med. Sci. Sports Exerc.*, **23**, 64–70

Nelson, J.F., Felicio, L.S., Randall, P.K., Sims, C. & Finch, C.E. (1982) A longitudinal study of estrous cyclicity in aging C57BL/6J mice: I. Cycle frequency, length and vaginal cytology. *Biol. Reprod.*, **27**, 327–339

Nelson, M.E., Fiatarone, M.A., Morganti, C.M., Trice, I., Greenberg, R.A. & Evans, W.J. (1994) Effects of high-intensity strength training on multiple risk factors for osteoporotic fractures. A randomized controlled trial. *JAMA*, **272**, 1909–1914

Nestler, J.E. (2000) Obesity, insulin, sex steroids and ovulation. *Int. J. Obes. Relat. Metab. Disord.*, **24 Suppl. 2**, S71–S73

Neugut, A.I., Lee, W.C., Garbowski, G.C., Waye, J.D., Forde, K.A., Treat, M.R. & Fenoglio-Preiser, C. (1991) Obesity and colorectal adenomatous polyps. *J. Natl Cancer Inst.*, **83**, 359–361

Neugut, A.I., Terry, M.B., Hocking, G., Mosca, L., Garbowski, G.C., Forde, K.A., Treat, M.R. & Waye, J. (1996) Leisure and occupational physical activity and risk of colorectal adenomatous polyps. *Int. J. Cancer*, **68**, 744–748

Newberne, P.M., Bueche, D., Suphiphat, V., Schrager, T.F. & Sahaphong, S. (1990) The influence of pre- and postnatal caloric intake on colon carcinogenesis. *Nutr. Cancer*, **13**, 165–173

Newcomb, P.A., Klein, R., Klein, B.E., Haffner, S., Mares-Perlman, J., Cruickshanks, K.J. & Marcus, P.M. (1995) Association of dietary and life-style factors with sex hormones in postmenopausal women. *Epidemiology*, **6**, 318–321

Newman, S.C., Lees, A.W. & Jenkins, H.J. (1997) The effect of body mass index and oestrogen receptor level on survival of breast cancer patients. *Int. J. Epidemiol.*, **26**, 484–490

Ng, E.H., Gao, F., Ji, C.Y., Ho, G.H. & Soo, K.C. (1997) Risk factors for breast carcinoma in Singaporean Chinese women: the role of central obesity. *Cancer*, **80**, 725–731

Ng, E.H., Ji, C.Y., Tan, P.H., Lin, V., Soo, K.C. & Lee, K.O. (1998) Altered serum levels of insulin-like growth-factor binding proteins in breast cancer patients. *Ann. Surg. Oncol.*, **5**, 194–201

Nguyen, U.N., Mougin, F., Simon-Rigaud, M.L., Rouillon, J.D., Marguet, P. & Regnard, J. (1998) Influence of exercise duration on serum insulin-like growth factor and its binding proteins in athletes. *Eur. J. Appl. Physiol.*, **78**, 533–537

Nicklas, B.J., Ryan, A.J., Treuth, M.M., Harman, S.M., Blackman, M.R., Hurley, B.F. & Rogers, M.A. (1995) Testosterone, growth hormone and IGF-I responses to acute and chronic resistive exercise in men aged 55-70 years. *Int. J. Sports Med.*, **16**, 445–450

Niedhammer, I., Bugel, I., Bonenfant, S., Goldberg, M. & Leclerc, A. (2000) Validity of self-reported weight and height in the French GAZEL cohort. *Int. J. Obes. Relat. Metab. Disord.*, **24**, 1111–1118

Nieman, D.C. (1994) Exercise, upper respiratory tract infection, and the immune system. *Med. Sci. Sports Exerc.*, **26**, 128–139

Nieman, D.C. (1997) Exercise immunology: practical applications. *Int. J. Sports Med.*, **18 Suppl. 1**, S91–S100

Nieman, D.C. & Pedersen, B.K. (1999) Exercise and immune function. Recent developments. *Sports Med.*, **27**, 73–80

Nieman, D.C., Nehlsen-Cannarella, S.L., Markoff, P.A., Balk-Lamberton, A.J., Yang, H., Chritton, D.B., Lee, J.W. & Arabatzis, K. (1990) The effects of moderate exercise training on natural killer cells and acute upper respiratory tract infections. *Int. J. Sports Med.*, **11**, 467–473

Nieman, D.C., Henson, D.A., Gusewitch, G., Warren, B.J., Dotson, R.C., Butterworth, D.E. & Nehlsen-Cannarella, S.L. (1993) Physical activity and immune function in elderly women. *Med. Sci. Sports Exerc.*, **25**, 823–831

Nieman, D.C., Buckley, K.S., Henson, D.A., Warren, B.J., Suttles, J., Ahle, J.C., Simandle, S., Fagoaga, O.R. & Nehlsen-Cannarella, S.L. (1995) Immune function in marathon runners versus sedentary controls. *Med. Sci. Sports Exerc.*, **27**, 986–992

Nieman, D.C., Nehlsen-Cannarella, S.I., Henson, D.A., Butterworth, D.E., Fagoaga, O.R., Warren, B.J. & Rainwater, M.K. (1996) Immune response to obesity and moderate weight loss. *Int. J. Obes. Relat. Metab. Disord.*, **20**, 353–360

Nieman, D.C., Nehlsen-Cannarella, S.L., Fagoaga, O.R., Henson, D.A., Utter, A., Davis, J.M., Williams, F. & Butterworth, D.E. (1998) Influence of mode and carbohydrate on the cytokine response to heavy exertion. *Med. Sci. Sports Exerc.*, **30**, 671–678

Niwa, K., Imai, A., Hashimoto, M., Yokoyama, Y., Mori, H., Matsuda, Y. & Tamaya, T. (2000) A case-control study of uterine endometrial cancer of pre- and post-menopausal women. *Oncol. Rep.*, **7**, 89–93

Norrish, A.E., McRae, C.U., Holdaway, I.M. & Jackson, R.T. (2000) Height-related risk factors for prostate cancer. *Br. J. Cancer*, **82**, 241–245

Nyholm, H.C., Nielsen, A.L., Lyndrup, J., Dreisler, A., Hagen, C. & Haug, E. (1993) Plasma oestrogens in postmenopausal women with endometrial cancer. *Br. J. Obstet. Gynaecol.*, **100**, 1115–1119

Nyomba, B.L., Berard, L. & Murphy, L.J. (1997) Free insulin-like growth factor I (IGF-I) in healthy subjects: relationship with IGF-binding proteins and insulin sensitivity. *J. Clin. Endocrinol. Metab.*, **82**, 2177–2181

O'Dea, J.P., Wieland, R.G., Hallberg, M.C., Llerena, L.A., Zorn, E.M. & Genuth, S.M. (1979) Effect of dietary weight loss on sex steroid binding, sex steroids, and gonadotropins in obese postmenopausal women. *J. Lab. Clin. Med.*, **93**, 1004–1008

Ögren, M., Hedberg, M., Berglund, G., Borgström, A. & Janzon, L. (1996) Risk of pancreatic carcinoma in smokers enhanced by weight gain. Results from 10-year follow-up of the Malmö preventive Project Cohort Study. *Int. J. Pancreatol.*, **20**, 95–101

Okano, G., Suzuki, M., Kojima, M., Sato, Y., Lee, S.J., Okamura, K., Noriyasu, S., Doi, T., Shimomura, Y., Fushiki, T. & Shimizu, S. (1999) Effect of timing of meal intake after squat exercise training on bone formation in the rat hindlimb. *J. Nutr. Sci. Vitaminol. (Tokyo)*, **45**, 543–552

Oleshansky, M.A., Zoltick, J.M., Herman, R.H., Mougey, E.H. & Meyerhoff, J.L. (1990) The influence of fitness on neuroendocrine responses to exhaustive treadmill exercise. *Eur. J. Appl. Physiol.*, **59**, 405–410

Oliveria, S.A., Kohl, H.W., III, Trichopoulos, D. & Blair, S.N. (1996) The association between cardiorespiratory fitness and prostate cancer. *Med. Sci. Sports Exerc.*, **28**, 97–104

O'Loughlin, J., Paradis, G., Meshefedjian, G. & Gray-Donald, K. (2000) A five-year trend of increasing obesity among elementary schoolchildren in multiethnic, low-income, inner-city neighborhoods in Montreal, Canada. *Int. J. Obes. Relat. Metab. Disord.*, **24**, 1176–1182

Olson, S.H., Trevisan, M., Marshall, J.R., Graham, S., Zielezny, M., Vena, J.E., Hellmann, R. & Freudenheim, J.L. (1995) Body mass index, weight gain, and risk of endometrial cancer. *Nutr. Cancer*, **23**, 141–149

Olson, S.H., Vena, J.E., Dorn, J.P., Marshall, J.R., Zielezny, M., Laughlin, R. & Graham, S. (1997) Exercise, occupational activity, and risk of endometrial cancer. *Ann. Epidemiol.*, **7**, 46–53

O'Mara, B.A., Byers, T. & Schoenfeld, E. (1985) Diabetes mellitus and cancer risk: a multisite case-control study. *J. Chronic. Dis.*, **38**, 435–441

Ornish, D., Brown, S.E., Scherwitz, L.W., Billings, J.H., Armstrong, W.T., Ports, T.A., McLanahan, S.M., Kirkeeide, R.L., Brand, R.J. & Gould, K.L. (1990) Can lifestyle changes reverse coronary heart disease? The Lifestyle Heart Trial. *Lancet*, **336**, 129-133

Oscai, L.B. & Holloszy, J.O. (1970) Weight reduction in obese rats by exercise or food restriction: effect on the heart. *Am. J. Physiol.*, **219**, 327–330

Oster, M.H., Fielder, P.J., Levin, N. & Cronin, M.J. (1995) Adaptation of the growth hormone and insulin-like growth factor-I axis to chronic and severe calorie or protein malnutrition. *J. Clin. Invest.*, **95**, 2258–2265

Østerlind, A., Tucker, M.A., Stone, B.J. & Jensen, O.M. (1988) The Danish case-control study of cutaneous malignant melanoma. III. Hormonal and reproductive factors in women. *Int. J. Cancer*, **42**, 821–824

Owen, N., Leslie, E., Salmon, J. & Fotheringham, M.J. (2000) Environmental determinants of physical activity and sedentary behavior. *Exerc. Sport Sci. Rev.*, **28**, 153–158

Owens, J.F., Matthews, K.A., Wing, R.R. & Kuller, L.H. (1992) Can physical activity mitigate the effects of aging in middle-aged women? *Circulation*, **85**, 1265–1270

Owusu, W., Willett, W., Ascherio, A., Spiegelman, D., Rimm, E., Feskanich, D. & Colditz, G. (1998) Body anthropometry and the risk of hip and wrist fractures in men: results from a prospective study. *Obes. Res.*, **6**, 12–19

Paffenbarger, R.S., Jr, Kampert, J.B. & Chang, H.G. (1980) Characteristics that predict risk of breast cancer before and after the menopause. *Am. J. Epidemiol.*, **112**, 258–268

Paffenbarger, R.S., Jr, Wing, A.L., Hyde, R.T. & Jung, D.L. (1983) Physical activity and incidence of hypertension in college alumni. *Am. J. Epidemiol.*, **117**, 245-257

Paffenbarger, R.S., Jr, Hyde, R.T. & Wing, A.L. (1987) Physical activity and incidence of cancer in diverse populations: a preliminary report. *Am. J. Clin. Nutr.*, **45**, 312–317

Paffenbarger, R.S., Jr, Lee, I.M. & Wing, A.L. (1992) The influence of physical activity on the incidence of site-specific cancers in college alumni. *Adv. Exp. Med. Biol.*, **322**, 7–15

Paffenbarger, R.S., Jr Hyde, R.T., Wing, A.L., Lee, I.M., Jung, D.L. & Kampert, J.B. (1993) The association of changes in physical-activity level and other lifestyle characteristics with mortality among men. *New Engl. J. Med.*, **328**, 538–545

Pamuk, E.R., Williamson, D.F., Madans, J., Serdula, M.K., Kleinman, J.C. & Byers, T. (1992) Weight loss and mortality in a national cohort of adults, 1971-1987. *Am. J. Epidemiol.*, **136**, 686-697

Pamuk, E.R., Williamson, D.F., Serdula, M.K., Madans, J. & Byers, T.E. (1993) Weight loss and subsequent death in a cohort of U.S. adults. *Ann. Intern. Med.*, **119**, 744–748

Pan, D.A., Lillioja, S., Kriketos, A.D., Milner, M.R., Baur, L.A., Bogardus, C., Jenkins, A.B. & Storlien, L.H. (1997a) Skeletal muscle triglyceride levels are inversely related to insulin action. *Diabetes*, **46**, 983–988

Pan, X.R., Li, G.W., Hu, Y.H., Wang, J.X., Yang, W.Y., An, Z.X., Hu, Z.X., Lin, J., Xiao, J.Z., Cao, H.B., Liu, P.A., Jiang, X.G., Jiang, Y.Y., Wang, J.P., Zheng, H., Zhang, H., Bennett, P.H. & Howard, B.V. (1997b) Effects of diet and exercise in preventing NIDDM in people with impaired glucose tolerance. The Da Qing IGT and Diabetes Study. *Diabetes Care*, **20**, 537–544

Parazzini, F., La Vecchia, C., Negri, E., Fasoli, M. & Cecchetti, G. (1988) Risk factors for adenocarcinoma of the cervix: a case-control study. *Br. J. Cancer*, **57**, 201–204

Parazzini, F., Moroni, S., La Vecchia, C., Negri, E., dal Pino, D. & Bolis, G. (1997) Ovarian cancer risk and history of selected medical conditions linked with female hormones. *Eur. J. Cancer*, **33**, 1634–1637

Parazzini, F., La Vecchia, C., Negri, E., Riboldi, G.L., Surace, M., Benzi, G., Maina, A. & Chiaffarino, F. (1999) Diabetes and endometrial cancer: an Italian case-control study. *Int. J. Cancer*, **81**, 539–542

Parker, D.R., Gonzalez, S., Derby, C.A., Gans, K.M., Lasater, T.M. & Carleton, R.A. (1997) Dietary factors in relation to weight change among men and women from two southeastern New England communities. *Int. J. Obes. Relat. Metab. Disord.*, **21**, 103–109

Parslov, M., Lidegaard, O., Klintorp, S., Pedersen, B., Jonsson, L., Eriksen, P.S. & Ottesen, B. (2000) Risk factors among young women with endometrial cancer: a Danish case-control study. *Am. J. Obstet. Gynecol.*, **182**, 23–29

Pashko, L.L. & Schwartz, A.G. (1992) Reversal of food restriction-induced inhibition of mouse skin tumor promotion by adrenalectomy. *Carcinogenesis*, **13**, 1925–1928

Pashko, L.L. & Schwartz, A.G. (1996) Inhibition of 7,12-dimethylbenz[a]anthracene-induced lung tumorigenesis in A/J mice by food restriction is reversed by adrenalectomy. *Carcinogenesis*, **17**, 209–212

Pasquali, R., Casimirri, F., Venturoli, S., Paradisi, R., Mattioli, L., Capelli, M., Melchionda, N. & Labò, G. (1983) Insulin resistance in patients with polycystic ovaries: its relationship to body weight and androgen levels. *Acta Endocrinol. (Copenh.)*, **104**, 110–116

Pasquali, R., Antenucci, D., Melchionda, N., Fabbri, R., Venturoli, S., Patrono, D. & Capelli, M. (1987) Sex hormones in obese premenopausal women and their relationships to body fat mass and distribution, B cell function and diet composition. *J. Endocrinol. Invest.*, **10**, 345–350

Pasquali, R., Antenucci, D., Casimirri, F., Venturoli, S., Paradisi, R., Fabbri, R., Balestra, V., Melchionda, N. & Barbara, L. (1989) Clinical and hormonal characteristics of obese amenorrheic hyperandrogenic women before and after weight loss. *J. Clin. Endocrinol. Metab.*, **68**, 173–179

Pasquali, R., Casimirri, F., Platè, L. & Capelli, M. (1990) Characterization of obese women with reduced sex hormone-binding globulin concentrations. *Horm. Metab. Res.*, **22**, 303–306

Pasquali, R., Casimirri, F., Cantobelli, S., Melchionda, N., Morselli Labate, A.M., Fabbri, R., Capelli, M. & Bortoluzzi, L. (1991) Effect of obesity and body fat distribution on sex hormones and insulin in men. *Metabolism*, **40**, 101–104

Pasquali, R., Casimirri, F., Venturoli, S., Antonio, M., Morselli, L., Reho, S., Pezzoli, A. & Paradisi, R. (1994) Body fat distribution has weight-independent effects on clinical, hormonal, and metabolic features of women with polycystic ovary syndrome. *Metabolism*, **43**, 706–713

Pasquali, R., Casimirri, F., De Iasio, R., Mesini, P., Boschi, S., Chierici, R., Flamia, R., Biscotti, M. & Vicennati, V. (1995) Insulin testosterone and sex hormone-binding globulin concentrations in adult normal weight and obese men. *J. Clin. Endocrinol. Metab.*, **80**, 654–658

Pasquali, R., Vicennati, V., Bertazzo, D., Casimirri, F., Pascal, G., Tortelli, O. & Morselli Labate, A.M. (1997a) Determinants of sex hormone-binding globulin blood concentrations in premenopausal and postmenopausal women with different estrogen status. Virgilio-Menopause-Health Group. *Metabolism*, **46**, 5–9

Pasquali, R., Casimirri, F. & Vicennati, V. (1997b) Weight control and its beneficial effect on fertility in women with obesity and polycystic ovary syndrome. *Hum. Reprod.*, **12 Suppl. 1**, 82–87

Pate, R.R., Pratt, M., Blair, S.N., Haskell, W.L., Macera, C.A., Bouchard, C., Buchner, D., Ettinger, W., Heath, G.W., King, A.C., Kriska, A., Leon, A.S., Marcus, B.H., Morris, J., Paffenbarger, R.S., Jr, Patrick, K., Pollock, M.L., Rippe, J.M., Sallis, J. & Wilmore, J.H. (1995) Physical activity and public health. A recommendation from the Centers for Disease Control and Prevention and the American College of Sports Medicine. *JAMA*, **273**, 402–407

Pathak, D.R. & Whittemore, A.S. (1992) Combined effects of body size, parity, and menstrual events on breast cancer incidence in seven countries. *Am. J. Epidemiol.*, **135**, 153–168

Patton, G.C., Selzer, R., Coffey, C., Carlin, J.B. & Wolfe, R. (1999) Onset of adolescent eating disorders: population based cohort study over 3 years. *BMJ*, **318**, 765–768

Pavlou, K.N., Krey, S. & Steffee, W.P. (1989) Exercise as an adjunct to weight loss and maintenance in moderately obese subjects. *Am. J. Clin. Nutr.*, **49**, 1115–1123

Peacock, S.L., White, E., Daling, J.R., Voigt, L.F. & Malone, K.E. (1999) Relation between obesity and breast cancer in young women. *Am. J. Epidemiol.*, **149**, 339–346

Pedersen, B.K., Bruunsgaard, H., Ostrowski, K., Krabbe, K., Hansen, H., Krzywkowski, K., Toft, A., Søndergaard, S.R., Petersen, E.W., Ibfelt, T. & Schjerling, P. (2000) Cytokines in aging and exercise. *Int. J. Sports Med.*, **21 Suppl. 1**, S4–S9

Peltonen, M., Huhtasaari, F., Stegmayr, B., Lundberg, V. & Asplund, K. (1998) Secular trends in social patterning of cardiovascular risk factor levels in Sweden. The Northern Sweden MONICA Study 1986–1994. Multinational Monitoring of Trends and Determinants in Cardiovascular Disease. *J. Intern. Med.*, **244**, 1–9

Penn, I. (1994) Depressed immunity and the development of cancer. *Cancer Detect. Prev.*, **18**, 241–252

Penttilä, T.L., Koskinen, P., Penttilä, T.A., Anttila, L. & Irjala, K. (1999) Obesity regulates bioavailable testosterone levels in women with or without polycystic ovary syndrome. *Fertil. Steril.*, **71**, 457–461

Pereira, M.A., FitzGerald, S.J., Gregg, E.W., Joswiak, M.L., Ryan, W.J., Suminski, R.R., Utter, A.C. & Zmuda, J.M. (1997) A collection of physical activity questionnaires for health-related research. *Med. Sci. Sports Exerc.*, **29**, S1–205

Perri, M.G., McAdoo, W.G., McAllister, D.A., Lauer, J.B. & Yancey, D.Z. (1986) Enhancing the efficacy of behavior therapy for obesity: effects of aerobic exercise and a multicomponent maintenance program. *J. Consult. Clin. Psychol.*, **54**, 670–675

Perri, M.G., McAllister, D.A., Gange, J.J., Jordan, R.C., McAdoo, G. & Nezu, A.M. (1988) Effects of four maintenance programs on the long-term management of obesity. *J. Consult. Clin. Psychol.*, **56**, 529–534

Perri, M.G., Martin, A.D., Leermakers, E.A., Sears, S.F. & Notelovitz, M. (1997) Effects of group- versus home-based exercise in the treatment of obesity. *J. Consult. Clin. Psychol.*, **65**, 278–285

Perseghin, G., Price, T.B., Petersen, K.F., Roden, M., Cline, G.W., Gerow, K., Rothman, D.L. & Shulman, G.I. (1996) Increased glucose transport-phosphorylation and muscle glycogen synthesis after exercise training in insulin-resistant subjects. *New Engl. J. Med.*, **335**, 1357–1362

Pescatello, L.S., Fargo, A.E., Leach, C.N., Jr & Scherzer, H.H. (1991) Short-term effect of dynamic exercise on arterial blood pressure. *Circulation*, **83**, 1557–1561

Peters, E.M. (1997) Exercise, immunology and upper respiratory tract infections. *Int. J. Sports Med.*, **18 Suppl. 1**, S69–S77

Peters, R.K., Garabrant, D.H., Yu, M.C. & Mack, T.M. (1989) A case-control study of occupational and dietary factors in colorectal cancer in young men by subsite. *Cancer Res.*, **49**, 5459–5468

Peters, E.T., Seidell, J.C., Menotti, A., Aravanis, C., Dontas, A., Fidanza, F., Karvonen, M., Nedeljkovic, S., Nissinen, A., Buzina, R., Bloemberg, B. & Kromhout, D. (1995) Changes in body weight in relation to mortality in 6441 European middle-aged men: the Seven Countries Study. *Int. J. Obes. Relat. Metab. Disord.*, **19**, 862–868

Petrek, J.A., Peters, M., Cirrincione, C., Rhodes, D. & Bajorunas, D. (1993) Is body fat topography a risk factor for breast cancer? *Ann. Intern. Med.*, **118**, 356–362

Petridou, E., Syrigou, E., Toupadaki, N., Zavitsanos, X., Willett, W. & Trichopoulos, D. (1996) Determinants of age at menarche as early life predictors of breast cancer risk. *Int. J. Cancer*, **68**, 193–198

Petridou, E., Roukas, K.I., Dessypris, N., Aravantinos, G., Bafaloukos, D., Efraimidis, A., Papacharalambous, A., Pektasidis, D., Rigatos, G. & Trichopoulos, D. (1997) Baldness and other correlates of sex hormones in relation to testicular cancer. *Int. J. Cancer*, **71**, 982–985

Petridou, E., Papadiamantis, Y., Markopoulos, C., Spanos, E., Dessypris, N. & Trichopoulos, D. (2000) Leptin and insulin growth factor I in relation to breast cancer (Greece). *Cancer Causes Control*, **11**, 383–388

Peyrat, J.P., Bonneterre, J., Hecquet, B., Vennin, P., Louchez, M.M., Fournier, C., Lefebvre, J. & Demaille, A. (1993) Plasma insulin-like growth factor-1 (IGF-1) concentrations in human breast cancer. *Eur. J. Cancer*, **29A**, 492–497

Pfeilschifter, J., Scheidt-Nave, C., Leidig-Bruckner, G., Woitge, H.W., Blum, W.F., Wuster, C., Haack, D. & Ziegler, R. (1996) Relationship between circulating insulin-like growth factor components and sex hormones in a population-based sample of 50- to 80-year-old men and women. *J. Clin. Endocrinol. Metab.*, **81**, 2534–2540

Pike, M.C., Krailo, M.D., Henderson, B.E., Casagrande, J.T. & Hoel, D.G. (1983) 'Hormonal' risk factors, 'breast tissue age' and the age-incidence of breast cancer. *Nature*, **303**, 767–770

Pinto, B.M. & Maruyama, N.C. (1999) Exercise in the rehabilitation of breast cancer survivors. *Psychooncology*, **8**, 191–206

Pintor, C., Genazzani, A.R., Puggioni, R., Carboni, G., Faedda, A., Pisano, E., Orani, S., Fanni, T., D'Ambrogio, G. & Corda, R. (1980) Effect of weight loss on adrenal androgen plasma levels in obese prepubertal girls. In: Genazzani, A.R. (ed.), *Adrenal Androgens*, New York, Raven Press, pp. 259–266

Pishdad, G.R. (1996) Overweight and obesity in adults aged 20–74 in southern Iran. *Int. J. Obes. Relat. Metab. Disord.*, **20**, 963–965

Pi-Sunyer, F.X. (1999) Comorbidities of overweight and obesity: current evidence and research issues. *Med. Sci. Sports Exerc.*, **31**, S602–S608

Platz, E.A., Giovannucci, E., Rimm, E.B., Curhan, G.C., Spiegelman, D., Colditz, G.A. & Willett, W.C. (1998) Retrospective analysis of birth weight and prostate cancer in the Health Professionals Follow-up Study. *Am. J. Epidemiol.*, **147**, 1140–1144

Plymate, S.R., Jones, R.E., Matej, L.A. & Friedl, K.E. (1988) Regulation of sex hormone binding globulin (SHBG) production in Hep G2 cells by insulin. *Steroids*, **52**, 339–340

Poehlman, E.T. & Copeland, K.C. (1990) Influence of physical activity on insulin-like growth factor-I in healthy younger and older men. *J. Clin. Endocrinol. Metab.*, **71**, 1468–1473

Poehlman, E.T., Rosen, C.J. & Copeland, K.C. (1994) The influence of endurance training on insulin-like growth factor-1 in older individuals. *Metabolism*, **43**, 1401–1405

Poehlman, E.T., Toth, M.J., Fishman, P.S., Vaitkevicius, P., Gottlieb, S.S., Fisher, M.L. & Fonong, T. (1995) Sarcopenia in aging humans: the impact of menopause and disease. *J. Gerontol. A Biol. Sci. Med. Sci.*, **50**, Spec. No., 73–77

Poehlman, E.T., Turturro, A., Bodkin, N., Cefalu, W., Heymsfield, S., Holloszy, J., Kemnitz, J. (2001) Caloric restriction mimetics: physical activity and body composition changes. *J. Gerontol. A Biol. Sci. Med. Sci.*, (in press)

Poetschke, H.L., Klug, D.B., Perkins, S.N., Wang, T.T., Richie, E.R. & Hursting, S.D. (2000) Effects of calorie restriction on thymocyte growth, death and maturation. *Carcinogenesis*, **21**, 1959–1964

Pollak, M. (2000) Insulin-like growth factor physiology and cancer risk. *Eur. J. Cancer*, **36**, 1224–1228

Pollak, M., Beamer, W. & Zhang, J.C. (1998) Insulin-like growth factors and prostate cancer. *Cancer Metastasis Rev.*, **17**, 383–390

Pollard, M. & Luckert, P.H. (1985) Tumorigenic effects of direct- and indirect-acting chemical carcinogens in rats on a restricted diet. *J. Natl Cancer Inst.*, **74**, 1347–1349

Pollard, M., Luckert, P.H. & Pan, G.Y. (1984) Inhibition of intestinal tumorigenesis in methylazoxymethanol-treated rats by dietary restriction. *Cancer Treat. Rep.*, **68**, 405–408

Pollard, M., Luckert, P.H. & Snyder, D. (1989) Prevention of prostate cancer and liver tumors in L-W rats by moderate dietary restriction. *Cancer*, **64**, 686–690

Pollock, M.L., Carroll, J.F., Graves, J.E., Leggett, S.H., Braith, R.W., Limacher, M. & Hagberg, J.M. (1991) Injuries and adherence to walk/jog and resistance training programs in the elderly. *Med. Sci. Sports Exerc.*, **23**, 1194–1200

Pols, M.A., Peeters, P.H., Bueno-de-Mesquita, H.B., Ocké, M.C., Wentink, C.A., Kemper, H.C. & Collette, H.J. (1995) Validity and repeatability of a modified Baecke questionnaire on physical activity. *Int. J. Epidemiol.*, **24**, 381–388

Pols, M.A., Peeters, P.H., Ocké, M.C., Slimani, N., Bueno-de-Mesquita, H.B. & Collette, H.J. (1997) Estimation of reproducibility and relative validity of the questions included in the EPIC physical activity questionnaire. *Int. J. Epidemiol.*, **26 Suppl. 1**, S181–S189

Popkin, B.M. & Doak, C.M. (1998) The obesity epidemic is a worldwide phenomenon. *Nutr. Rev.*, **56**, 106–114

Poretsky, L., Cataldo, N.A., Rosenwaks, Z. & Giudice, L.C. (1999) The insulin-related ovarian regulatory system in health and disease. *Endocr. Rev.*, **20**, 535–582

Pories, W.J., Swanson, M.S., MacDonald, K.G., Long, S.B., Morris, P.G., Brown, B.M., Barakat, H.A., deRamon, R.A., Israel, G., Dolezal, J.M. & Dohm, L. (1995) Who would have thought it? An operation proves to be the most effective therapy for adult-onset diabetes mellitus. *Ann. Surg.*, **222**, 339-352

Potischman, N., Hoover, R.N., Brinton, L.A., Siiteri, P., Dorgan, J.F., Swanson, C.A., Berman, M.L., Mortel, R., Twiggs, L.B., Barrett, R.J., Wilbanks, G.D., Persky, V. & Lurain, J.R. (1996) Case-control study of endogenous steroid hormones and endometrial cancer. *J. Natl Cancer Inst.*, **88**, 1127–1135

Potter, J.D. (1996) Nutrition and colorectal cancer. *Cancer Causes Control*, **7**, 127–146

Potter, J.D., Bostick, R.M., Grandits, G.A., Fosdick, L., Elmer, P., Wood, J., Grambsch, P. & Louis, T.A. (1996) Hormone replacement therapy is associated with lower risk of adenomatous polyps of the large bowel: the Minnesota Cancer Prevention Research Unit Case-Control Study. *Cancer Epidemiol.*

Biomarkers Prev., **5**, 779–784

Pouliot, M.C., Després, J.P., Lemieux, S., Moorjani, S., Bouchard, C., Tremblay, A., Nadeau, A. & Lupien, P.J. (1994) Waist circumference and abdominal sagittal diameter: best simple anthropometric indexes of abdominal visceral adipose tissue accumulation and related cardiovascular risk in men and women. *Am. J. Cardiol.*, **73**, 460–468

Poulos, J.E., Leggett-Frazier, N., Khazanie, P., Long, S., Sportsman, R., MacDonald, K. & Caro, J.F. (1994) Circulating insulin-like growth factor I concentrations in clinically severe obese patients with and without NIDDM in response to weight loss. *Horm. Metab. Res.*, **26**, 478–480

Pour, P.M., Permert, J., Mogaki, M., Fujii, H. & Kazakoff, K. (1993) Endocrine aspects of exocrine cancer of the pancreas. Their patterns and suggested biologic significance. *Am. J. Clin. Pathol.*, **100**, 223–230

Powell, K.E., Thompson, P.D., Caspersen, C.J. & Kendrick, J.S. (1987) Physical activity and the incidence of coronary heart disease. *Annu. Rev. Public Health*, **8**, 253–287

Pratt, M., Macera, C.A. & Blanton, C. (1999) Levels of physical activity and inactivity in children and adults in the United States: current evidence and research issues. *Med. Sci. Sports Exerc.*, **31**, S526–S533

Prentice, A.M. & Jebb, S.A. (1995) Obesity in Britain: gluttony or sloth? *BMJ*, **311**, 437–439

Prentice, R., Thompson, D., Clifford, C., Gorbach, S., Goldin, B. & Byar, D. (1990) Dietary fat reduction and plasma estradiol concentration in healthy postmenopausal women. The Women's Health Trial Study Group. *J. Natl Cancer Inst.*, **82**, 129–134

Preston-Martin, S., Jin, F., Duda, M.J. & Mack, W.J. (1993) A case-control study of thyroid cancer in women under age 55 in Shanghai (People's Republic of China). *Cancer Causes Control*, **4**, 431–440

Prineas, R.J., Folsom, A.R., Zhang, Z.M., Sellers, T.A. & Potter, J. (1997) Nutrition and other risk factors for renal cell carcinoma in postmenopausal women. *Epidemiology*, **8**, 31–36

Prior, G. (1999) Physical activity. In: Erens, B. & Primatesta, P., eds, *Health Survey for England: Cardiovascular Disease '98*, London, The Stationery Office, pp. 181–219

Province, M.A., Hadley, E.C., Hornbrook, M.C., Lipsitz, L.A., Miller, J.P., Mulrow, C.D., Ory, M.G., Sattin, R.W., Tinetti, M.E. & Wolf, S.L. (1995) The effects of exercise on falls in elderly patients. A preplanned meta-analysis of the FICSIT Trials. Frailty and Injuries: Cooperative Studies of Intervention Techniques. *JAMA*, **273**, 1341–1347

Pugeat, M. & Ducluzeau, P.H. (1999) Insulin resistance, polycystic ovary syndrome and metformin. *Drugs*, **58 Suppl. 1**, 41–46

Pugeat, M., Crave, J.C., Elmidani, M., Nicolas, M.H., Garoscio-Cholet, M., Lejeune, H., Dechaud, H. & Tourniaire, J. (1991) Pathophysiology of sex hormone binding globulin (SHBG): relation to insulin. *J. Steroid Biochem. Mol. Biol.*, **40**, 841–849

Pukkala, E., Poskiparta, M., Apter, D. & Vihko, V. (1993) Life-long physical activity and cancer risk among Finnish female teachers. *Eur. J. Cancer Prev.*, **2**, 369–376

Purdie, D., Green, A., Bain, C., Siskind, V., Ward, B., Hacker, N., Quinn, M., Wright, G., Russell, P. & Susil, B. (1995) Reproductive and other factors and risk of epithelial ovarian cancer: an Australian case-control study. Survey of Women's Health Study Group. *Int. J. Cancer*, **62**, 678–684

Putnam, S.D., Cerhan, J.R., Parker, A.S., Bianchi, G.D., Wallace, R.B., Cantor, K.P., & Lynch, C.F. (2000) Lifestyle and anthropometric risk factors for prostate cancer in a cohort of Iowa men. *Ann. Epidemiol.*, **10**, 361–369

Pyne, D.B., Baker, M.S., Fricker, P.A., McDonald, W.A., Telford, R.D. & Weidemann, M.J. (1995) Effects of an intensive 12-wk training program by elite swimmers on neutrophil oxidative activity. *Med. Sci. Sports Exerc.*, **27**, 536–542

Raastad, T., Bjoro, T. & Hallén, J. (2000) Hormonal responses to high- and moderate-intensity strength exercise. *Eur. J. Appl. Physiol.*, **82**, 121–128

Radak, Z., Sasvari, M., Nyakas, C., Taylor, A.W., Ohno, H., Nakamoto, H. & Goto, S. (2000) Regular training modulates the accumulation of reactive carbonyl derivatives in mitochondrial and cytosolic fractions of rat skeletal muscle. *Arch. Biochem. Biophys.*, **383**, 114–118

Radziuk, J. & Pye, S. (1999) The role of the liver in insulin action and resistance. In: Reaven, G.M. & Laws, A., eds, *Insulin Resistance*, Totowa, NJ, Humana Press, pp. 197–231

Randle, P.J. (1998) Regulatory interactions between lipids and carbohydrates: the glucose fatty acid cycle after 35 years. *Diabetes Metab. Rev.*, **14**, 263–283

Rao, G., Xia, E., Nadakavukaren, M.J. & Richardson, A. (1990) Effect of dietary restriction on the age-dependent changes in the expression of antioxidant enzymes in rat liver. *J. Nutr.*, **120**, 602–609

Rasheed, P., Abou-Hozaifa, B.M. & Khan, A. (1994) Obesity among young Saudi female adults: a prevalence study on medical and nursing students. *Public Health*, **108**, 289–294

Rasmussen, M.H., Frystyk, J., Andersen, T., Breum, L., Christiansen, J.S. & Hilsted, J. (1994) The impact of obesity, fat distribution, and energy restriction on insulin-like growth factor-1 (IGF-1), IGF-binding protein-3, insulin, and growth hormone. *Metabolism*, **43**, 315–319

Rasmussen, M.H., Hvidberg, A., Juul, A., Main, K.M., Gotfredsen, A., Skakkebaek, N.E. & Hilsted, J. (1995) Massive weight loss restores 24-hour growth hormone release profiles and serum insulin-like growth factor-I levels in obese subjects. *J. Clin. Endocrinol. Metab.*, **80**, 1407–1415

Rasmussen, M.H., Ho, K.K., Kjems, L. & Hilsted, J. (1996) Serum growth hormone-binding protein in obesity: effect of a short-term, very low calorie diet and diet-induced weight loss. *J. Clin. Endocrinol. Metab.*, **81**, 1519–1524

Raso, E., Timar, J. & Lapis, K. (1992) Development and characterization of a sex-dependent metastatic preputial gland adeno-carcinoma in human tumor-bearing immuno-suppressed F344 rats. *Carcinogenesis*, **13**, 1281–1284

Rauh, M.J., Hovell, M.F., Hofstetter, C.R., Sallis, J.F. & Gleghorn, A. (1992) Reliability and validity of self-reported physical activity in Latinos. *Int. J. Epidemiol.*, **21**, 966–971

Rauramaa, R., Salonen, J.T., Kukkonen-Harjula, K., Seppänen, K., Seppälä, E., Vapaatalo, H. & Huttunen, J.K. (1984) Effects of mild physical exercise on serum lipoproteins and metabolites of arachidonic acid: a controlled randomised trial in middle aged men. *Br. Med. J. (Clin. Res. Ed.)*, **288**, 603–606

Rauramaa, R., Salonen, J.T., Seppänen, K., Salonen, R., Venäläinen, J.M., Ihanainen, M. & Rissanen, V. (1986) Inhibition of platelet aggregability by moderate-intensity physical exercise: a randomized clinical trial in overweight men. *Circulation*, **74**, 939–944

Rauscher, G.H., Mayne, S.T. & Janerich, D.T. (2000) Relation between body mass index and lung cancer risk in men and women never and former smokers. *Am. J. Epidemiol.*, **152**, 506–513

Ravussin, E. & Gautier, J.F. (1999) Metabolic predictors of weight gain. *Int. J. Obes. Relat. Metab. Disord.*, **23 Suppl. 1**, 37–41

Recker, R.R., Davies, K.M., Hinders, S.M., Heaney, R.P., Stegman, M.R. & Kimmel, D.B. (1992) Bone gain in young adult women. *JAMA*, **268**, 2403–2408

Reddy Avula, C.P., Muthukumar, A. & Fernandes, G. (1999) Calorie restriction increases Fas/Fas-ligand expression and apoptosis in murine splenic lymphocytes. *FEBS Lett.*, **458**, 231–235

Reddy, B.S., Wang, C.X. & Maruyama, H. (1987) Effect of restricted caloric intake on azoxymethane-induced colon tumor incidence in male F344 rats. *Cancer Res.*, **47**, 1226–1228

Reddy, B.S., Sugie, S. & Lowenfels, A. (1988) Effect of voluntary exercise on azoxymethane-induced colon carcinogenesis in male F344 rats. *Cancer Res.*, **48**, 7079–7081

Reeder, B.A., Angel, A., Ledoux, M., Rabkin, S.W., Young, T.K. & Sweet, L.E. (1992) Obesity and its relation to cardiovascular disease risk factors in Canadian adults. Canadian Heart Health Surveys Research Group. *CMAJ*, **146**, 2009–2019

Regensteiner, J.G., Mayer, E.J., Shetterly, S.M., Eckel, R.H., Haskell, W.L., Marshall, J.A., Baxter, J. & Hamman, R.F. (1991) Relationship between habitual physical activity and insulin levels among nondiabetic men and women. San Luis Valley Diabetes Study. *Diabetes Care*, **14**, 1066–1074

Rencken, M.L., Chesnut, C.H. & Drinkwater, B.L. (1996) Bone density at multiple skeletal sites in amenorrheic athletes. *JAMA*, **276**, 238–240

Renehan, A.G., Jones, J., Potten, C.S., Shalet, S.M. & O'Dwyer, S.T. (2000a) Elevated serum insulin-like growth factor (IGF)-II and IGF binding protein-2 in patients with colorectal cancer. *Br. J. Cancer*, 83, 1344–1350

Renehan, A.G., Painter, J.E., O'Halloran, D., Atkin, W.S., Potten, C.S., O'Dwyer, S.T. & Shalet, S.M. (2000b) Circulating insulin-like growth factor II and colorectal adenomas. *J. Clin. Endocrinol. Metab.*, 85, 3402–3408

Reynolds, M.W., Fredman, L., Langenberg, P. & Magaziner, J. (1999) Weight, weight change, mortality in a random sample of older community-dwelling women. *J. Am. Geriatr. Soc*, 47, 1409-1414

Rhee, K., Bresnahan, W., Hirai, A., Hirai, M. & Thompson, E.A. (1995) c-Myc and cyclin D3 (CcnD3) genes are independent targets for glucocorticoid inhibition of lymphoid cell proliferation. *Cancer Res.*, 55, 4188–4195

Rhind, S.G., Shek, P.N., Shinkai, S. & Shephard, R.J. (1994) Differential expression of interleukin-2 receptor alpha and beta chains in relation to natural killer cell subsets and aerobic fitness. *Int. J. Sports Med.,* 15, 911–918

Rhind, S.G., Shek, P.N., Shinkai, S. & Shephard, R.J. (1996) Effects of moderate endurance exercise and training on in vitro lymphocyte proliferation, interleukin-2 (IL-2) production, and IL-2 receptor expression. *Eur. J. Appl. Physiol.*, 74, 348–360

Rhoads, G.G. & Kagan, A. (1983) The relation of coronary disease, stroke, and mortality to weight in youth and in middle age. *Lancet*, 1, 492–495

Riboli, E. & Kaaks, R. (1997) The EPIC Project: rationale and study design. European Prospective Investigation into Cancer and Nutrition. *Int. J. Epidemiol.*, 26 **Suppl. 1**, S6–S14

Richardson, M.T., Leon, A.S., Jacobs, D.R., Jr, Ainsworth, B.E. & Serfass, R. (1994) Comprehensive evaluation of the Minnesota Leisure Time Physical Activity Questionnaire. *J. Clin. Epidemiol.*, 47, 271–281

Richardson, M.T., Ainsworth, B.E., Wu, H.C., Jacobs, D.R., Jr & Leon, A.S. (1995) Ability of the Atherosclerosis Risk in Communities (ARIC)/Baecke Questionnaire to assess leisure-time physical activity. *Int. J. Epidemiol.*, 24, 685–693

Rimm, E.B., Stampfer, M.J., Giovannucci, E., Ascherio, A., Spiegelman, D., Colditz, G.A. & Willett, W.C. (1995) Body size and fat distribution as predictors of coronary heart disease among middle-aged and older US men. *Am. J. Epidemiol.*, 141, 1117–1127

Rippe, J.M., Price, J.M., Hess, S.A., Kline, G., DeMers, K.A., Damitz, S., Kreidieh, I. & Freedson, P. (1998) Improved psychological well-being, quality of life, and health practices in moderately overweight women participating in a 12-week structured weight loss program. *Obes Res.*, 6, 208-218

Risch, H.A. (1998) Hormonal etiology of epithelial ovarian cancer, with a hypothesis concerning the role of androgens and progesterone. *J. Natl Cancer Inst.*, 90, 1774–1786

Rissanen, A.M., Heliovaara, M., Knekt, P., Reunanen, A. & Aromaa, A. (1991) Determinants of weight gain and overweight in adult Finns. *Eur. J. Clin. Nutr.*, 45, 419–430

Rivara, F.P., Grossman, D.C. & Cummings, P. (1997a) Injury prevention. First of two parts. *New Engl. J. Med.*, 337, 543–548

Rivara, F.P., Grossman, D.C. & Cummings, P. (1997b) Injury prevention. Second of two parts. *New Engl. J. Med.*, 337, 613–618

Rizza, R.A., Mandarino, L.J. & Gerich, J.E. (1982) Effects of growth hormone on insulin action in man. Mechanisms of insulin resistance, impaired suppression of glucose production, and impaired stimulation of glucose utilization. *Diabetes*, 31, 663–669

Robinson, T.N. (1999) Reducing children's television viewing to prevent obesity: a randomized controlled trial. *JAMA*, 282, 1561–1567

Robinson, S., Kiddy, D., Gelding, S.V., Willis, D., Niththyananthan, R., Bush, A., Johnston, D.G. & Franks, S. (1993) The relationship of insulin insensitivity to menstrual pattern in women with hyperandrogenism and polycystic ovaries. *Clin. Endocrinol. (Oxf.)*, 39, 351–355

Robson, P.J., Blannin, A.K., Walsh, N.P., Castell, L.M. & Gleeson, M. (1999) Effects of exercise intensity, duration and recovery on *in vitro* neutrophil function in male athletes. *Int. J. Sports Med.*, 20, 128–135

Rockhill, B., Willett, W.C., Hunter, D.J., Manson, J.E., Hankinson, S.E., Spiegelman, D. & Colditz, G.A. (1998) Physical activity and breast cancer risk in a cohort of young women. *J. Natl Cancer Inst.*, 90, 1155–1160

Rockhill, B., Willett, W.C., Hunter, D.J., Manson, J.E., Hankinson, S.E. & Colditz, G.A. (1999) A prospective study of recreational physical activity and breast cancer risk. *Arch. Intern. Med.*, 159, 2290–2296

Roebuck, B.D., McCaffrey, J. & Baumgartner, K.J. (1990) Protective effects of voluntary exercise during the postinitiation phase of pancreatic carcinogenesis in the rat. *Cancer Res.*, 50, 6811–6816

Roebuck, B.D., Baumgartner, K.J. & MacMillan, D.L. (1993) Caloric restriction and intervention in pancreatic carcinogenesis in the rat. *Cancer Res.*, 53, 46–52

Roelen, C.A., de Vries, W.R., Koppeschaar, H.P., Vervoorn, C., Thijssen, J.H. & Blankenstein, M.A. (1997) Plasma insulin-like growth factor-I and high affinity growth hormone-binding protein levels increase after two weeks of strenuous physical training. *Int. J. Sports Med.*, 18, 238–241

Rojdmark, S. (1987) Increased gonadotropin responsiveness to gonadotropin-releasing hormone during fasting in normal subjects. *Metabolism*, 36, 21–26

Ron, E., Kleinerman, R.A., Boice, J.D., LiVolsi, V.A., Flannery, J.T. & Fraumeni, J.F., Jr (1987) A population-based case-control study of thyroid cancer. *J. Natl Cancer Inst.*, 79, 1–12

Rose, D.P., Boyar, A.P., Cohen, C. & Strong, L.E. (1987) Effect of a low-fat diet on hormone levels in women with cystic breast disease. I. Serum steroids and gonadotropins. *J. Natl Cancer Inst.*, 78, 623–626

Rose, D.P., Connolly, J.M., Chlebowski, R.T., Buzzard, I.M. & Wynder, E.L. (1993) The effects of a low-fat dietary intervention and tamoxifen adjuvant therapy on the serum estrogen and sex hormone-binding globulin concentrations of postmenopausal breast cancer patients. *Breast Cancer Res. Treat.*, 27, 253–262

Rosen, C.J. (1999) Serum insulin-like growth factors and insulin-like growth factor-binding proteins: clinical implications. *Clin. Chem.*, 45, 1384–1390

Rosenfield, R.L. (1999) Ovarian and adrenal function in polycystic ovary syndrome. *Endocrinol. Metab. Clin. North Am.*, 28, 265–293

Rosengren, A., Eriksson, H., Larsson, B., Svärdsudd, K., Tibblin, G., Welin, L. & Wilhelmsen, L. (2000) Secular changes in cardiovascular risk factors over 30 years in Swedish men aged 50: the study of men born in 1913, 1923, 1933 and 1943. *J. Intern. Med.*, **247**, 111–118

Rosenthal, M.B., Barnard, R.J., Rose, D.P., Inkeles, S., Hall, J. & Pritikin, N. (1985) Effects of a high-complex-carbohydrate, low-fat, low-cholesterol diet on levels of serum lipids and estradiol. *Am. J. Med.*, **78**, 23–27

Ross, R.J. (2000) GH, IGF-I and binding proteins in altered nutritional states. *Int. J. Obes. Relat. Metab. Disord.*, **24 Suppl. 2**, S92–S95

Ross, R.K., Shimizu, H., Paganini-Hill, A., Honda, G. & Henderson, B.E. (1987) Case-control studies of prostate cancer in blacks and whites in southern California. *J. Natl Cancer Inst.*, **78**, 869–874

Ross, J.A., Potter, J.D. & Severson, R.K. (1993) Platelet-derived growth factor and risk factors for colorectal cancer. *Eur. J. Cancer Prev.*, **2**, 197–210

Ross, R.K., Pike, M.C., Coetzee, G.A., Reichardt, J.K., Yu, M.C., Feigelson, H., Stanczyk, F.Z., Kolonel, L.N. & Henderson, B.E. (1998) Androgen metabolism and prostate cancer: establishing a model of genetic susceptibility. *Cancer Res.*, **58**, 4497–4504

Ross, R., Dagnone, D., Jones, P.J., Smith, H., Paddags, A., Hudson, R. & Janssen, I. (2000a) Reduction in obesity and related comorbid conditions after diet-induced weight loss or exercise-induced weight loss in men. A randomized, controlled trial. *Ann. Intern. Med.*, **133**, 92–103

Ross, R.K., Paganini-Hill, A., Wan, P.C. & Pike, M.C. (2000b) Effect of hormone replacement therapy on breast cancer risk: estrogen versus estrogen plus progestin. *J. Natl Cancer Inst.*, **92**, 328–332

Rossing, M.A., Voigt, L.F., Wicklund, K.G. & Daling, J.R. (2000) Reproductive factors and risk of papillary thyroid cancer in women. *Am. J. Epidemiol.*, **151**, 765–772

Rudolf, M.C., Sahota, P., Barth, J.H. & Walker, J. (2001) Increasing prevalence of obesity in primary school children: cohort study. *BMJ*, **322**, 1094–1095

Ruggeri, B.A., Klurfeld, D.M., Kritchevsky, D. & Furlanetto, R.W. (1989) Caloric restriction and 7,12-dimethylbenz(a)anthracene-induced mammary tumor growth in rats: alterations in circulating insulin, insulin-like growth factors I and II, and epidermal growth factor. *Cancer Res.*, **49**, 4130–4134

Rush, H.P. & Kline, B.E. (1944) The effect of exercise on the growth of mouse tumor. *Cancer Res.*, **4**, 116–118

Russell, D.G. & Wilson, N.C. (1991) *Life in New Zealand Commission Report.* Volume I: *Executive Overview,* Dunedin, University of Otago, pp. 1–28

Russell, J.B., Mitchell, D., Musey, P.I. & Collins, D.C. (1984) The relationship of exercise to anovulatory cycles in female athletes: hormonal and physical characteristics. *Obstet. Gynecol.*, **63**, 452–456

Russo, A., Franceschi, S., La Vecchia, C., Dal Maso, L., Montella, M., Conti, E., Giacosa, A., Falcini, F. & Negri, E. (1998) Body size and colorectal-cancer risk. *Int. J. Cancer*, **78**, 161–165

Rutanen, E.M. (1998) Insulin-like growth factors in endometrial function. *Gynecol. Endocrinol.*, **12**, 399–406

Rutanen, E.M., Pekonen, F., Nyman, T. & Wahlström, T. (1993) Insulin-like growth factors and their binding proteins in benign and malignant uterine diseases. *Growth Regul.*, **3**, 74–77

Rutanen, E.M., Nyman, T., Lehtovirta, P., Ämmälä, M. & Pekonen, F. (1994) Suppressed expression of insulin-like growth factor binding protein-1 mRNA in the endometrium: a molecular mechanism associating endometrial cancer with its risk factors. *Int. J. Cancer*, **59**, 307–312

Sabroe, S. & Olsen, J. (1998) Perinatal correlates of specific histological types of testicular cancer in patients below 35 years of age: a case-cohort study based on midwives' records in Denmark. *Int. J. Cancer*, **78**, 140–143

Sahi, T., Paffenbarger, R.S., Jr, Hsieh, C.C. & Lee,. I.M. (1998) Body mass index, cigarette smoking, and other characteristics as predictors of self-reported, physician-diagnosed gallbladder disease in male college alumni. *Am. J. Epidemiol.*, **147**, 644-651

Saitoh, H., Kamoda, T., Nakahara, S., Hirano, T. & Nakamura, N. (1998) Serum concentrations of insulin, insulin-like growth factor(IGF)-I, IGF binding protein (IGFBP)-1 and -3 and growth hormone binding protein in obese children: fasting IGFBP-1 is suppressed in normoinsulinaemic obese children. *Clin. Endocrinol. (Oxf.)*, **48**, 487–492

Salih, M.A., Herbert, D.C. & Kalu, D.N. (1993) Evaluation of the molecular and cellular basis for the modulation of thyroid C-cell hormones by aging and food restriction. *Mech. Ageing Dev.*, **70**, 1–21

Sallis, J.F. & Saelens, B.E. (2000) Assessment of physical activity by self-report: status, limitations, and future directions. *Res. Q. Exerc. Sport*, **71**, 1–14

Sallis, J.F., Haskell, W.L., Wood, P.D., Fortmann, S.P., Rogers, T., Blair, S.N. & Paffenbarger, R.S., Jr. (1985) Physical activity assessment methodology in the Five-City Project. *Am. J. Epidemiol.*, **121**, 91–106

Sallis, J.F., Bauman, A. & Pratt, M. (1998) Environmental and policy interventions to promote physical activity. *Am. J. Prev. Med.*, **15**, 379–397

Salmon, J., Bauman, A., Crawford, D., Timperio, A. & Owen, N. (2000) The association between television viewing and overweight among Australian adults participating in varying levels of leisure-time physical activity. *Int. J. Obes. Relat. Metab. Disord.*, **24**, 600–606

Sanderson, M., Williams, M.A., Malone, K.E., Stanford, J.L., Emanuel, I., White, E. & Daling, J.R. (1996) Perinatal factors and risk of breast cancer. *Epidemiology*, **7**, 34–37

Sandler, R.S., Pritchard, M.L. & Bangdiwala, S.I. (1995) Physical activity and the risk of colorectal adenomas. *Epidemiology*, **6**, 602–606

Sandvik, L., Erikssen, J., Thaulow, E., Erikssen, G., Mundal, R. & Rodahl, K. (1993) Physical fitness as a predictor of mortality among healthy, middle-aged Norwegian men. *New Engl. J. Med.*, **328**, 533–537

Saris, W.H. (1998) Fit, fat and fat free: the metabolic aspects of weight control. *Int. J. Obes. Relat. Metab. Disord.*, **22 Suppl. 2**, S15–S21

Sarkar, N.H., Fernandes, G., Telang, N.T., Kourides, I.A. & Good, R.A. (1982) Low-calorie diet prevents the development of mammary tumors in C3H mice and reduces circulating prolactin level, murine mammary tumor virus expression, and proliferation of mammary alveolar cells. *Proc. Natl Acad. Sci. USA*, **79**, 7758–7762

Scaglione, R., Averna, M.R., Dichiara, M.A., Barbagallo, C.M., Mazzola, G., Montalto, G., Licata, G. & Notarbartolo, A. (1991) Thyroid function and release of thyroid-stimulating hormone and prolactin from the pituitary in human obesity. *J. Int. Med. Res.*, **19**, 389–394

Scanga, C.B., Verde, T.J., Paolone, A.M., Andersen, R.E. & Wadden, T.A. (1998) Effects of weight loss and exercise training on natural killer cell activity in obese women. *Med. Sci. Sports Exerc.*, **30**, 1666–1671

Scarpelli, D.G. (1988) Comparative histopathology of the development of selected neoplasms of the liver, pancreas, and urinary bladder in rodents. *Environ. Health Perspect.*, **77**, 83–92

Schaefer, E.J., Lichtenstein, A.H., Lamon-Fava, S., McNamara, J.R., Schaefer, M.M., Rasmussen, H. & Ordovas, J.M. (1995) Body weight and low-density lipoprotein cholesterol changes after consumption of a low-fat ad libitum diet. *JAMA*, **274**, 1450–1455

Schairer, C., Lubin, J., Troisi, R., Sturgeon, S., Brinton, L. & Hoover, R. (2000) Estrogen-progestin replacement and risk of breast cancer. *JAMA*, **284**, 691–694

Schapira, D.V., Kumar, N.B., Lyman, G.H., Cavanagh, D., Roberts, W.S. & LaPolla, J. (1991) Upper-body fat distribution and endometrial cancer risk. *JAMA*, **266**, 1808–1811

Schatzkin, A., Lanza, E., Corle, D., Lance, P., Iber, F., Caan, B., Shike, M., Weissfeld, J., Burt, R., Cooper, M.R., Kikendall, J.W. & Cahill, J. (2000) Lack of effect of a low-fat, high-fiber diet on the recurrence of colorectal adenomas. Polyp Prevention Trial Study Group. *New Engl. J. Med.*, **342**, 1149–1155

Scheett, T.P., Mills, P.J., Ziegler, M.G., Stoppani, J. & Cooper, D.M. (1999) Effect of exercise on cytokines and growth mediators in prepubertal children. *Pediatr. Res.*, **46**, 429–434

Schenkein, D.P. & Schwartz, R.S. (1997) Neoplasms and transplantation—trading swords for plowshares. *New Engl. J. Med.*, **336**, 949–950

Schildkraut, J.M., Schwingl, P.J., Bastos, E., Evanoff, A. & Hughes, C. (1996) Epithelial ovarian cancer risk among women with polycystic ovary syndrome. *Obstet. Gynecol.*, **88**, 554–559

Schmidt, W., Doré, S., Hilgendorf, A., Strauch, S., Gareau, R. & Brisson, G.R. (1995) Effects of exercise during normoxia and hypoxia on the growth hormone-insulin-like growth factor I axis. *Eur. J. Appl. Physiol.*, **71**, 424–430

Schoeller, D.A., Shay, K. & Kushner, R.F. (1997) How much physical activity is needed to minimize weight gain in previously obese women? *Am. J. Clin. Nutr.*, **66**, 551–556

Schoen, R.E., Tangen, C.M., Kuller, L.H., Burke, G.L., Cushman, M., Tracy, R.P., Dobs, A. & Savage, P.J. (1999) Increased blood glucose and insulin, body size, and incident colorectal cancer. *J. Natl Cancer Inst.*, **91**, 1147–1154

Schulz, N., Propst, F., Rosenberg, M.P., Linnoila, R.I., Paules, R.S., Kovatch, R., Ogiso, Y. & Vande Woude, G. (1992) Pheochromocytomas and C-cell thyroid neoplasms in transgenic c-mos mice: a model for the human multiple endocrine neoplasia type 2 syndrome. *Cancer Res.*, **52**, 450–455

Schulz, T.F., Boshoff, C.H. & Weiss, R.A. (1996) HIV infection and neoplasia. *Lancet*, **348**, 587–591

Schuurman, A.G., Goldbohm, R.A., Dorant, E. & van den Brandt, P.A. (2000) Anthropometry in relation to prostate cancer risk in the Netherlands cohort study. *Am. J. Epidemiol.*, **6**, 541–549

Schwartz, R.S. (1990) Exercise training in the treatment of diabetes mellitus in elderly patients. *Diabetes Care*, **14**, 77–85

Schwartz, R.S., Shuman, W.P., Larson, V., Cain, K.C., Fellingham, G.W., Beard, J.C., Kahn, S.E., Stratton, J.R., Cerqueira, M.D. & Abrass, I.B. (1991) The effect of intensive endurance exercise training on body fat distribution in young and older men. *Metabolism*, **40**, 545–551

Schwarz, A.J., Brasel, J.A., Hintz, R.L., Mohan, S. & Cooper, D.M. (1996) Acute effect of brief low- and high-intensity exercise on circulating insulin-like growth factor (IGF) I, II, and IGF-binding protein-3 and its proteolysis in young healthy men. *J. Clin. Endocrinol. Metab.*, **81**, 3492–3497

Sea, M.M., Fong, W.P., Huang, Y. & Chen, Z.Y. (2000) Weight cycling-induced alteration in fatty acid metabolism. *Am. J. Physiol. Regul. Integr. Comp. Physiol.*, **279**, R1145-R1155

Seidell, J.C. (1998) Dietary fat and obesity: an epidemiologic perspective. *Am. J. Clin. Nutr.*, **67**, 546S–550S

Seidell, J.C. (2001) The epidemiology of obesity. In: Björntorp, P., ed., *International Textbook of Obesity*, Chichester, John Wiley, pp. 23–29

Seidell, J.C. & Visscher, T.L. (2000) Body weight and weight change and their health implications for the elderly. *Eur. J. Clin. Nutr.*, **54, Suppl. 3**, S33–S39

Seidell, J.C., Oosterlee, A., Deurenberg, P., Hautvast, J.G. & Ruijs, J.H. (1988) Abdominal fat depots measured with computed tomography: effects of degree of obesity, sex, and age. *Eur. J. Clin. Nutr.*, **42**, 805–815

Seidell, J.C., Björntorp, P., Sjöström, L., Kvist, H. & Sannerstedt, R. (1990a) Visceral fat accumulation in men is positively associated with insulin, glucose, and C-peptide levels, but negatively with testosterone levels. *Metabolism*, **39**, 897–901

Seidell, J.C., Cigolini, M., Charzewska, J., Ellsinger, B.M., Di Biase, G., Björntorp, P., Hautvast, J.G., Contaldo, F., Szostak, V. & Scuro, L.A. (1990b) Androgenicity in relation to body fat distribution and metabolism in 38-year-old women — the European Fat Distribution Study. *J. Clin. Epidemiol.*, **43**, 21–34

Seidell, J.C., Verschuren, W.M. & Kromhout, D. (1995) Prevalence and trends of obesity in The Netherlands 1987–1991. *Int. J. Obes. Relat. Metab. Disord.*, **19**, 924–927

Seidell, J.C., Verschuren, W.M., van Leer, E.M. & Kromhout, D. (1996) Overweight, underweight, and mortality. A prospective study of 48,287 men and women. *Arch. Intern. Med.*, **156**, 958–963

Seidell, J.C., Visscher, T.L. & Hoogeveen, R.T. (1999) Overweight and obesity in the mortality rate data: current evidence and research issues. *Med. Sci. Sports Exerc.*, **31**, S597-S601

Seilkop, S.K. (1995) The effect of body weight on tumor incidence and carcinogenicity testing in B6C3F1 mice and F344 rats. *Fundam. Appl. Toxicol.*, **24**, 247–259

Sellers, T.A., Kushi, L.H., Potter, J.D., Kaye, S.A., Nelson, C.L., McGovern, P.G. & Folsom, A.R. (1992) Effect of family history, body-fat distribution, and reproductive factors on the risk of postmenopausal breast cancer. *New Engl. J. Med.*, **326**, 1323–1329

Seng, J.E., Gandy, J., Turturro, A., Lipman, R., Bronson, R.T., Parkinson, A., Johnson, W., Hart, R.W. & Leakey, J.E. (1996) Effects of caloric restriction on expression of testicular cytochrome P450 enzymes associated with the metabolic activation of carcinogens. *Arch. Biochem. Biophys.*, **335**, 42–52

Senie, R.T., Rosen, P.P., Rhodes, P., Lesser, M.L. & Kinne, D.W. (1992) Obesity at diagnosis of breast carcinoma influences duration of disease-free survival. *Ann. Intern. Med.*, **116**, 26–32

Sesso, H.D., Paffenbarger, R.S., Jr & Lee, I.M. (1998) Physical activity and breast cancer risk in the College Alumni Health Study (United States). *Cancer Causes Control*, **9**, 433–439

Severson, R.K., Grove, J.S., Nomura, A.M. & Stemmermann, G.N. (1988) Body mass and prostatic cancer: a prospective study. *BMJ*, **297**, 713–715

Severson, R.K., Nomura, A.M., Grove, J.S. & Stemmermann, G.N. (1989) A prospective analysis of physical activity and cancer. *Am. J. Epidemiol.,* **130**, 522–529

Shamoon, H., Hendler, R. & Sherwin, R.S. (1981) Synergistic interactions among antiinsulin hormones in the pathogenesis of stress hyperglycemia in humans. *J. Clin. Endocrinol. Metab.,* **52**, 1235–1241

Sheldon, W.G., Bucci, T., Blackwell, B. & Turturro, A. (1996) Effect of *ad libitum* feeding and 40% feed restriction on body weight, longevity, and neoplasms in B6C3F$_1$, C57BL6, and B6D2F$_1$ mice. In: Mohr, U., Dungworth, D., Capen, C., Carlton, W., Sundberg, J. & Ward, J., eds, *Pathology of the Aging Mouse*, Washington DC, ILSI Press, pp. 21–26

Shephard, R.J. & Shek, P.N. (1995) Cancer, immune function, and physical activity. *Can. J. Appl. Physiol.*, **20**, 1–25

Shephard, R.J. & Shek, P.N. (1998) Associations between physical activity and susceptibility to cancer: possible mechanisms. *Sports Med.*, **26**, 293–315

Sherr, C.J. (2000) The Pezcoller lecture: cancer cell cycles revisited. *Cancer Res.,* **60**, 3689–3695

Shibata, A., Mack, T.M., Paganini-Hill, A., Ross, R.K. & Henderson, B.E. (1994) A prospective study of pancreatic cancer in the elderly. *Int. J. Cancer*, **58**, 46–49

Shigenaga, M.K., Hagen, T.M. & Ames, B.N. (1994) Oxidative damage and mitochondrial decay in aging. *Proc. Natl Acad. Sci. USA*, **91**, 10771–10778

Shimokawa, I. & Higami, Y. (1999) A role for leptin in the antiaging action of dietary restriction: a hypothesis. *Aging (Milano)*, **11**, 380–382

Shimokawa, I., Yu, B.P. & Masoro, E.J. (1991) Influence of diet on fatal neoplastic disease in male Fischer 344 rats. *J. Gerontol.*, **46**, B228–B232

Shimokawa, I., Higami, Y., Yu, B.P., Masoro, E.J. & Ikeda, T. (1996) Influence of dietary components on occurrence of and mortality due to neoplasms in male F344 rats. *Aging (Milano)*, **8**, 254–262

Shimokawa, I., Higami, Y., Okimoto, T., Tomita, M. & Ikeda, T. (1997) Effect of somatostatin-28 on growth hormone response to growth hormone-releasing hormone – impact of aging and lifelong dietary restriction. *Neuroendocrinology*, **65**, 369–376

Shinchi, K., Kono, S., Honjo, S., Todoroki, I., Sakurai, Y., Imanishi, K., Nishikawa, H., Ogawa, S., Katsurada, M. & Hirohata, T. (1994) Obesity and adenomatous polyps of the sigmoid colon. *Jpn J. Cancer Res*, **85**, 479–484

Shoff, S.M. & Newcomb, P.A. (1998) Diabetes, body size, and risk of endometrial cancer. *Am. J. Epidemiol.,* **148**, 234–240

Shoff, S.M., Newcomb, P.A., Trentham-Dietz, A., Remington, P.L., Mittendorf, R., Greenberg, E.R. & Willett, W.C. (2000) Early-life physical activity and postmenopausal breast cancer: effect of body size and weight change. *Cancer Epidemiol. Biomarkers Prev.,* **9**, 591–595

Shoupe, D., Kumar, D.D. & Lobo, R.A. (1983) Insulin resistance in polycystic ovary syndrome. *Am. J. Obstet. Gynecol.*, **147**, 588–592

Shu, X.O., Gao, Y.T., Yuan, J.M., Ziegler, R.G. & Brinton, L.A. (1989) Dietary factors and epithelial ovarian cancer. *Br. J. Cancer*, **59**, 92–96

Shu, X.O., Brinton, L.A., Zheng, W., Gao, Y.T., Fan, J. & Fraumeni, J.F., Jr (1991) A population-based case-control study of endometrial cancer in Shanghai, China. *Int. J. Cancer*, **49**, 38–43

Shu, X.O., Brinton, L.A., Zheng, W., Swanson, C.A., Hatch, M.C., Gao, Y.T. & Fraumeni, J.F., Jr (1992) Relation of obesity and body fat distribution to endometrial cancer in Shanghai, China. *Cancer Res.*, **52**, 3865–3870

Shu, X.O., Hatch, M.C., Zheng, W., Gao, Y.T. & Brinton, L.A. (1993) Physical activity and risk of endometrial cancer. *Epidemiology*, **4**, 342–349

Siconolfi, S.F., Lasater, T.M., Snow, R.C. & Carleton, R.A. (1985) Self-reported physical activity compared with maximal oxygen uptake. *Am. J. Epidemiol.*, **122**, 101–105

Siiteri, P.K. (1987) Adipose tissue as a source of hormones. *Am. J. Clin. Nutr.*, **45**, 277–282

Sikand, G., Kondo, A., Foreyt, J.P., Jones, P.H. & Gotto, A.M. (1988) Two-year follow-up of patients treated with a very-low-calorie diet and exercise training. *J. Am. Diet. Assoc.*, **88**, 487–488

Silver, J.R. (1993) Spinal injuries in sports in the UK. *Br. J. Sports Med.*, **27**, 115–120

Silverman, D.T., Swanson, C.A., Gridley, G., Wacholder, S., Greenberg, R.S., Brown, L.M., Hayes, R.B., Swanson, G.M., Schoenberg, J.B., Pottern, L.M., Schwartz, A.G., Fraumeni, J.F., Jr & Hoover, R.N. (1998) Dietary and nutritional factors and pancreatic cancer: a case-control study based on direct interviews. *J. Natl Cancer Inst.,* **90**, 1710–1719

Silverman, D.T., Schiffman, M., Everhart, J., Goldstein, A., Lillemoe, K.D., Swanson, G.M., Schwartz, A.G., Brown, L.M., Greenberg, R.S., Schoenberg, J.B., Pottern, L.M., Hoover, R.N. & Fraumeni, J.F., Jr (1999) Diabetes mellitus, other medical conditions and familial history of cancer as risk factors for pancreatic cancer. *Br. J. Cancer*, **80**, 1830–1837

Simons-Morton, D.G., Calfas, K.J., Oldenburg, B. & Burton, N.W. (1998) Effects of interventions in health care settings on physical activity or cardiorespiratory fitness. *Am. J. Prev. Med.*, **15**, 413–430

Singh, P.N. & Lindsted, K.D. (1998) Body mass and 26-year risk of mortality from specific diseases among women who never smoked. *Epidemiology*, **9**, 246–254

Singh, P. & Rubin, N. (1993) Insulin-like growth factors and binding proteins in colon cancer. *Gastroenterology*, **105**, 1218–1237

Singh, A., Hamilton-Fairley, D., Koistinen, R., Seppala, M., James, V.H., Franks, S. & Reed, M.J. (1990) Effect of insulin-like growth factor-type I (IGF-I) and insulin on the secretion of sex hormone binding globulin and IGF-I binding protein (IBP-I) by human hepatoma cells. *J. Endocrinol.*, **124**, R1–R3

Singh, R.B., Rastogi, S.S., Verma, R., Laxmi, B., Singh, R., Ghosh, S. & Niaz, M.A. (1992) Randomised controlled trial of cardioprotective diet in patients with recent acute myocardial infarction: results of one year follow up. *BMJ*, **304**, 1015-1019

Sinha, D.K., Gebhard, R.L. & Pazik, J.E. (1988) Inhibition of mammary carcinogenesis in rats by dietary restriction. *Cancer Lett.*, **40**, 133–141

Sinzinger, H. & Virgolini, I. (1988) Effects of exercise on parameters of blood coagulation, platelet function and the prostaglandin system. *Sports Med.*, **6**, 238–245

Sjöström, L., Rissanen, A., Andersen, T., Boldrin, M., Golay, A., Koppeschaar, H.P. & Krempf, M. (1998) Randomised placebo-controlled trial of orlistat for weight loss and prevention of weight regain in obese patients. European Multicentre Orlistat Study Group. *Lancet*, **352**, 167–172

Sjöström, C.D., Lissner, L., Wedel, H. & Sjöström, L. (1999) Reduction in incidence of diabetes, hypertension and lipid disturbances after intentional weight loss induced by bariatric surgery: the SOS Intervention Study. *Obes. Res.*, **7**, 477–484

Sjöström, C.D., Peltonen, M., Wedel, H. & Sjöström, L. (2000) Differentiated long-term effects of intentional weight loss on diabetes and hypertension. *Hypertension*, **36**, 20–25

Skender, M.L., Goodrick, G.K., Del Junco, D.J., Reeves, R.S., Darnell, L., Gotto, A.M. & Foreyt, J.P. (1996) Comparison of 2-year weight loss trends in behavioral treatments of obesity: diet, exercise, and combination interventions. *J. Am. Diet. Assoc.*, **96**, 342–346

Slabber, M., Barnard, H.C., Kuyl, J.M., Dannhauser, A. & Schall, R. (1994) Effects of a low-insulin-response, energy-restricted diet on weight loss and plasma insulin concentrations in hyperinsulinemic obese females. *Am. J. Clin. Nutr.*, **60**, 48–53

Slattery, M.L. & Jacobs, D.R. Jr (1995) Assessment of ability to recall physical activity of several years ago. *Ann. Epidemiol.*, **5**, 292–296

Slattery, M.L., Schumacher, M.C., Smith, K.R., West, D.W. & Abd-Elghany, N. (1988) Physical activity, diet, and risk of colon cancer in Utah. *Am. J. Epidemiol.*, **128**, 989–999

Slattery, M.L., Edwards, S.L., Ma, K.N., Friedman, G.D. & Potter, J.D. (1997a) Physical activity and colon cancer: a public health perspective. *Ann. Epidemiol.*, **7**, 137–145

Slattery, M.L., Potter, J., Caan, B., Edwards, S., Coates, A., Ma, K.N. & Berry, T.D. (1997b) Energy balance and colon cancer—beyond physical activity. *Cancer Res.*, **57**, 75–80

Slattery, M.L., Benson, J., Berry, T.D., Duncan, D., Edwards, S.L., Caan, B.J. & Potter, J.D. (1997c) Dietary sugar and colon cancer. *Cancer Epidemiol. Biomarkers Prev.*, **6**, 677–685

Slattery, M.L., Edwards, S.L., Boucher, K.M., Anderson, K. & Caan, B.J. (1999) Lifestyle and colon cancer: an assessment of factors associated with risk. *Am. J. Epidemiol.*, **150**, 869–877

Smith, S.R. & Zachwieja, J.J. (1999) Visceral adipose tissue: a critical review of intervention strategies. *Int. J. Obes. Relat. Metab. Disord.*, **23**, 329-335

Smith, C.P., Archibald, H.R., Thomas, J.M., Tarn, A.C., Williams, A.J., Gale, E.A. & Savage, M.O. (1988) Basal and stimulated insulin levels rise with advancing puberty. *Clin. Endocrinol. (Oxf.)*, **28**, 7–14

Smith, W.J., Underwood, L.E. & Clemmons, D.R. (1995) Effects of caloric or protein restriction on insulin-like growth factor-I (IGF-I) and IGF-binding proteins in children and adults. *J. Clin. Endocrinol. Metab.*, **80**, 443–449

Sobal, J. & Stunkard, A.J. (1989) Socioeconomic status and obesity: a review of the literature. *Psychol. Bull.*, **105**, 260-275

Sohal, R.S., Agarwal, S., Candas, M., Forster, M.J. & Lal, H. (1994a) Effect of age and caloric restriction on DNA oxidative damage in different tissues of C57BL/6 mice. *Mech. Ageing Dev.*, **76**, 215–224

Sohal, R.S., Ku, H.H., Agarwal, S., Forster, M.J. & Lal, H. (1994b) Oxidative damage, mitochondrial oxidant generation and antioxidant defenses during aging and in response to food restriction in the mouse. *Mech. Ageing Dev.*, **74**, 121–133

Sonnenschein, E., Toniolo, P., Terry, M.B., Bruning, P.F., Kato, I., Koenig, K.L. & Shore, R.E. (1999) Body fat distribution and obesity in pre- and postmenopausal breast cancer. *Int. J. Epidemiol.*, **28**, 1026–1031

Sönnichsen, A.C., Lindlacher, U., Richter, W.O. & Schwandt, P. (1990) Obesity, body fat distribution and the incidence of breast, cervical, endometrial and ovarian carcinomas. *Dtsch. Med. Wochenschr.*, **115**, 1906–1910

Sørensen, H.T., Sabroe, S., Gillman, M., Rothman, K.J., Madsen, K.M., Fischer, P. & Sørensen, T.I. (1997) Continued increase in prevalence of obesity in Danish young men. *Int. J. Obes.*, **21**, 712–714

Sorkin, J.D., Muller, D. & Andres, R. (1994) Body mass index and mortality in Seventh-day Adventist men. A critique and re-analysis. *Int. J. Obes. Relat. Metab. Disord.*, **18**, 752-754

Soygür, T., Küpeli, B., Aydos, K., Küpeli, S., Arikan, N. & Müftüoglu, Y.Z. (1996) Effect of obesity on prostatic hyperplasia: its relation to sex steroid levels. *Int. Urol. Nephrol.*, **28**, 55–59

Spady, T.J., McComb, R.D. & Shull, J.D. (1999) Estrogen action in the regulation of cell proliferation, cell survival, and tumorigenesis in the rat anterior pituitary gland. *Endocrine*, **11**, 217–233

Spiegelman, D., Israel, R.G., Bouchard, C. & Willett, W.C. (1992) Absolute fat mass, percent body fat, and body-fat distribution: which is the real determinant of blood pressure and serum glucose? *Am. J. Clin. Nutr.*, **55**, 1033–1044

Srivastava, A. & Kreiger, N. (2000) Relation of physical activity to risk of testicular cancer. *Am. J. Epidemiol.*, **151**, 78–87

Srivastava, V.K., Tilley, R.D., Hart, R.W. & Busbee, D.L. (1991) Effect of dietary restriction on the fidelity of DNA polymerases in aging mice. *Exp. Gerontol.*, **26**, 453–466

Stallone, D.D. (1994) The influence of obesity and its treatment on the immune system. *Nutr. Rev.*, **52**, 37–50

Stallone, D.D., Stunkard, A.J., Zweiman, B., Wadden, T.A. & Foster, G.D. (1994) Decline in delayed-type hypersensitivity response in obese women following weight reduction. *Clin. Diagn. Lab. Immunol.*, **1**, 202–205

Stamler, R., Stamler, J., Riedlinger, W.F., Algera, G. & Roberts, R.H. (1978) Weight and blood pressure. Findings in hypertension screening of 1 million Americans. *JAMA*, **240**, 1607–1610

Stam-Moraga, M.C., Kolanowski, J., Dramaix, M., De Henauw, S., De Bacquer, D., De Backer, G. & Kornitzer, M.D. (1998) Trends in the prevalence of obesity among Belgian men at work, 1977–1992. *Int. J. Obes. Relat. Metab. Disord.*, **22**, 988–992

Stanczyk, F.Z. (1997) Steroid hormones. In: Lobo, R.A., Mishell, D.R., Jr, Paulson, R.J. & Shoupe, D., eds, *Infertility, Contraception, and Reproductive Endocrinology*, Oxford, Blackwell Science, pp. 46–66

Stanik, S. & Marcus, R. (1980) Insulin secretion improves following dietary control of plasma glucose in severely hyperglycemic obese patients. *Metabolism*, **29**, 346–350

Stanik, S., Dornfeld, L.P., Maxwell, M.H., Viosca, S.P. & Korenman, S.G. (1981) The effect of weight loss on reproductive hormones in obese men. *J. Clin. Endocrinol. Metab.*, **53**, 828–832

Stanley, W.C. & Connett, R.J. (1991) Regulation of muscle carbohydrate metabolism during exercise. *FASEB J.*, **5**, 2155–2159

Stattin, P., Bylund, A., Rinaldi, S., Biessy, C., Déchaud, H., Stenman, U.H., Egevad, L., Riboli, E., Hallmans, G. & Kaaks, R. (2000) Plasma insulin-like growth factor-I, insulin-like growth factor-binding proteins, and prostate cancer risk: a prospective study. *J. Natl Cancer Inst.*, **92**, 1910–1917

Stattin, P., Soderberg, S., Hallmans, G., Bylund, A., Kaaks, R., Stenman, U.H., Bergh, A. & Olsson, T. (2001) Leptin is associated with increased prostate cancer risk: a nested case-referent study. *J. Clin. Endocrinol. Metab.*, **86**, 1341–1345

Steenland, K., Nowlin, S. & Palu, S. (1995) Cancer incidence in the National Health and Nutrition Survey I. Follow-up data: diabetes, cholesterol, pulse and physical activity. *Cancer Epidemiol. Biomarkers Prev.*, **4**, 807–811

Steinbach, G., Kumar, S.P., Reddy, B.S., Lipkin, M. & Holt, P.R. (1993) Effects of caloric restriction and dietary fat on epithelial cell proliferation in rat colon. *Cancer Res.*, **53**, 2745–2749

Steindorf, K., Tobiasz-Adamczyk, B., Popiela, T., Jedrychowski, W., Penar, A., Matyja, A. & Wahrendorf, J. (2000) Combined risk assessment of physical activity and dietary habits on the development of colorectal cancer. A hospital-based case-control study in Poland. *Eur. J. Cancer Prev.*, **9**, 309–316

Stene-Larsen, G., Weberg, R., Froyshov-Larsen, I., Bjortuft, O., Hoel, B. & Berstad, A. (1988) Relationship of overweight to hiatus hernia and reflux oesophagitis. *Scand. J. Gastroenterol.*, **23**, 427–432

Stenius-Aarniala, B., Poussa, T., Kvarnstrom, J., Gronlund, E.L., Ylikahri, M. & Mustajoki, P. (2000) Immediate and long term effects of weight reduction in obese people with asthma: randomised controlled study. *BMJ*, **320**, 827–832

Stephens, T. (1988) Physical activity and mental health in the United States and Canada: evidence from four population surveys. *Prev. Med.*, **17**, 35–47

Stephens, T. & Caspersen, C.J. (1994) The demography of physical activity. In: Bouchard, C., Shephard, R.J. & Stephens, T., eds, *Physical Activity, Fitness, and Health: A Consensus of Current Knowledge*, Champaign, Human Kinetics Publishers, pp. 204–213

Sternfeld, B., Cauley, J., Harlow, S., Liu, G. & Lee, M. (2000) Assessment of physical activity with a single global question in a large, multiethnic sample of midlife women. *Am. J. Epidemiol.*, **152**, 678–687

Stessman, J., Maaravi, Y., Hammerman-Rozenberg, R. & Cohen, A. (2000) The effects of physical activity on mortality in the Jerusalem 70-Year-Olds Longitudinal Study. *J. Am. Geriatr. Soc.*, **48**, 499–504

Stevens, J. (2000) Impact of age on associations between weight and mortality. *Nutr. Rev.*, **58**, 129-137

Stevens, J., Keil, J.E., Waid, L.R. & Gazes, P.C. (1990) Accuracy of current, 4-year, and 28-year self-reported body weight in an elderly population. *Am. J. Epidemiol.*, **132**, 1156–1163

Stevens, J., Cai, J., Pamuk, E.R., Williamson, D.F., Thun, M.J. & Wood, J.L. (1998) The effect of age on the association between body-mass index and mortality. *New Engl. J. Med.*, **338**, 1-7

Stevens, V.J., Obarzanek, E., Cook, N.R., Lee, I.M., Appel, L.J., West, D.S., Milas, N.C., Mattfeldt-Beman, M., Belden, L., Bragg, C., Millstone, M., Raczynski, J., Brewer, A., Singh, B. & Cohen, J. (2001) Long-term weight loss and changes in blood pressure: results of the Trials of Hypertension Prevention, Phase II. *Ann. Intern. Med.*, **134**, 1–11

Stevenson, M.R., Hamer, P., Finch, C.F., Elliot, B. & Kresnow, M. (2000) Sport, age, and sex specific incidence of sports injuries in Western Australia. *Br. J. Sports Med.*, **34**, 188–194

Stewart, C.E. & Rotwein, P. (1996) Growth, differentiation, and survival: multiple physiological functions for insulin-like growth factors. *Physiol. Rev.*, **76**, 1005–1026

Stoll, B.A. (1999) Western nutrition and the insulin resistance syndrome: a link to breast cancer. *Eur. J. Clin. Nutr.*, **53**, 83–87

Strain, G.W., Zumoff, B., Kream, J., Strain, J.J., Deucher, R., Rosenfeld, R.S., Levin, J. & Fukushima, D.K. (1982) Mild hypogonadotropic hypogonadism in obese men. *Metabolism*, **31**, 871–875

Strain, G.W., Zumoff, B., Miller, L.K., Rosner, W., Levit, C., Kalin, M., Hershcopf, R.J. & Rosenfeld, R.S. (1988) Effect of massive weight loss on hypothalamic-pituitary-gonadal function in obese men. *J. Clin. Endocrinol. Metab.*, **66**, 1019–1023

Strain, G., Zumoff, B., Rosner, W. & Pi-Sunyer, X. (1994) The relationship between serum levels of insulin and sex hormone-binding globulin in men: the effect of weight loss. *J. Clin. Endocrinol. Metab.*, **79**, 1173–1176

Straus, D.S. (1994) Nutritional regulation of hormones and growth factors that control mammalian growth. *FASEB J.*, **8**, 6–12

Strom, B.L., Soloway, R.D., Rios-Dalenz, J.L., Rodriguez-Martinez, H.A., West, S.L., Kinman, J.L., Polansky, M. & Berlin, J.A. (1995) Risk factors for gallbladder cancer. An international collaborative case-control study. *Cancer*, **76**, 1747–1756

Stuart, G.R., Oda, Y., Boer, J.G. & Glickman, B.W. (2000) No change in spontaneous mutation frequency or specificity in dietary restricted mice. *Carcinogenesis*, **21**, 317–319

Stubbs, R.J., Ritz, P., Coward, W.A. & Prentice, A.M. (1995) Covert manipulation of the ratio of dietary fat to carbohydrate and energy density: effect on food intake and energy balance in free-living men eating ad libitum. *Am. J. Clin. Nutr.*, **62**, 330–337

Stunkard, A.J., Sørensen, T.I., Hanis, C., Teasdale, T.W., Chakraborty, R., Schull, W.J. & Schulsinger, F. (1986) An adoption study of human obesity. *New Engl. J. Med.*, **314**, 193–198

Sturgeon, S.R., Brinton, L.A., Berman, M.L., Mortel, R., Twiggs, L.B., Barrett, R.J. & Wilbanks, G.D. (1993) Past and present physical activity and endometrial cancer risk. *Br. J. Cancer*, **68**, 584–589

Sugden, M.C., Grimshaw, R.M. & Holness, M.J. (1999) Caloric restriction leads to regional specialisation of adipocyte function in the rat. *Biochim. Biophys. Acta*, **1437**, 202–213

Sugie, S., Reddy, B.S., Lowenfels, A., Tanaka, T. & Mori, H. (1992) Effect of voluntary exercise on azoxymethane-induced hepatocarcinogenesis in male F344 rats. *Cancer Lett.*, **63**, 67–72

Sugie, S., Tanaka, T., Mori, H. & Reddy, B.S. (1993) Effect of restricted caloric intake on the development of the azoxymethane-induced glutathione S-transferase placental form positive hepatocellular foci in male F344 rats. *Cancer Lett.*, **68**, 67–73

Suikkari, A.M., Koivisto, V.A., Rutanen, E.M., Yki-Järvinen, H., Karonen, S.L. & Seppälä, M. (1988) Insulin regulates the serum levels of low molecular weight insulin-like growth factor-binding protein. *J. Clin. Endocrinol. Metab.*, **66**, 266–272

Sung, J.F., Lin, R.S., Pu, Y.S., Chen, Y.C., Chang, H.C. & Lai, M.K. (1999) Risk factors for prostate carcinoma in Taiwan: a case-control study in a Chinese population. *Cancer*, **86**, 484–491

Suominen, H. (1993) Bone mineral density and long term exercise. An overview of cross-sectional athlete studies. *Sports Med.*, **16**, 316–330

Svendsen, O.L., Hassager, C. & Christiansen, C. (1995) The response to treatment of overweight in postmenopausal women is not related to fat distribution. *Int. J. Obes. Relat. Metab. Disord.*, **19**, 496–502

Swanson, C.A., Brinton, L.A., Taylor, P.R., Licitra, L.M., Ziegler, R.G. & Schairer, C. (1989) Body size and breast cancer risk assessed in women participating in the Breast Cancer Detection Demonstration Project. *Am. J. Epidemiol.*, **130**, 1133–1141

Swanson, C.A., Potischman, N., Wilbanks, G.D., Twiggs, L.B., Mortel, R., Berman, M.L., Barrett, R.J., Baumgartner, R.N. & Brinton, L.A. (1993) Relation of endometrial cancer risk to past and contemporary body size and body fat distribution. *Cancer Epidemiol. Biomarkers Prev.*, **2**, 321–327

Swanson, C.A., Coates, R.J., Schoenberg, J.B., Malone, K.E., Gammon, M.D., Stanford, J.L., Shorr, I.J., Potischman, N.A. & Brinton, L.A. (1996) Body size and breast cancer risk among women under age 45 years. *Am. J. Epidemiol.*, **143**, 698–706

Swerdlow, A.J., Huttly, S.R. & Smith, P.G. (1989) Testis cancer: post-natal hormonal factors, sexual behaviour and fertility. *Int. J. Cancer*, **43**, 549–553

Swinburn, B.A., Ley, S.J., Carmichael, H.E. & Plank, L.D. (1999) Body size and composition in Polynesians. *Int. J. Obes. Relat. Metab. Disord.*, **23**, 1178–1183

Sylvester, P.W., Aylsworth, C.F. & Meites, J. (1981) Relationship of hormones to inhibition of mammary tumor development by underfeeding during the "critical period" after carcinogen administration. *Cancer Res.*, **41**, 1384–1388

Sylvester, P.W., Aylsworth, C.F., Van Vugt, D.A. & Meites, J. (1982) Influence of underfeeding during the "critical period" or thereafter on carcinogen-induced mammary tumors in rats. *Cancer Res.*, **42**, 4943–4947

Syngal, S., Coakley, E.H., Willett, W.C., Byers, T., Williamson, D.F. & Colditz, G.A. (1999) Long-term weight patterns and risk for cholecystectomy in women. *Ann. Intern. Med.*, **130**, 471–477

Tagliaferro, A.R., Ronan, A.M., Meeker, L.D., Thompson, H.J., Scott, A.L. & Sinha, D. (1996) Cyclic food restriction alters substrate utilization and abolishes protection from mammary carcinogenesis female rats. *J. Nutr.*, **126**, 1398–1405

Taguchi, T., Kishikawa, H., Motoshima, H., Sakai, K., Nishiyama, T., Yoshizato, K., Shirakami, A., Toyonaga, T., Shirontani, T., Araki, E. & Shichiri, M. (2000) Involvement of bradykinin in acute exercise-induced increase of glucose uptake and GLUT-4 translocation in skeletal muscle: studies in normal and diabetic humans and rats. *Metabolism*, **49**, 920–930

Taioli, E., Barone, J. & Wynder, E.L. (1995) A case-control study on breast cancer and body mass. The American Health Foundation—Division of Epidemiology. *Eur. J. Cancer*, **31A**, 723–728

Talamini, R., La Vecchia, C., Decarli, A., Negri, E. & Franceschi, S. (1986) Nutrition, social factors and prostatic cancer in a Northern Italian population. *Br. J. Cancer*, **53**, 817–821

Talamini, R., Baron, A.E., Barra, S., Bidoli, E., La Vecchia, C., Negri, E., Serraino, D. & Franceschi, S. (1990) A case-control study of risk factors for renal cell cancer in northern Italy. *Cancer Causes Control*, **1**, 125–131

Tanaka, T., Maesaka, H. & Suwa, S. (1985) Changes in somatomedin activity in anorexia nervosa. *Endocrinol. Jpn*, **32**, 891–897

Tanaka, K., Inoue, S., Numata, K., Okazaki, H., Nakamura, S. & Takamura, Y. (1990) Very-low-calorie diet-induced weight reduction reverses impaired growth hormone secretion response to growth hormone-releasing hormone, arginine, and L-dopa in obesity. *Metabolism*, **39**, 892–896

Tanaka, S., Inoue, S., Isoda, F., Waseda, M., Ishihara, M., Yamakawa, T., Sugiyama, A., Takamura, Y. & Okuda, K. (1993) Impaired immunity in obesity: suppressed but reversible lymphocyte responsiveness. *Int. J. Obes. Relat. Metab. Disord.*, **17**, 631–636

Tang, R., Wang, J.Y., Lo, S.K. & Hsieh, L.L. (1999) Physical activity, water intake and risk of colorectal cancer in Taiwan: a hospital-based case-control study. *Int. J. Cancer*, **82**, 484–489

Tannenbaum, A. (1945) The dependence of tumor formation on the degree of caloric restriction. *Cancer Res.*, **5**, 609–615

Tannenbaum, A. & Silverstone, H. (1953) Nutrition in relation to cancer. *Adv. Cancer Res.*, **1**, 451–501

Tannenbaum, G.S., Guyda, H.J. & Posner, B.I. (1983) Insulin-like growth factors: a role in growth hormone negative feedback and body weight regulation via brain. *Science*, **220**, 77–79

Tao, S.C., Yu, M.C., Ross, R.K. & Xiu, K.W. (1988) Risk factors for breast cancer in Chinese women of Beijing. *Int. J. Cancer*, **42**, 495–498

Tavani, A., Braga, C., La Vecchia, C., Conti, E., Filiberti, R., Montella, M., Amadori, D., Russo, A. & Franceschi, S. (1999) Physical activity and risk of cancers of the colon and rectum: an Italian case-control study. *Br. J. Cancer*, **79**, 1912–1916

Tavani, A., Gallus, S., La Vecchia, C., Dal Maso, L., Negri, E., Pelucchi, C., Montella, M., Conti, E., Carbone, A. & Franceschi, S. (2001) Physical activity and risk of ovarian cancer: An Italian case-control study. *Int. J. Cancer*, **91**, 407–411

Taylor, H.L., Jacobs, D.R., Jr, Schucker, B., Knudsen, J., Leon, A.S. & Debacker, G. (1978) A questionnaire for the assessment of leisure time physical activities. *J. Chronic Dis.*, **31**, 741–755

Taylor, C.B., Coffey, T., Berra, K., Iaffaldano, R., Casey, K. & Haskell, W.L. (1984) Seven-day activity and self-report compared to a direct measure of physical activity. *Am. J. Epidemiol.*, **120**, 818–824

Taylor, C.B., Fortmann, S.P., Flora, J., Kayman, S., Barrett, D.C., Jatulis, D. & Farquhar, J.W. (1991) Effect of long-term community health education on body mass index. The Stanford Five-City Project. *Am. J. Epidemiol.*, **134**, 235–249

Taylor, C.B., Jatulis, D.E., Winkleby, M.A., Rockhill, B.J. & Kraemer, H.C. (1994) Effects of life-style on body mass index change. *Epidemiology*, **5**, 599–603

Taylor, A., Lipman, R.D., Jahngen-Hodge, J., Palmer, V., Smith, D., Padhye, N., Dallal, G.E., Cyr, D.E., Laxman, E., Shepard, D., Morrow, F., Salomon, R., Perrone, G., Asmundsson, G., Meydani, M., Blumberg, J., Mune, M., Harrison, D., Archer, J. & Shigenaga, M.K. (1995) Dietary calorie restriction in the Emory mouse: effects on lifespan, eye lens cataract prevalence and progression, levels of ascorbate, glutathione, glucose, and glycohemoglobin, tail collagen breaktime, DNA and RNA oxidation, skin integrity, fecundity, and cancer. *Mech. Ageing Dev.*, **79**, 33–57

Taylor, W.C., Baranowski, T. & Young, D.R. (1998) Physical activity interventions in low-income, ethnic minority, and populations with disability. *Am. J. Prev. Med.*, **15**, 334–343

Tchernof, A., Després, J.P., Bélanger, A., Dupont, A., Prud'homme, D., Moorjani, S., Lupien, P.J. & Labrie, F. (1995) Reduced testosterone and adrenal C_{19} steroid levels in obese men. *Metabolism*, **44**, 513–519

Tegelman, R., Johansson, C., Hemmingsson, P., Eklöf, R., Carlström, K. & Pousette, A. (1990) Endogenous anabolic and catabolic steroid hormones in male and female athletes during off season. *Int. J. Sports Med.*, **11**, 103–106

Telama, R. & Yang, X. (2000) Decline of physical activity from youth to young adulthood in Finland. *Med. Sci. Sports Exerc.*, **32**, 1617–1622

Terry, P., Baron, J.A., Weiderpass, E., Yuen, J., Lichtenstein, P. & Nyrén, O. (1999) Lifestyle and endometrial cancer risk: a cohort study from the Swedish Twin Registry. *Int. J. Cancer*, **82**, 38–42

Thissen, J.P., Ketelslegers, J.M. & Underwood, L.E. (1994) Nutritional regulation of the insulin-like growth factors. *Endocr. Rev.*, **15**, 80–101

Thomas, J., Bertrand, H., Stacy, C. & Herlihy, J.T. (1993) Long-term caloric restriction improves baroreflex sensitivity in aging Fischer 344 rats. *J. Gerontol.*, **48**, B151–B155

Thomas, H.V., Reeves, G.K. & Key, T.J. (1997) Endogenous estrogen and postmenopausal breast cancer: a quantitative review. *Cancer Causes Control*, **8**, 922–928

Thompson, H.J. (1997) Effects of physical activity and exercise on experimentally-induced mammary carcinogenesis. *Breast Cancer Res. Treat.*, **46**, 135–141

Thompson, H.J., Ronan, A.M., Ritacco, K.A., Tagliaferro, A.R. & Meeker, L.D. (1988) Effect of exercise on the induction of mammary carcinogenesis. *Cancer Res.*, **48**, 2720-2723

Thompson, M.M., Garland, C., Barrett-Connor, E., Khaw, K.T., Friedlander, N.J. & Wingard, D.L. (1989a) Heart disease risk factors, diabetes, and prostatic cancer in an adult community. *Am. J. Epidemiol.*, **129**, 511–517

Thompson, H.J., Ronan, A.M., Ritacco, K.A. & Tagliaferro, A.R. (1989b) Effect of type and amount of dietary fat on the enhancement of rat mammary tumorigenesis by exercise. *Cancer Res.*, **49**, 1904–1908

Thompson, H.J., Strange, R. & Schedin, P.J. (1992) Apoptosis in the genesis and prevention of cancer. *Cancer Epidemiol. Biomarkers Prev.*, **1**, 597–602

Thompson, H.J., Westerlind, K.C., Snedden, J., Briggs, S. & Singh, M. (1995) Exercise intensity dependent inhibition of 1-methyl-1-nitrosourea induced mammary carcinogenesis in female F-344 rats. *Carcinogenesis*, **16**, 1783–1786

Thomsen, B.L., Ekstrom, C.T. & Sørensen, T.I. (1999) Development of the obesity epidemic in Denmark: cohort, time and age effects among boys born 1930–1975. *Int. J. Obes. Relat. Metab. Disord.*, **23**, 693–701

Thun, M.J., Calle, E.E., Namboodiri, M.M., Flanders, W.D., Coates, R.J., Byers, T., Boffetta, P., Garfinkel, L. & Heath, C.W., Jr (1992) Risk factors for fatal colon cancer in a large prospective study. *J. Natl Cancer Inst.*, **84**, 1491–1500

Thune, I. & Lund, E. (1994) Physical activity and the risk of prostate and testicular cancer: a cohort study of 53,000 Norwegian men. *Cancer Causes Control*, **5**, 549–556

Thune, I. & Lund, E. (1996) Physical activity and risk of colorectal cancer in men and women. *Br. J. Cancer*, **73**, 1134–1140

Thune, I. & Lund, E. (1997) The influence of physical activity on lung-cancer risk: A prospective study of 81,516 men and women. *Int. J. Cancer*, **70**, 57–62

Thune, I., Olsen, A., Albrektsen, G. & Tretli, S. (1993) Cutaneous malignant melanoma: association with height, weight and body-surface area. A prospective study in Norway. *Int. J. Cancer*, **55**, 555–561

Thune, I., Brenn, T., Lund, E. & Gaard, M. (1997) Physical activity and the risk of breast cancer. *New Engl. J. Med.*, **336**, 1269–1275

Thune, I., Njølstad, I., Løchen, M.L. & Førde, O.H. (1998) Physical activity improves the metabolic risk profiles in men and women: the Tromsø Study. *Arch. Intern. Med.*, **158**, 1633–1640

Thurman, J.D., Bucci, T.J., Hart, R.W. & Turturro, A. (1994) Survival, body weight, and spontaneous neoplasms in *ad libitum*-fed and food-restricted Fischer-344 rats. *Toxicol. Pathol.*, **22**, 1–9

Tibblin, G., Eriksson, M., Cnattingius, S. & Ekbom, A. (1995) High birthweight as a predictor of prostate cancer risk. *Epidemiology*, **6**, 423–424

Tibblin, G., Adlerberth, A., Lindstedt, G. & Björntorp, P. (1996) The pituitary-gonadal axis and health in elderly men: a study of men born in 1913. *Diabetes*, **45**, 1605–1609

Tikkanen, H.O., Hämäläinen, E., Sarna, S., Adlercreutz, H. & Härkönen, M. (1998) Associations between skeletal muscle properties, physical fitness, physical activity and coronary heart disease risk factors in men. *Atherosclerosis*, **137**, 377–389

Tischler, A.S., Sheldon, W. & Gray, R. (1996) Immunohistochemical and morphological characterization of spontaneously occurring pheochromocytomas in the aging mouse. *Vet. Pathol.*, **33**, 512–520

Tomatis, L., ed. (1990) *Cancer: Causes, Occurrence and Control* (IARC Scientific Publications No. 100), Lyon, International Agency for Research on Cancer, pp. 97–107

Toniolo, P., Bruning, P.F., Akhmedkhanov, A., Bonfrer, J.M., Koenig, K.L., Lukanova, A., Shore, R.E. & Zeleniuch-Jacquotte, A. (2000) Serum insulin-like growth factor-I and breast cancer. *Int. J. Cancer*, **88**, 828–832

Toode, K., Viru, A. & Eller, A. (1993) Lipolytic actions of hormones on adipocytes in exercise-trained organisms. *Jpn J. Physiol.*, **43**, 253–258

Torjesen, P.A., Birkeland, K.I., Anderssen, S.A., Hjermann, I., Holme, I. & Urdal, P. (1997) Lifestyle changes may reverse development of the insulin resistance syndrome. The Oslo Diet and Exercise Study: a randomized trial. *Diabetes Care*, **20**, 26–31

Törnberg, S.A. & Carstensen, J.M. (1994) Relationship between Quetelet's index and cancer of breast and female genital tract in 47,000 women followed for 25 years. *Br. J. Cancer*, **69**, 358–361

Tran, Z.V. & Weltman, A. (1985) Differential effects of exercise on serum lipid and lipoprotein levels seen with changes in body weight. A meta-analysis. *JAMA*, **254**, 919–924

Travers, S.H., Jeffers, B.W., Bloch, C.A., Hill, J.O. & Eckel, R.H. (1995) Gender and Tanner stage differences in body composition and insulin sensitivity in early pubertal children. *J. Clin. Endocrinol. Metab.*, **80**, 172–178

Trentham-Dietz, A., Newcomb, P.A., Storer, B.E., Longnecker, M.P., Baron, J., Greenberg, E.R. & Willett, W.C. (1997) Body size and risk of breast cancer. *Am. J. Epidemiol.*, **145**, 1011–1019

Trentham-Dietz, A., Newcomb, P.A., Egan, K.M., Titus-Ernstoff, L., Baron, J.A., Storer, B.E., Stampfer, M. & Willett, W.C. (2000) Weight change and risk of postmenopausal breast cancer (United States). *Cancer Causes Control*, **11**, 533–542

Tretli, S. (1989) Height and weight in relation to breast cancer morbidity and mortality. A prospective study of 570,000 women in Norway. *Int. J. Cancer*, **44**, 23–30

Tretli, S. & Magnus, K. (1990) Height and weight in relation to uterine corpus cancer morbidity and mortality. A follow-up study of 570,000 women in Norway. *Int. J. Cancer*, **46**, 165–172

Tretli, S. & Robsahm, T.E. (1999) Height, weight and cancer of the oesophagus and stomach: a follow-up study in Norway. *Eur. J. Cancer Prev.*, **8**, 115–122

Tretli, S., Haldorsen, T. & Ottestad, L. (1990) The effect of pre-morbid height and weight on the survival of breast cancer patients. *Br. J. Cancer*, **62**, 299–303

Troisi, R., Potischman, N., Hoover, R.N., Siiteri, P. & Brinton, L.A. (1997) Insulin and endometrial cancer. *Am. J. Epidemiol.*, **146**, 476–482

Troy, L.M., Hunter, D.J., Manson, J.E., Colditz, G.A., Stampfer, M.J. & Willett, W.C. (1995) The validity of recalled weight among younger women. *Int. J. Obes. Relat. Metab. Disord.*, **19**, 570–572

Tudor-Smith, C., Nutbeam, D., Moore, L. & Catford, J. (1998) Effects of the Heartbeat Wales programme over five years on behavioural risks for cardiovascular disease: quasi-experimental comparison of results from Wales and a matched reference area. *BMJ*, **316**, 818–822

Tung, H.T., Tsukuma, H., Tanaka, H., Kinoshita, N., Koyama, Y., Ajiki, W., Oshima, A. & Koyama, H. (1999) Risk factors for breast cancer in Japan, with special attention to anthropometric measurements and reproductive history. *Jpn J. Clin. Oncol.*, **29**, 137–146

Tuomilehto, J., Lindstrom, J., Eriksson, J.G., Valle, T.T., Hamalainen, H., Ilanne-Parikka, P., Keinanen-Kiukaanniemi, S., Laakso, M., Louheranta, A., Rastas, M., Salminen, V., Uusitupa, M.; Finnish Diabetes Prevention Study Group (2001) Prevention of type 2 diabetes mellitus by changes in lifestyle among subjects with impaired glucose tolerance. *New Engl. J. Med.*, **344**, 1343–1350

Turcato, E., Zamboni, M., De Pergola, G., Armellini, F., Zivelonghi, A., Bergamo-Andreis, I.A., Giorgino, R. & Bosello, O. (1997) Interrelationships between weight loss, body fat distribution and sex hormones in pre- and postmenopausal obese women. *J. Intern. Med.*, **241**, 363–372

Turturro, A., Duffy, P.H. & Hart, R.W. (1993) Modulation of toxicity by diet and dietary macronutrient restriction. *Mutat. Res.*, **295**, 151–164

Turturro, A., Duffy, P. & Hart, R. (1995) The effect of caloric modulation on toxicity studies. In: Hart, R., Neuman, D. & Robertson, R., eds, *Dietary Restriction: Implications for the Design and Interpretation of Toxicity and Carcinogenicity Studies*, Washington, DC, ILSI Press, pp. 79–98

Turturro, A., Duffy, P., Hart, R. & Allaben, W.T. (1996) Rationale for the use of dietary control in toxicity studies – B6C3F1 mouse. *Toxicol. Pathol.*, **24**, 769–775

Turturro, A., Hass, B.S., Hart, R. & Allaben, W.T. (1998) Body weight impact on spontaneous and agent-induced diseases in chronic bioassays. *Int. J. Toxicol.*, **17**, 79–100

Turturro, A., Witt, W.W., Lewis, S., Hass, B.S., Lipman, R.D. & Hart, R.W. (1999) Growth curves and survival characteristics of the animals used in the Biomarkers of Aging Program. *J. Gerontol. A Biol. Sci. Med. Sci.*, **54**, B492–B501

Turturro, A., Hass, B.S. & Hart, R.W. (2000) Does caloric restriction induce hormesis? *Hum. Exp. Toxicol.*, **19**, 320–329

Tutton, P.J. & Barkla, D.H. (1980) Influence of prostaglandin analogues on epithelial cell proliferation and xenograft growth. *Br. J. Cancer*, **41**, 47–51

Tvede, N., Kappel, M., Halkjaer-Kristensen, J., Galbo, H. & Pedersen, B.K. (1993) The effect of light, moderate and severe bicycle exercise on lymphocyte subsets, natural and lymphokine activated killer cells, lymphocyte proliferative response and interleukin 2 production. *Int. J. Sports Med.*, **14**, 275–282

Tymchuk, C.N., Tessler, S.B., Aronson, W.J. & Barnard, R.J. (1998) Effects of diet and exercise on insulin, sex hormone-binding globulin, and prostate-specific antigen. *Nutr. Cancer*, **31**, 127–131

Ueji, M., Ueno, E., Osei-Hyiaman, D., Takahashi, H. & Kano, K. (1998) Physical activity and the risk of breast cancer: a case-control study of Japanese women. *J. Epidemiol.*, **8**, 116–122

Uitenbroek, D.G. (1993) Seasonal variation in leisure time physical activity. *Med. Sci. Sports Exerc.*, **25**, 755–760

Uitenbroek, D.G. (1996) Sports, exercise, and other causes of injuries: results of a population survey. *Res. Q. Exerc. Sport*, **67**, 380–385

UK Testicular Cancer Study Group (1994a) Social, behavioural and medical factors in the aetiology of testicular cancer: results from the UK study. *Br. J. Cancer*, **70**, 513–520

UK Testicular Cancer Study Group (1994b) Aetiology of testicular cancer: association with congenital abnormalities, age at puberty, infertility, and exercise. *BMJ*, **308**, 1393–1399

UKPDS Group (1990) UK Prospective Diabetes Study 7: response of fasting plasma glucose to diet therapy in newly presenting type II diabetic patients. *Metabolism*, **39**, 905–912

Unger, R. & Foster, D.W. (1998) Diabetes mellitus. In: Wilson, J.D. & Foster, D.W., eds, *Williams Textbook of Endocrinology*, Philadelphia, W.B. Saunders, pp. 1255–1333

Unterman, T.G. (1993) Insulin-like growth factor binding protein-1: identification, purification, and regulation in fetal and adult life. *Adv. Exp. Med. Biol.*, **343**, 215–226

Ursin, G., London, S., Stanczyk, F.Z., Gentzschein, E., Paganini-Hill, A., Ross, R.K. & Pike, M.C. (1999) Urinary 2-hydroxyestrone/16α-hydroxyestrone ratio and risk of breast cancer in postmenopausal women. *J. Natl Cancer Inst.*, **91**, 1067–1072

US Department of Health and Human Services (1996) *Physical Activity and Health: a Report of the Surgeon General*, Atlanta, Centers for Disease Control and Prevention. National Center for Chronic Disease Prevention and Health Promotion

US Department of Labor (1993) *Selected Characteristics of Occupations Defined in the Revised Dictionary of Occupational Titles*, Washington, US Government Printing Office

Utell, M.J. & Looney, R.J. (1995) Environmentally induced asthma. *Toxicol. Lett.*, **82–83**, 47–53

Vague, J. (1956) The degree of masculine differentiation of obesities: a factor determining predisposition to diabetes, atherosclerosis, gout and uric calculous disease. *Am. J. Clin. Nutr.*, **4**, 20–34

van Baak, M.A. & Borghouts, L.B. (2000) Relationships with physical activity. *Nutr. Rev.*, **58**, S16–S18

van Dale, D., Saris, W.H. & ten Hoor, F. (1990) Weight maintenance and resting metabolic rate 18–40 months after a diet/-exercise treatment. *Int. J. Obes.*, **14**, 347–359

van den Brandt, P.A., Spiegelman, D., Yaun, S.S., Adami, H.O., Beeson, L., Folsom, A.R., Fraser, G., Goldbohm, R.A., Graham, S., Kushi, L., Marshall, J.R., Miller, A.B., Rohan, T., Smith-Warner, S.A., Speizer, F.E., Willett, W.C., Wolk, A. & Hunter, D.J. (2000) Pooled analysis of prospective cohort studies on height, weight, and breast cancer risk. *Am. J. Epidemiol.*, **152**, 514–527

Van Gaal, L.F., Wauters, M.A., Peiffer, F.W. & De Leeuw, I.H. (1998) Sibutramine and fat distribution: is there a role for pharmacotherapy in abdominal/visceral fat reduction? *Int. J. Obes. Relat. Metab. Disord.*, **22 Suppl. 1**, S38–S40

Van Itallie, T.B. (1985) Health implications of overweight and obesity in the United States. *Ann. Intern. Med.*, **103**, 983-988

van Leeuwen, F.E. & Rookus, M.A. (1989) The role of exogenous hormones in the epidemiology of breast, ovarian and endometrial cancer. *Eur. J. Cancer Clin. Oncol.*, **25**, 1961–1972

van Mechelen, W. (1992) Running injuries. A review of the epidemiological literature. *Sports Med.*, **14**, 320–335

van Mechelen, W., Twisk, J.W., Post, G.B., Snel, J. & Kemper, H.C. (2000) Physical activity of young people: the Amsterdam Longitudinal Growth and Health Study. *Med. Sci. Sports Exerc.*, **32**, 1610–1616

Vatten, L.J. & Kvinnsland, S. (1992) Prospective study of height, body mass index and risk of breast cancer. *Acta Oncol.*, **31**, 195–200

Vatten, L.J., Foss, O.P. & Kvinnsland, S. (1991) Overall survival of breast cancer patients in relation to preclinically determined total serum cholesterol, body mass index, height and cigarette smoking: a population-based study. *Eur. J. Cancer*, **27**, 641–646

Vaughan, T.L., Davis, S., Kristal, A. & Thomas, D.B. (1995) Obesity, alcohol, and tobacco as risk factors for cancers of the esophagus and gastric cardia: adenocarcinoma versus squamous cell carcinoma. *Cancer Epidemiol. Biomarkers Prev.*, **4**, 85–92

Vaz de Almeida, M.D., Graca, P., Afonso, C., D'Amicis, A., Lappalainen, R. & Damkjaer, S. (1999) Physical activity levels and body weight in a nationally representative sample in the European Union. *Public Health Nutr.*, **2**, 105–113

Veierod, M.B., Laake, P. & Thelle, D.S. (1997) Dietary fat intake and risk of prostate cancer: a prospective study of 25,708 Norwegian men. *Int. J. Cancer*, **73**, 634–638

Veldhuis, J.D., Iranmanesh, A., Ho, K.K., Waters, M.J., Johnson, M.L. & Lizarralde, G. (1991) Dual defects in pulsatile growth hormone secretion and clearance subserve the hyposomatotropism of obesity in man. *J. Clin. Endocrinol. Metab.*, **72**, 51–59

Veldhuis, J.D., Urban, R.J., Lizarralde, G., Johnson, M.L. & Iranmanesh, A. (1992) Attenuation of luteinizing hormone secretory burst amplitude as a proximate basis for the hypoandrogenism of healthy aging in men. *J. Clin. Endocrinol. Metab.*, **75**, 707–713

Veldhuis, J.D., Iranmanesh, A., Evans, W.S., Lizarralde, G., Thorner, M.O. & Vance, M.L. (1993) Amplitude suppression of the pulsatile mode of immunoradiometric luteinizing hormone release in fasting-induced hypoandrogenemia in normal men. *J. Clin. Endocrinol. Metab.*, **76**, 587–593

Veldhuis, J.D., Liem, A.Y., South, S., Weltman, A., Weltman, J., Clemmons, D.A., Abbott, R., Mulligan, T., Johnson, M.L., Pincus, S., Straume, M. & Iranmanesh, A. (1995) Differential impact of age, sex steroid hormones, and obesity on basal *versus* pulsatile growth hormone secretion in men as assessed in an ultrasensitive chemiluminescence assay. *J. Clin. Endocrinol. Metab.*, **80**, 3209–3222

Vena, J.E., Graham, S., Zielezny, M., Brasure, J. & Swanson, M.K. (1987) Occupational exercise and risk of cancer. *Am. J. Clin. Nutr.*, **45**, 318–327

Verloop, J., Rookus, M.A., van der Kooy, K. & van Leeuwen, F.E. (2000) Physical activity and breast cancer risk in women aged 20-54 years. *J. Natl Cancer Inst.*, **92**, 128–135

Vermeulen, A. (1996) Decreased androgen levels and obesity in men. *Ann. Med.*, **28**, 13–15

Vermeulen, A., Kaufman, J.M., Deslypere, J.P. & Thomas, G. (1993) Attenuated luteinizing hormone (LH) pulse amplitude but normal LH pulse frequency, and its relation to plasma androgens in hypogonadism of obese men. *J. Clin. Endocrinol. Metab.*, **76**, 1140–1146

Vermeulen, A., Kaufman, J.M. & Giagulli, V.A. (1996) Influence of some biological indexes on sex hormone-binding globulin and androgen levels in aging or obese males. *J. Clin. Endocrinol. Metab.*, **81**, 1821–1826

Verreault, R., Brisson, J., Deschênes, L. & Naud, F. (1989) Body weight and prognostic indicators in breast cancer. Modifying effect of estrogen receptors. *Am. J. Epidemiol.*, **129**, 260–268

Vihko, V.J., Apter, D.L., Pukkala, E.I., Oinonen, M.T., Hakulinen, T.R. & Vihko, R.K. (1992) Risk of breast cancer among female teachers of physical education and languages. *Acta Oncol.*, **31**, 201–204

Villeneuve, P.J., Johnson, K.C., Kreiger, N. & Mao, Y. (1999) Risk factors for prostate cancer: results from the Canadian National Enhanced Cancer Surveillance System. The Canadian Cancer Registries Epidemiology Research Group. *Cancer Causes Control*, **10**, 355–367

Vitiello, M.V., Wilkinson, C.W., Merriam, G.R., Moe, K.E., Prinz, P.N., Ralph, D.D., Colasurdo, E.A. & Schwartz, R.S. (1997) Successful 6-month endurance training does not alter insulin-like growth factor-I in healthy older men and women. *J. Gerontol. A Biol. Sci. Med. Sci.*, **52**, M149–M154

Vogelstein, B., Fearon, E.R., Hamilton, S.R., Kern, S.E., Preisinger, A.C., Leppert, M., Nakamura, Y., White, R., Smits, A.M. & Bos, J.L. (1988) Genetic alterations during colorectal-tumor development. *New Engl. J. Med.*, **319**, 525–532

Volk, M.J., Pugh, T.D., Kim, M., Frith, C.H., Daynes, R.A., Ershler, W.B. & Weindruch, R. (1994) Dietary restriction from middle age attenuates age-associated lymphoma development and interleukin 6 dysregulation in C57BL/6 mice. *Cancer Res.*, **54**, 3054–3061

Vuori, I.M. (2001) Dose-response of physical activity and low back pain, osteoarthritis, and osteoporosis. *Med. Sci. Sports Exerc.*, **33**, S551–S586

Waaler, H.T. (1984) Height, weight and mortality; the Norwegian experience. *Acta Med. Scand.*, Suppl., **679**,1–56

Waaler, H.T. (1988) Hazard of obesity—the Norwegian experience. *Acta Med. Scand.*, Suppl., **723**, 17–21

Wabitsch, M., Hauner, H., Heinze, E., Böckmann, A., Benz, R., Mayer, H. & Teller, W. (1995) Body fat distribution and steroid hormone concentrations in obese adolescent girls before and after weight reduction. *J. Clin. Endocrinol. Metab.*, **80**, 3469–3475

Wabitsch, M., Blum, W.F., Muche, R., Heinze, E., Haug, C., Mayer, H. & Teller, W. (1996) Insulin-like growth factors and their binding proteins before and after weight loss and their associations with hormonal and metabolic parameters in obese adolescent girls. *Int. J. Obes. Relat. Metab. Disord.*, **20**, 1073–1080

Wadden, T.A. & Stunkard, A.J. (1993) Psychosocial consequences of obesity and dieting. In: Stunkard, A.J. & Wadden, T.A., eds, *Obesity: Theory and Therapy,* New York, Raven Press, pp. 163-178

Wadden, T.A., Vogt, R.A., Foster, G.D. & Anderson, D.A. (1998) Exercise and the maintenance of weight loss: 1-year follow-up of a controlled clinical trial. *J. Consult. Clin. Psychol.*, **66**, 429–433

Wajchenberg, B.L., Giannella-Neto, D., Lerario, A.C., Marcondes, J.A. & Ohnuma, L.Y. (1988) Role of obesity and hyperinsulinemia in the insulin resistance of obese subjects with the clinical triad of polycystic ovaries, hirsutism and acanthosis nigricans. *Horm. Res.*, **29**, 7–13

Waldstreicher, J., Santoro, N.F., Hall, J.E., Filicori, M. & Crowley, W.F., Jr (1988) Hyperfunction of the hypothalamic-pituitary axis in women with polycystic ovarian disease: indirect evidence for partial gonadotroph desensitization. *J. Clin. Endocrinol. Metab.*, **66**, 165–172

Walker, K.Z., Piers, L.S., Putt, R.S., Jones, J.A. & O'Dea, K. (1999) Effects of regular walking on cardiovascular risk factors and body composition in normoglycemic women and women with type 2 diabetes. *Diabetes Care*, **22**, 555–561

Wallace, J.D., Cuneo, R.C., Baxter, R., Orskov, H., Keay, N., Pentecost, C., Dall, R., Rosen, T., Jorgensen, J.O., Cittadini, A., Longobardi, S., Sacca, L., Christiansen, J.S., Bengtsson, B.A. & Sonksen, P.H. (1999) Responses of the growth hormone (GH) and insulin-like growth factor axis to exercise, GH administration, and GH withdrawal in trained adult males: a potential test for GH abuse in sport. *J. Clin. Endocrinol. Metab.*, **84**, 3591–3601

Waller, B.F. & Roberts, W.C. (1980) Sudden death while running in conditioned runners aged 40 years or over. *Am. J. Cardiol.*, **45**, 1292–1300

Wang, H.S. & Chard, T. (1999) IGFs and IGF-binding proteins in the regulation of human ovarian and endometrial function. *J. Endocrinol.*, **161**, 1–13

Wang, J.T., Ho, L.T., Tang, K.T., Wang, L.M., Chen, Y.D. & Reaven, G.M. (1989) Effect of habitual physical activity on age-related glucose intolerance. *J. Am. Geriatr. Soc.*, **37**, 203–209

Wang, Q.S., Ross, R.K., Yu, M.C., Ning, J.P., Henderson, B.E. & Kimm, H.T. (1992) A case-control study of breast cancer in Tianjin, China. *Cancer Epidemiol. Biomarkers Prev.*, **1**, 435–439

Wang, J.S., Jen, C.J., Kung, H.C., Lin, L.J., Hsiue, T.R. & Chen, H.I. (1994) Different effects of strenuous exercise and moderate exercise on platelet function in men. *Circulation*, **90**, 2877–2885

Wannamethee, G. & Shaper, A.G. (1989) Body weight and mortality in middle aged British men: impact of smoking. *BMJ*, **299**, 1497–1502

Wannamethee, G. & Shaper, A.G. (1990) Weight change in middle-aged British men: implications for health. *Eur. J. Clin Nutr.*, **44**, 133-142

Wannamethee, S.G., Shaper, A.G., Whincup, P.H. & Walker, M. (2000) Characteristics of older men who lose weight intentionally or unintentionally. *Am. J. Epidemiol.*, **151**, 667–675

Wareham, N.J. & Rennie, K.L. (1998) The assessment of physical activity in individuals and populations: why try to be more precise about how physical activity is assessed? *Int. J. Obes. Relat. Metab. Disord.*, **22 Suppl. 2**, S30–S38

Warren, M. (1990) Metabolic factors and the onset of puberty. In: Grumbach, M., Sizonenko, P.C. & Aubert, M.L., eds, *Control of the Onset of Puberty,* Baltimore, Williams & Wilkins, pp. 553–573

Washburn, R.A., Smith, K.W., Goldfield, S.R. & McKinlay, J.B. (1991) Reliability and physiologic correlates of the Harvard Alumni Activity Survey in a general population. *J. Clin. Epidemiol.*, **44**, 1319–1326

Watson, R.R., Moriguchi, S., Jackson, J.C., Werner, L., Wilmore, J.H. & Freund, B.J. (1986) Modification of cellular immune functions in humans by endurance exercise training during β-adrenergic blockade with atenolol or propranolol. *Med. Sci. Sports Exerc.*, **18**, 95–100

Watts, N.B., Spanheimer, R.G., DiGirolamo, M., Gebhart, S.S., Musey, V.C., Siddiq, Y.K. & Phillips, L.S. (1990) Prediction of glucose response to weight loss in patients with non-insulin-dependent diabetes mellitus. *Arch. Intern. Med.*, **150**, 803–806

Weaver, J.U., Holly, J.M., Kopelman, P.G., Noonan, K., Giadom, C.G., White, N., Virdee, S. & Wass, J.A. (1990) Decreased sex hormone binding globulin (SHBG) and insulin-like growth factor binding protein (IGFBP-1) in extreme obesity. *Clin. Endocrinol. (Oxf.)*, **33**, 415–422

Weber, D.J., Rutala, W.A., Samsa, G.P., Bradshaw, S.E. & Lemon, S.M. (1986) Impaired immunogenicity of hepatitis B vaccine in obese persons. *New Engl. J. Med.*, **314**, 1393

Weber, R.V., Stein, D.E., Scholes, J. & Kral, J.G. (2000) Obesity potentiates AOM-induced colon cancer. *Dig. Dis. Sci.*, **45**, 890–895

Wei, M., Gibbons, L.W., Mitchell, T.L., Kampert, J.B., Lee, C.D. & Blair, S.N. (1999) The association between cardiorespiratory fitness and impaired fasting glucose and type 2 diabetes mellitus in men. *Ann. Intern. Med.*, **130**, 89-96

Weiderpass, E., Gridley, G., Nyrén, O., Ekbom, A., Persson, I. & Adami, H.O. (1997) Diabetes mellitus and risk of large bowel cancer. *J. Natl Cancer Inst.*, **89**, 660–661

Weiderpass, E., Partanen, T., Kaaks, R., Vainio, H., Porta, M., Kauppinen, T., Ojajärvi, A., Boffetta, P. & Malats, N. (1998) Occurrence, trends and environment etiology of pancreatic cancer. *Scand. J. Work Environ. Health*, **24**, 165–174

Weiderpass, E., Adami, H.O., Baron, J.A., Magnusson, C., Lindgren, A. & Persson, I. (1999a) Use of oral contraceptives and endometrial cancer risk (Sweden). *Cancer Causes Control*, **10**, 277–284

Weiderpass, E., Adami, H.O., Baron, J.A., Magnusson, C., Bergström, R., Lindgren, A., Correia, N. & Persson, I. (1999b) Risk of endometrial cancer following estrogen replacement with and without progestins. *J. Natl Cancer Inst.*, **91**, 1131–1137

Weiderpass, E., Persson, I., Adami, H.O., Magnusson, C., Lindgren, A. & Baron, J.A. (2000) Body size in different periods of life, diabetes mellitus, hypertension, and risk of postmenopausal endometrial cancer (Sweden). *Cancer Causes Control*, **11**, 185–192

Weiler, H.A., Wang, Z. & Atkinson, S.A. (1995) Dexamethasone treatment impairs calcium regulation and reduces bone mineralization in infant pigs. *Am. J. Clin. Nutr.*, **61**, 805–811

Weindruch, R. & Walford, R.L. (1982) Dietary restriction in mice beginning at 1 year of age: effect on life-span and spontaneous cancer incidence. *Science*, **215**, 1415–1418

Weindruch, R. & Walford, R.L. (1988) The retardation of ageing and disease by dietary restriction, New York, Charles C. Thomas

Weindruch, R., Walford, R.L., Fligiel, S. & Guthrie, D. (1986) The retardation of aging in mice by dietary restriction: longevity, cancer, immunity and lifetime energy intake. *J. Nutr.*, **116**, 641–654

Weindruch, R., Albanes, D. & Kritchevsky, D. (1991) The role of calories and caloric restriction in carcinogenesis. *Hematol. Oncol. Clin. North Am.*, **5**, 79–89

Weinstock, R.S., Dai, H. & Wadden, T.A. (1998) Diet and exercise in the treatment of obesity: effects of 3 interventions on insulin resistance. *Arch. Intern. Med.*, **158**, 2477–2483

Weiss, N.S., Cook, L.S., Farrow, D.C. & Rosenblatt, K.A. (1996) Ovarian cancer. In: Schottenfeld, D. & Fraumeni, J.F., Jr, eds, *Cancer Epidemiology and Prevention*, New York, Oxford University Press, pp. 1040–1057

Weiss, C., Seitel, G. & Bartsch, P. (1998) Coagulation and fibrinolysis after moderate and very heavy exercise in healthy male subjects. *Med. Sci. Sports Exerc.*, **30**, 246–251

Weraarchakul, N., Strong, R., Wood, W.G. & Richardson, A. (1989) The effect of aging and dietary restriction on DNA repair. *Exp. Cell Res.*, **181**, 197–204

Werner, H. & LeRoith, D. (1996) The role of the insulin-like growth factor system in human cancer. *Adv. Cancer Res.*, **68**, 183–223

West, D.W., Slattery, M.L., Robison, L.M., French, T.K. & Mahoney, A.W. (1991) Adult dietary intake and prostate cancer risk in Utah: a case-control study with special emphasis on aggressive tumors. *Cancer Causes Control*, **2**, 85–94

Westley, B.R. & May, F.E. (1994) Role of insulin-like growth factors in steroid modulated proliferation. *J. Steroid Biochem. Mol. Biol.*, **51**, 1–9

Westley, B.R., Clayton, S.J., Daws, M.R., Molloy, C.A. & May, F.E. (1998) Interactions between the oestrogen and insulin-like growth factor signalling pathways in the control of breast epithelial cell proliferation. *Biochem. Soc. Symp.*, **63**, 35–44

Wetter, T.J., Gazdag, A.C., Dean, D.J. & Cartee, G.D. (1999) Effect of calorie restriction on in vivo glucose metabolism by individual tissues in rats. *Am. J. Physiol.*, **276**, E728–E738

Wetterau, L.A., Moore, M.G., Lee, K.W., Shim, M.L. & Cohen, P. (1999) Novel aspects of the insulin-like growth factor binding proteins. *Mol. Genet. Metab.*, **68**, 161–181

Whaley, M.H. & Blair, S.N. (1995) Epidemiology of physical activity, physical fitness and coronary heart disease. *J. Cardiovasc. Risk*, **2**, 289–295

White, E., Jacobs, E.J. & Daling, J.R. (1996) Physical activity in relation to colon cancer in middle-aged men and women. *Am. J. Epidemiol.*, **144**, 42–50

Whittal, K.S. & Parkhouse, W.S. (1996) Exercise during adolescence and its effects on mammary gland development, proliferation, and nitrosomethylurea (NMU) induced tumorigenesis in rats. *Breast Cancer Res. Treat.*, **37**, 21–27

Whittal-Strange, K.S., Chadan, S., Parkhouse, W.S. & Chadau, S. (1998) Exercise during puberty and NMU induced mammary tumorigenesis in rats. *Breast Cancer Res. Treat.*, **47**, 1–8

Whittemore, A.S. (1993) Personal characteristics relating to risk of invasive epithelial ovarian cancer in older women in the United States. *Cancer*, **71**, 558–565

Whittemore, A.S., Paffenbarger, R.S., Jr, Anderson, K. & Lee, J.E. (1985) Early precursors of site-specific cancers in college men and women. *J. Natl Cancer Inst.*, **74**, 43–51

Whittemore, A.S., Wu-Williams, A.H., Lee, M., Zheng, S., Gallagher, R.P., Jiao, D.A., Zhou, L., Wang, X.H., Chen, K., Jung, D., Teh, C.Z., Chengde, L., Yao, X.J., Paffenbarger, R.S., Jr & Henderson, B.E. (1990) Diet, physical activity, and colorectal cancer among Chinese in North America and China. *J. Natl Cancer Inst.*, **82**, 915–926

Whittemore, A.S., Kolonel, L.N., Wu, A.H., John, E.M., Gallagher, R.P., Howe, G.R., Burch, J.D., Hankin, J., Dreon, D.M., West, D.W., Teh, C.Z. & Paffenbarger, R.S., Jr (1995) Prostate cancer in relation to diet, physical activity, and body size in blacks, whites, and Asians in the United States and Canada. *J. Natl Cancer Inst.*, **87**, 652–661

WHO Consultation on Obesity (1998) Global prevalence and secular trends in obesity. In: *Obesity. Preventing and Managing the Global Epidemic*, Geneva, WHO, pp. 17–40

WHO Expert Committee (1995) *Physical Status. The Use and Interpretation of Anthropometry*, Geneva, WHO

Wideman, L., Weltman, J.Y., Shah, N., Story, S., Veldhuis, J.D. & Weltman, A. (1999) Effects of gender on exercise-induced growth hormone release. *J. Appl. Physiol.*, **87**, 1154–1162

Wideroff, L., Gridley, G., Mellemkjaer, L., Chow, W.H., Linet, M., Keehn, S., Borch-Johnsen, K. & Olsen, J.H. (1997) Cancer incidence in a population-based cohort of patients hospitalized with diabetes mellitus in Denmark. *J. Natl Cancer Inst.*, **89**, 1360–1365

Wijnhoven, B.P., Siersema, P.D., Hop, W.C., van Dekken, H. & Tilanus, H.W. (1999) Adenocarcinomas of the distal oesophagus and gastric cardia are one clinical entity. Rotterdam Oesophageal Tumour Study Group. *Br. J. Surg.*, **86**, 529–535

Wilhelmsen, L., Tibblin, G., Aurell, M., Bjure, J., Ekström-Jodal, B. & Grimby, G. (1976) Physical activity, physical fitness and risk of myocardial infarction. *Adv. Cardiol.*, **18**, 217–230

Will, J.C., Galuska, D.A., Vinicor, F. & Calle, E.E. (1998) Colorectal cancer: another complication of diabetes mellitus? *Am. J. Epidemiol.*, **147**, 816–825

Willamson, D.F., Madans, J., Pamuk, E., Flegal, K.M., Kendrick, J.S., Serdula, M.K.. (1994) A prospective study of childbearing and 10-year weight gain in US white women 25 to 45 years of age. *Int. J. Obesity*, **18**, 561–569

Willett, W. (1998) *Nutritional Epidemiology* (Monographs in Epidemiology and Biostatistics, Vol. 30), New York, Oxford University Press

Willett, W.C., Browne, M.L., Bain, C., Lipnick, R.J., Stampfer, M.J., Rosner, B., Colditz, G.A., Hennekens, C.H. & Speizer, F.E. (1985) Relative weight and risk of breast cancer among premenopausal women. *Am. J. Epidemiol.*, **122**, 731–740

Willett, W.C., Manson, J.E., Stampfer, M.J., Colditz, G.A., Rosner, B., Speizer, F.E. & Hennekens, C.H. (1995) Weight, weight change, and coronary heart disease in women. Risk within the 'normal' weight range. *JAMA*, **273**, 461–465

Williams, P.T. (1997) Relationship of distance run per week to coronary heart disease risk factors in 8283 male runners. The National Runners' Health Study. *Arch. Intern. Med.*, **157**, 191-198

Williams, C.M., Maunder, K. & Theale, D. (1989) The effect of a low-fat diet on luteal-phase prolactin and oestradiol concentrations and erythrocyte phospholipids in normal pre-menopausal women. *Br. J. Nutr.*, **61**, 651–661

Williams, N.I., Bullen, B.A., McArthur, J.W., Skrinar, G.S. & Turnbull, B.A. (1999) Effects of short-term strenuous endurance exercise upon corpus luteum function. *Med. Sci. Sports Exerc.*, **31**, 949–958

Williamson, D.F. & Pamuk, E.R. (1993) The association between weight loss and increased longevity. A review of the evidence. *Ann. Intern. Med.*, **119**, 731-736

Williamson, D.F., Madans, J., Anda, R.F., Kleinman, J.C., Kahn, H.S. & Byers, T. (1993) Recreational physical activity and ten-year weight change in a US national cohort. *Int. J. Obes. Relat. Metab. Disord.*, **17**, 279–286

Williamson, D.F., Madans, J., Pamuk, E., Flegal, K.M., Kendrick, J.S. & Serdula, M.K. (1994) A prospective study of childbearing and 10-year weight gain in US white women 25 to 45 years of age. *Int. J. Obes. Relat. Metab. Disord.*, **18**, 561–569

Williamson, D.F., Pamuk, E., Thun, M., Flanders, D., Byers, T. & Heath, C. (1995) Prospective study of intentional weight loss and mortality in never-smoking overweight US white women aged 40-64 years. *Am. J. Epidemiol.*, **141**, 1128-1141

Williamson, D.F., Pamuk, E., Thun, M., Flanders, D., Byers, T. & Heath, C. (1999) Prospective study of intentional weight loss and mortality in overweight white men aged 40-64 years. *Am. J. Epidemiol.*, **149**, 491-503

Williamson, D.F., Thompson, T.J., Thun, M., Flanders, D., Pamuk, E. & Byers, T. (2000) Intentional weight loss and mortality among overweight individuals with diabetes. *Diabetes Care*, **23**, 1499–1504

Willich, S.N., Lewis, M., Lowel, H., Arntz, H.R., Schubert, F. & Schroder, R. (1993) Physical exertion as a trigger of acute myocardial infarction. Triggers and Mechanisms of Myocardial Infarction Study Group. *New Engl. J. Med.*, **329**, 1684–1690

Wing, R.R. (1999) Physical activity in the treatment of the adulthood overweight and obesity: current evidence and research issues. *Med. Sci. Sports Exerc.*, **31**, S547–S552

Wing, R.R., Epstein, L.H., Marcus, M.D. & Kupfer, D.J. (1984) Mood changes in behavioral weight loss programs. *J. Psychosom. Res.*, **28**, 189-196

Wing, R.R., Koeske, R., Epstein, L.H., Nowalk, M.P., Gooding, W. & Becker, D. (1987) Long-term effects of modest weight loss in type II diabetic patients. *Arch. Intern. Med.*, **147**, 1749-1753

Wing, R.R., Marcus, M.D., Salata, R., Epstein, L.H., Miaskiewicz, S. & Blair, E.H. (1991) Effects of a very-low-calorie diet on long-term glycemic control in obese type 2 diabetic subjects. *Arch. Intern. Med.*, **151**, 1334–1340

Wing, R.R., Jeffery, R.W., Burton, L.R., Thorson, C., Kuller, L.H. & Folsom, A.R. (1992) Change in waist-hip ratio with weight loss and its association with change in cardiovascular risk factors. *Am. J. Clin. Nutr.*, **55**, 1086–1092

Wing, R.R., Venditti, E., Jakicic, J.M., Polley, B.A. & Lang, W. (1998) Lifestyle intervention in overweight individuals with a family history of diabetes. *Diabetes Care*, **21**, 350–359

Wolf, A.M., Hunter, D.J., Colditz, G.A., Manson, J.E., Stampfer, M.J., Corsano, K.A., Rosner, B., Kriska, A. & Willett, W.C. (1994) Reproducibility and validity of a self-administered physical activity questionnaire. *Int. J. Epidemiol.*, **23**, 991–999

Wolk, A. & Rössner, S. (1995) Effects of smoking and physical activity on body weight: developments in Sweden between 1980 and 1989. *J. Intern. Med.*, **237**, 287–291

Wolk, A., Mantzoros, C.S., Andersson, S.O., Bergström, R., Signorello, L.B., Lagiou, P., Adami, H.O. & Trichopoulos, D. (1998) Insulin-like growth factor 1 and prostate cancer risk: a population-based, case-control study. *J. Natl Cancer Inst.*, **90**, 911–915

Wong, Y.C. & Wang, Y.Z. (2000) Growth factors and epithelial-stromal interactions in prostate cancer development. *Int. Rev. Cytol.*, **199**, 65–116

Woods, J.A., Davis, J.M., Kohut, M.L., Ghaffar, A., Mayer, E.P. & Pate, R.R. (1994) Effects of exercise on the immune response to cancer. *Med. Sci. Sports Exerc.*, **26**, 1109–1115

Woods, J.A., Davis, J.M., Smith, J.A. & Nieman, D.C. (1999) Exercise and cellular innate immune function. *Med. Sci. Sports Exerc.*, **31**, 57–66

World Cancer Research Fund (1997) *Food, Nutrition and the Prevention of Cancer: A Global Perspective*, London, WCRF

Wu, A.H., Paganini-Hill, A., Ross, R.K. & Henderson, B.E. (1987) Alcohol, physical activity and other risk factors for colorectal cancer: a prospective study. *Br. J. Cancer*, **55**, 687–694

Wu, X., Yu, H., Amos, C.I., Hong, W.K. & Spitz, M.R. (2000) Joint effect of insulin-like growth factors and mutagen sensitivity in lung cancer risk. *J. Natl Cancer Inst.*, **92**, 737–743

Wynder, E.L., Escher, G.C. & Mantel, N. (1966) An epidemiological investigation of cancer of the endometrium. *Cancer*, **19**, 489–520

Wynder, E.L., Mabuchi, K. & Whitmore, W.F., Jr (1971) Epidemiology of cancer of the prostate. *Cancer*, **28**, 344–360

Wyshak, G. & Frisch, R.E. (2000) Breast cancer among former college athletes compared to non-athletes: a 15-year follow-up. *Br. J. Cancer*, **82**, 726–730

Yaari, S. & Goldbourt, U. (1998) Voluntary and involuntary weight loss: associations with long term mortality in 9,228 middle-aged and elderly men. *Am. J. Epidemiol.*, **148**, 546–555

Yaktine, A.L., Vaughn, R., Blackwood, D., Duysen, E. & Birt, D.F. (1998) Dietary energy restriction in the SENCAR mouse: elevation of glucocorticoid hormone levels but no change in distribution of glucocorticoid receptor in epidermal cells. *Mol. Carcinog.*, **21**, 62–69

Yee, D. & Lee, A.V. (2000) Crosstalk between the insulin-like growth factors and estrogens in breast cancer. *J. Mammary Gland Biol. Neoplasia*, **5**, 107–115

Yee, D., Paik, S., Lebovic, G.S., Marcus, R.R., Favoni, R.E., Cullen, K.J., Lippman, M.E. & Rosen, N. (1989) Analysis of insulin-like growth factor I gene expression in malignancy: evidence for a paracrine role in human breast cancer. *Mol. Endocrinol.*, **3**, 509–517

Yong, L.C., Brown, C.C., Schatzkin, A. & Schairer, C. (1996) Prospective study of relative weight and risk of breast cancer: the Breast Cancer Detection Demonstration Project follow-up study, 1979 to 1987-1989. *Am. J. Epidemiol.*, **143**, 985–995

Yoshida, K., Inoue, T., Nojima, K., Hirabayashi, Y. & Sado, T. (1997) Calorie restriction reduces the incidence of myeloid leukemia induced by a single whole-body radiation in C3H/He mice. *Proc. Natl Acad. Sci. USA*, **94**, 2615–2619

Young, D.R., Haskell, W.L., Taylor, C.B. & Fortmann, S.P. (1996) Effect of community health education on physical activity knowledge, attitudes, and behavior. The Stanford Five-City Project. *Am. J. Epidemiol.*, **144**, 264–274

Youngman, L.D., Park, J.Y. & Ames, B.N. (1992) Protein oxidation associated with aging is reduced by dietary restriction of protein or calories. *Proc. Natl Acad. Sci USA*, **89**, 9112–9116

Ytterstad, B. (1996) The Harstad injury prevention study: the epidemiology of sports injuries. An 8 year study. *Br. J. Sports Med.*, **30**, 64–68

Yu, H. & Berkel, H. (1999) Insulin-like growth factors and cancer. *J. La State Med. Soc.*, **151**, 218–223

Yu, H. & Rohan, T. (2000) Role of the insulin-like growth factor family in cancer development and progression. *J. Natl Cancer Inst.*, **92**, 1472–1489

Yu, H., Spitz, M.R., Mistry, J., Gu, J., Hong, W.K. & Wu, X. (1999) Plasma levels of insulin-like growth factor-I and lung cancer risk: a case-control analysis. *J. Natl Cancer Inst.*, **91**, 151–156

Yuan, J.M., Castelao, J.E., Gago-Dominguez, M., Ross, R.K. & Yu, M.C. (1998) Hypertension, obesity and their medications in relation to renal cell carcinoma. *Br. J. Cancer*, **77**, 1508–1513

Yu-Poth, S., Zhao, G., Etherton, T., Naglak, M., Jonnalagadda, S. & Kris-Etherton, P.M. (1999) Effects of the National Cholesterol Education Program's Step I and Step II dietary intervention programs on cardiovascular disease risk factors: a meta-analysis. *Am. J. Clin. Nutr.*, **69**, 632–646

Zaadstra, B.M., Seidell, J.C., Van Noord, P.A., te Velde, E.R., Habbema, J.D., Vrieswijk, B. & Karbaat, J. (1993) Fat and female fecundity: prospective study of effect of body fat distribution on conception rates. *BMJ*, **306**, 484–487

Zainal, T.A., Oberley, T.D., Allison, D.B., Szweda, L.I. & Weindruch, R. (2000) Caloric restriction of rhesus monkeys lowers oxidative damage in skeletal muscle. *FASEB J.*, **14**, 1825–1836

Zamboni, M., Armellini, F., Turcato, E., Todesco, T., Bissoli, L., Bergamo-Andreis, I.A. & Bosello, O. (1993) Effect of weight loss on regional body fat distribution in premenopausal women. *Am. J. Clin. Nutr.*, **58**, 29–34

Zatonski, W.A., Lowenfels, A.B., Boyle, P., Maisonneuve, P., Bueno de Mesquita, H.B., Ghadirian, P., Jain, M., Przewozniak, K., Baghurst, P., Moerman, C.J., Simard, A., Howe, G.R., McMichael, A.J., Hsieh, C.C. & Walker, A.M. (1997) Epidemiologic aspects of gallbladder cancer: a case-control study of the SEARCH Program of the International Agency for Research on Cancer. *J. Natl Cancer Inst.*, **89**, 1132–1138

Zhang, S., Folsom, A.R., Sellers, T.A., Kushi, L.H. & Potter, J.D. (1995) Better breast cancer survival for postmenopausal women who are less overweight and eat less fat. The Iowa Women's Health Study. *Cancer*, **76**, 275–283

Zhang, Z.F., Kurtz, R.C., Sun, M., Karpeh, M., Yu, G.P., Gargon, N., Fein, J.S., Georgopoulos, S.K. & Harlap, S. (1996) Adenocarcinomas of the esophagus and gastric cardia: medical conditions, tobacco, alcohol, and socioeconomic factors. *Cancer Epidemiol. Biomarkers Prev.*, **5**, 761-768

Zhang, J., Wu, G., Chapkin, R.S. & Lupton, J.R. (1998) Energy metabolism of rat colonocytes changes during the tumorigenic process and is dependent on diet and carcinogen. *J. Nutr.*, **128**, 1262–1269

Zheng, T., Boyle, P., Willett, W.C., Hu, H., Dan, J., Evstifeeva, T.V., Niu, S. & MacMahon, B. (1993a) A case-control study of oral cancer in Beijing, People's Republic of China. Associations with nutrient intakes, foods and food groups. *Eur. J. Cancer B, Oral Oncol.*, **29B**, 45–55

Zheng, W., Shu, X.O., McLaughlin, J.K., Chow, W.H., Gao, Y.T. & Blot, W.J. (1993b) Occupational physical activity and the incidence of cancer of the breast, corpus uteri, and ovary in Shanghai. *Cancer*, **71**, 3620–3624

Zhu, P., Frei, E., Bunk, B., Berger, M.R. & Schmähl, D. (1991) Effect of dietary calorie and fat restriction on mammary tumor growth and hepatic as well as tumor glutathione in rats. *Cancer Lett.*, **57**, 145–152

Zhu, Z., Haegele, A.D. & Thompson, H.J. (1997) Effect of caloric restriction on pre-malignant and malignant stages of mammary carcinogenesis. *Carcinogenesis*, **18**, 1007–1012

Zhu, Z., Jiang, W. & Thompson, H.J. (1999a) Effect of energy restriction on tissue size regulation during chemically induced carcinogenesis. *Carcinogenesis*, **20**, 1721–1726

Zhu, Z., Jiang, W. & Thompson, H.J. (1999b) Effect of energy restriction on the expression of cyclin D1 and p27 during premalignant and malignant stages of chemically induced mammary carcinogenesis. *Mol. Carcinog.*, **24**, 241–245

Ziegler, R.G., Hoover, R.N., Nomura, A.M., West, D.W., Wu, A.H., Pike, M.C., Lake, A.J., Horn-Ross, P.L., Kolonel, L.N., Siiteri, P.K. & Fraumeni, J.F., Jr (1996) Relative weight, weight change, height, and breast cancer risk in Asian-American women. *J. Natl Cancer Inst.*, **88**, 650–660

Zimmet, P. (2000) Globalization, coca-colonization and the chronic disease epidemic: can the Doomsday scenario be averted? *J. Intern. Med.*, **247**, 301–310

Zmuda, J.M., Thompson, P.D. & Winters, S.J. (1996) Exercise increases serum testosterone and sex hormone-binding globulin levels in older men. *Metabolism*, **45**, 935–939

Zoratti, R. (1998) A review on ethnic differences in plasma triglycerides and high-density-lipoprotein cholesterol: is the lipid pattern the key factor for the low coronary heart disease rate in people of African origin? *Eur. J. Epidemiol.*, **14**, 9–21

Zumoff, B., Strain, G.W., Miller, L.K., Rosner, W., Senie, R., Seres, D.S. & Rosenfeld, R.S. (1990) Plasma free and non-sex-hormone-binding-globulin-bound testosterone are decreased in obese men in proportion to their degree of obesity. *J. Clin. Endocrinol. Metab.*, **71**, 929–931

Glossary

Weight control Weight control is widely defined as approaches to maintain body weight, including both *prevention of weight gain* and *weight loss.*

Body mass index Body mass index (BMI) is a measure of body mass relative to height, calculated as weight (kg) divided by height squared (m^2).

Healthy weight A healthy weight level for adults is defined as a body mass index within the range 18.5 to 24.9 kg/m^2 (WHO Expert Committee, 1995).

Overweight A body mass index within the range 25.0–29.9 kg/m^2 (WHO Expert Committee, 1995).

Obesity An increase in body weight beyond the limits of skeletal and physical requirements, as a result of excessive accumulation of fat in the body. A person is defined as obese if he or she has a body mass index of 30.0 kg/m^2 or over (WHO Expert Committee, 1995).

Energy Energy is measured in kilojoules and usually expressed as the quantity consumed or expended in a 24-hour period. Energy was previously expressed as calories (1 cal = 4.2 J).

Energy balance Energy balance corresponds to the equivalence between the energy consumed in diet and the energy expended to maintain basal metabolism, physiological functions of the body and physical activities. This is operationally defined as stable body composition.

Basal metabolic rate The amount of energy (in kilojoules per 24 hours) required to maintain the essential body functions in absolute resting and fasting conditions.

Fat-free body mass The portion of body weight that is not adipose tissue, consisting primarily of muscle, bone and water.

Physical activity Any bodily movement that is produced by contraction of skeletal muscle and that increases energy expenditure above resting levels.

Maximal oxygen consumption The highest rate of oxygen consumed during exercise. It is usually expressed as multiples of resting oxygen consumption, in MET (see below).

Maximal heart rate The highest heart rate achieved during maximal exercise. An estimate can be obtained using the formula 220 minus age.

Metabolic equivalent (MET) Represents the metabolic rate associated with seated rest and is set at 3.5 millilitres of oxygen consumed per kilogram body mass per minute.

Physical activity Physical inactivity or sedentary behaviour is a state in which body movement is minimal and energy expenditure approximates resting metabolic rate.

Physical fitness A set of attributes that people have or achieve that relates to the ability to perform physical activity.

Intensity of physical activity	The energy cost of the level of physical activity that is performed. This has been defined in three ways:

- Absolute intensity pertains to the rate of oxygen consumption (or energy expenditure) associated with participation in activity. This can be defined as oxygen consumed during the activity, and is often expressed as multiples of METs.

- Relative intensity compares the oxygen consumption associated with an activity relative to an individual's maximal oxygen consumption. An activity entailing a given oxygen consumption will have a higher relative intensity for persons with lower maximal consumption. For example, the relative intensity would be higher among older adults compared with younger adults because of the decline in maximal oxygen consumption associated with age.

- Subjective intensity is based on an individual's perception of physiological cues such as increased breathing, heart rate and sweating, each of which can increase with increasing metabolic demands of physical activity.

Light physical activity	Activity of an intensity of about 25–44% relative to a person's maximal oxygen consumption or 30–49% of maximal heart rate. Examples include walking at a normal pace for a woman aged 30 years but, because of his lower maximal oxygen consumption, walking slowly for a man aged 65 years (US Department of Health and Human Services, 1996).
Moderate physical activity	Activity of an intensity of about 45–59% relative to a person's maximal oxygen consumption or 50–69% of maximal heart rate. Examples include carrying and stacking wood for a man aged 25 years, but fast walking for a woman aged 45 years (DHHS, 1996).
Vigorous physical activity	Activity of an intensity of at least 60% relative to a person's maximal oxygen consumption or 70% of maximal heart rate. Examples include jogging for a woman aged 35 years, but brisk walking for a man aged 65 years (US Department of Health and Human Services, 1996).
Meal feeding	A laboratory animal's 24-hour allotment of food, divided into two or more portions. Each portion is provided to the animal at a specified time during a 24 hour period.
Cyclic feeding	An experimental design in which animals are provided a limited amount of diet for a speci-fied time, usually days or weeks, followed by a period during which the animals are given access to food *ad libitum*. This pattern of feeding may be repeated. This feeding regimen has also been referred to as energy cycling or patterned calorie restriction.
Diet restriction	Feeding experimental animals with less of the control diet and therefore reducing all constituents of the diet. These diets are sometimes supplemented with some of the micronutrients that the investigator does not want to reduce. Such diets can be semi-purified or cereal-based. It is not possible to supplement all minor constituents in a cereal-based diet because they are not defined.
Food restriction	Identical to diet restriction (see above).
Energy restriction	A dietary protocol in which energy intake is selectively reduced while protein and all micro-con-stituents (including micronutrients) are fed at the same level in the control and energy-restricted groups. Energy restriction is generally accomplished by selectively removing carbohydrate and/or fat, and is often referred to as calorie restriction.

Sources of Figures

Figure 1	Working Group
Figure 2	Working Group
Figure 3	Working Group
Figure 4	Working Group
Figure 5	IARC
Figure 6	SIPA Press, Paris, France
Figure 7	Working Group
Figure 8	Permission from Antero Aaltonen, Kerava, Finland
Figure 9	SIPA Press, Paris, France
Figure 10	SIPA Press, Paris, France
Figure 11	Working Group
Figure 12	Working Group
Figure 13	Working group
Figure 14	Working Group
Figure 15	Working Group
Figure 16	Permission from Antero Aaltonen, Kerava, Finland
Figure 17	Permission from Antero Aaltonen, Kerava, Finland
Figure 18	Working Group
Figure 19	Working Group
Figure 20	Working Group
Figure 21	Permission from Antero Aaltonen, Kerava, Finland
Figure 22	SIPA Press, Paris, France
Figure 23	NIEHS, USA
Figure 24	NIEHS, USA
Figure 25	SIPA Press, Paris, France
Figure 26	Working Group
Figure 27	Working Group (Permission from JNCI)
Figure 28	Working Group
Figure 29	Working Group
Figure 30	Working Group
Figure 31	SIPA Press, Paris, France
Figure 32	Permission from Zhaogang Wang, China
Page 206.	SIPA Press, Paris, France

Cover illustrations
Permission from Zhaogang Wang, China, Antero Aaltonen, Finland and Eric Lucas, IARC

Working Procedures for the *IARC Handbooks of Cancer Prevention*

The prevention of cancer is one of the key objectives of the International Agency for Research on Cancer (IARC). This may be achieved by avoiding exposures to known cancer-causing agents, by increasing host defences through immunization or chemoprevention or by modifying lifestyle. The aim of the series of *IARC Handbooks of Cancer Prevention* is to evaluate scientific information on agents and interventions that may reduce the incidence of or mortality from cancer.

Scope

Cancer-preventive strategies embrace chemical, immunological, dietary and behavioural interventions that may retard, block or reverse carcinogenic processes or reduce underlying risk factors. The term 'chemoprevention' is used to refer to interventions with pharmaceuticals, vitamins, minerals and other chemicals to reduce cancer incidence. The *IARC Handbooks* address the efficacy, safety and mechanisms of cancer-preventive strategies and the adequacy of the available data, including those on timing, dose, duration and indications for use.

Preventive strategies can be applied across a continuum of: (1) the general population; (2) subgroups with particular predisposing host or environmental risk factors, including genetic susceptibility to cancer; (3) persons with precancerous lesions; and (4) cancer patients at risk for second primary tumours. Use of the same strategies or agents in the treatment of cancer patients to control the growth, metastasis and recurrence of tumours is considered to be patient management, not prevention, although data from clinical trials may be relevant when making a *Handbooks* evaluation.

Objective

The objective of the *Handbooks* programme is the preparation of critical reviews and evaluations of evidence for cancer-prevention and other relevant properties of a wide range of potential cancer-preventive agents and strategies by international working groups of experts. The resulting *Handbooks* may also indicate when additional research is needed.

The *Handbooks* may assist national and international authorities in devising programmes of health promotion and cancer prevention and in making benefit–risk assessments. The evaluations of IARC working groups are scientific judgements about the available evidence for cancer-preventive efficacy and safety. No recommendation is given with regard to national and international regulation or legislation, which are the responsibility of individual governments and/or other international authorities.

Working Groups

Reviews and evaluations are formulated by international working groups of experts convened by the IARC. The tasks of each group are: (1) to ascertain that all appropriate data have been collected; (2) to select the data relevant for the evaluation on the basis of scientific merit; (3) to prepare accurate summaries of the data to enable the reader to follow the reasoning of the Working Group; (4) to evaluate the significance of the available data from human studies and experimental models on cancer-preventive activity, and other beneficial effects and also on adverse effects; and (5) to evaluate data relevant to the understanding of the mechanisms of preventive activity.

Approximately 13 months before a working group meets, the topics of the *Handbook* are announced, and participants are selected by IARC staff in consultation with other experts. Subsequently, relevant clinical, experimental and human data are collected by the IARC from all available sources of published information. Representatives of producer or consumer associations may assist in the preparation of sections on production and use, as appropriate.

Working Group participants who contributed to the considerations and evaluations within a particular *Handbook* are listed, with their addresses, at the beginning of each publication. Each participant serves as an individual scientist and not as a representative of any organization, government or industry. In addition, scientists nominated by national and international agencies, industrial associations and consumer and/or environmental organizations may be invited as observers. IARC staff involved in the preparation of the *Handbooks* are listed.

About eight months before the meeting, the material collected is sent to meeting participants to prepare sections for the first drafts of the *Handbooks*. These are then compiled by IARC staff and sent, before the meeting, to all participants of the Working Group for review. There is an opportunity to return the compiled specialized sections of the draft to the experts, inviting preliminary comments, before the complete first-draft document is distributed to all members of the Working Group.

Data for Handbooks

The *Handbooks* do not necessarily cite all of the literature on the agent or strategy being evaluated. Only those data considered by the Working Group to be relevant to making the evaluation are included. In principle, meeting abstracts and other reports that do not provide sufficient detail upon which to base an assessment of their quality are not considered.

With regard to data from toxicological, epidemiological and experimental studies and from clinical trials, only reports that have been published or accepted for publication in the openly available scientific literature are reviewed by the Working Group. In certain instances, government agency reports that have undergone peer review and are widely available are considered. Exceptions may be made on an ad-hoc basis to include unpublished reports that are in their final form and publicly available, if their inclusion is considered pertinent to making a final evaluation. In the sections on chemical and physical properties, on production, on use, on analysis and on human exposure, unpublished sources of information may be used.

The available studies are summarized by the Working Group. In general, numerical findings are indicated as they appear in the original report; units are converted when necessary for easier comparison. The Working Group may conduct additional analyses of the published data and use them in their assessment of the evidence. Important aspects of a study, directly impinging on its interpretation, are brought to the attention of the reader.

Criteria for selection of topics for evaluation

Agents, classes of agents and interventions to be evaluated in the *Handbooks* are selected on the basis of one or more of the following criteria.
- The available evidence suggests potential for significantly reducing the incidence of cancers.
- There is a substantial body of human, experimental, clinical and/or mechanistic data suitable for evaluation.
- The agent is in widespread use and of putative protective value, but of uncertain efficacy and safety.
- The agent shows exceptional promise in experimental studies but has not been used in humans.
- The agent is available for further studies of human use.

Evaluation of cancer-preventive agents

A wide range of findings must be taken into account before a particular agent can be recognized as preventing cancer and a systematized approach to data presentation has been adopted for *Handbooks* evaluations.

Characteristics of the agent or intervention

Chemical identity and other definitive information (such as genus and species of plants) are given as appropriate. Data relevant to identification, occurrence and biological activity are included. Technical products of chemicals, including trade names, relevant specifications and information on composition and impurities.

Preventive interventions can be broad, community-based interventions, or interventions targeted to individuals (counselling, behavioural, chemopreventive).

Occurrence, trends, analysis
Occurrence

Information on the occurrence of an agent in the environment is obtained from monitoring and surveillance in occupational environments, air, water, soil, foods and animal and human tissues. When available, data on the generation, persistence and bioaccumulation of the agent are included. For interventions, data on prevalence are supplied. The data on the prevalence of a factor (e.g., overweight) in different populations are collected as widely as possible.

Production and use

The dates of first synthesis and of first commercial production of a chemical or mixture are provided, the dates of first reported occurrence. In addition, methods of synthesis used in past and present commercial production and methods of production that may give rise to various impurities are described. For interventions, the dates of first mention of their use are given.

Data on the production, international trade and uses and applications of agents are obtained for representative regions. In the case of drugs, mention of their therapeutic applications does not necessarily represent current practice, nor does it imply judgement as to their therapeutic efficacy.

If an agent is used as a prescribed or over-the-counter pharmaceutical product, then the type of person receiving the product in terms of health status, age, sex and medical condition being treated are described. For non-pharmaceutical agents, particularly those taken because of cultural traditions, the characteristics of use or exposure and the relevant populations are described. In all cases, quantitative data, such as dose–response relationships, are considered to be of special importance.

Metabolism of and metabolic responses to the agent or metabolic consequences of an intervention

In evaluating the potential utility of a suspected cancer-preventive agent or strategy, a number of different properties, in addition to direct effects upon cancer incidence, are described and weighed. Furthermore, as many of the data leading to an evaluation are expected to come from studies in experimental animals, information that facilitates interspecies extrapolation is particularly important; this includes metabolic, kinetic and genetic data. Whenever possible, quantitative data, including information on dose, duration and potency, are considered.

Information is given on absorption, distribution (including placental transfer), metabolism and excretion in humans and experimental animals. Kinetic properties within the target species may affect the interpretation and extrapolation of dose–response relationships, such as blood concentrations, protein binding, tissue concentrations, plasma half-lives and elimination rates. Comparative information on the relationship between use or exposure and the dose that reaches the target site may be of particular importance for extrapolation between species. Studies that indicate the metabolic pathways and fate of an agent in humans and experimental animals are summarized, and data on humans and experimental animals are compared when possible. Observations are made on inter-individual variations and relevant metabolic polymorphisms. Data indicating long-term accumulation in human tissues are included. Physiologically based pharmacokinetic models and their parameter values are relevant and are included whenever they are available. Information on the fate of the compound within tissues and cells (transport, role of cellular receptors, compartmentalization, binding to macromolecules) is given.

The metabolic consequences of interventions are described.

Genotyping will be used increasingly, not only to identify subpopulations at increased or decreased risk for cancers but also to characterize variation in the biotransformation of and responses to cancer-preventive agents. This subsection can include effects of the compound on gene expression, enzyme induction or inhibition, or pro-oxidant status, when such data are not described elsewhere. It covers data obtained in humans and experimental animals, with particular attention to effects of long-term use and exposure.

Cancer-preventive effects
Human studies
Types of study considered
Human data are derived from experimental and non-experimental study designs and are focused on cancer, precancer or intermediate biological end-points. The experimental designs include randomized controlled trials and short-term experimental studies; non-experimental designs include cohort, case–control and cross-sectional studies.

Cohort and case–control studies relate individual use of, or exposure to, the agent or invervention under study to the occurrence of cancer in individuals and provide an estimate of relative risk (ratio of incidence or mortality in those exposed to incidence or mortality in those not exposed) as the main measure of association. Cohort and case–control studies follow an observational approach, in which the use of, or exposure to, the agent is not controlled by the investigator.

Intervention studies are experimental in design — that is, the use of, or exposure to, the agent or intervention is assigned by the investigator. The intervention study or clinical trial is the design that can provide the strongest and most direct evidence of a protective or preventive effect; however, for practical and ethical reasons, such studies are limited to observation of the effects among specifically defined study subjects of interventions of 10 years or fewer, which is relatively short when compared with the overall lifespan.

Intervention studies may be undertaken in individuals or communities and may or may not involve randomization to use or exposure. The differences between these designs is important in relation to analytical methods and interpretation of findings.

In addition, information can be obtained from reports of correlation (ecological) studies and case series; however, limitations inherent in these approaches usually mean that such studies carry limited weight in the evaluation of a preventive effect.

Quality of studies considered
The *Handbooks* are not intended to summarize all published studies. The Working Group considers the following aspects: (1) the relevance of the study; (2) the appropriateness of the design and analysis to the question being asked; (3) the adequacy and completeness of the presentation of the data; and (4) the degree to which chance, bias and confounding may have affected the results.

Studies that are judged to be inadequate or irrelevant to the evaluation are generally omitted. They may be mentioned briefly, particularly when the information is considered to be a useful supplement to that in other reports or when it provides the only data available. Their inclusion does not imply acceptance of the adequacy of the study design, nor of the analysis and interpretation of the results, and their limitations are outlined.

Assessment of the cancer-preventive effect at different doses and durations
The Working Group gives special attention to quantitative assessment of the preventive effect of the agent under study, by assessing data from studies at different doses. The Working Group also addresses issues of timing and duration of use or exposure. Such quantitative assessment is important to clarify the circumstances under which a preventive effect can be achieved, as well as the dose at which a toxic effect has been shown.

Criteria for a cancer-preventive effect.
After summarizing and assessing the individual studies, the Working Group makes a judgement concerning the evidence that the agent or intervention in question prevents cancer in humans. In making the judgement, the Working Group considers several criteria for each relevant cancer site.

Evidence of protection derived from intervention studies of good quality is particularly informative. Evidence of a substantial and significant reduction in risk, including a 'dose'–response relationship, is more likely to indicate a real effect. Nevertheless, a small effect, or an effect without a dose–response relationship, does not imply lack of real benefit and may be important for public health if the cancer is common.

Evidence is frequently available from different types of study and is evaluated as a whole. Findings that are replicated in several studies of the same design or using different approaches are more likely to provide evidence of a true protective effect than isolated observations from single studies.

The Working Group evaluates possible explanations for inconsistencies across studies, including differences in use of, or exposure to, the agent, differences in the underlying risk of cancer and metabolism and genetic differences in the population.

The results of studies judged to be of high quality are given more weight. Note is taken of both the applicability of preventive action to several cancers and of possible differences in activity, including contradictory findings, across cancer sites.

Data from human studies (as well as from experimental models) that suggest plausible mechanisms for a cancer-preventive effect are important in assessing the overall evidence.

The Working Group may also determine whether, on aggregate, the evidence from human studies is consistent with a lack of preventive effect.

Experimental models
Experimental animals
Animal models are an important component of research into cancer prevention. They provide a means of identifying effective compounds, of carrying out fundamental investigations into their mechanisms of action, of determining how they can be used optimally, of evaluating toxicity and, ultimately, of providing an information base for developing intervention trials in humans. Models that permit evaluation of the effects of cancer-preventive agents on the occurrence of cancer in most major organ sites are available. Major groups of animal models include: those in which cancer is produced by the administration of chemical or physical carcinogens; those involving genetically engineered animals; and those in which tumours develop spontaneously. Most cancer-preventive agents investigated in such studies can be placed into one of three categories: compounds that prevent molecules from reaching or reacting with critical target sites (blocking agents); compounds that decrease the sensitivity of target tissues to carcinogenic stimuli; and compounds that prevent evolution of the neoplastic process (suppressing agents). There is increasing interest in the use of combinations of agents as a means of improving efficacy and minimizing toxicity. Animal models are useful in evaluating such combinations. The development of optimal strategies for human intervention trials can be facilitated by the use of animal models that mimic the neoplastic process in humans.

Specific factors to be considered in such experiments are: (1) the temporal requirements of administration of the cancer-preventive agents; (2) dose–response effects; (3) the site-specificity of cancer-preventive activity; and (4) the number and structural diversity of carcinogens whose activity can be reduced by the agent being evaluated.

An important variable in the evaluation of the cancer-preventive response is the time and the duration of administration of the agent or intervention in relation to any carcinogenic treatment, or in transgenic or other experimental models in which no carcinogen is administered. Furthermore, concurrent administration of a cancer-preventive agent may result in a decreased incidence of tumours in a given organ and an increase in another organ of the same animal. Thus, in these experiments it is important that multiple organs be examined.

For all these studies, the nature and extent of impurities or contaminants present in the cancer-preventive agent or agents being evaluated are given when available. For experimental studies of mixtures, consideration is given to the possibility of changes in the physico-chemical properties of the test substance during collection, storage, extraction, concentration and delivery. Chemical and toxicological interactions of the components of mixtures may result in nonlinear dose–response relationships.

As certain components of commonly used diets of experimental animals are themselves known to have cancer-preventive activity, particular consideration should be given to the interaction between the diet and the apparent effect of the agent or intervention being studied. Likewise, restriction of diet may be important. The appropriateness of the diet given relative to the composition of human diets may be commented on by the Working Group.

Qualitative aspects. An assessment of the experimental prevention of cancer involves several considerations of qualitative importance, including: (1) the experimental conditions under which the test was performed (route and schedule of exposure, species, strain, sex and age of animals studied, duration of the exposure, and duration of the study); (2) the consistency of the results, for example across species and target organ(s); (3) the stage or stages of the neoplastic process, from preneoplastic lesions and benign tumours to malignant neoplasms, studied and (4) the possible role of modifying factors.

Considerations of importance to the Working Group in the interpretation and evaluation of a particular study include: (1) how clearly the agent was defined and, in the case of mixtures, how adequately the sample composition was reported; (2) the composition of the diet and the stability of the agent in the diet; (3) whether the source, strain and quality of the animals was reported; (4) whether the dose and schedule of treatment with the known carcinogen were appropriate in assays of combined treatment; (5) whether the doses of the cancer-preventive agent were adequately monitored; (6) whether the agent(s) was absorbed, as shown by blood concentrations; (7) whether the survival of treated animals was similar to that of controls; (8) whether the body and organ weights of treated animals were similar to those of controls; (9) whether there were adequate numbers of animals, of appropriate age, per group; (10) whether animals of each sex were used, if appropriate; (11) whether animals were allocated randomly to groups; (12) whether appropriate respective controls were used; (13) whether the duration of the experiment was adequate; (14) whether there was adequate statistical analysis; and (15) whether the data were adequately reported. If available, recent data on the incidence of specific tumours in historical controls, as well as in concurrent controls, are taken into account in the evaluation of tumour response.

Quantitative aspects. The probability that tumours will occur may depend on the species, sex, strain and age of the animals, the dose of carcinogen (if any),

the dose of the agent and the route and duration of exposure. A decreased incidence and/or decreased multiplicity of neoplasms in adequately designed studies provides evidence of a cancer-preventive effect. A dose-related decrease in incidence and/or multiplicity further strengthens this association.

Statistical analysis. Major factors considered in the statistical analysis by the Working Group include the adequacy of the data for each treatment group: (1) the initial and final effective numbers of animals studied and the survival rate; (2) body weights; and (3) tumour incidence and multiplicity. The statistical methods used should be clearly stated and should be the generally accepted techniques refined for this purpose. In particular, the statistical methods should be appropriate for the characteristics of the expected data distribution and should account for interactions in multifactorial studies. Consideration is given as to whether the appropriate adjustment was made for differences in survival.

In-vitro models
Cell systems *in vitro* contribute to the early identification of potential cancer-preventive agents and to elucidation of mechanisms of cancer prevention. A number of assays in prokaryotic and eukaryotic systems are used for this purpose. Evaluation of the results of such assays includes consideration of: (1) the nature of the cell type used; (2) whether primary cell cultures or cell lines (tumorigenic or nontumorigenic) were studied; (3) the appropriateness of controls; (4) whether toxic effects were considered in the outcome; (5) whether the data were appropriately summated and analysed; (6) whether appropriate quality controls were used; (7) whether appropriate concentration ranges were used; (8) whether adequate numbers of independent measurements were made per group; and (9) the relevance of the end-points, including inhibition of

mutagenesis, morphological transformation, anchorage-independent growth, cell–cell communication, calcium tolerance and differentiation.

Intermediate biomarkers
Other types of study include experiments in which the end-point is not cancer but a defined preneoplastic lesion or tumour-related intermediate biomarker.

The observation of effects on the occurrence of lesions presumed to be preneoplastic or the emergence of benign or malignant tumours may aid in assessing the mode of action of the presumed cancer-preventive agent or intervention. Particular attention is given to assessing the reversibility of these lesions and their predictive value in relation to cancer development.

Mechanisms of cancer prevention
Data on mechanisms can be derived from both human studies and experimental models. For a rational implementation of cancer-preventive measures, it is essential not only to assess protective end-points but also to understand the mechanisms by which the agents or interventions exert their anticarcinogenic action. Information on the mechanisms of cancer-preventive activity can be inferred from relationships between chemical structure and biological activity, from analysis of interactions between agents and specific molecular targets, from studies of specific end-points *in vitro*, from studies of the inhibition of tumorigenesis *in vivo*, from the effects of modulating intermediate biomarkers, and from human studies. Therefore, the Working Group takes account of data on mechanisms in making the final evaluation of cancer prevention.

Several classifications of mechanisms have been proposed, as have several systems for evaluating them. Cancer-preventive agents may act at several distinct levels. Their action may be: (1) extracellular, for example, inhibiting the uptake or endogenous formation of carcinogens, or forming complexes with, diluting and/or deactivating carcinogens; (2) intracellular, for example, trapping carcinogens in non-target cells, modifying transmembrane transport, modulating metabolism, blocking reactive molecules, inhibiting cell replication or modulating gene expression or DNA metabolism; or (3) at the level of the cell, tissue or organism, for example, affecting cell differentiation, intercellular communication, proteases, signal transduction, growth factors, cell adhesion molecules, angiogenesis, interactions with the extracellular matrix, hormonal status and the immune system.

Many cancer-preventive agents are known or suspected to act by several mechanisms, which may operate in a coordinated manner and allow them a broader spectrum of anticarcinogenic activity. Therefore, multiple mechanisms of action are taken into account in the evaluation of cancer-prevention.

Beneficial interactions, generally resulting from exposure to inhibitors that work through complementary mechanisms, are exploited in combined cancer-prevention. Because organisms are naturally exposed not only to mixtures of carcinogenic agents but also to mixtures of protective agents, it is also important to understand the mechanisms of interactions between inhibitors.

Other beneficial effects

An expanded description is given, when appropriate, of the efficacy of the agent in the maintenance of a normal healthy state and the treatment of particular diseases. Information on the mechanisms involved in these activities is described. Reviews, rather than individual studies, may be cited as references.

The physiological functions of agents such as vitamins and micronutrients can be described briefly, with reference to reviews. Data on the therapeutic effects of drugs approved for clinical use are summarized.

Toxic effects

Toxic effects are of particular importance in the case of agents or interventions that may be used widely over long periods in healthy populations. Data are given on acute and chronic toxic effects, such as organ toxicity, increased cell proliferation, immunotoxicity and adverse endocrine effects. Some agents or interventions may have both carcinogenic and anticarcinogenic activities. If the agent has been evaluated within the *IARC Monographs on the Evaluation of Carcinogenic Risks to Humans*, that evaluation is accepted, unless significant new data have appeared that may lead the Working Group to reconsider the evidence. If the agent occurs naturally or has been in clinical use previously, the doses and durations used in cancer-prevention trials are compared with intakes from the diet, in the case of vitamins, and previous clinical exposure, in the case of drugs already approved for human use. When extensive data are available, only summaries are presented; if adequate reviews are available, reference may be made to these. If there are no relevant reviews, the evaluation is made on the basis of the same criteria as are applied to epidemiological studies of cancer. Differences in response as a consequence of species, sex, age and genetic variability are presented when the information is available.

Data demonstrating the presence or absence of adverse effects in humans are included; equally, lack of data on specific adverse effects is stated clearly.

Information is given on carcinogenicity, immunotoxicity, neurotoxicity, cardiotoxicity, haematological effects and toxicity to other target organs. Specific case reports in humans and any previous clinical data are noted. Other biochemical effects thought to be relevant to adverse effects are mentioned.

The results of studies of genetic and related effects in mammalian and non-mammalian systems *in vivo* and *in vitro* are summarized. Information on whether DNA damage occurs via direct interaction with the agent or via indirect mechanisms (e.g. generation of free radicals) is included, as is information on other genetic effects such as mutation, recombination, chromosomal damage, aneuploidy, cell immortalization and transformation, and effects on cell–cell communication. The presence and toxicological significance of cellular receptors for the cancer-preventive agent are described.

Structure–activity relationships that may be relevant to the evaluation of the toxicity of an agent are described.

Summary of data

In this section, the relevant human and experimental data are summarized. Inadequate studies are generally not included but are identified in the preceding text.

Recommendations

During the evaluation process, it is likely that opportunities for further research will be identified. These are clearly stated, with the understanding that the areas are recommended for future investigation. It is made clear that these research opportunities are identified in general terms on the basis of the data currently available.

Recommendations for public health action are listed, based on the analysis of the existing scientific data.

Evaluation

Evaluations of the strength of the evidence for cancer-preventive activity and carcinogenic effects from studies in humans and experimental models are made, using standard terms. These terms may also be applied to other beneficial and adverse effects, when indicated. When appropriate, reference is made to specific organs and populations.

It is recognized that the criteria for these evaluation categories, described below, cannot encompass all factors that may be relevant to an evaluation of cancer-preventive activity. In considering all the relevant scientific data, the Working Group may assign the agent or intervention to a higher or lower category than a strict interpretation of these criteria would indicate.

Cancer-preventive activity

The evaluation categories refer to the strength of the evidence that an agent or intervention prevents cancer. The evaluations may change as new information becomes available.

Evaluations are inevitably limited to the cancer sites, conditions and levels of exposure and length of observation covered by the available studies. An evaluation of degree of evidence, whether for an agent or intervention, is limited to the materials tested, as defined physically, chemically or biologically, or to the intensity or frequency of an intervention. When agents are considered by the Working Group to be sufficiently closely related, they may be grouped for the purpose of a single evaluation of degree of evidence.

Information on mechanisms of action is taken into account when evaluating the strength of evidence in humans and in experimental animals, as well as in assessing the consistency of results between studies in humans and experimental models.

Cancer-preventive activity in humans

The evidence relevant to cancer prevention in humans is classified into one of the following categories.

- *Sufficient evidence of cancer-preventive activity*

The Working Group considers that a causal relationship has been established between use of the agent or intervention and the prevention of human cancer in studies in which chance, bias

and confounding could be ruled out with reasonable confidence.

- *Limited evidence of cancer-preventive activity*

The data suggest a reduced risk for cancer with use of the agent or intervention but are limited for making a definitive evaluation either because chance, bias or confounding could not be ruled out with reasonable confidence or because the data are restricted to intermediary biomarkers of uncertain validity in the putative pathway to cancer.

- *Inadequate evidence of cancer-preventive activity*

The available studies are of insufficient quality, consistency or statistical power to permit a conclusion regarding a cancer-preventive effect of the agent or intervention, or no data on the prevention of cancer in humans are available.

- *Evidence suggesting lack of cancer-preventive activity*

Several adequate studies of use or exposure to the agent or intervention are mutually consistent in not showing a preventive effect.

The strength of the evidence for any carcinogenic effect is assessed in parallel.

Both cancer-preventive activity and carcinogenic effects are identified and, when appropriate, tabulated by organ site. The evaluation also cites the population subgroups concerned, specifying age, sex, genetic or environmental predisposing risk factors and the relevance of precancerous lesions.

Cancer-preventive activity in experimental animals

Evidence for cancer prevention in experimental animals is classified into one of the following categories.

- *Sufficient evidence of cancer-preventive activity*

The Working Group considers that a causal relationship has been established between the agent or intervention and a decreased incidence and/or multiplicity of neoplasms.

- *Limited evidence of cancer-preventive activity*

The data suggest a cancer-preventive effect but are limited for making a definitive evaluation because, for example, the evidence of cancer prevention is restricted to a single experiment, the agent or intervention decreases the incidence and/or multiplicity only of benign neoplasms or lesions of uncertain neoplastic potential or there is conflicting evidence.

- *Inadequate evidence of cancer-preventive activity*

The studies cannot be interpreted as showing either the presence or absence of a preventive effect because of major or quantitative limitations (unresolved questions regarding the adequacy of the design, conduct or interpretation of the study), or no data on cancer prevention in experimental animals are available.

- *Evidence suggesting lack of cancer-preventive activity*

Adequate evidence from conclusive studies in several models shows that, within the limits of the tests used, the agent or intervention does not prevent cancer.

Overall evaluation

Finally, the body of evidence is considered as a whole, and summary statements are made that emcompass the effects of the agent or intervention in humans with regard to cancer-preventive activity and other beneficial effects or adverse effects, as appropriate.

Available in the same series:

IARC Handbooks of Cancer Prevention:

Volume 1   Non-Steroidal Anti-inflammatory Drugs (NSAIDs)
Volume 2   Carotenoids
Volume 3   Vitamin A
Volume 4   Retinoids
Volume 5   Sunscreens

These books can be ordered from:

IARC*Press*
150 Cours Albert Thomas
69372 Lyon cedex 08
France
Fax: + 33 4 72 73 83 02

IARC*Press*
WHO Office
Suite 480
1775 K Street
Washington DC 20006
USA
Fax: + 1 202 223 1782

Oxford University Press
Walton Street
Oxford OX2 6DP
UK
Fax: + 44 1865 267782